Molecular Nutrition

Molecular Nutrition

Vitamins

Edited by

VINOOD B. PATEL, PHD, FHEA, FRSC
School of Life Sciences,
University of Westminster,
London, United Kingdom

ELSEVIER

ACADEMIC PRESS
An imprint of Elsevier

Academic Press is an imprint of Elsevier
125 London Wall, London EC2Y 5AS, United Kingdom
525 B Street, Suite 1650, San Diego, CA 92101, United States
50 Hampshire Street, 5th Floor, Cambridge, MA 02139, United States
The Boulevard, Langford Lane, Kidlington, Oxford OX5 1GB, United Kingdom

British Library Cataloguing-in-Publication Data
A catalogue record for this book is available from the British Library

Library of Congress Cataloging-in-Publication Data
A catalog record for this book is available from the Library of Congress

ISBN: 978-0-12-811907-5

For Information on all Academic Press publications
visit our website at https://www.elsevier.com/books-and-journals

Publisher: Charlotte Cockle
Acquisition Editor: Megan R. Ball
Editorial Project Manager: Redding Morse
Production Project Manager: Vignesh Tamil
Cover Designer: Miles Hitchen

Typeset by MPS Limited, Chennai, India

Contents

List of Contributors

Andrea Aghi
Department of Medicine, Clinica Medica 1, University of Padova, Padova, Italy

Mourad Akdad
Department of Biology, Faculty of Sciences and Technology, FSTE, Errachidia, Morocco

Emmanuel Andres
Department of Internal Medicine, Diabetes and Metabolic Diseases, Hôpitaux Universitaires de Strasbourg, Strasbourg, France; EA 3072 "Mitochondrie, Stress oxydant et Protection musculaire", Université de Strasbourg, Strasbourg, France

Desirée Bartolini
Department of Pharmaceutical Science, University of Perugia, Laboratory of Clinical Biochemistry and Nutrition, Perugia, Italy

Paula Brandão
Department of Chemistry/CICECO, University of Aveiro, Portugal

Allison Bridges
Department of Biochemistry and Molecular Biology, Augusta University, Augusta, GA, United States

Paola Casanello
Department of Obstetrics, Department of Neonatology, School of Medicine, Pontificia Universidad Católica de Chile, Santiago, Chile

Erika Castaño-Moreno
Laboratory of Nutrition and Metabolic Regulation, Human Nutrition Unit, Institute of Nutrition and Food Technology (INTA), University of Chile, Santiago, Chile

S.G. Chailyan
H Buniatian Institute of Biochemistry, National Academy of Science of Armenia, Yerevan, Armenia

Paola Ciceri
Renal Research Laboratory, Department of Nephrology, Dialysis and Renal Transplant, Fondazione Ca' Granda IRCCS, Ospedale Maggiore Policlinico, Milan, Italy

Ferruccio Conte
Renal Division, Renal Division and Laboratory of Experimental Nephrology, ASST Santi Paolo e Carlo, Dipartimento di Scienze della Salute, S. Paolo Hospital, Department of Health Sciences, University of Milan, Milan, Italy

Mario Cozzolino
Renal Division, Renal Division and Laboratory of Experimental Nephrology, ASST Santi Paolo e Carlo, Dipartimento di Scienze della Salute, S. Paolo Hospital, Department of Health Sciences, University of Milan, Milan, Italy

Gabriele Cruciani
Department of Chemistry, Biology and Biotechnology, University of Perugia, Perugia, Italy

John Cunningham
University College London, London, United Kingdom

Nassim Dali-Youcef
Laboratory of General and Specialized Biochemistry, Hôpitaux Universitaires de Strasbourg, Strasbourg, France; Department of Molecular Science, University Hospital of Strasbourg, University of Strasbourg, Strasbourg, France

Danyel Bueno Dalto
Sherbrooke Research and Development Centre, Agriculture and Agri-Food Canada, Sherbrooke, QC, Canada

K.E. Danielyan
H Buniatian Institute of Biochemistry, National Academy of Science of Armenia, Yerevan, Armenia

Domenica De Santis
Department of Medicine, School of Medicine, University of Verona, Verona, Italy

Venkata Satish Dontaraju
Internal Medicine, Rockford Memorial Hospital, Rockford, IL, United States

Venkateshwara Dronamraju
College of Pharmacy, University of Louisiana at Monroe, Monroe, LA, United States

Bachir El Bouhali
Department of Biology, Faculty of Sciences and Technology, FSTE, Errachidia, Morocco

Joshua T. Emmerson
Department of Neuroscience, Carleton University, Ottawa, ON, Canada

Jakub Fichna
Department of Biochemistry, Faculty of Medicine, Medical University of Lodz, Lodz, Poland

Simonetta Friso
Department of Medicine, School of Medicine, University of Verona, Verona, Italy

Maria Fusaro
National Research Council (CNR) – Institute of Clinical Physiology (IFC), Pisa, Italy; Department of Medicine, University of Padova, Padova, Italy

Roberta Galarini
Istituto Zooprofilattico Sperimentale dell'Umbria e delle Marche "Togo Rosati", Perugia, Italy

Andrea Galassi
Renal Division, Renal Division and Laboratory of Experimental Nephrology, ASST Santi Paolo e Carlo, Dipartimento di Scienze della Salute, S. Paolo Hospital, Department of Health Sciences, University of Milan, Milan, Italy

Francesco Galli
Department of Pharmaceutical Science, University of Perugia, Laboratory of Clinical Biochemistry and Nutrition, Perugia, Italy

Maurizio Gallieni
Nephrology and Dialysis Unit, Department of Clinical and Biomedical Sciences 'Luigi Sacco', University of Milan, Milan, Italy

Andreas Geier
Division of Hepatology, Department of Internal Medicine II, University Hospital Würzburg, Würzburg, Germany

Antimo Gioiello
Department of Pharmaceutical Science, University of Perugia, Laboratory of Clinical Biochemistry and Nutrition, Perugia, Italy

Danilo Giusepponi
Istituto Zooprofilattico Sperimentale dell'Umbria e delle Marche "Togo Rosati", Perugia, Italy

Cláudio M. Gomes
Biosystems and Integrative Sciences Institute, Faculdade de Ciências, Universidade de Lisboa, and Departamento de Química e Bioquímica, Faculdade de Ciências, Universidade de Lisboa, Lisboa, Portugal

Álisson de Carvalho Gonçalves
Laboratory of Experimental Nutrition, Federal University of Triangulo Mineiro, Uberaba, Brazil

Samuel Guieu
Department of Chemistry/QOPNA/CICECO, University of Aveiro, Portugal

Shin-ichiro Hagiwara
Department of Pediatric Gastroenterology, Nutrition and Endocrinology, Osaka Medical Center and Research Institute for Maternal and Child Health, Osaka, Japan

Ghazaleh Hajiluian
Department of Nutrition, School of Public Health, Iran University of Medical Sciences, Tehran, Iran

Bárbara J. Henriques
Biosystems and Integrative Sciences Institute, Faculdade de Ciências, Universidade de Lisboa, and Departamento de Química e Bioquímica, Faculdade de Ciências, Universidade de Lisboa, Lisboa, Portugal

Giorgio Iervasi
National Research Council (CNR) – Institute of Clinical Physiology (IFC), Pisa, Italy

Nafisa M. Jadavji
Department of Neuroscience, Carleton University, Ottawa, ON, Canada; Department of Biomedical Sciences, Midwestern University, Glendale, AZ, United States

Daniel Jahn
Hepatology Research Laboratory, Division of Hepatology, Department of Internal Medicine II, University Hospital Würzburg, Würzburg, Germany

Magdalena Jankowska
Department of Nephrology, Transplantology and Internal Medicine, Medical University of Gdansk, Gdansk, Poland

O Karmin
Department of Animal Science, University of Manitoba, Winnipeg, MB, Canada; Department of Physiology and Pathophysiology, University of Manitoba, Winnipeg, MB, Canada; Laboratory of Integrative Biology, St. Boniface Hospital Research Centre, Winnipeg, MB, Canada

Norihisa Kato
Graduate School of Integrated Sciences for Life, Hiroshima University, Higashi-Hiroshima, Japan

Farid Khallouki
Department of Biology, Faculty of Sciences and Technology, FSTE, Errachidia, Morocco

Jerzy Kruk
Department of Plant Physiology and Biochemistry, Faculty of Biochemistry, Biophysics and Biotechnology, Jagiellonian University, Kraków, Poland

Thanutchaporn Kumrungsee
Graduate School of Integrated Sciences for Life, Hiroshima University, Higashi-Hiroshima, Japan

Dmytro Labudzinskyi
Department of Biochemistry of Vitamins and Coenzymes, Palladin Institute of Biochemistry of National Academy of Sciences of Ukraine, Kyiv, Ukraine

Antonio Simone Laganà
Department of Obstetrics and Gynecology, "Filippo Del Ponte" Hospital, University of Insubria, Varese, Italy

Olha Lisakovska
Department of Biochemistry of Vitamins and Coenzymes, Palladin Institute of Biochemistry of National Academy of Sciences of Ukraine, Kyiv, Ukraine

Miguel Llanos
Laboratory of Nutrition and Metabolic Regulation, Human Nutrition Unit, Institute of Nutrition and Food Technology (INTA), University of Chile, Santiago, Chile

Francesco Locatelli
Division of Nephrology and Dialysis, A. Manzoni Hospital, Lecco, Italy

Rita Marinelli
Department of Pharmaceutical Science, University of Perugia, Laboratory of Clinical Biochemistry and Nutrition, Perugia, Italy

Jean-Jacques Matte
Sherbrooke Research and Development Centre, Agriculture and Agri-Food Canada, Sherbrooke, QC, Canada

Anna Mazanova
Department of Biochemistry of Vitamins and Coenzymes, Palladin Institute of Biochemistry of National Academy of Sciences of Ukraine, Kyiv, Ukraine

Maria Cristina Mereu
Nephrologist Independent Researcher, Cagliari, Italy

Maria C. Millan-Linares
Cell Biology Unit, Instituto de la Grasa, CSIC, Seville, Spain

Mahira Moftah
Department of Neuroscience, Carleton University, Ottawa, ON, Canada

Sergio Montserrat-de la Paz
Department of Medical Biochemistry, Molecular Biology, and Immunology, School of Medicine, University of Seville, Seville, Spain

Gnanasekar Munirathinam
Department of Biomedical Sciences, University of Illinois-College of Medicine, Rockford, IL, United States

Sushmita Mustafi
John P. Hussman Institute for Human Genomics, Miller School of Medicine, University of Miami, Miami, FL, United States

Siti Syairah Mohd Mutalip
Department of Pharmaceutical Life Sciences, Faculty of Pharmacy, Universiti Teknologi MARA (UiTM), Selangor, Malaysia

Maria C. Naranjo
Department of Food Technology, School of Agricultural and Forest Engineering, University of Lleida, Lleida, Spain

Beatrycze Nowicka
Department of Plant Physiology and Biochemistry, Faculty of Biochemistry, Biophysics and Biotechnology, Jagiellonian University, Kraków, Poland

Robert Wyn Owen
Division of Chemopreventive Oncology, German Cancer Research Center, Heidelberg, Germany

Yuliya Parkhomenko
Department of Vitamins and Coenzymes Biochemistry, A.V. Palladin Institute of Biochemistry of the National Academy of Sciences of Ukraine, Kyiv, Ukraine

Reyna Peñailillo
Laboratory of Nutrition and Metabolic Regulation, Human Nutrition Unit, Institute of Nutrition and Food Technology (INTA), University of Chile, Santiago, Chile

Raúl Piñuñuri
School of Nutrition and Dietetics, Faculty of Health, University of Bernardo O'Higgins, Santiago, Chile

Francesca Pizzolo
Department of Medicine, School of Medicine, University of Verona, Verona, Italy

Mario Plebani
Department of Medicine, University of Padova, Laboratory Medicine Unit, Padova, Italy

Marc Poirot
Cancer Research Center of Toulouse, Team Cholesterol Metabolism and Therapeutic Innovations, UMR 1037 INSERM-University of Toulouse, Toulouse, France

Guilherme Vannucchi Portari
Health Institute, Department of Nutrition, Federal University of Triangulo Mineiro, Uberaba, Brazil

Puttur D. Prasad
Department of Biochemistry and Molecular Biology, Augusta University, Augusta, GA, United States

Victor R. Preedy
Diabetes & Nutritional Sciences Division, School of Medicine, King's College London, London, United Kingdom

Mina Yamazaki Price
Division of Critical Care, Medicine and Surgery, Department of Therapies, Royal Free Hospital, Royal Free London NHS Foundation Trust, London, United Kingdom

Zoya Protasova
Department of Vitamins and Coenzymes Biochemistry, A.V. Palladin Institute of Biochemistry of the National Academy of Sciences of Ukraine, Kyiv, Ukraine

Pragya Rajpurohit
Department of Biochemistry and Molecular Biology, Augusta University, Augusta, GA, United States

Gianluca Rizzo
Independent Researcher, Messina, Italy

Ana María Ronco
Laboratory of Nutrition and Metabolic Regulation, Human Nutrition Unit, Institute of Nutrition and Food Technology (INTA), University of Chile, Santiago, Chile

Bartolomeo Sebastiani
Department of Chemistry, Biology and Biotechnology, University of Perugia, Perugia, Italy

Farzad Shidfar
Department of Nutrition, School of Public Health, Iran University of Medical Sciences, Tehran, Iran

Ihor Shymanskyi
Department of Biochemistry of Vitamins and Coenzymes, Palladin Institute of Biochemistry of National Academy of Sciences of Ukraine, Kyiv, Ukraine

Victoria Sid
Department of Physiology and Pathophysiology, University of Manitoba, Winnipeg, MB, Canada; Laboratory of Integrative Biology, St. Boniface Hospital Research Centre, Winnipeg, MB, Canada

Sandrine Silvente-Poirot
Cancer Research Center of Toulouse, Team Cholesterol Metabolism and Therapeutic Innovations, UMR 1037 INSERM-University of Toulouse, Toulouse, France

Yaw L. Siow
Department of Physiology and Pathophysiology, University of Manitoba, Winnipeg, MB, Canada; Agriculture and Agri-Food Canada, Canadian Centre for Agri-Food Research in Health and Medicine, Winnipeg, MB, Canada; Innovative Therapy Research Laboratory, St. Boniface Hospital Research Centre, Winnipeg, MB, Canada

Lydia Siragusa
Molecular Horizon, Perugia, Italy

Luiz Ricardo Soldi
Laboratory of Experimental Nutrition, Federal University of Triangulo Mineiro, Uberaba, Brazil

Andrea Stucchi
Renal Division, Renal Division and Laboratory of Experimental Nephrology, ASST Santi Paolo e Carlo, Dipartimento di Scienze della Salute, S. Paolo Hospital, Department of Health Sciences, University of Milan, Milan, Italy

Takashi Suda
Department of Immunology and Molecular Biology, Cancer Research Institute, Kanazawa University, Kanazawa, Japan

Sofya Suidasari
Graduate School of Integrated Sciences for Life, Hiroshima University, Higashi-Hiroshima, Japan

Paul William Sylvester
College of Pharmacy, University of Louisiana at Monroe, Monroe, LA, United States

Agata Szymaszkiewicz
Department of Biochemistry, Faculty of Medicine, Medical University of Lodz, Lodz, Poland

Renata Szymańska
Department of Medical Physics and Biophysics, Faculty of Physics and Applied Computer Science, AGH University of Science and Technology, Kraków, Poland

Kiran Thakur
Associate Professor, School of Food Science and Engineering, Hefei University of Technology, Hefei, People's Republic of China

Muthusamy Thangaraju
Department of Biochemistry and Molecular Biology, Augusta University, Augusta, GA, United States

Sudhir Kumar Tomar
Principal Scientist, Dairy Microbiology, ICAR-National Dairy Research Institute, Karnal, Haryana, India

Pierangelo Torquato
Department of Pharmaceutical Science, University of Perugia, Laboratory of Clinical Biochemistry and Nutrition, Perugia, Italy

Agnieszka Trela
Department of Medical Physics and Biophysics, Faculty of Physics and Applied Computer Science, AGH University of Science and Technology, Kraków, Poland

Giovanni Tripepi
Clinical Epidemiology and Physiopathology of Renal Diseases and Hypertension, CNR, Institute of Clinical Physiology, Reggio Calabria, Italy

Silvia Udali
Department of Medicine, School of Medicine, University of Verona, Verona, Italy

Mykola Veliky
Department of Biochemistry of Vitamins and Coenzymes, Palladin Institute of Biochemistry of National Academy of Sciences of Ukraine, Kyiv, Ukraine

Smita Vinjamuri
Department of Biomedical Sciences, University of Illinois-College of Medicine, Rockford, IL, United States

Andriy Vovk
Department of Bioorganic Mechanisms, V.P. Kukhar Institute of Bioorganic Chemistry and Petrochemistry of the National Academy of Sciences of Ukraine, Kyiv, Ukraine

Gaofeng Wang
John P. Hussman Institute for Human Genomics, Dr. John T. Macdonald Foundation Department of Human Genetics, Sylvester Comprehensive Cancer Center, Miller School of Medicine, University of Miami, Miami, FL, United States

Zhao-Jun Wei
Professor, School of Food Science and Engineering, Hefei University of Technology, Hefei, People's Republic of China

Connie W.H. Woo
Department of Pharmacology and Pharmacy, Li Ka Shing Faculty of Medicine, University of Hong Kong, Hong Kong, SAR, China

Noriyuki Yanaka
Graduate School of Integrated Sciences for Life, Hiroshima University, Higashi-Hiroshima, Japan

Martina Zaninotto
Department of Medicine, University of Padova, Laboratory Medicine Unit, Padova, Italy

Peipei Zhang
State Key Laboratory of Cellular Stress Biology, School of Medicine & School of Life Science, Xiamen University, Xiamen, Fujian, China

Mikołaj Świerczyński
Department of Biochemistry, Faculty of Medicine, Medical University of Lodz, Lodz, Poland

Series Preface

In this series on Molecular Nutrition, the editors of each book aim to disseminate important material pertaining to molecular nutrition in its broadest sense. The coverage ranges from molecular aspects to whole organs, and the impact of nutrition or malnutrition on individuals and whole communities. It includes concepts, policy, preclinical studies, and clinical investigations relating to molecular nutrition. The subject areas include molecular mechanisms, polymorphisms, SNPs, genome-wide analysis, genotypes, gene expression, genetic modifications, and many other aspects. Information given in the Molecular Nutrition series relates to national, international, and global issues.

A major feature of the series that sets it apart from other texts is the initiative to bridge the transintellectual divide so that it is suitable for novices and experts alike. It embraces traditional and nontraditional formats of nutritional sciences in different ways. Each book in the series has both overviews and detailed and focused chapters. Molecular Nutrition is designed for nutritionists, dieticians, educationalists, health experts, epidemiologists, and health-related professionals such as chemists. It is also suitable for students, graduates, postgraduates, researchers, lecturers, teachers, and professors. Contributors are national or international experts, many of whom are from world-renowned institutions or universities. It is intended to be an authoritative text covering nutrition at the molecular level.

V.R. Preedy
Series Editor

Preface

In this book *Molecular Nutrition: Vitamins* we focus on *Vitamins*. In total there are 13 vitamins which are essential constituents of the diet. Vitamins are classified as either fat soluble (A, D, E, and K) or water soluble (B_1, B_2, B_3, B_5, B_6, B_7 B_9, B_{12}, and C) and are termed as micronutrients due to the low quantities required in the diet. The majority of vitamins, except for vitamin D and small amounts of B_3, need to be obtained from the diet, and thus inadequate intake can lead to deficiencies. The most common deficiencies in the United States are of vitamin B_6, vitamin B_{12}, vitamin C, folic acid, and vitamin D, with the deficiency subject to variation depending on the ethnic group, gender, and age of the person. Furthermore, the quantity of vitamin required from the diet varies quite significantly between vitamins from micrograms to milligrams.

Vitamins are an important field to study within Molecular Nutrition as vitamins are pivotal to numerous biochemical and genetic pathways. For example, vitamin B_{12}, also known as cobalamin, is important for DNA synthesis, nerve health, amino acids, and fatty acids metabolism, and together with vitamin B_9 (folate), is central to red blood cell maturation. Vitamin B_3 (niacin) is a precursor of the coenzymes nicotinamide adenine dinucleotide and nicotinamide adenine dinucleotide phosphate, which are key to metabolic pathways. Similarly, vitamin B_2 (riboflavin) is a component of flavin nucleotides that are essential for respiration.

There are many conditions that develop due to inadequate vitamin intake from the diet. For example, thiamine deficiency (vitamin B_1) can lead to memory loss, as seen in Wernicke/Korsakoff syndrome and in chronic alcoholics; acute and chronic pancreatitis and chronic liver disease leads to a disruption in fat absorption, which affects the absorption of fat-soluble vitamins; the lack of folate can lead to anemia and during pregnancy developmental disorders in newborns. More recently vitamins have been studied due to their therapeutic properties as highlighted throughout this book. Thus this text is relevant to nutritionists and nutrition researchers as vitamins are integral to human health and metabolic pathways, are components of enzymes, and can aid in the treatment of a wide range of conditions.

This book, *Molecular Nutrition: Vitamins*, contains three sections. In *Part 1* there is coverage of nutrition and vitamins in terms of general aspects, and their contribution to the diet. In *Part 2* there is coverage on vitamin B_2 and mitochondrial energy; the use of folate in liver disease; vitamin K and treatment of prostate cancer; the preventive properties of vitamin B_6 in inflammation; niacin and hyperlipidemia; molecular and nutritional aspects of vitamin E; vitamins in chronic kidney disease; vitamin B_{12} malabsorption; vitamin D and diabetes mellitus; and vitamin C and Alzheimer disease. *Part 3* covers the epigenetics of vitamins; gene expression; and the role of vitamins in transcriptional and transcriptome regulation.

The Editor

PART I

General and Introductory Aspects

CHAPTER 1

Reference dietary requirements of vitamins in different stages of life

Mina Yamazaki Price[1] and Victor R. Preedy[2]
[1]Division of Critical Care, Medicine and Surgery, Department of Therapies, Royal Free Hospital, Royal Free London NHS Foundation Trust, London, United Kingdom
[2]Diabetes & Nutritional Sciences Division, School of Medicine, King's College London, London, United Kingdom

Contents

Molecular Nutrition
DOI: https://doi.org/10.1016/B978-0-12-811907-5.00002-6

Key facts of vitamins

- Vitamins are organic compounds and usually present naturally in food items in very small amounts.
- Each vitamin has highly specific roles in normal physiological functions and metabolism including growth, development, and maintenance.
- Humans require minute amounts of vitamins to meet physiological needs but are unable to endogenously synthesize adequate amounts. Therefore it is essential to obtain vitamins from food items.
- A severe and prolonged insufficient dietary intake of specific vitamins can cause specific deficiency syndromes. For example, beriberi is a disorder caused by thiamin (vitamin B1) deficiency. Symptoms of beriberi include peripheral neuropathy, muscle pain, and weakness.
- Vitamins are commonly classified under the umbrella of "micronutrients" in contrast to "macronutrients" (i.e., carbohydrate, protein, and fat).

Summary points

- Currently 13 substances are recognized as vitamins. They can be categorized into two groups according to their solubilities, namely fat-soluble and water-soluble vitamins.
- Fat-soluble vitamins are vitamins A, D, E, and K. Water-soluble vitamins are thiamin (vitamin B1), riboflavin (vitamin B2), niacin (vitamin B3), vitamin B6 (pyridoxine), vitamin B12 (cobalamin), folate (vitamin B9), vitamin C, pantothenic acid, and biotin.
- For each vitamin, reference dietary requirements have been derived, though the amounts and age categories vary differ between countries.
- Differences in dietary and nutrient patterns in different populations, even within the same country, influence overall vitamin intake and thus determine whether reference dietary requirements are met.
- There are various challenges between different age groups for meeting vitamin B12 reference dietary requirements. On the other hand, it is less challenging to meet vitamin K reference dietary requirements across different populations.

Definitions of words and terms

- *Micronutrient*: A chemical element required in very small amounts in living organisms to maintain normal physiological functions. It is often used in contrast to macronutrients (i.e., dietary carbohydrates, proteins, and fats).

- *Endogenously synthesized*: Substances that are produced or synthesized within an organism rather than provided by nutrition.
- *Metabolic activation*: The chemical reactions of a relatively inert substance to a more biologically active form within living organisms.
- *Biopotency*: A measure of the capacity and/or ability of a substance such as nutrients including vitamins to have a specified biochemical action in living organisms.
- *Essential nutrients*: Nutrients required for normal physiological functions including growth, reproduction, and maintaining good health that cannot be synthesized at all or in sufficient quantities within a living organism; hence they are required to be provided by nutritional means.
- *Free radical*: A molecule having an unpaired electron which makes it extremely reactive. It can be generated within a living organism as a result of normal biological processes as well as introduced by environmental factors such as exposure to ultraviolet sunlight and smoking.
- *Oxidative stress*: A disturbance in the balance between the production of free radicals and antioxidant defenses within a living organism. Therefore the host is unable to detoxify their harmful effects. Oxidative stress is believed to be a causal factor in various conditions including aging, age-related diseases such as Alzheimer disease, macular degeneration, cataract formation, cardiovascular diseases, and cancers.

Abbreviations

AI	Adequate intake
CoA	Coenzyme A
COMA	Committee on Medical Aspects of Food Policy
DRI	Dietary reference intake
DRV	Dietary reference value
NAD	Nicotinamide adenine nucleotide
NADP	Nicotinamide adenine dinucleotide phosphate
RDA	Recommended dietary allowance
RNI	Reference nutrient intake

1.1 Introduction

Vitamins are essential for life and have highly specific roles for the maintenance of normal physiological function including growth and development. The vitamins do not constitute structural components in cells nor contribute to energy needs. However, they are used for the efficient homeostatic control of cells, metabolic pathways, and developmental processes. For example, they are involved in metabolic activation as enzyme cofactors or contribute to the production of other components in cells. They are required in very small amounts, hence the vitamins are classified under the umbrella of "micronutrients."

Vitamins are not endogenously synthesized in adequate amounts in humans to meet normal physiological needs. Vitamins are organic compounds and naturally occur in food items. Of course for every generalization there are exceptions. For example, vitamin K2 can be synthesized endogenously although in the Western diet most of the vitamin K is derived from plant foods in the form of vitamin K1 (Yamazaki Price and Preedy, 2018).

This chapter describes the various vitamins, their requirements, and very briefly their physiological roles. We use the nomenclature of vitamins as described in the report of the Panel on Dietary Reference Values of the Committee on Medical Aspects of Food Policy (COMA) (DH, 1991).

Currently 13 substances are recognized as vitamins. They can be categorized into two groups according to their solubilities, namely fat-soluble and water-soluble vitamins.

Fat-soluble vitamins are vitamins A, D, E, and K. Water-soluble vitamins are thiamin (vitamin B1), riboflavin (vitamin B2), niacin (vitamin B3), vitamin B6 (pyridoxine), vitamin B12 (cobalamin), folate (vitamin B9), vitamin C, pantothenic acid, and biotin.

The realization of vitamins as essential nutrients occurred at the beginning of the 20th century after decades of studying associations between diseases and certain types of diet among specific populations. An example of such an association includes scurvy in seamen during the 14th century (months of diet principally based on dried and salted foods) and beriberi in Asian populations in the 19th century (surviving on polished "white" rice) (Combs and McClung, 2017). Since then, particularly since the early 1980s, the scientific knowledge and understanding of each vitamin's functions have been dramatically expanded. Thus the increasing understanding of their physiological roles and the effects of deficiencies on human health and well-being (including the diversity of syndromes associated with deficiencies) has become more evident. Advances in evidence-based research have led to an improved knowledge of vitamin requirements and the development of dietary guidelines to ensure adequacy.

This chapter reviews the reference requirements of 13 vitamins for different stages of life for the United States and the United Kingdom. However, it is important to mention from the outset of this review that different countries have their own nomenclature. As a generalization to cover the United States and the United Kingdom we use the term "reference dietary requirements." Later on we define specific terms used in the United States and United Kingdom.

1.2 Reference dietary requirements

Reference dietary requirements are the amounts of nutrients that individuals and populations need to consume in order to minimize the risk of deficiency or excess: overall achieving optimal health and prevention of disease.

The reference dietary requirements apply to healthy individuals and populations. The requirements for one nutrient presuppose that the requirements of other nutrients have been met. Furthermore, reference dietary requirements assume that intake is via the oral route in food. In other words they cannot be used for artificial support regimes such as total parenteral nutrition (DH, 1991).

Reference dietary requirements potentially have four uses as follows:

1. assessing individuals;
2. determining at risk subgroups or subpopulations;
3. prescribing diets; and
4. food labeling (DH, 1991).

There is limited scientific support behind the values for the specific reference dietary requirements across age ranges, gender, and physiological status. However, where relevant and possible, these values include an allowance for bioavailability and utilization (WHO and FAO, 2004).

In the United Kingdom, the reference dietary requirements are termed dietary reference values (DRVs). For other countries, for example, in the United States, these values are termed as dietary reference intakes (DRIs), which are essentially equivalent to the DRVs used in the United Kingdom. Definitions of the reference dietary requirements for the United Kingdom and the United States are described in Table 1.1.

Below we briefly describe the roles of the various vitamins. With a limited text it is impossible to cover all of the detailed aspects of the vitamins and the reader is referred to individual chapters within this book.

Table 1.1 Definitions of reference dietary intakes (DRIs) for the United States and the United Kingdom.

United States	Definition
Adequate intakes (AIs)	A recommended average daily nutrient intake level based on observed or experimentally determined approximations or estimates of mean nutrient intake by a group (or groups) of apparently healthy people. An AI is used when the recommended dietary allowance cannot be determined.
Dietary reference intakes (DRIs)	A set of nutrient-based reference values that are quantitative estimates of nutrient intakes to be used for planning and assessing diets for healthy people. DRIs expand on the periodic reports called recommended dietary allowances (RDAs), which were first published by the Institute of Medicine in 1941.
Estimated average requirements (EAR)	The average daily nutrient intake level estimated to meet the requirements of half the healthy individuals in a particular life stage and sex group.
Recommended dietary allowances (RDA)	The average daily dietary intake level that is sufficient to meet the nutrient requirements of nearly all (97%–98%) healthy individuals in a particular life stage and sex group.
Tolerable upper intake levels (UL)	The highest average daily nutrient intake level likely to pose no risk of adverse health effects for nearly all individuals in a particular life stage and sex group. As intake increases above the UL, the potential risk of adverse health effects increases.
United Kingdom	**Definition**
Dietary reference values (DRV)	A term used to cover LRNI, EAR, RNI, and safe intake.
Estimated average requirement (EAR)	Estimated average requirement of a group of people for energy or protein or a vitamin or mineral. About half will usually need more than the EAR, and half less.
Lower reference nutrient intake (LRNI)	LRNI for protein or a vitamin or mineral. An amount of the nutrient that is enough for only the few people in a group who have low needs.
Reference nutrient intake (RNI)	RNI for protein or a vitamin or mineral. An amount of the nutrient that is enough, or more than enough, for about 97% of people in a group. If average intake of a group is at RNI, then the risk of deficiency in the group is very small.
Safe intake (SI)	A term used to indicate the intake or range of intakes of a nutrient for which there is not enough information to estimate RNI, EAR, or LRNI. It is an amount that is enough for almost everyone but not so large as to cause undesirable effects.

Source: For the United States, adapted from Office of Disease Prevention and Health Promotion (ODPHP), 2015. 2015–2020 Dietary Guidelines for Americans. <http://health.gov/dietaryguidelines/2015/guidelines/> (accessed 8.04.18.) (ODPHP, 2015); for the United Kingdom, adapted from Department of Health (DH), 1991. Dietary Reference Values for Food Energy and Nutrients for the United Kingdom. The Stationary Office (TSO), Norwich.

1.3 Fat-soluble vitamins

1.3.1 Vitamin A

Vitamin A is vital for embryonic development, differentiation of tissues, growth, epithelial integrity, red blood cell production, reproduction, immune function, and the visual system (Imdad et al., 2017). Vitamin A comes in two forms, namely retinol (preformed vitamin A) and provitamin A carotenoids. Retinol (mostly in the form of retinyl esters) occurs naturally in animal foods and has 100% bioavailability (i.e., completely absorbed) (Combs and McClung, 2017). In contrast, carotenoids (mostly in the form of β-carotene), which occur in plant foods, have much less bioavailability. Not all carotenoids have provitamin A activity. After the consideration of the physiological efficacy of in vivo conversion of carotenoids to retinol and intestinal absorption capacity, currently the widely accepted conversion values in a normal mixed diet are 6 μg β-carotene to 1 μg retinol (DH, 1991). Commonly, reference dietary requirements are expressed in retinol equivalent (μg). Table 1.2 shows the vitamin A reference dietary requirements for the United States and the United Kingdom.

1.3.2 Vitamin D

Ergocalciferol (vitamin D2) and cholecalciferol (vitamin D3) are the two major forms of vitamin D. Vitamin D has a crucial role in maintaining the normal mineralization of bones and teeth, muscle contraction, nerve conduction, and general cellular function in all parts of the body. This is achieved by the role of vitamin D in plasma calcium homeostasis (WHO and FAO, 2004). More recently, it has been suggested that the role of vitamin D may go beyond calcium homeostasis. These other roles include the possible inhibition of cancer progression and certain autoimmune diseases, and there are also positive effects on the cardiovascular, dermatological, and immune systems (Christakos et al., 2014). Humans, with modest sun exposure, are able to produce sufficient vitamin D endogenously from sterols in the body by the action of ultraviolet light on the skin. Hence vitamin D is often called the "sunshine vitamin" (Combs and McClung, 2017).

Vitamin D is distributed sparsely in dietary sources and is present in very low amounts. It is considered that the diet provides approximately 20% of vitamin D so the remainder must come from sunlight (Borel et al., 2015). However the respective contributions of vitamin D from the diet and via sunlight will depend on a number of factors including

Table 1.2 Vitamin A reference dietary requirements for the Unites States and the United Kingdom.

Life stage group	Male (μg/day)	Female (μg/day)
United States		
0–6 months	400*	400*
6–12 months	500*	500*
1–3 years	300	300
4–8 years	400	400
9–13 years	600	600
14–18 years	900	700
19–30 years	900	700
31–50 years	900	700
51–70 years	900	700
>70 years	900	700
Pregnancy 14–18 years	–	750
19–30 years	–	770
31–50 years	–	770
Lactation 14–18 years	–	1200
19–30 years	–	1300
31–50 years	–	1300
United Kingdom		
0–3 months	350	350
4–6 months	350	350
7–9 months	350	350
10–12 months	350	350
1–3 years	400	400
4–6 years	400	400
7–10 years	500	500
11–14 years	600	600
15–18 years	700	600
19–50 years	700	600
>50 years	700	600
Pregnancy	–	700
Lactation 0–4 months	–	950
>4 months	–	950

Data show reference dietary requirements of vitamin A for the United States and the United Kingdom in μg retinol equivalent/day. For the United States, figures with an asterisk (*) are presented as adequate intakes (AIs). All other figures for the United States are presented as recommended dietary allowances (RDAs). For the United Kingdom, the name of the vitamin used in the table is based on the report by the Committee on Medical Aspects of Food Policy (COMA) (DH, 1991). All figures for the United Kingdom are presented as reference nutrient intakes (RNIs). Cells showing "–" indicate that there are no values for that particular life stage or gender.

Data from: For the United States, The National Academies of Sciences Engineering Medicine (NASEM), 2016. Dietary Reference Intakes Tables and Application. <http://www.nationalacademies.org/hmd/Activities/Nutrition/SummaryDRIs/DRI-Tables.aspx> (accessed 26.01.18.) (NASEM, 2016); for the United Kingdom, Department of Health (DH), 1991. Dietary Reference Values for Food Energy and Nutrients for the United Kingdom. The Stationary Office (TSO), Norwich.

geographical location, cultural characteristics of body coverage with clothes, and so on. Table 1.3 shows the vitamin D reference dietary requirements for the United States and the United Kingdom.

1.3.3 Vitamin K

Plant-derived phylloquinones (vitamin K1) and the bacterial-derived menaquinones (vitamin K2) are the two major forms of vitamin K (Yamazaki Price and Preedy, 2015, 2018). The primary role of vitamin K is its participation in hemostasis and this has been well established since the 1970s. Vitamin K is a cofactor for the posttranslational carboxylation of glutamyl residues in plasma-clotting protein factors II (prothrombin), VII, IX, and X in the coagulation cascade. The product of this process is γ-carboxyglutamyl residues which have an affinity for calcium. Proteins which require vitamin K for the formation of γ-carboxyglutamyl residues are called vitamin K−dependent proteins. Currently a total of 16 vitamin K−dependent proteins (including the aforementioned four involved in the coagulation cascade) are known. Thus the role of vitamin K is considered to go beyond hemostasis. For example, it is now known that vitamin K contributes to antiinflammatory activity, bone structure and function, glucose homeostasis, and vascular health. Vitamin K, particularly the plant-derived phylloquinones (vitamin K1), is widely distributed in the diet and clinical deficiency is almost nonexistent in general except for neonatal populations (Yamazaki Price and Preedy, 2018). Table 1.4 shows the vitamin K reference dietary requirements for the United States and the United Kingdom.

1.3.4 Vitamin E

Vitamin E, a family of eight homologues which consist of four tocopherol homologues (α-, β-, γ-, δ-) and four tocotrienols homologues (α-, β-, γ-, δ-), is entirely synthesized by plants. Additionally, synthetic forms are also commonly available. Among the vitamin E family, α-tocopherol has the highest biopotency. Therefore in human nutrition, vitamin E activity is expressed in α-tocopherol equivalents (Combs and McClung, 2017). The biological role of vitamin E is principally based on its antioxidant properties, especially in preventing lipid peroxidation. Cells are constantly exposed to free radicals which have the potential to cause oxidative stress and induce damage to biological systems and structures. Increased oxidative stress and lipid peroxidation are associated with a wide range of diseases including cardiovascular diseases, cancers, cataracts, macular

Table 1.3 Vitamin D reference dietary requirements for the United States and United Kingdom.

Life stage group	Male (μg/day)	Female (μg/day)
United States		
0–6 months	10*	10*
6–12 months	10*	10*
1–3 years	15	15
4–8 years	15	15
9–13 years	15	15
14–18 years	15	15
19–30 years	15	15
31–50 years	15	15
51–70 years	15	15
>70 years	20	20
Pregnancy 14–18 years	–	15
19–30 years	–	15
31–50 years	–	15
Lactation 14–18 years	–	15
19–30 years	–	15
31–50 years	–	15
United Kingdom		
0–3 months	8.5–10	8.5–10
4–6 months	8.5–10	8.5–10
7–9 months	8.5–10	8.5–10
10–12 months	8.5–10	8.5–10
1–4 years	10	10
5–6 years	10	10
7–10 years	10	10
11–14 years	10	10
15–18 years	10	10
19–50 years	10	10
>50 years	10	10
Pregnancy	–	10
Lactation 0–4 months	–	10
>4 months	–	10

Data show reference dietary requirements of vitamin D for the United States (in μg cholecalciferol/day) and the United Kingdom (in μg cholecalciferol and ergocalciferol/day). Data are presented as either RDA (United States) or RNI (United Kingdom). For the United States, figures with an asterisk (*) are presented as adequate intakes (AIs). Cells showing "–" indicate that there are no values for that particular life stage or gender. For both countries, figures are derived under the assumption of minimum sunlight exposure. For the United Kingdom, figures from 0 month to 3 years are presented as safe intakes (SIs). Figures for age 0–11 months for the United Kingdom are based on the concentration of vitamin D in infant formula. All other figures (i.e., aged 4 years and above, including pregnant and lactating women for the United Kingdom) are presented as RNIs. For other details, see Table 1.1 for definitions and the legend to Table 1.2.

Source: For the United States, The National Academies of Sciences Engineering Medicine (NASEM), 2016. Dietary Reference Intakes Tables and Application. <http://www.nationalacademies.org/hmd/Activities/Nutrition/SummaryDRIs/DRI-Tables.aspx> (accessed 26.01.18.) (NASEM, 2016); for the United Kingdom, Department of Health (DH), 1991. Dietary Reference Values for Food Energy and Nutrients for the United Kingdom. The Stationary Office (TSO), Norwich; Scientific Advisory Committee on Nutrition (SACN), 2016. SACN vitamin D and health report. <https://www.gov.uk/government/uploads/system/uploads/attachment_data/file/537616/SACN_Vitamin_D_and_Health_report.pdf> (accessed 19.03.18.) (SACN, 2016).

Table 1.4 Vitamin K reference dietary requirements for the United States and United Kingdom.

Life stage group	Male (μg/day)	Female (μg/day)
United States		
0–6 months	2	2
6–12 months	2.5	2.5
1–3 years	30	30
4–8 years	55	55
9–13 years	60	60
14–18 years	75	75
19–30 years	120	90
31–50 years	120	90
51–70 years	120	90
>70 years	120	90
Pregnancy 14–18 years	–	75
19–30 years	–	90
31–50 years	–	90
Lactation 14–18 years	–	75
19–30 years	–	90
31–50 years	–	90
United Kingdom		
0–11 months	10	10
19–50 years	68.8–71.5	59.0–59.9
>50 years	65.1–68.8	54.3–59.0

Data show reference dietary requirements of vitamin K for the United States and the United Kingdom in μg/day. For the United States, all figures are presented as AIs. Cells showing "–" indicate that there are no values for that particular life stage or gender. For the United Kingdom, all figures are presented as safe intakes. For the age 0–11 months, figures are based on the highest value for breast milk. All other figures are calculated based on 1 μg/body weight (kg)/day (DH, 1991) using reference weights for males 19–24 years, 71.5 kg, 25–34 years, 71.0 kg; 35–44 years, 69.7 kg; 45–50 years, 68.8 kg; 51–54 years, 68.8 kg; 55–64 years 68.3 kg; 65–74 years, 67.0 kg; over 75 years, 65.1 kg. For females, 19–24 years, 59.9 kg; 25–34 years, 59.7 kg; 45–50 years, 59.0 kg; 51–54 years, 59.0 kg; 55–64 years, 58.0 kg; 65–74 years, 57.2 kg; over 75 years, 54.3 kg (SACN, 2011). For the United Kingdom, for all life stages and both genders, there are no LRNIs, EARs, or RNIs. For other details, see Table 1.1 for definitions and the legend to Table 1.2.

Source: For the United States, The National Academies of Sciences Engineering Medicine (NASEM), 2016. Dietary Reference Intakes Tables and Application. <http://www.nationalacademies.org/hmd/Activities/Nutrition/SummaryDRIs/DRI-Tables.aspx> (accessed 26.01.18.) (NASEM, 2016); for the United Kingdom, Department of Health (DH), 1991. Dietary Reference Values for Food Energy and Nutrients for the United Kingdom. The Stationary Office (TSO), Norwich; Scientific Advisory Committee on Nutrition (SACN), 2011. Dietary Reference Values for energy. <https://www.gov.uk/government/uploads/system/uploads/attachment_data/file/339317/SACN_Dietary_Reference_Values_for_Energy.pdf> (accessed 23.03. 18.).

degeneration, and neurodegenerative diseases including Alzheimer disease (Azzi, 2018). Vitamin E is mainly located within the phospholipid bilayer of cell membranes. It then acts as a free radical scavenger, protecting cellular components such as polyunsaturated fatty acids, DNA, and low-density lipoprotein from lipid peroxidation (WHO and FAO, 2004). Consequently, vitamin E is believed to have protective effects in the aforementioned diseases. The primary dietary sources are vegetable oils. Table 1.5 shows the vitamin E reference dietary requirements for the United States and the United Kingdom.

Table 1.5 Vitamin E reference dietary requirements for the United States and United Kingdom.

Life stage group	Male (mg/day)	Female (mg/day)
United States		
0–6 months	4*	4*
6–12 months	5*	5*
1–3 years	6	6
4–8 years	7	7
9–13 years	11	11
14–18 years	15	15
19–30 years	15	15
31–50 years	15	15
51–70 years	15	15
>70 years	15	15
Pregnancy 14–18 years	–	15
19–30 years	–	15
31–50 years	–	15
Lactation 14–18 years	–	19
19–30 years	–	19
31–50 years	–	19
United Kingdom		
0–11 months	0.4	0.4
19–50 years	>4	>3
>50 years	>4	>3

Data show the reference dietary requirements of vitamin E for the United States (in mg α-tocopherol/day) and the United Kingdom (in mg/g polyunsaturated fatty acid/day for 0–11 months; in mg α-tocopherol/day for all other figures). For the United Kingdom, all figures are presented as Safe Intakes. For the United Kingdom, for all life stages and both genders, there are no LRNIs, EARs, or RNIs. Data are presented as RDA for the United States. For the United States, figures with an asterisk (*) are presented as adequate intakes (AIs). Cells showing "–" indicate that there are no values for that particular life stage or gender. For other details, see Table 1.1 for definitions and the legend to Table 1.2.

Source: For the United States, The National Academies of Sciences Engineering Medicine (NASEM), 2016. Dietary Reference Intakes Tables and Application. <http://www.nationalacademies.org/hmd/Activities/Nutrition/SummaryDRIs/DRI-Tables.aspx> (accessed 26.01.18.) (NASEM, 2016); for the United Kingdom, Department of Health (DH), 1991. Dietary Reference Values for Food Energy and Nutrients for the United Kingdom. The Stationary Office (TSO), Norwich.

1.4 Water-soluble vitamins

1.4.1 Thiamin (vitamin B1)

Thiamin (thiamin pyrophosphate is the metabolically functional form) has crucial roles as a cofactor for several enzymes participating in intermediary metabolism (DH, 1991; WHO and FAO, 2004). Thiamin is equally spelled as *thiamine* in many text books. Thiamin also has roles in neural function as it is involved in the synthesis of neurotransmitters (Kerns et al., 2015). Beriberi, polyneuritis, and Wernicke-Korsakoff syndrome are established diseases of thiamin deficiency. General physiological signs of thiamin deficiency include severe decreases in appetite, a decrease in growth, bradycardia, and muscular weakness. Thiamin is widely distributed in dietary sources, for example, grains, vegetables, fruits, meats, fishes, legumes, dairy products, and eggs but mostly in low concentrations.

Thiamin is not evenly distributed in grains and has a higher concentration in the germ. Therefore those who consume refined grains (e.g., polished rice and white wheat where the germ has been removed), in relatively large proportions, may be vulnerable to thiamin deficiency. Obese people may be highly susceptible to thiamin deficiency due to the poor quality of their diet (Kerns et al., 2015). Table 1.6 shows the thiamin reference dietary requirements for the United States and the United Kingdom.

1.4.2 Riboflavin (vitamin B2)

Riboflavin is found in two major forms, namely flavin mononucleotide and flavin adenine dinucleotide. It has essential roles in the intermediary metabolism of macronutrients and numerous oxidative processes to provide cellular antioxidant protection with its coenzyme functions (Combs and McClung, 2017). Because riboflavin is involved in numerous biological pathways, deficiency states manifest themselves in a variety of clinical conditions. For example, general symptoms (e.g., loss of appetite and depressed growth), dermal (e.g., cheilosis, angular stomatitis, and dermatitis), neural (e.g., ataxia and paralysis), and vascular (e.g., anemia) disorders are well-established consequences of riboflavin deficiency. Furthermore, riboflavin has roles in the metabolism of vitamin B6, folate, vitamin B12, and other vitamins. Thus some of the clinical manifestations (e.g., pregnancy complications and cognitive impairments) of riboflavin deficiency are also the result of combinations of complex deficiencies (Thakur et al., 2017). Riboflavin is ubiquitously distributed, that is, can be found in all

Table 1.6 Thiamin (vitamin B1) reference dietary requirements for the United States and United Kingdom.

Life stage group	Male (mg/day)	Female (mg/day)
United States		
0–6 months	0.2*	0.2*
6–12 months	0.3*	0.3*
1–3 years	0.5	0.5
4–8 years	0.6	0.6
9–13 years	0.9	0.9
14–18 years	1.2	1.0
19–30 years	1.2	1.1
31–50 years	1.2	1.1
51–70 years	1.2	1.1
>70 years	1.2	1.1
Pregnancy 14–18 years	–	1.4
19–30 years	–	1.4
31–50 years	–	1.4
Lactation 14–18 years	–	1.4
19–30 years	–	1.4
31–50 years	–	1.4
United Kingdom		
0–3 months	0.2	0.2
4–6 months	0.2	0.2
7–9 months	0.2	0.2
10–12 months	0.3	0.3
1–3 years	0.5	0.5
4–6 years	0.7	0.7
7–10 years	0.7	0.7
11–14 years	0.9	0.7
15–18 years	1.1	0.8
19–50 years	1.0	0.8
>50 years	0.9	0.8
Pregnancy	–	0.9
Lactation 0–4 months	–	1.0
>4 months	–	1.0

Data show reference dietary requirements of thiamin (vitamin B1) for the United States and the United Kingdom in mg/day. For the United Kingdom, the figure for pregnancy is only applied to the last trimester. Data are presented as either RDA (United States) or RNI (United Kingdom). For the United States, figures with an asterisk (*) are presented as adequate intakes (AIs). Cells showing "–" indicate that there are no values for that particular life stage or gender. For other details, see Table 1.1 for definitions and the legend to Table 1.2.

Source: For the United States, The National Academies of Sciences Engineering Medicine (NASEM), 2016. Dietary Reference Intakes Tables and Application. <http://www.nationalacademies.org/hmd/Activities/Nutrition/SummaryDRIs/DRI-Tables.aspx> (accessed 26.01.18.) (NASEM, 2016); for the United Kingdom (Department of Health (DH), 1991. Dietary Reference Values for Food Energy and Nutrients for the United Kingdom. The Stationary Office (TSO), Norwich).

main food groups (i.e., cereals, meats, fishes, dairy products, eggs, fruits, and vegetables). Therefore in general, a balanced diet should be sufficient to meet reference dietary requirements. In spite of this, riboflavin deficiency is not uncommon even in developed countries. For example, it is well recognized that people with alcoholism are vulnerable to riboflavin deficiency due to inadequate diets. In addition, subclinical riboflavin deficiency is widespread in other cohorts including the elderly population due to their limited dietary variations and decreased dietary intake. Table 1.7 shows the riboflavin reference dietary requirements for the United States and the United Kingdom.

1.4.3 Niacin (vitamin B3)

Niacin (vitamin B3) is the generic descriptor of pyridine-3-carbolylic acid and its derivatives. It has two major metabolically active forms, namely nicotinic acid and nicotinamide (Combs and McClung, 2017). Niacin is the precursor of the pyridine nucleotides, nicotinamide adenine nucleotides (NAD), and nicotinamide adenine dinucleotide phosphate (NADP). NAD and NADP are coenzymes for numerous dehydrogenases, and take part in oxidation and reduction reactions in vivo. Thus niacin is essential in all aspects of metabolism including DNA repair and the synthesis of steroid hormones. Niacin deficiency manifests in a variety of organs. It often prominently manifests in the form of skin inflammation with exposure to sunlight, with a great resemblance to sunburn (e.g., cracking and peeling), which is known as pellagra. Pellagra may also present with other conditions such as diarrhea (as a result of damage to the gastrointestinal tract) and illnesses including depression and dementia (as a result of neurodegenerative processes). Furthermore, niacin deficiency is also associated with other psychiatric conditions such as schizophrenia (Xu and Jiang, 2015). Importantly, metabolically active niacin can be synthesized in vivo from one of the essential amino acids, tryptophan. The widely accepted conversion is that 1 mg of dietary niacin equates to 60 mg tryptophan. Therefore high-protein-containing foods such as meat, fish, and dairy products are considered good dietary sources of performed niacin. Niacin is also present in a wide variety of foods including cereals, vegetable, fruits, and nuts. Table 1.8 shows the niacin reference dietary requirements for the United States and the United Kingdom.

Table 1.7 Riboflavin (vitamin B2) reference dietary requirements for the United States and United Kingdom.

Life stage group	Male (mg/day)	Female (mg/day)
United States		
0–6 months	0.3*	0.3*
6–12 months	0.4*	0.4*
1–3 years	0.5	0.5
4–8 years	0.6	0.6
9–13 years	0.9	0.9
14–18 years	1.3	1.0
19–30 years	1.3	1.1
31–50 years	1.3	1.1
51–70 years	1.3	1.1
>70 years	1.3	1.1
Pregnancy 14–18 years	–	1.4
19–30 years	–	1.4
31–50 years	–	1.4
Lactation 14–18 years	–	1.6
19–30 years	–	1.6
31–50 years	–	1.6
United Kingdom		
0–3 months	0.4	0.4
4–6 months	0.4	0.4
7–9 months	0.4	0.4
10–12 months	0.4	0.4
1–3 years	0.6	0.6
4–6 years	0.8	0.8
7–10 years	1.0	1.0
11–14 years	1.2	1.1
15–18 years	1.3	1.1
19–50 years	1.3	1.1
>50 years	1.3	1.1
Pregnancy	–	1.4
Lactation 0–4 months	–	1.5
>4 months	–	1.5

Data show reference dietary requirements of riboflavin (vitamin B2) for the United States and the United Kingdom in mg/day. Data are presented as either RDA (United States) or RNI (United Kingdom). For the United States, figures with an asterisk (*) are presented as adequate intakes (AIs). Cells showing "–" indicate that there are no values for that particular life stage or gender. For other details, see Table 1.1 for definitions and the legend to Table 1.2.

Source: For the United States, The National Academies of Sciences Engineering Medicine (NASEM), 2016. Dietary Reference Intakes Tables and Application. <http://www.nationalacademies.org/hmd/Activities/Nutrition/SummaryDRIs/DRI-Tables.aspx> (accessed 26.01.18.) (NASEM, 2016); for the United Kingdom, Department of Health (DH), 1991. Dietary Reference Values for Food Energy and Nutrients for the United Kingdom. The Stationary Office (TSO), Norwich.

Table 1.8 Niacin (vitamin B3) reference dietary requirements for the United States and United Kingdom.

Life stage group	Male (mg/day)	Female (mg/day)
United States		
0–6 months	2*	2*
6–12 months	4*	4*
1–3 years	6	6
4–8 years	8	8
9–13 years	12	12
14–18 years	16	14
19–30 years	16	14
31–50 years	16	14
51–70 years	16	14
>70 years	16	14
Pregnancy 14–18 years	–	18
19–30 years	–	18
31–50 years	–	18
Lactation 14–18 years	–	17
19–30 years	–	17
31–50 years	–	17
United Kingdom		
0–3 months	4.1	3.8
4–6 months	4.3	3.9
7–9 months	4.6	4.3
10–12 months	5.0	4.7
1–3 years	6.5	6.0
4–6 years	9.8	9.1
7–10 years	12.0	11.4
11–14 years	15.5	14.4
15–18 years	19.9	16.1
19–50 years	17.0–18.3	13.9–14.4
>50 years	15.1–17.0	12.1–13.9
Pregnancy	–	15.1–17.4
Lactation 0–4 months	–	21.7–24.6
>4 months	–	21.7–24.6

Data show reference dietary requirements of niacin (vitamin B3) for the United States (for 0–6 months in preformed niacin, for all other figures in niacin equivalents) and the United Kingdom (niacin equivalents) in mg/day. For the United Kingdom, figures are calculated based on niacin equivalents per 4.184 MJ (DH, 1991) using energy reference values for males 0–3 months, 2.6 MJ; 4–6 months, 2.7 MJ; 7–9 months 2.9 MJ; 10–12 months 3.2 MJ; 1–3 years, 4.1 MJ; 4–6 years 6.2 MJ; 7–10 years, 7.6 MJ; 11–14 years, 9.8 MJ; 15–18 years 12.6 MJ; 19–24 years, 11.6 MJ, 25–34 years, 11.5 MJ; 35–44 years, 11.0 MJ; 45–54 years, 10.8 MJ; 55–64 years 10.8 MJ; 65–74 years, 9.8 MJ; over 75 years, 9.6 MJ. For females, 0–3 months, 2.4 MJ; 4–6 months, 2.5 MJ; 7–9 months 2.7 MJ; 10–12 months 3.0 MJ; 1–3 years, 3.8 MJ; 4–6 years 5.8 MJ; 7–10 years, 7.2 MJ; 11–14 years, 9.1 MJ; 15–18 years 10.2 MJ; 19–24 years, 9.1 MJ, 25–34 years, 9.1 MJ; 35–44 years, 8.8 MJ; 45–54 years, 8.8 MJ; 55–64 years 8.7 MJ; 65–74 years, 8.0 MJ; over 75 years, 7.7 MJ. For pregnancy, an increment in 0.8 MJ/day is added only during the last trimester (applied to the ages between 15 and 50 years) (SACN, 2011). For lactation, an increment of 1.38 MJ/day is added only for the first 6 months (applied age 15–50 years) (DH, 1991). Data are presented as either RDA (United States) or RNI (United Kingdom). For the United States, figures with an asterisk (*) are presented as adequate intakes (AIs). Cells showing "–" indicate that there are no values for that particular life stage or gender. For other details, see Table 1.1 for definitions and the legend to Table 1.2.

Source: For the United States, The National Academies of Sciences Engineering Medicine (NASEM), 2016. Dietary Reference Intakes Tables and Application. <http://www.nationalacademies.org/hmd/Activities/Nutrition/SummaryDRIs/DRI-Tables.aspx> (accessed 26.01.18.) (NASEM, 2016); for the United Kingdom, Department of Health (DH), 1991. Dietary Reference Values for Food Energy and Nutrients for the United Kingdom. The Stationary Office (TSO), Norwich; Scientific Advisory Committee on Nutrition (SACN), 2011. Dietary Reference Values for energy. <https://www.gov.uk/government/uploads/system/uploads/attachment_data/file/339317/SACN_Dietary_Reference_Values_for_Energy.pdf> (accessed 23.03. 18.).

1.4.4 Vitamin B6 (pyridoxine)

Vitamin B6 is the generic descriptor for pyridoxine, pyridoxal, pyridoxamine (they are interconvertible in vivo), and their 5′-phosptates (i.e., pridoxal-5-phosphate, 4-prydoxic acid, and pyridoxine hydrochloride). The metabolically active form is prydoxal-5-phosphate. It acts as a carbonyl-reactive coenzyme in a number of metabolic pathways, including amino acid and lipid metabolism, tryptophan—niacin conversion, gluconeogenesis, and neurotransmitter synthesis (Combs and McClung, 2017). Vitamin B6 is widely distributed in dietary sources. Additionally, gut microflora synthesize vitamin B6, although the contribution to human nutrition is likely not significant. For dietary sources vitamin B6 is found in greatest concentrations in meats, whole-grain products, and vegetables and nuts. Vitamin B6 is often present as the prydoxal-5-β-D-glycosides in dietary plant sources. It has low bioavailability and its presence may reduce the bioavailability of coingested free pyridoxine. Clinical deficiency of vitamin B6 alone is uncommon but most generally occurs in conjunction with the deficiency of other B vitamins. However, specific vitamin B6 deficiency cases, for example, anemia due to vitamin B6 deficiency post pancreaticoduodenectomy, have been reported in the literature (Yasuda et al., 2015). Table 1.9 shows the vitamin B6 reference dietary requirements for the United States and the United Kingdom.

1.4.5 Folate (vitamin B9)

Folate is the generic descriptor for folic acid (pteroyl glutamic acid) derivatives. Folates have important roles in various catabolic and biosynthetic reactions by transferring one-carbon units from donor molecules. Folates are involved in amino acid and nucleotide metabolism and methylation reactions. For example, folates have an essential role in normal embryogenesis by supporting cell division. It is well established that adequate dietary intake of folate, including supplementation in early pregnancy, can significantly lower the risk of neural tube defects at birth. Furthermore, impaired biosynthesis of DNA as a result of folate deficiency can cause clinical symptoms of megaloblastic anemia, alopecia, achromotrichia, and neuropathy (Laird et al., 2018). Folates are widely available in dietary sources of plant and animal origins. Dairy products, green leafy vegetables, yeast extract, and liver are rich sources in the human diet (Combs and McClung, 2017). However, the bioavailability of naturally occurring folates is considered generally poor compared to synthetic folic acid,

Table 1.9 Vitamin B6 (pyridoxine) reference dietary requirements for the United States and United Kingdom.

Life stage group	Male (mg/day)	Female (mg/day)
United States		
0–6 months	0.1*	0.1*
6–12 months	0.3*	0.3*
1–3 years	0.5	0.5
4–8 years	0.6	0.6
9–13 years	1.0	1.0
14–18 years	1.3	1.2
19–30 years	1.3	1.3
31–50 years	1.3	1.3
51–70 years	1.7	1.5
>70 years	1.7	1.5
Pregnancy 14–18 years	–	1.9
19–30 years	–	1.9
31–50 years	–	1.9
Lactation 14–18 years	–	2.0
19–30 years	–	2.0
31–50 years	–	2.0
United Kingdom		
0–3 months	0.2	0.2
4–6 months	0.2	0.2
7–9 months	0.3	0.2
10–12 months	0.4	0.3
1–3 years	0.5	0.5
4–6 years	0.8	0.8
7–10 years	1.0	0.9
11–14 years	1.3	1.2
15–18 years	1.7	1.3
19–50 years	1.4–1.5	1.2
>50 years	1.3–1.4	1.0–1.2
Pregnancy	–	1.3–1.4
Lactation 0–4 months	–	1.3–1.5
>4 months	–	1.3–1.5

Data show reference dietary requirements of vitamin B6 (pyridoxine) for the United States and the United Kingdom in mg/day. For the United Kingdom, the RNI for vitamin B6 (pyridoxine) is 15 μg/g of dietary protein. Figures in the table are calculated based on 15 μg per reference protein intake values: reference protein intake values are calculated with the assumption that protein provides 14.7% of energy reference values (DH, 1991). For energy reference values see the legend to Table 1.8. Data are presented as either RDA (United States) or RNI (United Kingdom). For the United States, figures with an asterisk (*) are presented as adequate intakes (AIs). Cells showing "–" indicate that there are no values for that particular life stage or gender. For other details, see Table 1.1 for definitions and the legend to Table 1.2.

Source: For the United States, The National Academies of Sciences Engineering Medicine (NASEM), 2016. Dietary Reference Intakes Tables and Application. <http://www.nationalacademies.org/hmd/Activities/Nutrition/SummaryDRIs/DRI-Tables.aspx> (accessed 26.01.18.) (NASEM, 2016); for the United Kingdom, Department of Health (DH), 1991. Dietary Reference Values for Food Energy and Nutrients for the United Kingdom. The Stationary Office (TSO), Norwich; Scientific Advisory Committee on Nutrition (SACN), 2011. Dietary Reference Values for energy. <https://www.gov.uk/government/uploads/system/uploads/attachment_data/file/339317/SACN_Dietary_Reference_Values_for_Energy.pdf> (accessed 23.03.18.).

which is used in food fortification and supplements. Folate deficiency is common; elderly populations are known to be vulnerable. Folate deficiency in the elderly population is generally multifactorial, including decreased dietary folate intake, age-related impairments in absorption, comorbidities affecting folate metabolisms (e.g., small bowel diseases), and use of folic acid antagonist drugs (e.g., methotrexate) (Enderami et al., 2018). Table 1.10 shows the folate reference dietary requirements for the United States and the United Kingdom.

1.4.6 Vitamin B12 (cobalamin)

Vitamin B12 (cobalamin) is synthesized by certain microorganisms such as bacteria and algae (WHO and FAO, 2004). Therefore in human nutrition the main dietary sources are almost exclusively foods of animal origin (e.g., meats, dairy products, fish, and eggs). There are plant-based dietary vitamin B12 sources such as edible algae (e.g., seaweeds) and fermented soybean-based foods (i.e., tempe, possibly due to bacterial contamination during production), as well as fortified breakfast cereals (Watanabe et al., 2014). However, in general, vegetables, fruits, and grains do not contain vitamin B12. In animals, including humans, vitamin B12 serves as a coenzyme in two vitamin B12–dependent enzymes, namely methionine synthase and methylmalonyl-CoA mutase. These vitamin B12–dependent enzymes have crucial roles in amino acid and fatty acid metabolism and DNA synthesis. Methionine synthase also requires folate for its action. Therefore vitamin B12 deficiency results in the same syndromes as folate deficiency (i.e., megaloblastic anemia) (DH, 1991). Other consequences of vitamin B12 deficiency include peripheral neuropathy and neurological dysfunction (e.g., cognition) (Combs and McClung, 2017). Strict vegans may be vulnerable to vitamin B12 deficiency. Moreover, the elderly population is known to have a high risk of deficiency due to the increase in age-related decreased ability of absorption (i.e., gastric atrophy). Additionally, post intestinal surgery patients, including those who have undergone bariatric surgery or bowel resection, are also vulnerable to vitamin B12 deficiency due to their compromised absorption capacity. Table 1.11 shows the vitamin B12 reference dietary requirements for the United States and the United Kingdom.

Table 1.10 Folate (vitamin B9) reference dietary requirements for the United States and United Kingdom.

Life stage group	Male (μg/day)	Female (μg/day)
United States		
0–6 months	65*	65*
6–12 months	80*	80*
1–3 years	150	150
4–8 years	200	200
9–13 years	300	300
14–18 years	400	400
19–30 years	400	400
31–50 years	400	400
51–70 years	400	400
>70 years	400	400
Pregnancy 14–18 years	—	600
19–30 years	—	600
31–50 years	—	600
Lactation 14–18 years	—	500
19–30 years	—	500
31–50 years	—	500
United Kingdom		
0–3 months	50	50
4–6 months	50	50
7–9 months	50	50
10–12 months	50	50
1–3 years	70	70
4–6 years	100	100
7–10 years	150	150
11–14 years	200	200
15–18 years	200	200
19–50 years	200	200
>50 years	200	200
Pregnancy	—	300
Lactation 0–4 months	—	260
>4 months	—	260

Data show reference dietary requirements of folate (vitamin B9) for the United States (in dietary folate equivalents) and the United Kingdom in μg/day. Data are presented as either RDA (United States) or RNI (United Kingdom). For the United States, figures with an asterisk (*) are presented as adequate intakes (AIs). Cells showing "—" indicate that there are no values for that particular life stage or gender. For other details, see Table 1.1 for definitions and the legend to Table 1.2.
Source: For the United States, The National Academies of Sciences Engineering Medicine (NASEM), 2016. Dietary Reference Intakes Tables and Application. <http://www.nationalacademies.org/hmd/Activities/Nutrition/SummaryDRIs/DRI-Tables.aspx> (accessed 26.01.18) (NASEM, 2016); for the United Kingdom, Department of Health (DH), 1991. Dietary Reference Values for Food Energy and Nutrients for the United Kingdom. The Stationary Office (TSO), Norwich.

Table 1.11 Vitamin B12 (cobalamin) reference dietary requirements for the United States and United Kingdom.

Life stage group	Male (μg/day)	Female (μg/day)
United States		
0–6 months	0.4*	0.4*
6–12 months	0.5*	0.5*
1–3 years	0.9	0.9
4–8 years	1.2	1.2
9–13 years	1.8	1.8
14–18 years	2.4	2.4
19–30 years	2.4	2.4
31–50 years	2.4	2.4
51–70 years	2.4	2.4
>70 years	2.4	2.4
Pregnancy 14–18 years	–	2.6
19–30 years	–	2.6
31–50 years	–	2.6
Lactation 14–18 years	–	2.8
19–30 years	–	2.8
31–50 years	–	2.8
United Kingdom		
0–3 months	0.3	0.3
4–6 months	0.3	0.3
7–9 months	0.4	0.4
10–12 months	0.4	0.4
1–3 years	0.5	0.5
4–6 years	0.8	0.8
7–10 years	1.0	1.0
11–14 years	1.2	1.2
15–18 years	1.5	1.5
19–50 years	1.5	1.5
>50 years	1.5	1.5
Pregnancy	–	2.0
Lactation 0–4 months	–	2.0
>4 months	–	2.0

Data show reference dietary requirements of vitamin B12 for the United States and the United Kingdom in μg/day. Data are presented as either RDA (United States) or RNI (United Kingdom). For the United States, figures with an asterisk (*) are presented as adequate intakes (AIs). Cells showing "–" indicate that there are no values for that particular life stage or gender. For other details, see Table 1.1 for definitions and the legend to Table 1.2.

Source: For the United States, The National Academies of Sciences Engineering Medicine (NASEM), 2016. Dietary Reference Intakes Tables and Application. <http://www.nationalacademies.org/hmd/Activities/Nutrition/SummaryDRIs/DRI-Tables.aspx> (accessed 26.01.18.) (NASEM, 2016); for the United Kingdom, Department of Health (DH), 1991. Dietary Reference Values for Food Energy and Nutrients for the United Kingdom. The Stationary Office (TSO), Norwich.

1.4.7 Vitamin C (ascorbic acid)

Vitamin C (ascorbic acid) is a metabolite of glucose and most living organisms are capable of de novo synthesis. However, a few species including humans are unable to do so due to a single enzyme deficiency (i.e., L-gulonolactone oxidase). Hence vitamin C is an essential dietary component for human nutrition. Vitamin C has important roles as an enzyme cofactor, modulator, or protective agent and antioxidant agent. Scurvy is a well-established consequence of vitamin C deficiency. Typical symptoms of scurvy, such as impaired wound healing, hemorrhage, and edema, commonly manifest as swollen bleeding gums (Combs and McClung, 2017). Vitamin C is widely distributed in plant- and animal-based foods. In particular, citrus, noncitrus soft fruits, and green leafy vegetables have high concentrations of vitamin C. Therefore the regularity of fruit and vegetable consumption can determine vitamin C status. Vitamin C is one of the most unstable nutrients, easily destroyed by oxygen, metal ions, increased pH, heat, or light (DH, 1991). This means there is a loss of vitamin C during storage and cooking processes. Hence suboptimal vitamin C status may not be uncommon and deficiency can be observed in specific cohorts, such as hospitalized patients, even in developed countries (Sharma et al., 2018). Table 1.12 shows the vitamin C reference dietary requirements for the United States and the United Kingdom.

1.4.8 Pantothenic acid

Pantothenic acid is ubiquitously available from both plant and animal dietary sources. The bioavailability of pantothenic acid is not well understood, the availability of a wide range of foods makes deficiency extremely rare. Pantothenic acid has essential functions in energy metabolism as a component of coenzyme A (CoA). The biological functions of CoA are ubiquitous, taking part in lipid synthesis and energy production pathways. More recently, it has been suggested that pantothenic acid may have a cardioprotective role by providing antiinflammatory effects through antioxidant properties (Jung et al., 2017). Pantothenic acid deficiency is relatively rare, though when it occurs it may exhibit signs in vital organs, including effects on the liver (e.g., steatosis) and the nervous system (e.g., paralysis), as well as general symptoms such as decreased appetite and fatigue (Combs and McClung, 2017). Table 1.13 shows the pantothenic

Table 1.12 Vitamin C reference dietary requirements for the United States and United Kingdom.

Life stage group	Male (mg/day)	Female (mg/day)
United States		
0–6 months	40*	40*
6–12 months	50*	50*
1–3 years	15	15
4–8 years	25	25
9–13 years	45	45
14–18 years	75	65
19–30 years	90	75
31–50 years	90	75
51–70 years	90	75
>70 years	90	75
Pregnancy 14–18 years	–	80
19–30 years	–	85
31–50 years	–	85
Lactation 14–18 years	–	115
19–30 years	–	120
31–50 years	–	120
United Kingdom		
0–3 months	25	25
4–6 months	25	25
7–9 months	25	25
10–12 months	25	25
1–3 years	30	30
4–6 years	30	30
7–10 years	30	30
11–14 years	35	35
15–18 years	40	40
19–50 years	40	40
>50 years	40	40
Pregnancy	–	50
Lactation 0–4 months	–	70
>4 months	–	70

Data show reference dietary requirements of vitamin C for the United States and the United Kingdom in mg/day. For the United Kingdom, the figure for pregnancy is only applied for the last trimester. Data are presented as either RDA (United States) or RNI (United Kingdom). For the United States, figures with an asterisk (*) are presented as adequate intakes (AIs). Cells showing "–" indicate that there are no values for that particular life stage or gender. For other details, see Table 1.1 for definitions and the legend to Table 1.2.

Source: For the United States, The National Academies of Sciences Engineering Medicine (NASEM), 2016. Dietary Reference Intakes Tables and Application. <http://www.nationalacademies.org/hmd/Activities/Nutrition/SummaryDRIs/DRI-Tables.aspx> (accessed 26.01.18.) (NASEM, 2016); for the United Kingdom, Department of Health (DH), 1991. Dietary Reference Values for Food Energy and Nutrients for the United Kingdom. The Stationary Office (TSO), Norwich.

Table 1.13 Pantothenic acid reference dietary requirements for the United States and United Kingdom.

Life stage group	Male (mg/day)	Female (mg/day)
United States		
0–6 months	1.7	1.7
6–12 months	1.8	1.8
1–3 years	2	2
4–8 years	3	3
9–13 years	4	4
14–18 years	5	5
19–30 years	5	5
31–50 years	5	5
51–70 years	5	5
>70 years	5	5
Pregnancy 14–18 years	—	6
19–30 years	—	6
31–50 years	—	6
Lactation 14–18 years	—	7
19–30 years	—	7
31–50 years	—	7
United Kingdom		
All life stages and gender: 3–7 mg/day		

Data show reference dietary requirements of pantothenic acid for the United States in mg/day. For the United Kingdom, for all life stages and both genders, there are no LRNIs, EARs, or RNIs. However, there are Safe Intakes which are between 3 and 7 mg/day for all life stages and both genders, including pregnant and lactating women (DH, 1991). For the United States, all figures are presented as adequate intakes (AIs). Cells showing "—" indicate that there are no values for that particular life stage or gender. For other details, see Table 1.1 for definitions and the legend to Table 1.2.
Source: For the United States, The National Academies of Sciences Engineering Medicine (NASEM), 2016. Dietary Reference Intakes Tables and Application. <http://www.nationalacademies.org/hmd/Activities/Nutrition/SummaryDRIs/DRI-Tables.aspx> (accessed 26.01.18.) (NASEM, 2016); for the United Kingdom, Department of Health (DH), 1991. Dietary Reference Values for Food Energy and Nutrients for the United Kingdom. The Stationary Office (TSO), Norwich.

acid reference dietary requirements for the United States and the United Kingdom.

1.4.9 Biotin

Biotin has functions as a cofactor within intermediary metabolism. Furthermore, it has metabolic functions as a regulator in cell metabolism, gene expression, the cell cycle, and as a substrate for the modification of proteins (Elahi et al., 2018). Biotinylation is the process whereby biotin is attached to proteins: for example, biotinylation is necessary for the biological activity of mammalian carboxylases. Biotin is widely distributed in food items. Furthermore, it is known to be synthesized in meaningful amounts by gut microflora in humans. Therefore in general, dietary biotin deficiency is considered extremely rare. Recently it was also suggested that biotin has a role in immune-mediated intestinal inflammation (Elahi et al., 2018). Table 1.14 shows the biotin reference dietary requirements for the United States and the United Kingdom.

Table 1.14 Biotin reference dietary requirements for the United States and United Kingdom.

Life stage group	Male (μg/day)	Female (μg/day)
United States		
0–6 months	5	5
6–12 months	6	6
1–3 years	8	8
4–8 years	12	12
9–13 years	20	20
14–18 years	25	25
19–30 years	30	30
31–50 years	30	30
51–70 years	30	30
>70 years	30	30
Pregnancy 14–18 years	–	30
19–30 years	–	30
31–50 years	–	30
Lactation 14–18 years	–	35
19–30 years	–	35
31–50 years	–	35
United Kingdom		
All life stages and gender: 10–200 μg/day		

Data show reference dietary requirements of biotin for the United States in μg/day. For the United States, all figures are presented as AIs. For the United Kingdom, for all life stages and both genders, there are no LRNIs, EARs, or RNIs. However, there are safe intakes. For the United Kingdom, the safe intakes are between 10 and 200 μg/day for all life stages and gender, including pregnant and lactating women (DH, 1991). Cells showing "–" indicate that there are no values for that particular life stage or gender. For other details, see Table 1.1 for definitions and the legend to Table 1.2.
Source: For the United States, The National Academies of Sciences Engineering Medicine (NASEM), 2016. Dietary Reference Intakes Tables and Application. <http://www.nationalacademies.org/hmd/Activities/Nutrition/SummaryDRIs/DRI-Tables.aspx> (accessed 26.01.18.) (NASEM, 2016); for the United Kingdom, Department of Health (DH), 1991. Dietary Reference Values for Food Energy and Nutrients for the United Kingdom. The Stationary Office (TSO), Norwich.

1.5 Challenges of meeting requirements

In the earlier sections, we have briefly described the functional roles of the vitamins. We have also tabulated their reference dietary requirements for the United States and the United Kingdom (Tables 1.2–1.14). The tables illustrate differences between data for the United States and United Kingdom with variable definitions and age categories for the same vitamins.

When studying the challenges of meeting reference dietary requirements, one needs to consider the number of variables that distinguish the two countries, such as food availability, food policies, and public health strategies. There are also different dietary patterns among particular cohorts due to ethnicity, religion, age, gender, social classes, regions, climates, etc. within the same country. These variables contribute to differences between groups and influence whether vitamin intakes achieve the reference dietary requirements (Jenab et al., 2009). Life stages also have an influence on whether or not reference dietary requirements are met. For example, the elderly population is well known to be vulnerable to vitamin B12 deficiency. Reference dietary requirements for the elderly population (over 70 years for the United States and over 50 years for the United Kingdom) are the same as younger adults (Table 1.11). However, for both countries, the prevalence of vitamin B12 deficiency could be as high as 20% for the population over 60 years old while the prevalence for those less than 60 years of age is around 6% (Hunt et al., 2014). As described in the earlier section, the main dietary sources of vitamin B12 are foods of animal origin, except for a few examples found in plant sources such as edible algae and fermented soybean-based foods. However, in general, these aforementioned plant sources are not commonly consumed or available in Western countries. Furthermore, elderly populations may experience general reduced overall dietary intake of animal products, therefore compromising vitamin B12 intake. Moreover, vitamin B12 has a complex absorption pathway and the aging process alters this. Gastric atrophy in aging reduces the ability of the gastric parietal cells to synthesize and secrete the intrinsic factor and gastric acid. Both are required for the enteric absorption of vitamin B12. Additionally, elderly populations are more commonly found to have multiple comorbidities and chronic diseases leading to polypharmacy. Common drugs prescribed for the elderly include proton pump inhibitors, H2-receptor antagonists, and antidiabetic drugs (metformin). These are known to be associated with reduced serum circulating vitamin B12 concentrations (Miller, 2018).

A recent study showed older adults living in long-term care institutions have a higher prevalence of vitamin B12 deficiency compared to the free-living older adults (Wong et al., 2015). The authors hypothesized that older adults living in the institutions are likely to have poorer health status in general compared to the free-living individuals and besides, vitamin B12 requirements could possibly become higher with aging (Wong et al., 2015).

Another example of the complexities of meeting requirements relates to vitamin K. The exact dietary requirements of vitamin K in numerical terms have not been fully established. This is due to (1) the lack of detailed information on the bioavailability of vitamin K from foods; (2) difficulties in establishing a causal link between plausible biomarkers of vitamin K deficiency and reproducible health outcome measures; (3) difficulties in inducing vitamin K deficiency through dietary deprivation alone; and (4) finding individuals who are vitamin K deficient via classical undernutrition studies. Vitamin K is also synthesized in the gastrointestinal tract by the gut microflora, which also contributes to the complications involved in establishing exact dietary requirements (Yamazaki Price and Preedy, 2018). Meeting the reference dietary requirements of vitamin K (i.e., adequate intakes for the United States and safe intakes for the United Kingdom, Table 1.4) is rarely problematic except for neonates. As vitamin K is ubiquitously distributed in nature most of the population meets reference dietary requirements despite differences in dietary and nutrient patterns.

Further detailed information relating to vitamins can be found elsewhere within this book.

References

Azzi, A., 2018. Many tocopherols, one vitamin E. Mol. Aspects Med. 61, 92–103. Available from: https://doi.org/10.1016/j.mam.2017.06.004.

Borel, P., Caillaud, D., Cano, N.J., 2015. Vitamin D bioavailability: state of the art. Crit. Rev. Food Sci. Nutr. 55 (9), 1193–1205. Available from: https://doi.org/10.1080/10408398.2012.688897.

Christakos, S., Seth, T., Wei, R., Veldurthy, V., Sun, C., Kim, K.I., et al., 2014. Vitamin D and health: beyond bone. MD Advis. 7 (3), 28–32.

Combs Jr., G.F., McClung, P.J., 2017. The Vitamins Fundamental Aspects in Nutrition and Health, fifth ed. Elsevier/Academic Press, London/San Diego.

Department of Health (DH), 1991. Dietary Reference Values for Food Energy and Nutrients for the United Kingdom. The Stationary Office (TSO), Norwich.

Elahi, A., Sabui, S., Narasappa, N.N., Agrawal, S., Lambrecht, N.W., Agrawal, A., et al., 2018. Biotin deficiency induces Th1- and Th17-mediated proinflammatory responses in human CD4(+) T lymphocytes via activation of the mTOR signaling pathway. J. Immunol. 200 (8), 2563–2570. Available from: https://doi.org/10.4049/jimmunol.1701200.

Enderami, A., Zarghami, M., Darvishi-Khezri, H., 2018. The effects and potential mechanisms of folic acid on cognitive function: a comprehensive review. Neurol. Sci. Available from: https://doi.org/10.1007/s10072-018-3473-4.

Hunt, A., Harrington, D., Robinson, S., 2014. Vitamin B12 deficiency. BMJ 349, g5226. Available from: https://doi.org/10.1136/bmj.g5226.

Imdad, A., Mayo-Wilson, E., Herzer, K., Bhutta, Z.A., 2017. Vitamin A supplementation for preventing morbidity and mortality in children from six months to five years of age. Cochrane Database Syst. Rev. 3, CD008524. Available from: https://doi.org/10.1002/14651858.CD008524.pub3.

Jenab, M., Salvini, S., van Gils, C.H., Brustad, M., Shakya-Shrestha, S., Buijsse, B., et al., 2009. Dietary intakes of retinol, beta-carotene, vitamin D and vitamin E in the European Prospective Investigation into Cancer and Nutrition Cohort. Eur. J. Clin. Nutr. 63 (Suppl. 4), S150–S178. Available from: https://doi.org/10.1038/ejcn.2009.79.

Jung, S., Kim, M.K., Choi, B.Y., 2017. The long-term relationship between dietary pantothenic acid (vitamin B5) intake and C-reactive protein concentration in adults aged 40 years and older. Nutr. Metab. Cardiovasc. Dis. 27 (9), 806–816. Available from: https://doi.org/10.1016/j.numecd.2017.05.008.

Kerns, J.C., Arundel, C., Chawla, L.S., 2015. Thiamin deficiency in people with obesity. Adv. Nutr. 6 (2), 147–153. Available from: https://doi.org/10.3945/an.114.007526.

Laird, E.J., O'Halloran, A.M., Carey, D., O'Connor, D., Kenny, R.A., Molloy, A.M., 2018. Voluntary fortification is ineffective to maintain the vitamin B12 and folate status of older Irish adults: evidence from the Irish Longitudinal Study on Ageing (TILDA). Br. J. Nutr. 120 (1), 111–120. Available from: https://doi.org/10.1017/s0007114518001356.

Miller, J.W., 2018. Proton pump inhibitors, H2-receptor antagonists, metformin, and vitamin B-12 deficiency: clinical implications. Adv. Nutr. 9 (4), 511s–518s. Available from: https://doi.org/10.1093/advances/nmy023.

Office of Disease Prevention and Health Promotion (ODPHP), 2015. 2015–2020 Dietary Guidelines for Americans. Available from <http://health.gov/dietaryguidelines/2015/guidelines/> (accessed 8.04.18.).

Scientific Advisory Committee on Nutrition (SACN), 2011. Dietary Reference Values for energy. Available from <https://www.gov.uk/government/uploads/system/uploads/attachment_data/file/339317/SACN_Dietary_Reference_Values_for_Energy.pdf> (accessed 23.03.18.).

Scientific Advisory Committee on Nutrition (SACN), 2016. SACN vitamin D and health report. Available from: <https://www.gov.uk/government/uploads/system/uploads/attachment_data/file/537616/SACN_Vitamin_D_and_Health_report.pdf> (accessed 19.03.18.).

Sharma, Y., Miller, M., Shahi, R., Doyle, A., Horwood, C., Hakendorf, P., et al., 2018. Vitamin C deficiency in Australian hospitalized patients: an observational study. Intern. Med. J. 49 (2), 189–196. Available from: https://doi.org/10.1111/imj.14030.

Thakur, K., Tomar, S.K., Singh, A.K., Mandal, S., Arora, S., 2017 Riboflavin and health: a review of recent human research. Crit. Rev. Food Sci. Nutr. 57 (17), 3650–3660. Available from: https://doi.org/10.1080/10408398.2016.1145104.

The National Academies of Sciences Engineering Medicine (NASEM), 2016. Dietary Reference Intakes Tables and Application. Available from: <http://www.nationalacademies.org/hmd/Activities/Nutrition/SummaryDRIs/DRI-Tables.aspx> (accessed 26.01.18.).

Watanabe, F., Yabuta, Y., Bito, T., Teng, F., 2014. Vitamin B(1)(2)-containing plant food sources for vegetarians. Nutrients 6 (5), 1861–1873. Available from: https://doi.org/10.3390/nu6051861.

Wong, C.W., Ip, C.Y., Leung, C.P., Leung, C.S., Cheng, J.N., Siu, C.Y., 2015. Vitamin B12 deficiency in the institutionalized elderly: a regional study. Exp. Gerontol. 69, 221–225. Available from: https://doi.org/10.1016/j.exger.2015.06.016.

World Health Organization (WHO) and Food and Agriculture Organization of the United Nations (FAO), 2004. Vitamin and Mineral Requirements in Human Nutrition, second ed. Available from: <http://apps.who.int/iris/bitstream/handle/10665/42716/9241546123.pdf;
jsessionid = CC8E98897EB8209FD3310D5D925FC830?sequence = 1> (accessed 08.04.18.).

Xu, X.J., Jiang, G.S., 2015. Niacin-respondent subset of schizophrenia—a therapeutic review. Eur. Rev. Med. Pharmacol. Sci. 19 (6), 988–997.

Yamazaki Price, M., Preedy, V., 2015. Urinary Markers in Nutritional Studies, General Methods in Biomarker Research and Their Applications. Springer Reference, London, pp. 547–566.

Yamazaki Price, M.Y., Preedy, V.R., 2018. Vitamin K status in nutritionally compromised circumstances. In: Preedy, V.R., Patel, V.B. (Eds.), Handbook of Famine, Starvation and Nutrient Deprivation: From Biology to Policy. Springer.

Yasuda, H., Fujiwara, N., Ishizaki, Y., Komatsu, N., 2015. Anemia attributed to vitamin B6 deficiency in post-pancreaticoduodenectomy patients. Pancreatology 15 (1), 81–83. Available from: https://doi.org/10.1016/j.pan.2014.12.001.

Further reading

National Diet and Nutrition Survey Results From Years 7 and 8 (combined) of the Rolling Programme, (2014/2015–2015/2016). Available from: <https://assets.publishing.service.gov.uk/government/uploads/system/uploads/attachment_data/file/699241/NDNS_results_years_7_and_8.pdf> (accessed 01.06.18.).

Scientific Advisory Committee on Nutrition (SACN), 2017. Update on folic acid. Available from: <https://assets.publishing.service.gov.uk/government/uploads/system/uploads/attachment_data/file/637111/SACN_Update_on_folic_acid.pdf> (accessed 13.07.17.).

Yamazaki Price, M.Y., Preedy, V.R., 2017. Dietary reference values. In: Preedy, V.R., Rajendram, R., Martin, C.R. (Eds.), Metabolism and Pathophysiology of Bariatric Surgery. Academic Press, London, pp. 399–417.

CHAPTER 2

Bioactive vitamin–metal compounds: other potential applications of vitamins

Paula Brandão[1] and Samuel Guieu[2]
[1]Department of Chemistry/CICECO, University of Aveiro, Portugal
[2]Department of Chemistry/QOPNA/CICECO, University of Aveiro, Portugal

Contents

Key facts of vitamin–metal complexes

1. Vitamins are naturally abundant and cheap building blocks, showing many modes of metal coordination.
2. They have been used as bioligands for the preparation of bioactive metal complexes exhibiting different architectures and a wide variety of biomedical applications.
3. Complexing a vitamin with a metal can dramatically change its bioactivity.
4. The biomedical applications of vitamins complexes, and mainly vitamins–metal–organic framework (MOFs), are still scarce.
5. Among all vitamins, vitamin B_3 and vitamin B_6 are good choices for the preparation of vitamin-based metal complexes.

Molecular Nutrition
DOI: https://doi.org/10.1016/B978-0-12-811907-5.00022-1

Summary points

1. This chapter focuses on the preparation and biomedical applications of vitamin–metal complexes and polymers.
2. Vitamins are an attractive class of organic bioligands containing a wide variety of binding modes to metals.
3. Vitamins are viewed as building blocks for the construction of metal compounds.
4. The combination of vitamins with metals can change their mode of action.
5. Vitamin-based compounds show biocompatibility and recyclability.
6. Some vitamin–metal complexes have demonstrated anticancer activities.
7. Metal–organic frameworks incorporating vitamins as ligands have been used for the slow release of therapeutic compounds in organisms.
8. Vitamins are excellent candidates to build multinuclear metal complexes with interesting magnetic and luminescent properties.

Abbreviations

MOFs	metal–organic frameworks
0D	zero dimension
1D	one dimension
2D	two dimension
3D	three dimension
NO	nitric oxide
PN	pyridoxine
PL	pyridoxal
PM	pyridoxamine
^{1}H NMR	proton nuclear magnetic resonance
DFT	density functional theory
Caco-2 cells	human colon adenocarcinoma cells
4T1 cells	mouse breast cancer cells

2.1 Introduction

Vitamins are organic molecules containing a variety of functional groups, such as carboxyl (–COOH), amino (–NH_2), and hydroxyl (–OH) groups. Their rich coordination chemistry (through the carboxylate, amino, hydroxyl groups and side chains) makes them an attractive class of organic linkers for the preparation of metal complexes and metal–organic framework (MOF) compounds. These classes of compounds are typically built by bridging metal centers with organic linkers possessing different dimensionalities: metal complex (0D), chains (1D), layers (2D), and MOFs—3D extended structures. Over the past decades, metal complexes and MOFs have had enormous success in relevant biological and medical applications such as anticancer drugs, imaging agents, and drug delivery (Zhang and Lippard, 2003; Zhou et al., 2010; McKinlay et al., 2010; Imaz et al., 2011; Anderson and Stylianou, 2017). This interest stimulated research into the synthesis of metal compounds with organic ligands showing low toxicity, which is a key requirement and still a challenge in metal compounds designed for biomedical application. In this context the vitamins are an attractive family of bioligands for the preparation of biocompounds. On the other hand, the researchers, considering the ability of vitamins to bind the metal in monodentate, bidentate, bidentate bridging, and tridentate-bridging coordination modes, have chosen these molecules as linkers to design novel metal compounds for biological and medical applications. Vitamins are an interesting linker to obtain biocompatible compounds and open alternative routes for the development of new biologically active materials. According to literature available, the more common vitamins used in material coordination chemistry are vitamins B_1, B_2, B_3, B_6, B_9, C, and a few examples of vitamins A and D. Fig. 2.1 illustrates the different coordination modes of some of those vitamins (Fig. 2.1).

2.2 Vitamin-based metal complexes

Cisplatin, *cis*-$[Pt(NH_3)_2Cl_2]$, is the paradigmatic example of a "small" transition metal complex which had been widely used as an antitumoral drug (Rosenberg et al., 1969; Jamieson and Lippard, 1999). However, its effectiveness was clouded by several undesirable side effects along with acquired drug resistance. These drawbacks have stimulated the research and the development of new anticancer drugs, based on different metals as well as on the use of natural linkers, with improved pharmacological properties. Because of their rich functional groups, vitamins could be an excellent alternative to prepare metal drugs to improve clinical effectiveness, to reduce toxicity, and to broaden the spectrum of activity in the biomedical field. Table 2.1 shows some examples of vitamin-based metal complexes and their applications.

Vitamin A_1, also called retinol, is a fat-soluble alcohol (Fig. 2.1) with important functions in several physiological processes such as the immune

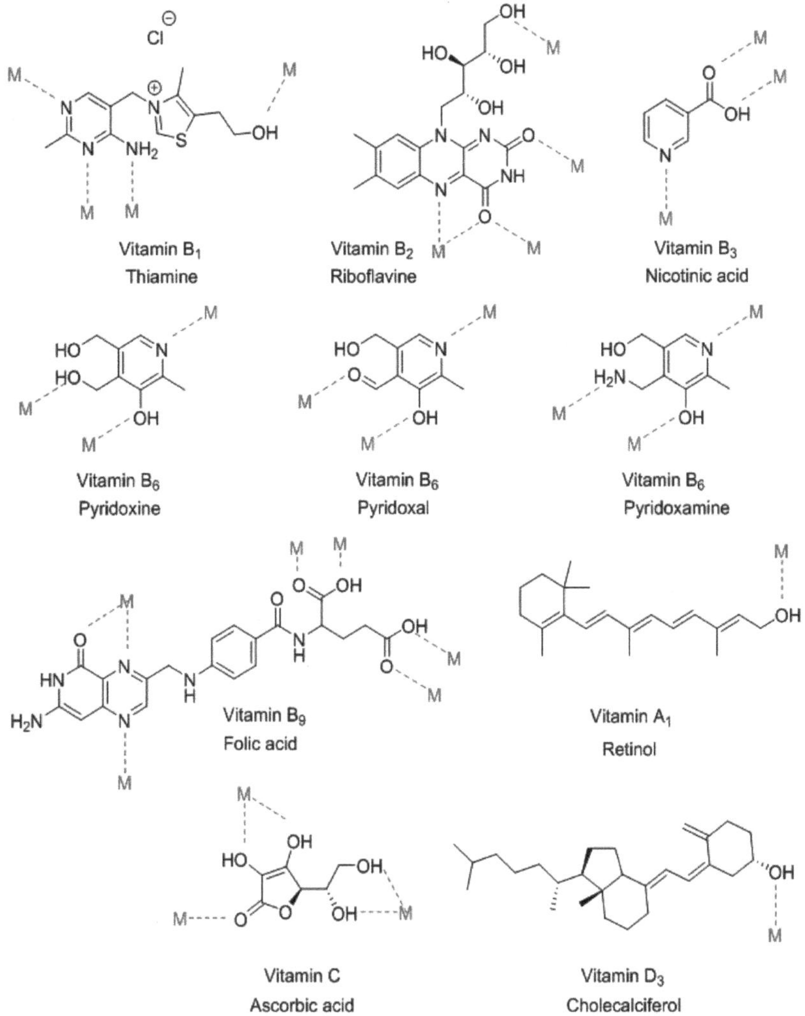

Figure 2.1 Different coordination modes of vitamins commonly used in coordination material chemistry.

system, vision, cell growth, cell proliferation, and reproduction. Sánchez-Guijo and Montero (2010) investigated the interaction of vitamin A_1 and the physiological relevant ions Na^+, Li^+, and K^+ in solution by using mass spectrometry. The preparation of these stable compounds highlights the coordination chemistry of vitamin A_1 and demonstrates the possibility of studying the interaction of vitamin A_1 with other metal ions.

Table 2.1 Some examples of metal-based vitamins and their biological application.

Metal	Vitamin	Biological application	Reference
Cobalt, nickel	B_3	Antibacterial	Verma and Bhojak (2017) (and references therein)
Iron, copper, nickel, zinc, palladium, cadmium, gold	B_3	Antimicrobial	Verma and Bhojak (2017) (and references therein)
Palladium, platinum, gold	B_3	Antitumor	Verma and Bhojak (2017) (and references therein)
Copper	B_3	Antitumor	Anacleto et al. (2017)
Copper, manganese, iron, nickel, cadmium	$B_3 + B_9$	Antitumor	Verma and Bhojak (2017) (and references therein)
Vanadium	B_6	Insulin-like activity	Casas et al. (2012) (and references therein)
Manganese	B_6	Hepatobiliary activity MRI contrast	Casas et al. (2012) (and references therein)
Nickel	B_6	CT−DNA interactions	Chylewska et al. (2017)
Lanthanum, yttrium, cerium, samarium	B_6	Antimicrobial	Refat et al. (2014)
Vanadium	B_9	Antioxidant	Refat et al. (2016)
Lead	B_9	Cellular Bioimaging	Zhao et al. (2013)
Tin	C	Antitumor antiinflammatory	Zumreoglu-Karan (2006) (and references therein)
Platinum	C	Antitumor	Hollis et al. (1985)

Vitamin B_1, also known as thiamine, is composed of an aminopyrimidine and a thiazole ring linked by a methylene bridge. The thiazole ring contains a methyl and an hydroxyethyl side chain. This biomolecule could act as monodentate, bidentate, bidentate-bridging metal coordination modes due to the presence of the aminopyrimidine ring and hydroxyl group (Fig. 2.1). In the literature, complexes of several metals (Hg, Cd, Zn, Pt, Pd, Cu, and Co) with vitamin B_1 have been described (Caira et al., 1974; Cramer et al., 1981, 1984, 1988; Adeyemo et al., 1987; Bencini and Borghi, 1987; Bau et al., 1988; Archibong et al., 1989; Aoki et al., 1990; Casas et al., 1995a; Hu et al., 2001). All these complexes show the metal coordinated to a nitrogen atom from the aminopyrimidine ring in a monodentate mode, and the metal coordination sphere is completed by water molecules, and chloride or bromide ions. Two other complexes with Mn and Cd are known in which the metal is coordinated to the same nitrogen atom and also to the oxygen atom from the hydroxyethyl group, producing dinuclear metal complexes (Hu., 1991; Casas et al., 1995b). Aoki et al. (1991) synthesized a cadmium thiamine polymeric structure with the octahedral Cd(II) bonded to thiamine through the hydroxyethyl oxygen and five thiocyanato ligands, one terminal and the others ones bridging. Despite the considerable number of vitamin B_1-based metal compounds synthesized and well-characterized, to the best of our knowledge no biological applications have been studied. The investigation of the applicability of these type of compounds in medicinal chemistry could be an interesting future work.

Vitamin B_2, also known as riboflavin, is one of the eight B-complex vitamins, and is an important antioxidant. Like other B vitamins, it plays a role in energy production in the body. In the literature only a few examples of vitamin B_2—metal complexes are reported (Malele et al., 2010; Refat et al., 2011). Malele et al. (2010) reported the synthesis and spectroscopic characterization of a vitamin B_2—molybdenum complex, suggesting that the Mo(V) coordinated to vitamin B_2 via the azomethine nitrogen atom of the pyrazine ring. Refat et al. (2011) described a series of vitamin B_2 and alkaline earth metal(II) complexes with a proposed structure of the type [M(vitamin $B_2)_2(X)_2$] where M = Mg(II), Ca(II), Sr(II) or Ba(II); X = Cl or NO_3. In the absence of single-crystal data for all these reported structures, the authors suggested, based on spectroscopic studies, that maybe the vitamin B_2 binds the metal in a bidentate feature through the azomethine nitrogen of the pyrazine ring and the C = O of the pyrimidine-2,4-dione. As mentioned above, vitamin B_2 exhibits antioxidant properties, but what about the metal compounds based on vitamin B_2? Nothing is reported in the literature. Bearing in mind that the functions of vitamins are synergistic, the combination of vitamin B_2 with metal might be of both scientific and pharmacological interest.

Vitamin B_3, also known as niacin or nicotinic acid, displays monodentate, bidentate, bidentate-bridging, and tridentate-bridging metal coordination modes due to the presence of a pyridyl and a carboxylate group, becoming a versatile ligand to design novel metal complexes (Fig. 2.1). Because of a wide variety of coordination possibilities, a huge number of metal—vitamin B_3 complexes have been prepared, and reviewed very recently by Verma and Bhojak (2017). As could be seen in this review, it is possible to prepare vitamin B_3 complexes with all the metal atoms present in the periodic table. These authors also focused on the different biological activities of some of these vitamin B_3 metal complexes, such as antibacterial, antifungal, antiviral, antitumor, antiinflammatory, etc.

In a paper recently published by Anacleto et. al. the synthesis and structural characterization of a series of Cu(I) and Cu(II)—vitamin B_3 metal complexes are investigated (Fig. 2.2). The antitumor capacity of the complexes was tested in vitro against a human cancer cell line, the colorectal adenocarcinoma (Caco-2) cell line, and showed better activity than the free ligand (Anacleto et al., 2017). Regarding all the investigations concerning vitamin B_3-based metal complexes, vitamin B_3 is an excellent choice as a bioligand for the development of new biologically active metallodrugs.

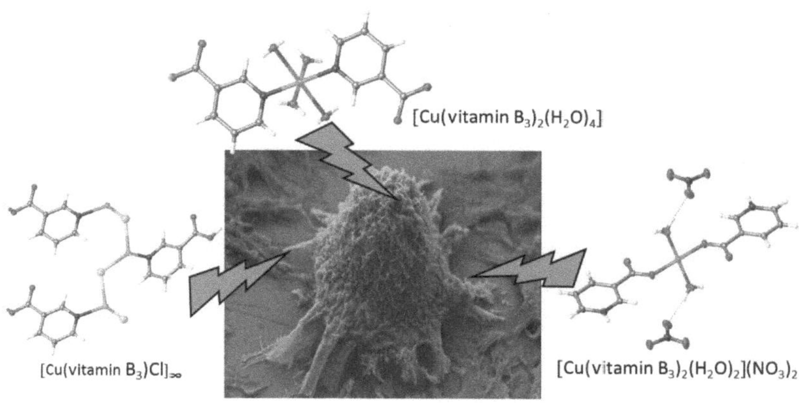

Figure 2.2 Vitamin B_3—copper compounds cytotoxicity against human colon adenocarcinoma Caco-2 cells (Anacleto et al., 2017).

Vitamin B_6 is a group of three naturally occurring water-soluble vitamers, the 3-hydroxy-2-methylpyridine derivatives pyridoxine (PN), pyridoxal (PL), and pyridoxamine (PM) (see Fig. 2.1). This group of natural ligands exhibits multiple different metal ion coordination sites through the oxymethyl oxygen, adjacent phenolate groups, as well as through the pyridine nitrogen, making them an excellent choice to develop new metal complexes with tailored architectures and potential biomedical applications. A review paper of Casas et al. (2012) describes the structural characterization of several vitamin B_6 complexes of different metals (Co, Cu, Fe, Zn, V, Pd, Pt, Ag, Sn, and U) and their uses as therapeutic agents. Chylewska et al. (2015) investigated the different binding modes of the three forms of vitamin B_6, PM, PN, and PL, with Cu(II) in aqueous solution. Chylewska et al. (2017) described the interaction of PM and PL with Ni(II) ions and their binding mode with CT-DNA. In the last decades lanthanide compounds have drawn much attention due to their biological and clinical significance. Refat et al. (2014) having this in mind as well the advantages of natural ligands such as vitamin B_6, prepared several PN lanthanide complexes (La(III), Sm(III), Ce(III), Y(III)), and studied their in vitro antimicrobial activity. Very recently Stouder et al. (2017) reported the structural characterization of PN lanthanide complexes of formula $[Ln(NO_2)_2(H_2O)(pyridoxine)_2]NO_3$, with Ln = Gd, Tb, Dy, Ho, and Er, and investigated the interaction of the PN gadolinium complex with DNA. The considerable number of vitamin B_6 metal complexes reported demonstrate that this vitamin is an interesting linker for the development of new biocompatible materials.

Vitamin B_9, known as folic acid, is an important vitamin which possesses many important biochemical properties. It is structurally composed of pteroic acid and glutamic acid connected via an amide linkage. This organic molecule contains two carboxylate groups which can work as a bidentate ligand binding to a single metal or alternatively as a bridging bidentate ligand coordinating to two metals or as a monodentate ligand (Fig. 2.1). In the literature we can find several studies on the complexation between vitamin B_9 and transition metal ions, such as Fe(III), Al(III), Cr(III), Cu(II), Mn(II), Co(II), Ni(II), Zn(II), Cd(II), and Hg(II). The authors suggested that vitamin B_9 acts as a bidentate ligand through both carboxylic groups (Abd et al., 2008; Fazary and Rajhi, 2015). Two other vitamin B_9 complexes with copper and iron, having the general formula $K_n[M(\text{vitamin } B_9)_2(H_2O)_2] \cdot xH_2O$, where (M = Cu(II) or Fe(III), $n = 2$ or 1, $x = 2$ or 3), were prepared by Hamed et al. (2009), and they investigated their absorption efficiency in blood. Refat and collaborators prepared a vitamin B_9 vanadium complex formulated as $[(VO)_2(\text{vitamin } B_9)(NH_4)_2(SO_4)_2]$ and studied its activity as antioxidant and its interaction with DNA. As observed for the other vitamin B_9 metal complexes, vanadium bound vitamin B_9 via the carboxylate groups in a bidentate fashion (Refat et al., 2016). Zhao et al. (2013) presented the synthesis and characterization of a 2D framework with vitamin B_9 and lead $[Pb\ (\text{vitamin } B_9)]\cdot 4H_2O$ which exhibits considerably higher fluorescence intensity compared to vitamin B_9. For this, vitamin B_9 binds Pb(II) ions in a bidentate mode and simultaneously acts as a bridging ligand (see Fig. 2.3). The lead vitamin B_9 compound is a promising fluorescent probe for cellular bioimaging. To obtain an ideal compound for biological imaging, the same authors investigated the possibility of replacing lead with iron because of its biocompatibility. The Fe–vitamin B_9 complex prepared is also effective as a fluorescent probe for cellular bioimaging. However, in the absence of single crystals of Fe–vitamin B_9, the authors cannot say much about the structure. The iron compound was structurally

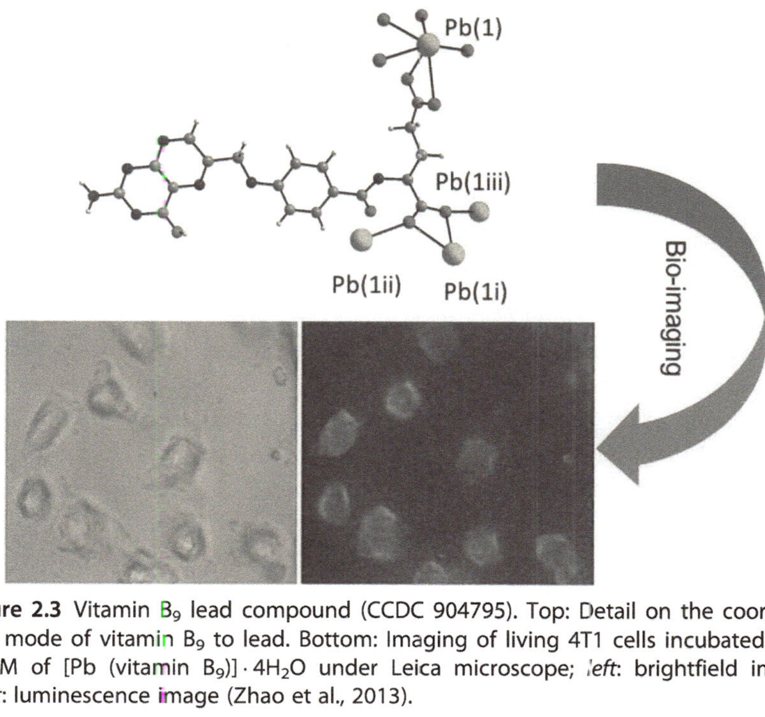

Figure 2.3 Vitamin B_9 lead compound (CCDC 904795). Top: Detail on the coordination mode of vitamin B_9 to lead. Bottom: Imaging of living 4T1 cells incubated with 10 μM of $[Pb\ (\text{vitamin } B_9)]\cdot 4H_2O$ under Leica microscope; *left*: brightfield image; *right*: luminescence image (Zhao et al., 2013).

characterized mainly by spectroscopy techniques. Nevertheless these results indicate that vitamin B_9-based metal compounds are of interest for therapeutic applications.

Vitamin C (L-ascorbic acid), with important biochemical properties, can bind metal ions in a monodentate and/or bidentate mode via the oxygen atoms from the hydroxyl and carbonyl groups (Fig. 2.1), which is strongly dependent on the pH of the solution and on the type of metal. In the literature there is a considerable amount of research on transition metal–vitamin C complexes, mainly in aqueous solution, summarized by Zumreoglu-Karan (2006). This review paper describes in detail the synthesis and characterization of vitamin C complexes with several transition metals (vanadium, chromium, iron, copper, zinc, titanium, tin, and platinum). Important aspects of the interactions between vitamin C and metal ions are evaluated, such as ligand binding mode, pH dependence, metal–ligand stoichiometry, type of metal, etc. In 2012 a series of aqueous complexes of titanium(IV) and vitamin C were studied under biological conditions by Buettner et al. (2012). Vitamin C–metal complexes are difficult to study experimentally because the ligand has multiple protonation and oxidation states, and because deoxygenation of the medium is important to avoid the irreversible oxidation of the vitamin, and the metal complex is often unstable in the solid phase. Only a few examples in solid phase are described and their structures have been solved by single-crystal X-ray diffraction, including with thallium and platinum as metals (Hughes, 1973; Hollis et al., 1985; Yuge and Miyamoto, 1996). The anticancer properties of the vitamin C platinum complexes with general formula *cis*-[Pt(RNH_2)-vitamin C] were investigated by Hollis et al. (1985). Because almost no single crystal is available, the proposed structures of these complexes are a subject of controversy, and consequently research in this area is still important for the elucidation of the coordination chemistry between vitamin C and metals and regarding their application in chelating therapy. Very recently Cesario et al. studied the complexation of Al (III) and Ni(II) with vitamin C under physiological conditions, using a combination of different techniques—potentiometric measurements, ^{1}H NMR spectroscopy, and DFT computation (Cesario et al., 2017).

Vitamin D, also known as cholecalciferol, is the sunshine vitamin that is produced by the body as a response to sun exposure; it can also be consumed in food or supplements. Mercê et al. (1998, 1999, 2003)determined the stability constants of vitamin D complexes involving Co(II), Ni (II), Cu(II), Mn(II), Fe(II), Fe(III), Zn(II), Al (III), Cd(II), Gd(III), and Pb

(II), by potentiometric study. The experimental studies suggested that the vitamin D metal complexes formed are of type ML, ML_2, and ML_3. Only for Fe(III) does the metal binds the vitamin D in a monodentate fashion through the hydroxyl group.

2.3 Vitamin-based metal–organic frameworks as delivery vehicles of therapeutic molecules

MOFs, typically built by bridging metal centers with organic linkers, have emerged as very interesting candidates in the field of functional materials. The ability to design MOFs with a specific function due to practically limitless combinations of metal ions and organic ligands has initiated extensive scientific investigation. To date the potential applications of MOFs have been examined in gas storage and separation, heterogeneous catalysis, magnetism, chemical sensing, imaging agents, and drug delivery (Horcajada et al., 2012; Furukawa et al., 2013; Ma and Perman, 2018; Suh et al., 2012; Kurmoo, 2009; Chen et al., 2010; Della Rocca and Lin, 2010). Among these applications, the delivery of biologically active molecules is particularly interesting. Recently more chemists have begun paying attention to biocompatible MOFs which have potential biomedical applications. So far, a considerable number of bio-MOFs have been reported (McKinlay et al., 2010; Imaz et al., 2011; Anderson and Stylianou, 2017). Vitamins have been proven to be excellent candidates as organic linkers to design biocompatible and biodegradable MOFs to be used as drug delivery vehicles. They can have different functionalities, the ability to bind the metals through multiple coordination sites, and their synergy with metals might be of both scientific and pharmacological interest. In the literature only a few examples of vitamin B_3–MOFs (3D) have been reported to date (Lu and Babb, 2001; Miller et al., 2010; Pinto et al., 2017). The first example described is a copper–vitamin B_3 [Cu (vitamin B_3)]$_n$ three-dimensional framework containing eight member rings and a small pore size, and because of that it is not suitable for drug delivery (Lu and Babb, 2001). Miller et al. in 2010 described the synthesis of a therapeutic 3D MOF denoted as BioMIL-1 containing nontoxic iron linked together through vitamin B_3, with the formula $[Fe_3(\mu_3\text{-}O)(\mu_2\text{-acetate})(\mu_3\text{-vitamin } B_3)_3(\mu_2\text{-vitamin } B_3)_2]$, which is itself the bioactive molecule to be delivered. The release of vitamin B_3 is reached through the degradation of the hybrid compound under physiological conditions, allowing delivery of the bioactive molecule (Miller et al., 2010).

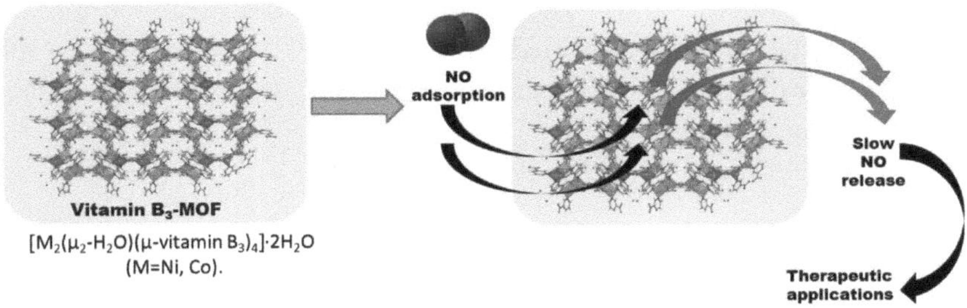

Figure 2.4 3D framework structure constructed from vitamin B$_3$ and Ni or Co, as potential delivery vehicles for therapeutic NO (Pinto et al., 2017).

Pinto et al. very recently synthesized two isostructural Co and Ni MOFs using vitamin B$_3$ (Fig. 2.3) as building blocks, with a formula of [M$_2$(μ$_2$-H$_2$O)(μ$_3$-vitamin B$_3$)$_2$(μ$_2$-vitamin B$_3$)$_2$]•2H$_2$O (M = Ni, Co). They contain two crystallographic distinct divalent metal centers connected by a bridging water and vitamin B$_3$ through a nitrogen atom from the pyridyl group and oxygen atoms belonging to the carboxylate group. These two vitamin−MOFs have the capability of storing and releasing NO in a slow and reversible manner and show low toxicity (Fig. 2.4) (Pinto et al., 2017). The Fe, Ni, and Co vitamin B$_3$−MOFs presented are excellent pointers for the development of other vitamin MOFs with potential biomedical applications.

2.4 Vitamin-based multinuclear metal compounds with magnetic, luminescent, and electrical properties

In the last decade the interest in the design of lanthanide compounds has increased, as well as lanthanide−transition metal compounds, because of their potential application in magnetism and luminescence. Vitamins as multifunctional ligands are excellent candidates for the construction of this type of compound. Among vitamins, vitamin B$_3$, containing two types of coordination atoms in which the carboxylate group favors the coordination to lanthanide ions and the nitrogen atom is likely to bond transition metal, leads to the construction of fascinating architectures combining different type of metals.

Liu et al. (2008) took advantage of vitamin B$_3$ as an excellent bridging ligand between lanthanide and transition metal ions to prepare four new 4d-4f coordination frameworks denoted as [Ag$_2$Ln(vitamin B$_3$)$_4$(H$_2$O)$_4$ · (ClO$_4$) · H$_2$O], [Ln = Eu (1), Gd (2)], [AgLn(vitamin

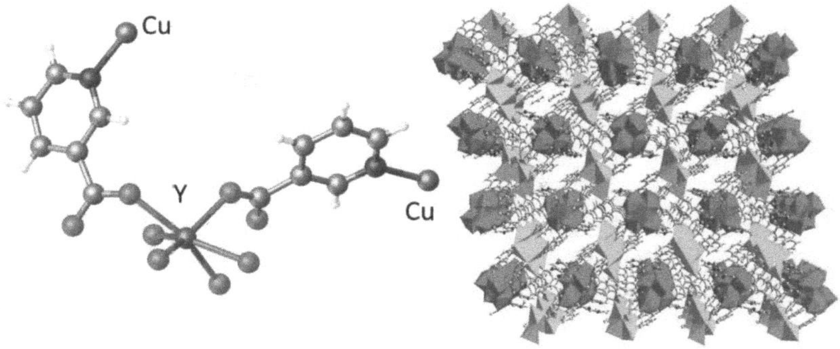

Figure 2.5 Structure details of the 3D yttrium–copper–organic framework (CCDC 660702) $Y_2Cu_2I_2(OH)_2(pca)_2(vitamin\ B_3)_2$; *left*: yttrium ions is bonded to vitamin B_3 through the oxygen atoms from the carboxylate groups and copper ion is connected to the vitamin via nitrogen atom; *right*: 3D heterometallic framework showing two distinct tetranuclear units of cubane $\{Y_4\}$and chair-like $\{Cu_4\}$(Cheng et al., 2008).

$B_3)_2$(oxalate)0.5$(H_2O)_2 \cdot (ClO_4) \cdot H_2O$], and [Ln = Tb (3), Yb (4)]. Cheng et al. using vitamin B_3 in combination with a second ligand, 2-pyrazinecarboxylic acid (pca), prepared three novel 3D lanthanide–transition metal structures of general formula $Ln_2Cu_2I_2(OH)_2(pca)_2(vitamin\ B_3)_2$ (Ln = Y, Er, and Yb). The three isostructural compounds are built from two distinct tetranuclear units of cubane {Ln4} and chair-like {Cu4} clusters, as can be observed in Fig. 2.5 (Cheng et al., 2008).

Zhang et al. (2009) prepared a vitamin B_3 Neodymium MOF [Nd $(C_7H_5NO_4)$(vitamin $B_3)(H_2O)$], showing a rare magnetic interaction between adjacent Nd(III) ions. In 2015 the syntheses, structures, and optical properties of two vitamin B_3-based Ln_{26} (Ln = Dy and Tb) three-dimensional frameworks with Ag and Cu transition metals were reported (Zhang et al., 2015).

A 3D framework Nickel(II) compound with azide and vitamin B_3 $[Ni_{1.5}(N_3)(nic)_2(Hnic)]_n$ with unusual magnetic properties has been described (Verma and Bhojak, 2017).

Vitamin B_6, as mentioned previously, contains a wide variety of coordination possibilities and is an interesting ligand for researchers who work on the preparation of multinuclear metal compounds. Nadia Marino et al. (2013) developed two tetranuclear compounds using vitamin B_6 in its PN form with formulas $[Mn_4(PN\text{-}H)_4(CH_3CO_2)_3Cl_2]$ $Cl \cdot 2CH_3OH \cdot 2H_2O$ and $[Cu_4(PN\text{-}H)_4Cl_2(H_2O)_2]Cl_2$, with interesting magnetic properties. The overall results indicate that among all the vitamins, vitamin B_3 and vitamin B_6 are good choices for the preparation of multinuclear metal compounds.

2.5 Summary

The success of vitamin-derived compounds is based on the diversity of the functional groups that can be connected with numerous metals, giving rise to the compound's biological compatibility and easy recyclability, which makes them attractive candidates for biomedical utilities. The vitamin–metal compounds described in this chapter are great examples of the value-added benefits of vitamins for their potential utility in medicine. Despite the tremendous interest in the preparation of biocompounds, the biomedical applications of vitamin complexes, and mainly vitamin–MOFs, is still poor. In this regard, and bearing in mind the examples of vitamin-based compounds previously presented, vitamins remain a great challenge as building blocks for the construction of biomaterials.

Acknowledgments

This work was developed within the scope of the projects CICECO-Aveiro Institute of Materials, POCI-01-0145-FEDER-007679 (FCT Ref. UID/CTM/50011/2013) and QOPNA research Unit (FCT Ref. UID/QUI/00062/2019), financed by national funds through the FCT/MEC and when appropriate cofinanced by FEDER under the PT2020 Partnership Agreement. S.G. also thanks the pAge project: Life-long protein aggregation (Centro-01–0145-FEDER-000003) for financial support.

References

Abd, E.M.G., Refat, M.S., El-Megharbel, S.M., 2008. Synthesis, spectroscopic and thermal characterization of some transition metal complexes of folic acid. Spectrochim. Acta Part A 70, 916–922.

Adeyemo, A., Oderinde, R., Turner, A., Shamim, A., 1987. Platinum(II) and palladium (II) complexes of vitamin B_1. Bulletin des Sociétés Chimiques Belges 96, 15–22.

Anacleto, B., Gomes, P., Correia-Branco, A., Silva, C., Martel, F., Brandão, P., 2017. Design, structural characterization and cytotoxic properties of copper (I) and copper (II) complexes formed by vitamin B_3 type. Polyhedron 138, 277–286.

Anderson, S.L., Stylianou, K.C., 2017. Biologically derived metal organic frameworks. Coord. Chem. Rev. 349, 102–128.

Aoki, K., Hu, N.H., Yamazaki, H.A., Adeyemo, O., 1990. Metal ion interactions with thiamine. Crystal structures of Co(thiamine)$Cl_3 \cdot 0.4H_2O$ and Zn(thiamine)$Br_3 \cdot 0.2H_2O$: metal bonding to the base. Inorg. Chim. Acta 175, 247–254.

Aoki, K., Yamazaki, H., Adeyemo, A., 1991. Metal ion interactions with vitamin B_1. Crystal structures of Zn(thiamine)$(SCN)_3$ having a metal-base bond and Cd(thiamine) $(SCN)_3$ having a metal-hydroxyethyl bond. Inorg. Chim. Acta 180, 117–124.
Archibong, E., Adeyemo, A., Aoki, K., Yamazaki, H., 1989. Thiamine-metal ion and thiamine-anion interactions. Crystal structure of Cu(thiamine)Br_2. Inorg. Chim. Acta 156, 77–83.
Bau, R., Hyun, Y.S., Lim, J., Choi, H.K., Yannopoulos, A., Hadjiliadis, N., 1988. The crystal structure of tetrahydrothiamine and its Co(II) complex. Inorg. Chim. Acta 150, 107–112.
Bencini, A., Borghi, E., 1987. Complexes of vitamin B_1 with transition metal ions. Crystal and molecular structure of Zn(thiamine)$Cl_3 \cdot 0.4H_2O$. Inorg. Chim. Acta 135, 85–91.
Buettner, K.M., Collins, J.M., Valentine, A.M., 2012. Titanium(IV) and vitamin C: aqueous complexes of a bioactive form of Ti(IV). Inorg. Chem. 51, 11030–11039.
Caira, M.R., Fazakerley, G.V., Linder, P.W., Nassimbeni, L.R., 1974. The crystal structure of the thiamine hydrochloride copper(II) complex. Acta Cryst. B30, 1660–1666.
Casas, J.S., Couce, M.D., Sordo, J., 2012. Coordination chemistry of vitamin B_6 and derivatives: a structural overview. Coord. Chem. Rev. 256, 3036–3062.
Casas, J.S., Castineras, A., Couce, M.D., Sánchez, A., Sordo, J., Varela, J.M., 1995a. The CdCl2/thiamine(vitamin B1) system: crystal structure and Spectroscopic properties of the new complex *trans*-[Cd(thiamine)$_2Cl_4$]. Polyhedron 14, 1825–1829.
Casas, J.S., Castellano, E.E., Couce, M.D., Sánchez, A., Sordo, J., Varela, J.M., et al., 1995b. Vitamin B_1: chemical interaction with $CdCl_2$ and in *vivo* effects on cadmium toxicity in rats. Crystal structure of [Cd(thiamine)$Cl_3]_2 \bullet 2H_2O$, a complex containing pyrimidine and cadmium hydroxyethyl bonds. Inorg. Chem. 34, 2430–2437.
Cesario, D., Furia, E., Mazzone, G., Beneduci, A., De Luca, G., Sicilia, E., 2017. Complexation of Al^{3+} and Ni^{2+} by *L*-ascorbic acid: an experimental and theoretical investigation. J. Phys. Chem. A 121, 9773–9781.
Chen, B., Xiang, S. Qian, G., 2010. Metal – organic frameworks with functional pores for recognition of small molecules. Acc. Chem. Res. 43, 1115–1124.
Cheng, J., Zheng, S., Liu, W., Yang, G., 2008. 3D lanthanide-transition-metal–organic frameworks constructed by two distinct tetranuclear units of cubane {Ln4} and chair-like{Cu4} clusters. CrystEngComm 10, 1047–1051.
Chylewska, A., Ogryzek, M., Chmurzyński, L., Makowski, M., 2015. Spectrophotometric, potentiometric, and conductometric studies of binary complex formation between copper(II) and three forms of vitamin B_6 in aqueous solutions. J. Coord. Chem. 68, 3761–3775.
Chylewska, A., Ogryzek, M., Chmurzyński, L., Makowski, M., 2017. Multi-analytical studies about physico-chemical properties of Ni(II)-vitamin B_6 coordination compounds and their CT-DNA interations. J. Molec. Liquids 243, 771–780.
Cramer, R.E., Maynard, R.B., Ibers, J.A., 1981. A metal ion complex of vitamin B_1: the preparation and structure of Cd(thiamine)$Cl_3 \bullet$0.6H2O. J. Am. Chem. Soc. 103, 76–81.
Cramer, R.E., Maynard, R.B., Evangelista, R.S., 1984. Synthesis and crystal structure of a Cu(I) complex of vitamin B_1, Cu(thiamine)Cl_2. J. Am. Chem. Soc. 106, 111–116.
Cramer, R.E., Kirkup, R.E., Carrie, M.J.J., 1988. The tetrachloroplatinate(2-)/thiamin system. Structures of a complex, Pt(thiamin)$Cl_3 \bullet H_2O$, and two salts, (Hthiamin) $(PtCl_4)$ and (Hthiamin)$_2(PtCl_4)(Cl)_2.2H_2O$. Inorg. Chem. 27, 123–130.
Della Rocca, J., Lin, W., 2010. Nanoscale metal-organic frameworks: magnetic resonance imaging contrast agents and beyond. Eur. J. Inorg. Chem. 3725–3734.
Fazary, A.E., Rajhi, A.Q., 2015. Complexation equilibria of vitamin B_9, glycine oligopeptides with Di-and trivalent metal ions. Asian J. Chem. 27, 3872–3876.

Furukawa, H., Cordova, K.E., O'Keeffe, M., Yaghi, O.M., 2013. The chemistry and applications of metal-organic frameworks. Science 341 (6149), 1230444.

Hamed, E., Attia, M.S., Bassiouny, K., 2009. Synthesis, spectroscopic and thermal characterization of copper(II) and iron(III) complexes of folic acid and their absorption efficiency in the blood. Bioinorg. Chem. Appl. 1–6. Article ID 979680.

Hollis, L.S., Amundsen, A.R., Stern, E.W., 1985. Synthesis, structure, and antitumour properties of platinum complexes of vitamin C. J. Am. Chem. Soc. 107, 274–276.

Horcajada, P., Gref, R., Baati, T., Allan, P.K., Maurin, G., Couvreur, P., et al., 2012. Metal-organic frameworks in biomedicine. Chem. Rev. 112, 1232–1268.

Hu, N.H., 1991. A novel metal-thiamine complex with a cyclic dimer formed by metal-bridged two thiamine ligands. Crystal structure of [Mn(thiamine) $Cl_2(H_2O)]_2[thiamine]_2Cl_4 \cdot 2H_2O$. Inorg. Chim. Acta 186, 209–214.

Hu, N.H., Aoki, K., Adeyemo, A.O., Wiliams, G.N., 2001. Metal ion and anion coordination in the thiamine–$[Pt^{II}(NO_2)_4]^{2-}$ system. Structures of a metal complex, $Pt(thiamine)(NO_2)_3$, and two salts, (H-thiamine)$[Pt(NO_2)_4] \cdot 2H_2O$ and (thiamine monophosphate)$_2$ $[Pt(NO_2)_4] \cdot 2H_2O$. Inorg. Chim. Acta 325, 9–19.

Hughes, D.L., 1973. Crystal structure of thallium(I) *L*-ascorbate. J. Chem. Soc. Dalton Trans. 2209–2215.

Imaz, I., Rubio-Martínez, M., An, J., Solé-Font, I., Rosi, N.L., Maspoch, D., 2011. Metal–biomolecule frameworks (MBioFs). Chem. Commun. 47, 7287–7302.

Jamieson, E.R., Lippard, S.J., 1999. Structure, recognition, and processing of cisplatin-DNA adducts. Chem. Rev. 99 (9), 2467–2498.

Kurmoo, M., 2009. Magnetic metal–organic frameworks. Chem. Soc. Rev. 38, 1353–1379.

Liu, Z., Qiu, Y., Li, Y., Deng, H., Zeller, M., 2008. Synthesis, structures and luminescent properties of 4d–4f heterometallic coordination frameworks based on lanthanide oxalate substructures with nicotinate bridging ligands. Polyhedron 27, 3493–3499.

Lu, J.Y., Babb, A.M., 2001. A new 3-D neutral framework coordination polymer constructed via square pyramidal binuclear Cu(II) and nicotinato ligand. Inorg. Chem. Commun. 4, 716–718.

Ma, S., Perman, J.A., 2018. Elaboration and Applications of Metal-organic Frameworks, vol. 2. World Scientific publishing Co. Pte. Ltd.

Malele, C.N., Ray, J., Jones Jr, W.E., 2010. Synthesis, characterization and spectroscopic study of riboflavin–molybdenum complex. Polyhedron 29, 749–756.

Marino, N., Armentano, D., Mastropietro, T.F., Julve, M., De Munno, G., Martínez-Lillo, J., 2013. Cubane-type Cu^{II}_4 and Mn^{II}_2 Mn^{III}_2 complexes based on pyridoxine: a versatile ligand for metal assembling. Inorg. Chem. 52, 11934–11943.

McKinlay, A.C., Morris, R.E., Horcajada, P., Férey, G., Gref, R., Couvreur, P., et al., 2010. BioMOFs: metal-organic frameworks for biological and medical applications. Angew. Chem., Int. Ed. 49, 6260–6266.

Mercê, A.L.R., Szpoganicz, B., Dutra, R.C., Khan, M.A., Do Thanh, X., Bouet, G., 1998. Potentiometric study of vitamin D_3 complexes with cobalt (II), nickel (II) and copper (II) in water-ethanol medium. J. Inorg. Biochem,. 71, 87–91.

Mercê, A.L.R., Szpoganicz, B., Dutra, R.C., Khan, M.A., Do Thanh, X., Bouet, G., 1999. Potentiometric study of vitamin D_3 complexes with manganese(II), iron(II), iron(Ill) and zinc(II) in water-ethanol medium. J. Inorg. Biochem. 73, 167–172.

Mercê, A.L.R., Yano, L.S., Dutra, R.C., Khan, M.A., Do Thanh, X., Bouet, G., 2003. Complexing power of vitamin D_3 toward various metals. Potentiometric studies of vitamin D3 complexes with Al^{3+}, Cd^{2+}, Gd^{3+} and Pb^{2+} ions in water–ethanol solution. J. Sol. Chem. 32, 1075–1085.

Miller, S.R., Heurtaux, D., Baati, T., Horcajada, P., Grenèche, J., Serre, C., 2010. Biodegradable therapeutic MOFs for the delivery of bioactive molecules. Chem. Commun. 46, 4526–4528.

Pinto, R.V., Antunes, F., Pires, J., Graça, V., Brandão, P., Pinto, M.L., 2017. Vitamin B_3 metal-organic frameworks as potential delivery vehicles for therapeutic nitric oxide. Acta Biomater. 51, 66–74.

Refat, M.S., Moussa, M.A.A., Mohamed, S.F., 2011. Synthesis, spectroscopic characterization, thermal analysis and electrical conductivity studies of Mg(II), Ca(II), Sr(II) and Ba(II) vitamin B_2 complexes. J. Molec. Struct. 994, 194–201.

Refat, M.S., Al-Azab, F.M., Al-Maydama, H.M.A., Amin, R.R., Jamil, Y.M.S., 2014. Synthesis and in vitro microbial evaluation of La(III), Ce(III), Sm(III) and Y(III) metal complexes of vitamin B_6 drug. Spectrochim. Acta Part A: Molec. Biomol. Spectrosc. 127, 196–215.

Refat, M.S., El-Megharbel, S.M., Kobeasy, M.I., Mahamoud, G.I., Al-Omar, M.A., Naglah, A.M., 2016. Synthesis, spectroscopic characterizations and biological activities of vanadyl(II) folate compound as a new anti-DNA damage and antioxidant agent. J. Molec. Liquids 220, 468–477.

Rosenberg, B., Van Camp, L., Trosko, J.E., Mansour, V.H., 1969. Platinum compounds: a new class of potent antitumour agents. Nature 222, 385–386.

Sánchez-Guijo, A., Montero, O., 2010. Stable ion complexes of vitamin A species (retinol) in solution as detected by mass spectrometry. Rapid Commun. Mass Spectrom. 24, 1161–1164.

Stouder, C.E., Warren, K.J., Perdue, O.F., Stewart, A.L., Padgett, C.W., Amonette, A.J., et al., 2017. Synthesis, characterization, computational study, and biological relevance of a family of isostructural, mononuclear Ln (Ln = Gd, Tb, Dy, Ho, Er) complexes containing pyridoxine, an essential ingredient of vitamin B6 enzyme. Inorg. Chim. Acta 46, 172–181.

Suh, M.P., Park, H.J , Prasad, T.K., Lim, D.W., 2012. Hydrogen storage in metal-organic frameworks. Chem. Rev. 112, 782–835.

Verma, S.K., Bhojak, N., 2017. A review on coordination behaviour and bioactivity of metal complexes of nicotinic acid and its derivatives. World J. Pharm. Pharmac. Sci. 6, 490–514.

Yuge, H., Miyamoto, T.K., 1996. New synthesis and crystal structures of platinum(II) *L*-ascorbate complexes. Chem. Lett. 25 (5), 375–376.

Zhang, C.X., Lippard, S.J., 2003. New metal complexes as potential therapeutics. Curr. Opin. Chem. Biol. 7, 481–489.

Zhang, D., Song, T., Wang, L., Shi, J., Xu, J., Wang, Y., et al., 2009. Hydrothermal synthesis, structure and rare ferromagnetic property of a 3-D Nd(III) metal–organic framework based on mixed pyridine-2,5-dicarboxylic acid/nicotinic acid ligands. Inorg. Chim. Acta 362, 299–302.

Zhang, Y., Huang, L., Miao, H., Wan, H.X., Mei, H., Liu, Y., et al., 2015. Hydrothermal synthesis, structure, and optical properties of two nanosized Ln26@CO3 (Ln = Dy and Tb) cluster-based lanthanide-transition-metal-organic-framework (Ln MOFs). Chem. Eu. J. 21, 3234–3241.

Zhao, F., Zhang, H. Hu, H., Zhang, G., Yang, K., Liu, R., et al., 2013. Lead–vitamin complex $[Pb(C_{19}H_{15}N_7O_6)] \cdot 4H_2O$ and its application in bioimaging. Inor. Chem. Comm. 29, 165–168.

Zhou, C.H., Zhang, Y.Y., Yan, C.Y., Wan, K., Gan, L.L., Shi, Y., 2010. Recent researches in metal supramolecular complexes as anticancer agents. Anti-Cancer Agents Med. Chem. 10, 371–395.

Zumreoglu-Karan, B., 2006. The coordination chemistry of vitamin C: an overview. Coord. Chem. Rev. 250, 2295–2307.

CHAPTER 3

Vitamin E: an overview

Farid Khallouki[1], Robert Wyn Owen[2], Mourad Akdad[1], Bachir El Bouhali[1], Sandrine Silvente-Poirot[3] and Marc Poirot[3]
[1]Department of Biology, Faculty of Sciences and Technology, FSTE, Errachidia, Morocco
[2]Division of Chemopreventive Oncology, German Cancer Research Center, Heidelberg, Germany
[3]Cancer Research Center of Toulouse, Team Cholesterol Metabolism and Therapeutic Innovations, UMR 1037 INSERM-University of Toulouse, Toulouse, France

Contents

Summary points

- This chapter focuses on vitamin E, which comprises a group of eight compounds including tocopherols and tocotrienols.
- Vitamin E components are produced by plants and are present in vegetable food and oils in various amounts.
- α-Tocopherol is the major lipid-soluble antioxidant found in human blood.
- α-Tocopherol is widely used as a dietary supplement all over the world.
- α-Tocopherol was proposed as a chemopreventive agent for various pathologies.
- Results from clinical studies showed evidence of possible interference by α-tocopherol with drugs.
- Diet supplementation with a high dose of α-tocopherol during some drug treatments, such as tamoxifen, is not recommended.

Molecular Nutrition
DOI: https://doi.org/10.1016/B978-0-12-811907-5.00001-4

Vitamin E is a fat-soluble vitamin discovered in 1922 at the University of Berkeley (California, United States) by Herbert Mclean Evans's group (Evans and Bishop, 1922). They were studying the impact of diet on rat reproduction. They found that pregnant female rats fed a minimal-fat diet showed fetal resorption and did not develop fetuses, suggesting that fats from the diet might be important for reproduction. They found that supplementation of this minimal-diet with a compound called "substance X," which is present in various foods, prevented the death of fetuses (Evans and Bishop, 1922). Substance X was later shown to be important for lactation (Evans, 1924) and male sterility by two independent groups (Evans, 1925; Evans and Burr, 1925; Sure, 1924). Sure (1924), Evans (1925), and Evans and Burr (1925) proposed that substance X should be named vitamin E, because vitamin D was attributed to the antirachitic factor described (McCollum et al., 1922) just 5 months before Evan's paper on substance X (Evans and Bishop, 1922). In 1935 Evans et al. achieved the isolation of vitamin E from wheat germ oil and established it was an alcohol, which they named "α-tocopherol" (α-TP) with a provisional molecular formula of $C_{29}H_{50}O_2$ (Evans et al., 1935). The name tocopherol came from the Greek words "tocos," which means "birth," and "pherein," which means "to bear." The chemical structure of α-TP was deciphered by Fernholz (1938). It consists of a trimethylated chromanol ring grafted to a saturated-phytyl side chain bearing three asymmetric carbon atoms (Fernholz, 1938). In the same year, Paul Karrer, a winner of the Nobel Prize for Chemistry, reported the first synthesis of the racemic α-TP from trimethylhydroquinone and phytylbromide using zinc chloride as a catalyst (Karrer et al., 1938). Subsequently, other isoforms, thereafter named TP homologues or tocotrienols (TT), have been extracted from many vegetable materials and in particular from vegetable oils. These include β-, γ-, and δ-TP, the latter being reported in 1947 (Stern et al., 1947). Both the isolation of all forms of TT and their chemical structures were reported in the 1960s (Pennock et al., 1964; Whittle et al., 1966). Vitamin E appears as colorless or pale yellow sticky oils which are found in most vegetable oils, and in nuts, seeds, and whole grains (Grilo et al., 2014; Khallouki et al., 2003).

3.1 Chemistry of vitamin E

Vitamin E components are fats that are soluble in lipoid solvents and weakly soluble in water. They are sensitive to light in the presence of air

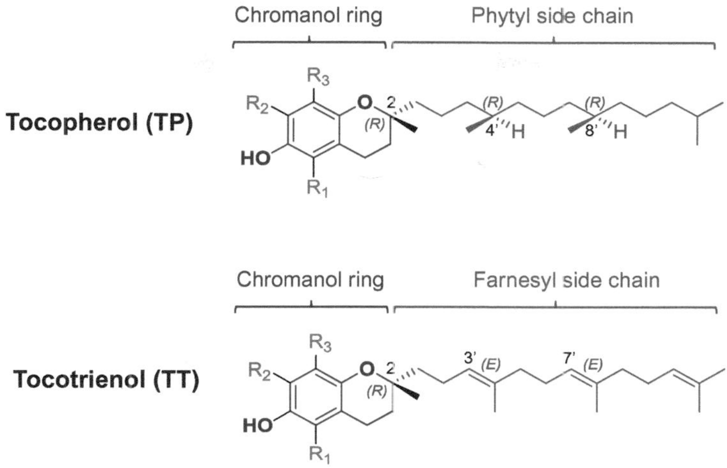

Figure 3.1 Chemical structure of vitamin E homologues. α-TP and α-TT: $R_1 = R_2 = R_3 = CH_3$; β-TP and β-TT: $R_1 = R_3 = CH_3$, $R_2 = H$; γ-TP and γ-TT: $R_1 = H$, $R_2 = R_3 = CH_3$; δ-TP and δ-TT: $R_1 = R_2 = H$, $R_3 = CH_3$. Chiral carbons are numbered. (*R*) indicates the stereochemistry of the asymmetric carbons. (*E*) indicates the *trans* geometry of the double bonds.

or other oxidants, and are easily transformed into tocopheryl-*p*-quinones, which makes vitamin E one of the most potent natural antioxidants (Niki and Noguchi, 2004).

Vitamin E components are bicyclic phenolic compounds grafted to an extended hydrocarbon side chain. They are composed of α-, β-, γ-, and δ-homologues differing by the number and sites of methyl substituents on the chroman ring for TP and TT. TP has an aliphatic C-16 phytyl side chain, which is replaced by an unsaturated farnesyl side chain in TT (Fig. 3.1). α-TP is the most abundant and biologically active form of vitamin E (Khallouki et al., 2015; Pennock et al., 1964).

The natural α-TP has a 2*R*, 4′*R*, and 8′*R* configuration (Fig. 3.1). Therefore its systematic name is (2R, 4′*R*, 8′*R*)-α-TP, formerly known as D-α-TP, the notation RRR-α-TP should also be used. Synthetically it can be obtained by condensation of trimethylhydroquinone with phytol to get a mixture of racemic TP (DellaPenna and Pogson, 2006). α-TP exists in an *R* configuration for the three asymmetric carbons. On the other hand, TT has only one chiral carbon with an *R* configuration, and two double bonds in a *trans* (*E*) geometry at C3′ and C7′(2*R*,3′*E*,7′*E*) (Pennock et al., 1964).

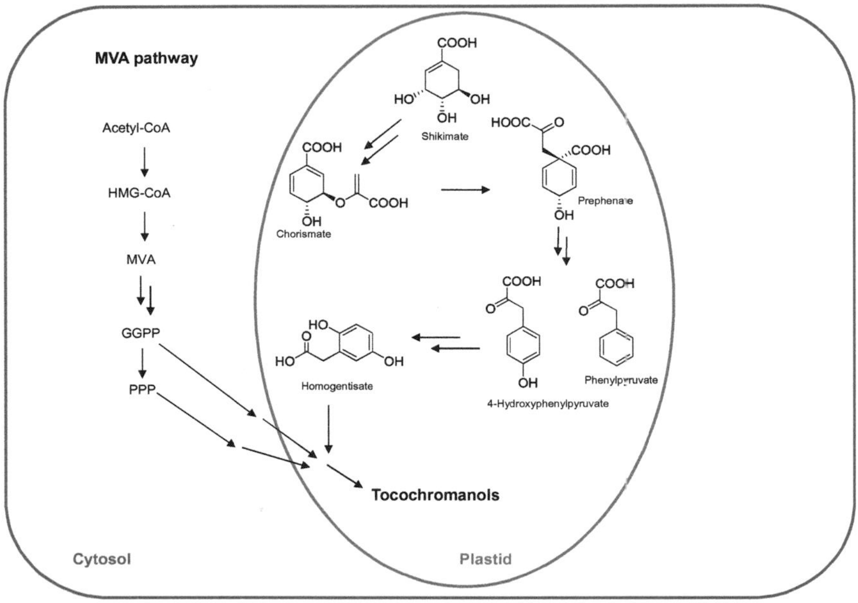

Figure 3.2 ***Biosynthesis of tocochromanols in plants.*** *GGPP*, Geranylgeranyl pyrophosphate; *MVA*, mevalonate.

3.2 Biosynthesis of vitamin E

The biosynthesis of tocochromanols (including TP and TT) has been well documented in photosynthetic and nonphotosynthetic organisms and is depicted in Fig. 3.2. The chromanol ring is derived from the shikimate pathways via the formation of homogentisic acid. The hydrophobic hydrocarbon side chain is produced from the mevalonate pathway via geranylgeranyl pyrophosphate or phytyl pyrophosphate to give TT and TPs, respectively (Mene-Saffrane, 2017).

3.3 Vitamin E components are phenolic antioxidants

Vitamin E's chromanol head group prevents harmful peroxidation events (Jiang, 2014) because of the presence of a phenol group (Foti, 2007). This is the first line mechanism of protection against polyunsaturated fatty acids peroxidation. This occurs through the transfer of the acidic H from the OH of vitamin E to peroxy radicals ROO$^{\bullet}$, and thus inhibiting the radical chain propagation within lipid domains (Peh et al., 2016; Yin et al., 2011). In addition, TP can trap other oxidizing reagents such as singlet oxygen, superoxide anion (Csallany and Ha, 1992), ozone (Liebler, 1993), peroxynitrite (Hogg et al., 1994), and nitrogen dioxide radicals (Cooney et al., 1995). Vitamin E deficiency is associated with an increase in circulating lipoperoxides (Richard et al., 1990), and inhibits in vivo lipoperoxidation (Peuchant et al., 1994). The inhibition of lipoperoxidation by vitamin E impacts on the cholesterol oxidation process by blocking sterol-5,6-epoxidation (Poirot and Silvente-Poirot, 2013).

3.4 Vitamin E oxidation products

The chemical nature of TP oxidation products depends on the reaction conditions that are used. This includes solvents, temperature, light, the physical state of the system, the oxygen pressure, the type of TP substrates, and their respective concentrations. TP components exhibit different oxidation potentials, which depend upon the acidity of their phenol group (Madeira et al., 2011). α-TP blocks the propagation step during lipid oxidation into hydroperoxides by donating its phenolic radical proton atom to a peroxyl radical. This reaction occurs at a very high rate and is faster than the reaction of polyunsaturated lipid with peroxy radicals (Niki et al., 1984). The TP form resonance-stabilized TP radicals (called tocopheryl semiquinone radicals), as depicted in Fig. 3.3, which do not propagate oxidation. The tocopheroxyl radical that is formed can combine with a peroxyl radical yielding an inactive, nonradical product. This affords 8α-substituted tocopherones, which rearrange into α-tocopherylquinone as the major oxidation product of α-TP. This reaction can form the side products C4/C5-epoxy-8-α-hydroperoxytocopherones and C7/C8-epoxy-8-α-hydroperoxytocopherones. These intermediates are precursors, after hydrolysis, of 5,6-epoxy-α-tocopherolquinone and 2,3-epoxy-α-tocopherolquinone, respectively, as minor oxidation products of α-TP (Brigelius-Flohe and Traber, 1999) (Fig. 3.3). In lipid systems, additional reactions can occur by self-coupling of the tocopheryloxy radicals to form dimers and trimers (Faustman et al., 1999; Liebler and Burr, 1992; Verleyen et al., 2001).

In plasma the weak concentration of α-tocopherylquinone found is due, in part, to its recycling through tocopheroxyl reductase activity. This reductase activity, which produces TP, was attributed to NADH-cytochrome b6-dependent enzymatic activity. Alternatively the reduction of α-tocopherylquinone into α-TP can be produced by a nonenzymatic mechanism involving ascorbate and dihydrolipoic acid (Traber, 1994).

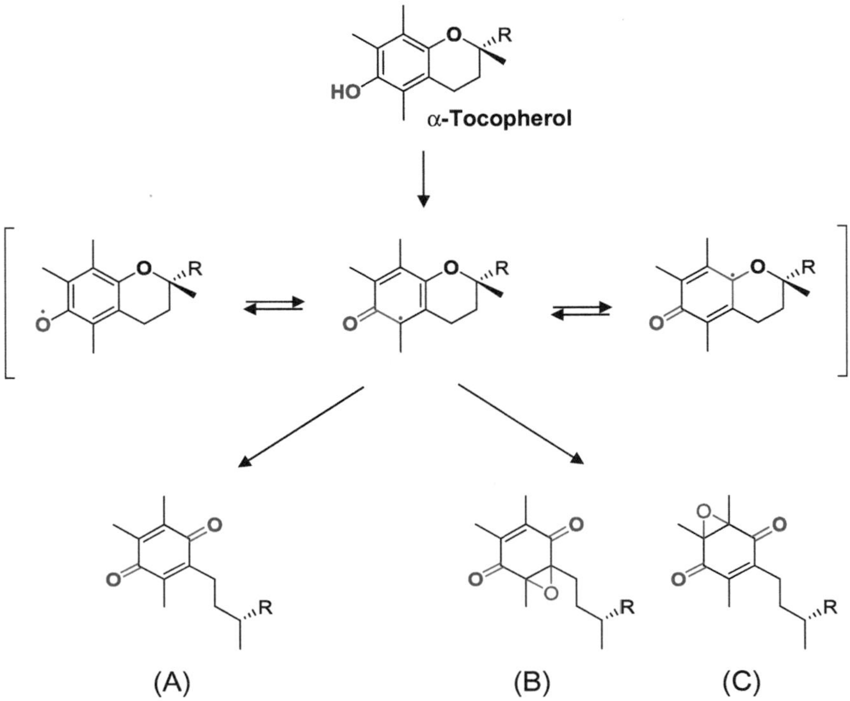

Figure 3.3 ***α-Tocopheroxyl radical and its resonance-stabilized forms in association of its main and major oxidation products*** α-tocopherylquinone (A), 2,3-epoxy-α-tocopherolquinone (B), and 5,6-epoxy-α-tocopherolquinone (C), R = $C_{16}H_{33}$.

3.5 Vitamin E and human pathologies

While earlier experiments established that vitamin E was essential for reproduction in rats (Evans, 1924, 1925; Evans and Bishop, 1922; Evans and Burr, 1925; Sure, 1924), it has never been established that vitamin E has a similar effect in humans (Khadangi and Azzi, 2018). However, deficiencies in vitamin E were linked to various human pathologies, such as bronchopulmonary dysplasia (Stone et al., 2018), emphysema (Pacht et al., 1986), and chronic alcoholism (von Herbay et al., 1994), and a complementation therapy with vitamin E was proposed to treat these diseases. Vitamin E complementation was also proposed in patients with abetalipoproteinemia, which is associated with intestinal fat malabsorption associated with a severe vitamin E deficiency (Cuerq et al., 2018).

Vitamin E deficiency was linked to chronic pancreatitis (Duggan et al., 2014), ulcerative colitis, such as inflammatory bowel diseases (Fabisiak et al., 2017), cystic fibrosis (Okebukola et al., 2017), and hereditary spherocytosis or Gaucher disease (Rachmilewitz et al., 1982). In Gaucher disease, it was proposed that lysosomal accumulation of glucocerebrosides stimulated phagocytes into a maintained "respiratory burst" with an excessive production of oxygen free radicals, resulting in a massive oxidation of vitamin E, eventually leading to its deficiency. Vitamin E deficiency has been observed in cases of neuromuscular disorders, polyneuropathy, and skeletal myopathy (Traber et al., 1987; Wysota et al., 2017).

3.6 Vitamin E and disease prevention

Dietary intake of antioxidants, such as vitamin E, through the consumption of fruits and vegetable has been proposed as a strategy to prevent aging, and degenerative diseases, such as cancer, cardiovascular diseases, sensory impairment, and a decline in the immune system (Liu, 2013). Clinical trials have not provided evidence to date that dietary supplementation with vitamin E prevents cardiovascular diseases or reduces mortality in middle-aged or elderly patients with heart diseases or risk factors for heart diseases (Brown and Crowley, 2005; Lonn et al., 2005). High dosage α-TP supplements may increase the risk of all-cause mortality and should be avoided (Miller et al., 2005). Dietary supplementation with vitamin E significantly increased the risk of prostate cancer among healthy men (Klein et al., 2011), while it was found that it significantly protected smokers from prostate cancer (Heinonen et al., 1998). Clinical evaluations of vitamin E on colon cancers have been inconsistent (Park et al., 2010; Wu et al., 2002) or showed a modestly association with a lower risk of colon cancer (Longnecker et al., 1992). No reduction in the incidence of lung cancer was observed among the male smokers who received vitamin E (Alpha-Tocopherol, 1994), while it was found to accelerate lung cancer progression in mice (Sayin et al., 2014). As observed for other cancers, the impact of vitamin E on breast cancer (BC) was inconsistent (Cuzick, 2017), although a recent pharmacogenomic study showed that vitamin E can be of benefit to a specific genetic variant of the catechol-O-methyltransferase (Hall et al., 2019). Additionally, vitamin E showed a positive outcome for nonalcoholic fatty liver diseases (Lavine et al., 2011; Sanyal et al., 2010) and Alzheimer's disease (Dysken et al., 2014).

3.7 Molecular targets for vitamin E

Beside the antioxidant action of vitamin E components, several molecular and pharmacological targets were identified for vitamin E components, and α-TP was shown to be a direct inhibitor of protein kinase C (Galli et al., 2017). Vitamin E was reported to modulate the lipoxygenation of arachidonic acid in leukocytes (Goetzl, 1980) and to inhibit the 5-lipoxygenase enzyme (Pein et al., 2018; Reddanna et al., 1985). On the other hand, TT, but not TP, was shown to inhibit cholesterol biosynthesis (Pearce et al., 1992) through the downregulation of the expression of the hydroxymethylglutaryl-coenzyme A reductase (HMGR) (Parker et al., 1993), which led to the blockage of the mevalonate pathway. The inhibition of HMGR blocks the neosynthesis of cholesterol and cell proliferation (Khallouki et al., 2015). TP and TT were shown to be ligands of the estrogen receptors (ER) and are phytoestrogens. δ-TP is the most potent of the series and stimulates the proliferation of BC cells in an ER-dependent manner, while TT homologues inhibit cell proliferation through the inhibition of the HMGR (Khallouki et al., 2015). Importantly, ER modulation was not observed with the corresponding quinonic oxidation product of δ-TP. This illustrates the importance of defining the molecular species of the vitamin E components that are responsible for the measured effects (Galli et al., 2017).

3.8 Interference of vitamin E with the pharmacological action of drugs

Laboratory as well as clinical studies showed that consumption of high-dose vitamin E supplements led to vitamin E—drug interactions in some cases, which may alter their pharmacological activities (Podszun and Frank, 2014). Several clinical studies have shown that chemotherapy and radiation therapy deplete antioxidants, such as α-TP, from tissues, which can be oxidized by free radicals (Moss, 2007). Although cellular and animal studies clearly highlighted possible interferences with various anticancer treatments, clinical studies were not that conclusive, but risks were identified in several cases (Podszun and Frank, 2014; Vernieri et al., 2018).

The case of tamoxifen (Tam) is an interesting one. Tam is a well-known drug used to treat and prevent ER-positive BC. The rational for its clinical use is that it blocks the mitogenic action of 17β-estradiol at the ER level (Jordan, 2006). Tam, however, displays a complex pharmacology and several other pharmacological targets were identified (Leignadier et al., 2017). Among them, the microsomal antiestrogen binding site (AEBS) is a high affinity site for Tam. The AEBS is a heterooligomeric complex composed of 3β-hydroxysterol-Δ8-Δ7-isomerase (D8D7I) and 3β-hydroxysterol-Δ7-reductase (DHCR7). It was found that D8DI and DHCR7 carried out the cholesterol-5,6-epoxide hydrolase (ChEH) enzymatic activity (de Medina et al., 2010; Silvente-Poirot and Poirot, 2012). The inhibition of the D8D7 by Tam leads to the accumulation of zymostenol which induces a protective autophagy in cancer cells (de Medina et al., 2009b,c; Leignadier et al., 2017; Poirot et al., 2012; Segala et al., 2017; Sola et al., 2013). On the other hand, Tam induces BC cell differentiation and death via the AEBS. Tam stimulates the lipoperoxidation in BC cells which leads to the production of cholesterol-5,6-epoxides (5,6-EC), and the inhibition of ChEH by Tam induces their accumulation in BC cells (Segala et al., 2013). Tam reactivates the lactation process that was lost during oncogenesis and that was shut down in BC cells. Tam induces the production of triacyl glycerol (TG), which is the major lipid found in milk (de Medina et al., 2009a,b; Payre et al., 2008) (Fig. 3.4).

Tam induces TG biosynthesis in hepatocytes through a mechanism independent of ER (Moya et al., 2010) but that may involve the AEBS, the liver being the richest source of AEBS (de Medina et al., 2010). The induction of BC cell differentiation and death by Tam is mediated by 5,6-EC. α-TP totally blocked 5,6-EC biosynthesis, cell differentiation, and death (Leignadier et al., 2017). This explains at the molecular level the earlier observations showing that α-TP inhibits cytotoxicity induced by Tam in BC cells (Mandlekar and Kong, 2001). Tam induces a reversible hypertriglyceridemia in patients, which was shown to be totally inhibited by α-TP (Babu et al., 2000). Together these observations showed that the protection against a side effect of Tam by α-TP may block Tam's anticancer action. This strongly suggests that diet supplementation with α-TP is not recommended for patients under Tam treatment (Fig. 3.5).

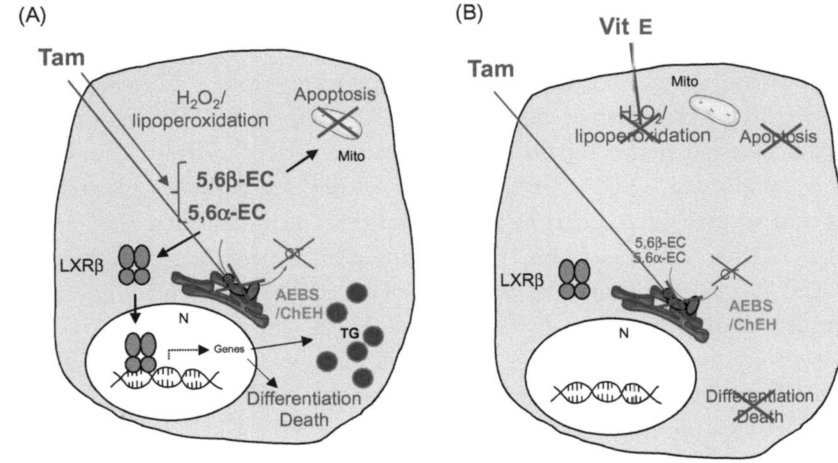

Figure 3.4 ***Vitamin E (Vit E, α-tocopherol) inhibits the induction by tamoxifen (Tam) in breast cancer (BC) cell differentiation and death.*** (A) Tam stimulates a lipoperoxidation-dependent cholesterol epoxidation that produces 5,6β-epoxycholesterol and 5,6α-epocholesterol (5,6β-EC and 5,6α-EC). 5,6β-EC and 5,6α-EC accumulate in BC cells due to the inhibition by Tam of the AEBS/ChEH complex. 5,6β-EC is the second messenger of Tam that induces apoptosis. 5,6α-EC is the second messenger of Tam that induces BC cell death and differentiation in an LXR-dependent manner. In particular Tam triggers triacyl glycerol (TG) biosynthesis and secretion by BC cells. (B) Vit E inhibits the lipoperoxidation-dependent cholesterol epoxidation and the production of 5,6-EC second messengers. Vit E inhibits totally the induction of call death and differentiation by Tam. *CT*, Cholestane-3β,5α,6β-triol; *H_2O_2*, hydrogen peroxide; *LXRβ*, liver-X-receptor β; *Mito*, mitochondria; *N*, nucleus.

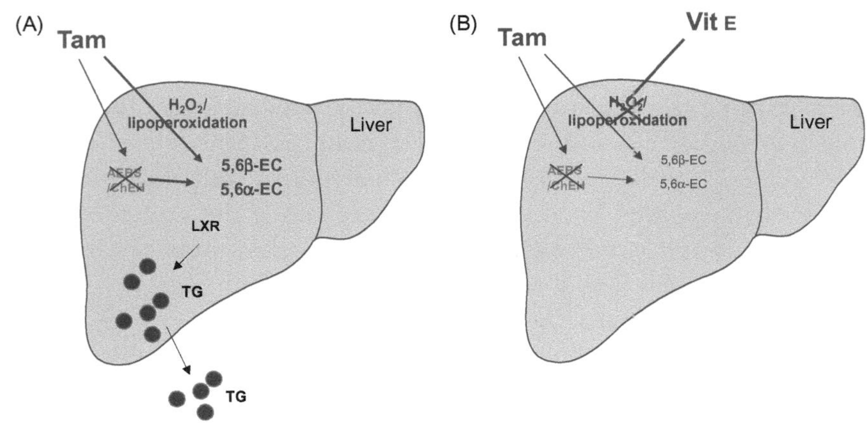

Figure 3.5 ***Vitamin E inhibits the Tam-dependent induction of hypertriglyceridemia.*** (A) Tam induces TG biosynthesis in hepatocytes via the production of 5,6α-EC as second messengers that activate LXR receptors. (B) Vitamin E blocks lipoperoxidation and the formation of 5,6α-EC and 5,6β-EC. This led to the inhibition of hepatosteatosis and hypertriglyceridemia induced by Tam.

3.9 Conclusion

Vitamins are very popular dietary supplements and were reported to be used by 50% adults in the United States for disease prevention (Kantor et al., 2016). They are also commonly used by cancer survivors (Marian, 2017). The present review highlights that it is important to define the molecular mechanism of bioactive substances. It shows that a high-dose dietary supplementation of α-TP can constitute a potential risk for cancer development and a risk of interference with the hormotherapy of BC, which is the most frequently diagnosed female cancer around the world. Even if recent epidemiological studies suggest that a higher pro plant-based diet is associated with a decreased risk of overall cancers (Kane-Diallo et al., 2018), that does not mean that this protective effect results from a single plant component, such as vitamin E.

References

Alpha-Tocopherol, B.C.C.P.S.G., 1994. The effect of vitamin E and beta carotene on the incidence of lung cancer and other cancers in male smokers. N. Engl. J. Med. 330, 1029–1035.

Babu, J.R., Sundravel, S., Arumugam, G., Renuka, R., Deepa, N., Sachdanandam, P., 2000. Salubrious effect of vitamin C and vitamin E on tamoxifen-treated women in breast cancer with reference to plasma lipid and lipoprotein levels. Cancer Lett. 151, 1–5.

Brigelius-Flohe, R., Traber, M.G., 1999. Vitamin E: function and metabolism. FASEB J. 13, 1145–1155.

Brown, B.G., Crowley, J., 2005. Is there any hope for vitamin E? JAMA 293, 1387–1390.

Cooney, R.V., Harwood, P.J., Franke, A.A., Narala, K , Sundström, A.-K., Berggren, P.-O., et al., 1995. Products of γ-tocopherol reaction with NO_2 and their formation in rat insulinoma (RINm5F) cells. Free Radic. Biol. Med. 19, 259–269.

Csallany, A.S., Ha, Y.L., 1992. α-Tocopherol oxidation mediated by superoxide anion (O^{2-}). I. Reactions in aprotic and protic conditions. Lipids 27, 195–200.

Cuerq, C., Henin, E., Restier, L., Blond, E., Drai, J., Marcais, C., et al., 2018. Efficacy of two vitamin E formulations in patients with abetalipoproteinemia and chylomicron retention disease. J. Lipid Res. 59, 1640–1648.

Cuzick, J., 2017. Preventive therapy for cancer. Lancet Oncol. 18, e472–e482.

de Medina, P., Paillasse, M.R., Payre, B., Silvente-Poirot, S., Poirot, M., 2009a. Synthesis of new alkylaminooxysterols with potent cell differentiating activities: identification of leads for the treatment of cancer and neurodegenerative diseases. J. Med. Chem. 52, 7765–7777.

de Medina, P., Payre, B., Boubekeur, N., Bertrand-Michel, J., Terce, F., Silvente-Poirot, S., et al., 2009b. Ligands of the antiestrogen-binding site induce active cell death and autophagy in human breast cancer cells through the modulation of cholesterol metabolism. Cell Death Differ. 16, 1372–1384.

de Medina, P., Silvente-Poirot, S., Poirot, M., 2009c. Tamoxifen and AEBS ligands induced apoptosis and autophagy in breast cancer cells through the stimulation of sterol accumulation. Autophagy 5, 1066–1067.
de Medina, P., Paillasse, M.R., Segala, G., Poirot, M., Silvente-Poirot, S., 2010. Identification and pharmacological characterization of cholesterol-5,6-epoxide hydrolase as a target for tamoxifen and AEBS ligands. Proc. Natl Acad. Sci. U.S.A. 107, 13520–13525.
DellaPenna, D., Pogson, B.J., 2006. Vitamin synthesis in plants: tocopherols and carotenoids. Annu. Rev. Plant Biol. 57, 711–738.
Duggan, S.N., Smyth, N.D., O'Sullivan, M., Feehan, S., Ridgway, P.F., Conlon, K.C., 2014. The prevalence of malnutrition and fat-soluble vitamin deficiencies in chronic pancreatitis. Nutr. Clin. Pract. 29, 348–354.
Dysken, M.W., Sano, M., Asthana, S., Vertrees, J.E., Pallaki, M., Llorente, M., et al., 2014. Effect of vitamin E and memantine on functional decline in Alzheimer disease: the TEAM-AD VA cooperative randomized trial. JAMA 311, 33–44.
Evans, H.M., 1924. Unique dietary needs for lactation. Science 60, 20–22.
Evans, H.M., 1925. Invariable occurrence of male sterility with dietaries lacking fat soluble vitamin E. Proc. Natl Acad. Sci. U.S.A. 11, 373–377.
Evans, H.M., Bishop, K.S., 1922. On the existence of a hitherto unrecognized dietary factor essential for reproduction. Science 56, 650–651.
Evans, H.M., Burr, G.O., 1925. The anti-sterility vitamine fat soluble E. Proc. Natl Acad. Sci. U.S.A. 11, 334–341.
Evans, H.M., Murphy, E.A., Archibald, R.C., Cornish, R.E., 1935. Preparation and properties of vitamin E concentrates. J. Biol. Chem. 108, 515–523.
Fabisiak, N., Fabisiak, A., Watala, C., Fichna, J., 2017. Fat-soluble vitamin deficiencies and inflammatory bowel disease: systematic review and meta-analysis. J. Clin. Gastroenterol. 51, 878–889.
Faustman, C., Liebler, D.C., McClure, T.D., Sun, Q., 1999. Alpha, beta-unsaturated aldehydes accelerate oxymyoglobin oxidation. J. Agric. Food Chem. 47, 3140–3144.
Fernholz, E., 1938. On the constitution of α-tocopherol. J. Am. Chem. Soc. 60, 700–705.
Foti, M.C., 2007. Antioxidant properties of phenols. J. Pharm. Pharmacol. 59, 1673–1685.
Galli, F., Azzi, A., Birringer, M., Cook-Mills, J.M., Eggersdorfer, M., Frank, J., et al., 2017. Vitamin E: emerging aspects and new directions. Free Radic. Biol. Med. 102, 16–36.
Goetzl, E.J., 1980. Vitamin E modulates the lipoxygenation of arachidonic acid in leukocytes. Nature 288, 183–185.
Grilo, E.C., Costa, P.N., Gurgel, C.S.S., Beserra, A.F., Almeida, F.N., Dimenstein, R., 2014. Alpha-tocopherol and gamma-tocopherol concentration in vegetable oils. Food Sci. Technol. 34, 379–385.
Hall, K.T., Buring, J.E., Mukamal, K.J., Vinayaga Moorthy, M., Wayne, P.M., Kaptchuk, T.J., et al., 2019. COMT and alpha-tocopherol effects in cancer prevention: gene-supplement interactions in two randomized clinical trials. J. Natl Cancer Inst.
Heinonen, O.P., Albanes, D., Virtamo, J., Taylor, P.R., Huttunen, J.K., Hartman, A.M., et al., 2019. Prostate cancer and supplementation with alpha-tocopherol and beta-carotene: incidence and mortality in a controlled trial. J. Natl Cancer Inst. 90, 440–446. in press, https://doi:10.1093/jnci/djy204.
Hogg, N., Joseph, J., Kalyanaraman, B., 1994. The oxidation of α-tocopherol and trolox by peroxynitrite. Arch. Biochem. Biophys. 314, 153–158.

Jiang, Q., 2014. Natural forms of vitamin E: metabolism, antioxidant, and anti-inflammatory activities and their role in disease prevention and therapy. Free Radic. Biol. Med. 72, 76–90.

Jordan, V.C., 2006. Tamoxifen (ICI46,474) as a targeted therapy to treat and prevent breast cancer. Br. J. Pharmacol. 147 (Suppl. 1), S269–276.

Kane-Diallo, A., Srour, B., Sellem, L., Deschasaux, M., Latino-Martel, P., Hercberg, S., et al., 2018. Association between a pro plant-based dietary score and cancer risk in the prospective NutriNet-sante cohort. Int. J. Cancer 143, 2168–2176.

Kantor, E.D., Rehm, C.D., Du, M., White, E., Giovannucci, E.L., 2016. Trends in dietary supplement use among US adults from 1999–2012. JAMA 316, 1464–1474.

Karrer, P., Fritzsche, H., Ringier, B.H., Salomon, H., 1938. Synthese des α-tocopherols. Helv. Chim. Acta 21, 820–825.

Khadangi, F., Azzi, A., 2018. Vitamin E—the next 100 years. IUBMB Life 71 (4), 411–415.

Khallouki, F., Younos, C., Soulimani, R., Oster, T., Charrouf, Z., Spiegelhalder, B., et al., 2003. Consumption of argan oil (Morocco) with its unique profile of fatty acids, tocopherols, squalene, sterols and phenolic compounds should confer valuable cancer chemopreventive effects. Eur. J. Cancer Prev. 12, 67–75.

Khallouki, F., de Medina, P., Caze-Subra, S., Bystricky, K., Balaguer, P., Poirot, M., et al., 2015. Molecular and biochemical analysis of the estrogenic and proliferative properties of vitamin E compounds. Front. Oncol. 5, 287.

Klein, E.A., Thompson, I.M., Tangen, C.M., Crowley, J.J., Lucia, M.S., Goodman, P.J., et al., 2011. Vitamin E and the risk of prostate cancer: the Selenium and Vitamin E Cancer Prevention Trial (SELECT). JAMA 306, 1549–1556.

Lavine, J.E., Schwimmer, J.B., Van Natta, M.L., Molleston, J.P., Murray, K.F., Rosenthal, P., et al., 2011. Effect of vitamin E or metformin for treatment of nonalcoholic fatty liver disease in children and adolescents: the TONIC Randomized Controlled Trial. JAMA 305, 1659–1668.

Leignadier, J., Dalenc, F., Poirot, M., Silvente-Poirot, S., 2017. Improving the efficacy of hormone therapy in breast cancer: the role of cholesterol metabolism in SERM-mediated autophagy, cell differentiation and death. Biochem. Pharmacol. 144, 18–28.

Liebler, D.C., 1993. The role of metabolism in the antioxidant function of vitamin E. Crit. Rev. Toxicol. 23, 147–169.

Liebler, D.C., Burr, J.A., 1992. Oxidation of vitamin E during iron-catalyzed lipid peroxidation: evidence for electron-transfer reactions of the tocopheroxyl radical. Biochemistry 31, 8278–8284.

Liu, R.H., 2013. Health-promoting components of fruits and vegetables in the diet. Adv. Nutr. 4, 384S–392S.

Longnecker, M.P., Martin-Moreno, J.M., Knekt, P., Nomura, A.M., Schober, S.E., Stahelin, H.B., et al., 1992. Serum alpha-tocopherol concentration in relation to subsequent colorectal cancer: pooled data from five cohorts. J Natl Cancer Inst. 84, 430–435.

Lonn, E., Bosch, J., Yusuf, S., Sheridan, P., Pogue, J., Arnold, J.M., et al., 2005. Effects of long-term vitamin E supplementation on cardiovascular events and cancer: a randomized controlled trial. JAMA 293, 1338–1347.

Madeira, P.J., Faddoul, M., Afonso, M.B., Vaz, P.D., Fernandez, M.T., Leal, J.P., 2011. On the way to understand antioxidants: chromanol and dimethoxyphenols gas-phase acidities. J. Mass Spectrom. 46, 640–648.

Mandlekar, S., Kong, A.N., 2001. Mechanisms of tamoxifen-induced apoptosis. Apoptosis 6, 469–477.

Marian, M.J., 2017. Dietary supplements commonly used by cancer survivors: are there any benefits? Nutr. Clin. Pract. 32, 607–627.

McCollum, E.V., Simmonds, N., Becker, J.E., Shipley, P.G., 1922. Studies on experimental rickets: XXI. An experimental demonstration of the existence of a vitamin which promotes calcium deposition. J. Biol. Chem. 53, 293–312.
Mene-Saffrane, L., 2017. Vitamin E biosynthesis and its regulation in plants. Antioxidants (Basel) 7. Available from: https://doi.org/10.3390/antiox7010002.
Miller, E.R., Pastor-Barriuso, R., Dalal, D., Riemersma, R.A., Appel, L.J., Guallar, E., 2005. Meta-analysis: high-dosage vitamin E supplementation may increase all-cause mortality. Ann. Intern. Med. 142, 37–46.
Moss, R.W., 2007. Do antioxidants interfere with radiation therapy for cancer? Integr. Cancer Ther. 6, 281–292.
Moya, M., Gomez-Lechon, M.J., Castell, J.V., Jover, R., 2010. Enhanced steatosis by nuclear receptor ligands: a study in cultured human hepatocytes and hepatoma cells with a characterized nuclear receptor expression profile. Chem. Biol. Interact. 184, 376–387.
Niki, E., Noguchi, N., 2004. Dynamics of antioxidant action of vitamin E. Acc. Chem. Res. 37, 45–51.
Niki, E., Saito, T., Kawakami, A., Kamiya, Y., 1984. Inhibition of oxidation of methyl linoleate in solution by vitamin E and vitamin C. J. Biol. Chem. 259, 4177–4182.
Okebukola, P.O., Kansra, S., Barrett, J., 2017. Vitamin E supplementation in people with cystic fibrosis. Cochrane Database Syst. Rev. 3.
Pacht, E.R., Kaseki, H., Mohammed, J.R., Cornwell, D.G., Davis, W.B., 1986. Deficiency of vitamin E in the alveolar fluid of cigarette smokers. Influence on alveolar macrophage cytotoxicity. J. Clin. Invest. 77, 789–796.
Park, Y., Spiegelman, D., Hunter, D.J., Albanes, D., Bergkvist, L., Buring, J.E., et al., 2010. Intakes of vitamins A, C, and E and use of multiple vitamin supplements and risk of colon cancer: a pooled analysis of prospective cohort studies. Cancer Causes Control 21, 1745–1757.
Parker, R.A., Pearce, B.C., Clark, R.W., Gordon, D.A., Wright, J.J., 1993. Tocotrienols regulate cholesterol production in mammalian cells by post-transcriptional suppression of 3-hydroxy-3-methylglutaryl-coenzyme A reductase. J. Biol. Chem. 268, 11230–11238.
Payre, B., de Medina, P., Boubekeur, N., Mhamdi, L., Bertrand-Michel, J., Terce, F., et al., 2008. Microsomal antiestrogen-binding site ligands induce growth control and differentiation of human breast cancer cells through the modulation of cholesterol metabolism. Mol. Cancer Ther. 7, 3707–3718.
Pearce, B.C., Parker, R.A., Deason, M.E., Qureshi, A.A., Wright, J.J., 1992. Hypocholesterolemic activity of synthetic and natural tocotrienols. J. Med. Chem. 35, 3595–3606.
Peh, H.Y., Tan, W.S., Liao, W., Wong, W.S., 2016. Vitamin E therapy beyond cancer: tocopherol versus tocotrienol. Pharmacol. Ther. 162, 152–169.
Pein, H., Ville, A., Pace, S., Temml, V., Garscha, U., Raasch, M., et al., 2018. Endogenous metabolites of vitamin E limit inflammation by targeting 5-lipoxygenase. Nat. Commun. 9, 3834.
Pennock, J.F., Hemming, F.W., Kerr, J.D., 1964. A reassessment of tocopherol in chemistry. Biochem. Biophys. Res. Commun. 17, 542–548.
Peuchant, E., Carbonneau, M.A., Dubourg, L., Thomas, M.J., Perromat, A., Vallot, C., et al., 1994. Lipoperoxidation in plasma and red blood cells of patients undergoing haemodialysis: vitamins A, E, and iron status. Free Radic. Biol. Med. 16, 339–346.
Podszun, M., Frank, J., 2014. Vitamin E–drug interactions: molecular basis and clinical relevance. Nutr. Res. Rev. 27, 215–231.
Poirot, M., Silvente-Poirot, S., 2013. Cholesterol-5,6-epoxides: chemistry, biochemistry, metabolic fate and cancer. Biochimie 95, 622–631.

Poirot, M., Silvente-Poirot, S., Weichselbaum, R.R., 2012. Cholesterol metabolism and resistance to tamoxifen. Curr. Opin. Pharmacol. 12, 683–689.
Rachmilewitz, E.A., Kornberg, A., Acker, M., 1982. Vitamin E deficiency due to increased consumption in beta-thalassemia and in Gaucher's disease. Ann. N.Y. Acad. Sci. 393, 336–347.
Reddanna, P., Rao, M.K., Reddy, C.C., 1985. Inhibition of 5-lipoxygenase by vitamin E. FEBS Lett. 193, 39–43.
Richard, C., Lemonnier, F., Thibault, M., Couturier, M., Auzepy, P., 1990. Vitamin E deficiency and lipoperoxidation during adult respiratory distress syndrome. Crit. Care Med. 18, 4–9.
Sanyal, A.J., Chalasani, N., Kowdley, K.V., McCullough, A., Diehl, A.M., Bass, N.M., et al., 2010. Pioglitazone, vitamin E, or placebo for nonalcoholic steatohepatitis. N. Engl. J. Med. 362, 1675–1685.
Sayin, V.I., Ibrahim, M.X., Larsson, E., Nilsson, J.A., Lindahl, P., Bergo, M.O., 2014. Antioxidants accelerate lung cancer progression in mice. Sci. Transl. Med. 6, 221ra215.
Segala, G., de Medina, P., Iuliano, L., Zerbinati, C., Paillasse, M.R., Noguer, E., et al., 2013. 5,6-Epoxy-cholesterols contribute to the anticancer pharmacology of tamoxifen in breast cancer cells. Biochem. Pharmacol. 86, 175–189.
Segala, G., David, M., de Medina, P., Poirot, M.C., Serhan, N., Vergez, F., et al., 2017. Dendrogenin A drives LXR to trigger lethal autophagy in cancers. Nat. Commun. 8, 1903.
Silvente-Poirot, S., Poirot, M., 2012. Cholesterol epoxide hydrolase and cancer. Curr. Opin. Pharmacol. 12, 696–703.
Sola, B., Poirot, M., de Medina, P., Bustany, S., Marsaud, V., Silvente-Poirot, S., et al., 2013. Antiestrogen-binding site ligands induce autophagy in myeloma cells that proceeds through alteration of cholesterol metabolism. Oncotarget 4, 911–922.
Stern, M.H., Robeson, C.D., Weisler, L., Baxter, J.G., 1947. δ-Tocopherol. I. Isolation from soybean oil and properties 1. J. Am. Chem. Soc. 69, 869–874.
Stone Jr., C.A., McEvoy, C.T., Aschner, J.L., Kirk, A., Rosas-Salazar, C., Cook-Mills, J. M., et al., 2018. Update on vitamin E and its potential role in preventing or treating bronchopulmonary dysplasia. Neonatology 113, 366–378.
Sure, B., 1924. Dietary requirements for reproduction: III. The existence of the reproductive dietary complex (vitamin E) in the ethereal extracts of yellow corn, wheat embryo, and hemp-seed. J. Biol. Chem. 62, 371–396.
Traber, M.G., 1994. Determinants of plasma vitamin E concentrations. Free Radic. Biol. Med 16, 229–239.
Traber, M.G., Sokol, R.J., Ringel, S.P., Neville, H.E., Thellman, C.A., Kayden, H.J., 1987. Lack of tocopherol in peripheral nerves of vitamin E-deficient patients with peripheral neuropathy. N. Engl. J. Med. 317, 262–265.
Verleyen, T., Verhe, R., Huyghebaert, A., Dewettinck, K., De Greyt, W., 2001. Identification of alpha-tocopherol oxidation products in triolein at elevated temperatures. J. Agric. Food Chem. 49, 1508–1511.
Vernieri, C., Nichetti, F., Raimondi, A., Pusceddu, S., Platania, M., Berrino, F., et al., 2018. Diet and supplements in cancer prevention and treatment: clinical evidences and future perspectives. Crit. Rev. Oncol. Hematol. 123, 57–73.
von Herbay, A., de Groot, H., Hegi, U., Stremmel, W., Strohmeyer, G., Sies, H., 1994. Low vitamin E content in plasma of patients with alcoholic liver disease, hemochromatosis and Wilson's disease. J. Hepatol. 20, 41–46.
Whittle, K.J., Dunphy, P.J., Pennock, J.F., 1966. The isolation and properties of delta-tocotrienol from *Hevea* latex. Biochem. J. 100, 138–145.

Wu, K., Willett, W.C., Chan, J.M., Fuchs, C.S., Colditz, G.A., Rimm, E.B., et al., 2002. A prospective study on supplemental vitamin E intake and risk of colon cancer in women and men. Cancer Epidemiol. Biomarkers Prev. 11, 1298–1304.
Wysota, B., Michael, S., Hiew, F.L., Dawson, C., Rajabally, Y.A., 2017. Severe but reversible neuropathy and encephalopathy due to vitamin E deficiency. Clin. Neurol. Neurosurg. 160, 19–20.
Yin, H., Xu, L., Porter, N.A., 2011. Free radical lipid peroxidation: mechanisms and analysis. Chem. Rev. 111, 5944–5972.

CHAPTER 4

Vitamin E: structure and forms

Renata Szymańska[1], Beatrycze Nowicka[2], Agnieszka Trela[1] and Jerzy Kruk[2]
[1]Department of Medical Physics and Biophysics, Faculty of Physics and Applied Computer Science, AGH University of Science and Technology, Kraków, Poland
[2]Department of Plant Physiology and Biochemistry, Faculty of Biochemistry, Biophysics and Biotechnology, Jagiellonian University, Kraków, Poland

Contents

Key facts of vitamin E

- Vitamin E is a collective term for isoprenoid chromanols, sharing a similar structure and properties but varying in biological activity in animals, mostly due to the differences in the efficiency of the uptake and transport.
- Vitamin E comprises tocopherols, tocotrienols, and some less widespread compounds, such as tocomonoenols, tocodienols, or plastochromanol.
- Due to the amphipathic properties, isoprenoid chromanols localize mostly in membranes. They can also be found in structures which function as lipid-storage or lipid-transport sites, such as plastoglobules, oil bodies, and lipoproteins.
- The most widespread form of vitamin E is α-tocopherol which occurs in the green parts of plants. It is also the vitamer displaying the highest

Molecular Nutrition
DOI: https://doi.org/10.1016/B978-0-12-811907-5.00021-X

vitamin E activity in humans. Another common form is γ-tocopherol, which often dominates in seed oils.

- The biosynthetic pathway of tocopherols occurs in most cyanobacteria and photosynthetic eukaryotes. The distribution of tocotrienols and tocomonoenols is considerably more limited.
- In higher plants the last steps of biosynthesis of isoprenoid chromanols take place in plastids.
- Isoprenoid chromanols, both in plants and in animals, function as lipid-soluble antioxidants eliminating reactive oxygen species.
- Besides antioxidant properties, isoprenoid chromanols are known to modulate membrane properties, as well as to participate in signal transduction and the regulation of gene expression.
- Depending on the nature of a sample, different solvents are used to extract vitamin E.
- The most frequently used method for vitamin E determination is high-pressure liquid chromatography (HPLC), both normal- and reverse-phase.
- The recommended dietary allowance (RDA) of vitamin E varies from 3 to 15 mg/day in different countries and depends on the age of a person.
- Vitamin E is an essential micronutrient for humans which determines the beneficial health outcomes.
- Vitamin E shows an impact on numerous diseases, such as immune system disorders, cancer, cardiovascular and neurodegenerative diseases.

Definition of words and terms

- *Amphipathic properties* are shown by compounds having both hydrophilic and hydrophobic parts of the molecule.
- *Antioxidants* are compounds that are able to quench and/or scavenge reactive oxygen species (ROS).
- *Lipid peroxidation* is the oxidative degradation of lipids. There are three known mechanisms of lipid peroxidation radical, enzymatic, and non-radical; the latter is caused by singlet oxygen and ozone which directly react with lipid molecules.
- *Oxidative stress* takes place when there is an imbalance between the generation and detoxification of ROS, resulting in the increase in ROS content in cells and/or tissues.
- *Quenching* is physical deactivation of an excited state of a molecule.

- *Reactive oxygen species (ROS)* are both radical and non-radical oxidizing agents, such as superoxide ($O_2^{\bullet -}$), hydroperoxyl ($HO_2^{\bullet}$), hydroxyl ($OH^{\bullet}$), alkoxyl ($RO_2^{\bullet}$) and peroxyl ($RO_2^{\bullet}$) radicals, as well as singlet oxygen ($^1O_2$), hydrogen peroxide (H_2O_2), hypochlorous acid (HOCl) and ozone (O_3).
- *Scavenging* is a process of deactivation of harmful compounds by direct chemical reaction of antioxidants with ROS.
- *Tocomonoenols* are isoprenoid chromanols containing side chains with one double bond.
- *Tocopherols* are isoprenoid chromanols with fully saturated side chains.
- *Tocotrienols* are isoprenoid chromanols with unsaturated side chains having three double bonds.
- *Vitamers* are a group of chemical compounds sharing a similar structure, chemical properties, and biological functions, that have a certain vitamin activity.
- *Vitamin E* is the collective term for isoprenoid chromanols, such as tocopherols and tocotrienols and other compounds of similar structure and biological activity.

Abbreviations

DMPBQ	2,3-dimethyl-6-phytyl-1,4-benzoquinone
DXP pathway	1-deoxy-D-xylulose-5-phosphate pathway
GGPP	geranylgeranyl pyrophosphate
HPLC	high-pressure liquid chromatography
HPT	homogentisate phytyltransferase
LDLs	low-density lipoproteins
MPBQ	2-methyl-6-phytyl-1,4-benzoquinone
MVA pathway	mevalonate pathway
PC-8	plastochromanol-8
PPP	phytyl pyrophosphate
PQH_2	plastoquinol
PUFAs	polyunsaturated fatty acids
RDA	recommended dietary allowance
RNS	reactive nitrogen species
ROS	reactive oxygen species
NP-HPLC	normal-phase high-pressure liquid chromatography
RP-HPLC	reversed-phase high-pressure liquid chromatography
TC	tocopherol cyclase
γ-TMT	γ-tocopherol methyltransferase
α-TTP	α-tocopherol transfer protein
VLDLs	very-low-density lipoproteins

4.1 Introduction

The term vitamin E encompasses compounds belonging to isoprenoid chromanols, such as tocopherols, tocotrienols, and some less known forms, like plastochromanol, tocomonoenols, tocodienols, and others (*see below*). The chromanol ring is a hydrophilic part of the molecule, while the isoprenoid side chain makes vitamin E lipid-soluble. Due to their amphipathic properties, these compounds occur mostly in the membranes (Szymańska et al., 2017). The classification and nomenclature of certain vitamers is based on the degree of saturation of the isoprenoid side chain and the pattern of ring substitution (Munné-Bosch and Alegre, 2002).

Among isoprenoid chromanols, tocopherols occur in plants in the highest amounts. The tocopherol biosynthetic pathway has evolved in cyanobacteria and later, due to the endosymbiotic origin of plastids, was inherited by photosynthetic eukaryotes. The most common vitamer is α-tocopherol, which usually dominates in green parts of higher plants. Another commonly occurring form is γ-tocopherol, abundant in seed oils of many plant species (Mène-Saffrané and DellaPenna, 2010). Tocotrienols can be found in seeds of some plants, primarily monocots (Munné-Bosch and Alegre, 2002), while the other forms, such as tocomonoenols and tocodienols, occur only in minor amounts in certain species (Szymańska and Kruk, 2018).

Animals cannot synthesize isoprenoid chromanols, therefore they need to acquire these compounds in diet. Vitamin E was discovered nearly a century ago by Evans and Bishop who observed that it was necessary for the reproduction of rats (Evans and Bishop, 1922). The name tocopherol is derived from Greek words "tokos" and "pherein" which mean to give birth, while the "-ol" ending was added to indicate the alcohol nature of the compound (Machlin and Brin, 1980). Particular isoprenoid chromanols vary in vitamin E activity, which is mostly because of the difference in the efficiency of the uptake and transport of certain vitamers. Not surprisingly, α-tocopherol is the vitamin displaying the most pronounced biological activity in animals (Szymańska et al., 2017). The specific functions of other isoprenoid chromanols in humans have been also postulated (Sen et al., 2006).

The main and the most recognized function of isoprenoid chromanols is their antioxidant action. These compounds are effective scavengers and quenchers of reactive oxygen species (ROS). In particular, they are known to protect membrane and storage lipids from lipid peroxidation

(Kruk et al., 2016). Isoprenoid chromanols are also known to modulate membrane properties and to participate in signal transduction and the regulation of gene expression (Szymańska et al., 2017).

4.2 Chemistry, biosynthesis, and occurrence of vitamin E

Vitamin E in its pure form is a colorless oily liquid, prone to oxidation in light, oxygen, and in the presence of some metal ions. It is water-insoluble, but soluble in organic solvents and vegetable oils (Peh et al., 2016). Chemical structures of tocopherols and tocotrienols are shown in Fig. 4.1. These two groups of isoprenoid chromanols differ by the saturation of the isoprenoid chain. A fully saturated phytyl-derived side chain is characteristic for tocopherols, whereas a geranylgeranyl-derived side chain with three double bonds is present in tocotrienols (Munné-Bosch and Alegre, 2002). The α-, β-, γ-, and δ-forms of tocopherols and tocotrienols differ by the position and number of methyl groups in the chromanol ring. In naturally occurring tocopherols there are three asymmetric carbon atoms, that is, C2 of the chromanol ring and C4′ and C8′ of the side chain. All of them show *R* configuration. The double bonds in the side chain of tocotrienols are in *all-trans* configuration (Dörmann, 2007). The biosynthesis of isoprenoid chromanols is stereospecific, whereas most methods of chemical synthesis result in all the possible eight tocopherol stereoisomers (Szymańska et al., 2017). If natural phytol is used for the synthesis, the equimolar mixture of two stereoisomers, differing in the substituents conformation at C2, is obtained. However, the stereoisomers other than the natural form have decreased biological activity (Kamal-Eldin and Appelqvist, 1996) (see also examples given in Section 4.5.1).

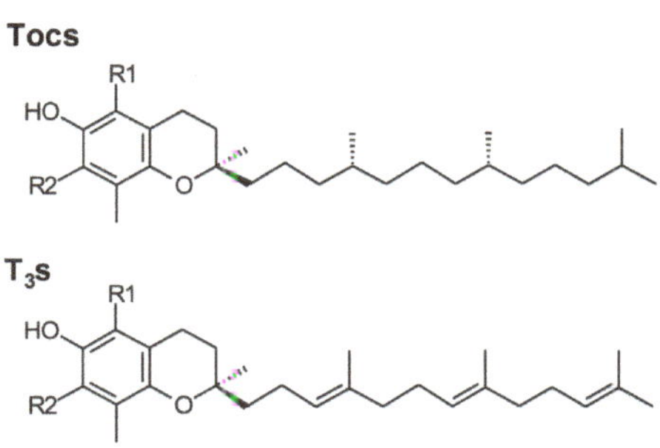

Form	R1	R2	MW
α-Toc	CH_3	CH_3	430.71
β-Toc	CH_3	H	416.68
γ-Toc	H	CH_3	416.68
δ-Toc	H	H	402.65
α-T_3	CH_3	CH_3	424.66
β-T_3	CH_3	H	410.63
γ-T_3	H	CH_3	410.63
δ-T_3	H	H	396.61

Figure 4.1 The structure of tocopherols and tocotrienols. Toc, tocopherol; T_3, tocotrienol.

The methods of stereospecific chemical synthesis of tocopherols have been developed later, but they are more elaborate (Szymańska et al., 2017). Commercially used vitamin E is in the form of acetate or succinate tocopherol esters. This modification improves their stability and in the case of succinate, also water solubility (Zingg and Azzi, 2004). The hydrophilic derivative of α-tocopherol also used in pharmaceuticals is called Trolox and contains a carboxyl group instead of a phytyl chain (Hosomi et al., 1997).

Other isoprenoid chromanols are shown in Fig. 4.2. They differ from tocopherols by the number of methyl groups in the chromanol ring, the side chain saturation, or length (Kruk et al., 2014; Szymańska and Kruk, 2018).

The chromanol ring is crucial for ROS and reactive nitrogen species (RNS) detoxification (Kruk et al., 2016; Sjoholm et al., 2000). The reaction of radical scavenging by tocopherols leads to the formation of tocopheroxyl radicals, which can be reduced back to tocopherols by ascorbic acid, ubiquinol, plastoquinol (PQH_2), or phenolic compounds. The scavenging of $^1O_2$ by α-tocopherol results in the formation of 8a-hydroperoxy-α-tocopherone (Fig. 4.3). This compound is unstable and can be reduced back to α-tocopherol by ascorbic acid or may be further oxidized to the stable form, α-tocopheryloquinone (Kruk et al., 2016). The

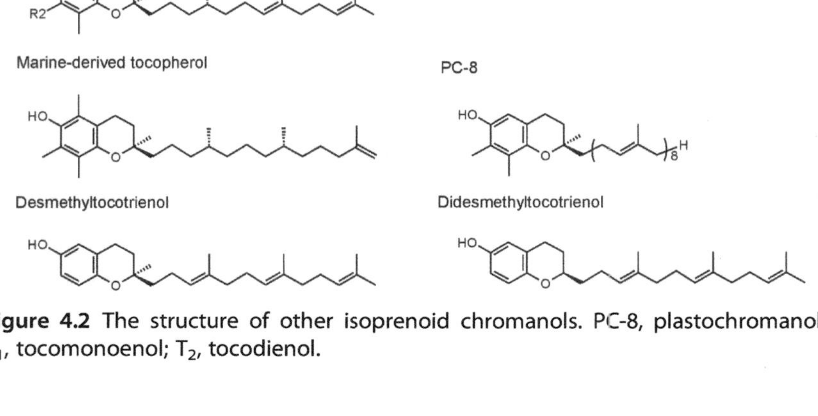

Figure 4.2 The structure of other isoprenoid chromanols. PC-8, plastochromanol-8; T_1, tocomonoenol; T_2, tocodienol.

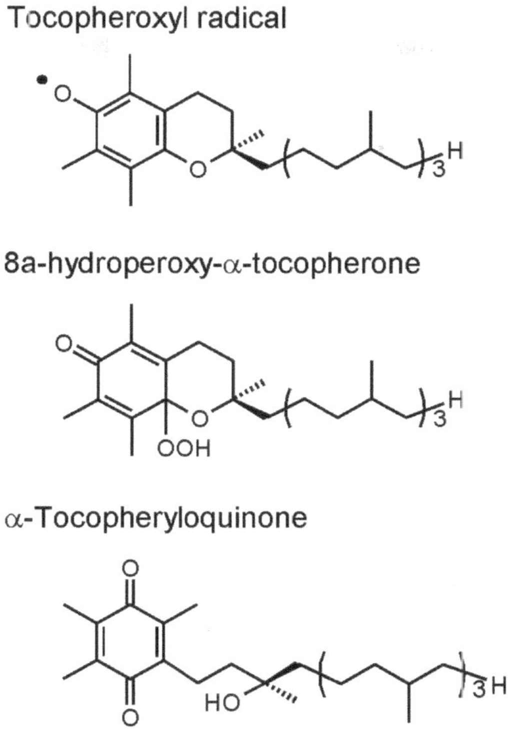

Figure 4.3 Naturally occurring products of the reaction of reactive oxygen species (ROS) with α-tocopherol.

aromatic ring of isoprenoid chromanols plays also a crucial role in $^1O_2$ quenching (Gruszka et al., 2008).

The biosynthetic pathway of tocopherols occurs in most cyanobacteria (Szymańska et al., 2017). Among the photosynthetic eukaryotes, higher plants are the most thoroughly examined group (Mène-Saffrané and DellaPenna, 2010). The pathway has been elucidated and is shown in Fig. 4.4.

The direct biosynthetic precursors of tocopherols are homogentisate (HGA) and phytyl pyrophosphate (PPP). In higher plants, HGA is derived from tyrosine (Bouvier et al., 2005), while PPP is a product of the reduction of geranylgeranyl pyrophosphate (GGPP), catalyzed by geranylgeranyl reductase. GGPP is synthesized via the condensation of two carbon precursors, dimethylallyl diphosphate and isopentenyl diphosphate (Bouvier et al., 2005). There are two known pathways for the synthesis of

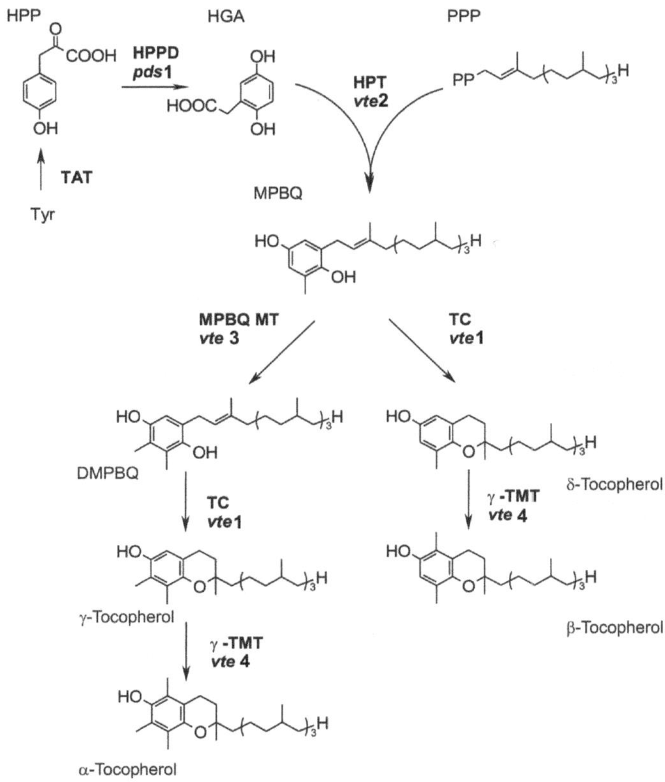

Figure 4.4 Tocopherol synthesis in cyanobacteria and higher plants. The mutants of genes encoding the enzymes in *Arabidopsis thaliana* are given in italics. DMPBQ, 2,3-dimethyl-6-phytyl benzoquinone; HGA, homogentisic acid; HPP, *p*-hydroxyphenylpyruvate; HPPD, *p*-hydroxyphenylpyruvate dioxygenase; HPT, homogentisate phytyltransferase; MPBQ, 2-methyl-6-phytyl benzoquinone; MPBQ MT, 2-methyl-6-phytyl benzoquinone methyltransferase; PPP, phytyl pyrophosphate; TAT, tyrosine aminotransferase; TC, tocopherol cyclase; γ-TMT, γ-tocopherol methyltransferase; Tyr, tyrosine.

these compounds: the 1-deoxy-D-xylulose-5-phosphate (DXP) pathway also known as the methylerythritol phosphate pathway, and the mevalonate (MVA) pathway. Cyanobacteria use the DXP pathway for the synthesis of isoprenoid precursors. In higher plants enzymes of the DXP pathway occur in plastids, while the MVA pathway is found in the cytoplasm. The experiments with the radiolabeled compounds showed that, at least in the case of overproduction of isoprenoid precursors in the cytoplasm, they can be transported to the chloroplast and incorporated into plastidic isoprenoids (Pellaud and Mène-Saffrané, 2017). Additionally, in plants phytol derived from the degradation of chlorophyll can be phosphorylated to the PPP by the kinase encoded by *VTE5* gene (Mène-Saffrané and DellaPenna, 2010). Presently, it is supposed that phytol recycling is the main source of the side chain precursor for tocopherol biosynthesis in leaves (Pellaud and Mène-Saffrané, 2017).

The first specific step for the tocochromanol biosynthetic pathway is the condensation of HGA and PPP. Another key reaction is cyclization, leading to the formation of the chromanol ring. It is worth mentioning that both tocopherol cyclase (TC) and γ-tocopherol methyltransferase (γ-TMT) do not have strict substrate specificity, which broadens the spectrum of their products (see in Fig. 4.4 how the sequence of certain head group modifications influences the vitamer produced) (Szymańska et al., 2017).

The biosynthesis of tocotrienols and tocomonoenols is analogous to that of tocopherols. In the case of tocotrienols the GGPP is the side chain precursor, used for the HGA prenylation catalyzed by homogentisate geranylgeranyl transferase. The subsequent cyclization and methylation reactions, leading to the formation of α-, β-, γ-, and δ-tocotrienol, are catalyzed by the same enzymes, which participate in the synthesis of tocopherols (Mène-Saffrané and DellaPenna, 2010). In the biosynthesis of tocomonoenols, the tetrahydrogeranylgeranyl pyrophosphate serves as a substrate for phytyltransferase instead of phytol, and the following steps proceed as in the case of tocopherol biosynthesis (Kruk et al., 2011; Pellaud et al., 2018). PQH_2-9, which is the reduced form of plastoquinone-9, the photosynthetic electron and proton carrier, can be also a substrate for TC. The cyclization of PQH_2-9 results in the formation of PC-8 (Szymańska and Kruk, 2010a).

In higher plants the final specific steps of tocopherols, tocotrienols, and PC-8 synthesis take place in plastids. Homogentisate phytyltransferase (HPT) and both methyltransferases are located in the inner envelope of chloroplasts, while TC occurs in plastoglobules, which are plastid storage sites for lipophilic compounds (Szymańska et al., 2017). On the other hand, the experiments on the photosynthetic protozoan *Euglena gracilis* suggest that in this organism the biosynthesis of α-tocopherol can occur both in chloroplasts and mitochondria (Kusmic et al., 1999).

Attempts of manipulation of tocopherol and tocotrienol biosynthesis in plants via genetic engineering have been carried out to enhance vitamin E synthesis or to increase the content of α-tocopherol in seed oils (Cahoon et al., 2003; DellaPenna, 2005; Wani et al., 2015).

Within plant cells isoprenoid chromanols are present mainly in the chloroplasts, both in the membranes (envelopes and thylakoids) and plastoglobules. The latter is the site where chromanols are accumulated and stored during stress acclimation and leaf senescence (Munné-Bosch and Alegre, 2002; Szymańska and Kruk, 2010a; Zbierzak et al., 2010). These compounds were also found in other types of plastids, such as chromoplasts and leucoplasts. The presence of isoprenoid chromanols in mitochondria, nucleus, vacuoles, and microsomal fractions has been also reported but needs to be verified (Munné-Bosch and Alegre, 2002). Tocochromanols stored in the seed cells are localized in leucoplasts and oleosomes. The latter can account for up to 40% of the total seed chromanol pool (Maeda et al., 2008).

In the green parts of higher plants, α-tocopherol is the predominant isoprenoid chromanol. This vitamer can be also found in nonphotosynthetic organs, such as flowers, fruits, roots, tubers, bulbs, and seeds, although its content is often lower than in leaves (Szymańska et al., 2017). γ-Tocopherol is usually present in leaves in minor amounts, but often it is the major vitamer present in the seed oils. Minor amounts of β- and δ-tocopherols may also occur in seeds. However, it needs to be emphasized that the composition of homologues in seeds depends on the species (Szymańska et al., 2017). Interestingly, γ-tocopherol and δ-tocopherol were also found in cuticular waxes of some species, such as those belonging to the genera *Rubus* and *Ginkgo* (Munné-Bosch and Alegre, 2002). Tocotrienols are present in seeds of some species, mostly monocots. They were also found in latex of the rubber tree and some fruits (Dunphy et al., 1965; Asensi-Fabado and Munné-Bosch, 2010). PC-8 has been identified in the leaves and seeds of many species (Kruk et al., 2014).

The contents of isoprenoid chromanols in various organs of plants and seed oils are shown in Tables 4.1 and 4.2, respectively. It should be emphasized that the content of isoprenoid chromanols also depends on the developmental stage of the plants and environmental conditions. Usually the chromanol content increases during leaf senescence and acclimation to stress conditions (Lushchak and Semchuk, 2012; Munné-Bosch, 2005; Szymańska et al., 2017).

Table 4.1 The content of tocochromanols in plant organs.

Plant species and organ	Total chromanol content (μg/g FW)	Major homologue (% of total chromanols)	Reference
		Leaves	
Arabidopsis thaliana leaves	10–20	90% α-Toc	Szymańska et al. (2017)
Lettuce leaves	7	55% α-Toc	Szymańska et al. (2017)
Parsley leaves	48.1	98% α-Toc	Szymańska and Kruk (2008)
Spinach leaves	30	63% α-Toc	Szymańska et al. (2017)
		Seeds	
A. thaliana seeds	200–300	95% γ-Toc	Szymańska et al. (2017)
Almonds	263	97% α-Toc	Saini and Keum (2016)
Corn seeds	60	75% γ-Toc	Szymańska et al. (2017)
Flaxseed	236	84% γ-Toc	Saini and Keum (2016)
Peas	160	64% α-Toc	Ryan et al. (2007)
Pistachio nuts	240	85% γ-Toc	Saini and Keum (2016)
Rice seeds	17	30% α-T_3	Szymańska et al. (2017)
Wheat seeds	50	56% β-T_3	Szymańska et al. (2017)
		Fruits	
Apple pulp	1–4	90% α-Toc	Chun et al. (2006)
Avocado pulp	15–31	84% α-Toc	Chun et al. (2006)
Banana pulp	1.5	87% α-Toc	Chun et al. (2006)
Cranberries	16	76% α-Toc	Chun et al. (2006)
Cucumber	1.6	50% α-T_3	Chun et al. (2006)
Gooseberries	8.4	87% α-Toc	Piironen et al. (1986)
Kiwi	14.5	90% α-Toc	Chun et al. (2006)
Raspberries	37	40% γ-Toc	Piironen et al. (1986)
Strawberries	4.1	68% α-Toc	Chun et al. (2006)
Tomatoes	6.8	78% α-Toc	Chun et al. (2006)
		Other	
Carrot roots	8.7	99% α-Toc	Chun et al. (2006)
Potato tubers	0.7	90% α-Toc	Szymańska et al. (2017)
Sweet potato tubers	3.6	70% α-Toc	Chun et al. (2006)

Toc, Tocopherol; T_3, tocotrienol.

Table 4.2 The content of tocochromanols in seed oils.

Plant-derived product	Total chromanol content (μg/g of oil)	Major homologue (% of total chromanols)	Reference
Barley oil	750–1500	50–60% α-T_3	Shahidi and de Camargo (2016)
Coconut palm oil	12	60% δ-Toc	Szymańska et al. (2017)
Corn seed oil	1000	70% γ-Toc	Szymańska et al. (2017)
Cottonseed oil	400–900	65%–75% α-Toc	Shahidi and de Camargo (2016)
Grapeseed oil	194	77% α-Toc	Herting and Drury (1963)
Linseed oil	595	96% γ-Toc	Shahidi and de Camargo (2016)
Olive oil	126	94% α-Toc	Szymańska et al. (2017)
Peanut oil	130–530	60% α-Toc	Shahidi and de Camargo (2016)
Rapeseed oil	570–770	65% γ-Toc	Shahidi and de Camargo (2016)
Rice bran oil	710	32% γ-T_3	Shahidi and de Camargo (2016)
Sesame oil	170–1070	50% γ-Toc	Shahidi and de Camargo (2016)
Soybean seed oil	1200	70% γ-Toc	Szymańska et al. (2017)
Sunflower seed oil	700	96% α-Toc	Szymańska et al. (2017)
Walnut oil	1608	37% γ-Toc	Szymańska et al. (2017)
Wheat germ oil	2700	47% α-Toc	Szymańska et al. (2017)

Toc, Tocopherol; *T_3*, tocotrienol.

4.3 Rare natural forms of vitamin E

Besides the well-known vitamin E forms, there are several related compounds of unknown function and/or origin. These are for example tocoenols, tocopherol acids, tocopherol phosphate, tocochromanol esters, and glycosides (Szymańska and Kruk, 2018). Novel tocochromanols are still being discovered. It is interesting that rare vitamin E forms usually show higher biological activity than tocopherols (Yamamoto et al., 2001). For example, PC-8, tocotrienols, tocoenols, and tocopherol acids are more efficient in ROS scavenging than tocopherols (Gruszka et al., 2008; Qureshi et al., 2000; Terashima et al., 1997). Moreover, these compounds show many physiological effects that are not shared with tocopherols. For example, tocotrienols are capable of reducing cholesterol levels and can be used as a preventive agent in cardiovascular diseases (CVDs) (Nesaretnam et al., 2012).

Examples of rare tocoenols are tocomonoenols, tocodienols, and desmethyltocotrienols. They are found in seed oils (palm and pumpkin seed oil), fruits (kiwi fruit), leaves (*Kalanchoe daigremontiana*, *Phaseolus coccineus*), as well as in animals (chum salmon eggs, fish, krill) (Szymańska and Kruk, 2018). Tocomonoenols and tocodienols are supposed to be additional antioxidants that protect cells against oxidative damage caused by strong illumination or cold stress (Yamamoto et al., 2001; Kruk et al., 2011). Desmethyl- and didesmethyl tocotrienols have strong cholesterol-lowering activity and were more effective in the inhibition of B16 melonoma cell proliferation than α-tocopherol (Qureshi et al., 2000).

The biosynthesis and metabolism of PC-8 was revealed recently (Szymańska and Kruk, 2010a; Kruk et al., 2014) 0–50 years after its discovery (Whittle et al., 1965). Besides PC-8, its hydroxy-derivative was found in *Arabidopsis thaliana* leaves (Szymańska and Kruk, 2010b). Hydroxy-plastochromanol is formed in vitro and in vivo under $^1O_2$ action and can be regarded as a natural indicator of singlet oxygen stress (Szymańska and Kruk, 2018). Flue-cured tobacco leaves are a source of an analogue of PC-8 — solanachromene (Rowland, 1958). This compound has an unsaturated double bond in the heterocyclic ring. Its presence and function in plant tissues needs to be confirmed and examined (Szymańska and Kruk, 2018).

α-Tocopherol phosphate is an example of tocochromanol esters, which was found in a variety of food and plant materials (Gianello et al., 2005). This water-soluble compound is a strong antioxidant in a hydrophilic environment. α-Tocopherol phosphate can serve as a signaling molecule within the cells. Moreover, it extends the use of natural vitamin E forms in many industrial branches (i.e., cosmetology, pharmacy, or medicine) (Gianello et al., 2005; Szymańska and Kruk, 2018).

The presented data indicate that the origin, biosynthesis, function, taxonomic distribution, and metabolism of uncommon vitamin E forms deserve intensive study.

4.4 Extraction, separation, and detection methods of vitamin E

Due to the nutritional importance of vitamin E, many analytical methods for the extraction and determination of tocochromanols have been developed. The most time-consuming step in the analysis of vitamin E is the sample preparation and it is also the main source of errors. Since tocopherols and tocotrienols are easily soluble and stable in organic solvents, the solvent extraction is the most widely used method to extract these compounds from various sources, i.e., plant materials, foods, biological fluids and tissues (Gimeno et al., 2000; Zaspel and Csallany, 1983; Desai, 1984). Depending on the nature of a sample, different solvents are used to extract vitamin E, but *n*-hexane is commonly applied (Ryynänen et al., 2004). Other solvents include, for example, acetone, methanol, ethanol, ethyl acetate, isooctane, chloroform, and isopropanol, as well as their mixtures (Szymańska et al., 2017).

Tocochromanols can be extracted from fresh, dried, or lyophilized samples. Before extraction, the material is usually mechanically disintegrated, that is, cut, milled, ground in a mortar, or homogenized in a blender (Szymańska et al., 2017). Vortexing, shaking, or sonication is also applied in order to improve the extractability of vitamin E from the sample matrix (Saini and Keum, 2016; Rupérez et al., 2001).

In some cases saponification is recommended prior to the extraction of vitamin E (Quek et al., 2007). This step facilities the disintegration of carbohydrates and proteins associated with tocopherols and tocotrienols, and releases these compounds by disrupting the sample matrix, which improves their chromatographic separation. Saponification is most frequently performed by heating with KOH, usually in methanol or ethanol (Rupérez et al., 2001) However, the saponification can result in the partial degradation of vitamin E compounds as they are relatively unstable in alkaline conditions and this should be taken into account during extraction procedures (Ryynänen et al., 2004; Xu, 2008).

Because tocochromanols are easily oxidized when exposed to the air and heat, it is also important to provide conditions that would protect vitamin E from degradation during extraction and storage. It is suggested to analyze the samples directly after preparation or to store them at low temperature in the dark. During sample preparation, vitamin E can also be protected by the use of antioxidants, e.g., ascorbic acid, pyrogallol, or butylated hydroxytoluene, either alone or in combination (Saini and Keum, 2016).

As a possible alternative to a traditional solvent extraction method, supercritical fluid or pressurized liquid extraction is also used. These techniques have gained popularity as they provide a shorter extraction time and a reduction in organic solvent consumption (Irakli et al., 2011).

After sample preparation procedures, the vitamin E compounds can be separated using various techniques. The method most commonly used for the separation of tocochromanols is high-pressure liquid chromatography (HPLC) with both normal (NP-HPLC) and reverse phase (RP-HPLC) (Delgado and Borges, 2006).

The separation of vitamin E homologues by NP-HPLC is based on the absorption in the stationary phase depending on the number of methyl substituents in the chromanol ring, which determines their polarity (Delgado and Borges, 2006). In NP-HPLC methods, the silica-based columns are preferred as stationary phases and mobile phases contain *n*-hexane, together with various organic modifiers, for example, 1,4-dioxane, *tert*-butyl methyl ether, diethyl ether, methanol, or isopropanol (Tsochatzis and Tzimou-Tsitouridou, 2015; Kamal-Eldin et al., 2000).

The normal-phase columns provide the separation of all vitamin E forms, whereas β- and γ-isomers are not effectively resolved in traditionally used reverse-phase columns. Apart from the possibility to separate both of these isomers, the advantage of NP-HPLC columns is also the compatibility with the organic solvents which allows the high solubility for lipids. In addition, this system tolerates high loads of lipids which are easy to wash out by nonpolar solvents. Therefore, the NP-HPLC system is successfully used for the direct analysis of oils and fats (Rupérez et al., 2001).

The main stationary phase used in RP-HPLC techniques is a C18-bonded silica column and the mobile phases usually contain methanol, water, acetonitrile, or isopropanol (Gruszka and Kruk, 2007; Tsochatzis and Tzimou-Tsitouridou, 2015). In RP-HPLC the separation of vitamin E compounds occurs according to the saturation of the isoprenoid side chain. The more saturated homologues have a stronger affinity for the stationary phase and they are retained longer (Rupérez et al., 2001).

Complete resolution of eight vitamin E compounds has not been obtained with conventionally used C18 RP-HPLC columns, as the β- and γ-isomers of tocopherols and tocotrienols are not easily separated. However, it is possible to separate these compounds with RP-HPLC using more specific columns, such as pentaflurophenyl (Górnaś et al., 2014) or C30-bonded silica (Gruszka and Kruk, 2007), which are nowadays commercially available. Nevertheless, when the separation of β- and γ-isomers is not the main aim of analysis, the C18 RP-HPLC systems are preferred as they have higher column stability, better reproducibility, and shorter analysis times. Moreover, RP-HPLC solvent systems are more environmentally friendly than those used in NP-HPLC (Gimeno et al., 2000). In addition, the RP-HPLC system provide a good separation of γ-tocopherol and PC-8, which is difficult to achieve using NP-HPLC, as these compounds have the same chromanol ring and differ only in the length of isoprenoid side chain (Szymańska et al., 2017). In some cases when samples with a more complicated vitamin E composition are analyzed, the use of both methods can be necessary.

Besides HPLC, the most common method used for the analysis of vitamin E is gas chromatography. However, the applicability of this technique is limited due to the necessity of sample derivatization which can result in the decomposition of vitamin E caused by the high temperature used in the process (Saini and Keum, 2016). Other techniques, such as thin-layer chromatography, nanoliquid chromatography, capillary electrochromatography, synchronous fluorescence spectroscopy, and Fourier transform infrared spectroscopy, have been also applied for the determination of vitamin E (Saini and Keum, 2016; Tsochatzis and Tzimou-Tsitouridou, 2015).

Detection methods used for the analysis of vitamin E include ultraviolet (UV), diode or photodiode assay (DAD or PDA), fluorescence, electrochemical (ED), evaporative light-scattering, as well as mass spectrometry (MS) detection (Irakli et al., 2011; Saini and Keum, 2016).

The absorption spectra of separated tocopherols and tocotrienols are easily obtained using DAD and UV detectors, however these systems show poor selectivity and sensitivity. The fluorescence detector is the most sensitive for the determination of vitamin E compounds due to their native fluorescence properties and this is the technique used for most of the biological samples (Saini and Keum, 2016). In fluorescence detection usually an excitation wavelength at 290 or 295 nm and an emission wavelength at 330 nm is applied, whereas absorption detection is performed at 292 or 295 nm (Szymańska et al., 2017). The ED, for example, pulse amperometric or coulometric, is also applied as a sensitive detector for tocochromanols analysis after HPLC separation, especially for their determination in blood and serum samples (Moreau and Lampi, 2012). However, ED is limited to RP-HPLC because the necessary electrolytes are miscible with aqueous mobile phases (Rupérez et al., 2001). MS is also used to detect the vitamin E homologues, although its use has not been significantly extended due to the ionization difficulty of nonpolar compounds and the high cost of this detection system (Delgado and Borges, 2006).

The vitamin E analysis procedure used by the authors of this chapter is based on RP-HPLC separation using a C18 column with a fluorescence detector set at an excitation wavelength of 295 nm and an emission wavelength of 330 nm. To analyze the tocopherols and tocotrienols, acetonitrile:methanol:water (72:8:1 v/v) is used with a flow rate of 1.5 mL/min, whereas to analyze the PC-8, methanol:hexane (340:20 v/v) is used at the same flow rate (Gruszka and Kruk, 2007; Szymańska and Kruk, 2010b).

4.5 Nutritional value of vitamin E

4.5.1 Vitamin E metabolism in humans

Vitamin E is not synthesized by humans, thus it must be obtained in the diet. Its absorption strictly depends on lipids uptake. Within the blood vitamin E is transported in a form of lipoprotein (Fig. 4.5) (Szymańska et al., 2017). Lipoprotein hydrolysis leads to the release of vitamin E followed by its absorption by cells. From all the absorbed vitamin E forms, only α-tocopherol is preferentially recognized and used. This is due to the presence of a hepatic 32 kDa α-tocopherol transfer protein (α-TTP) and tocopherol-associated proteins, which selectively bind α-tocopherol (Traber and Atkinson, 2007). While α-TTP has a high affinity to natural

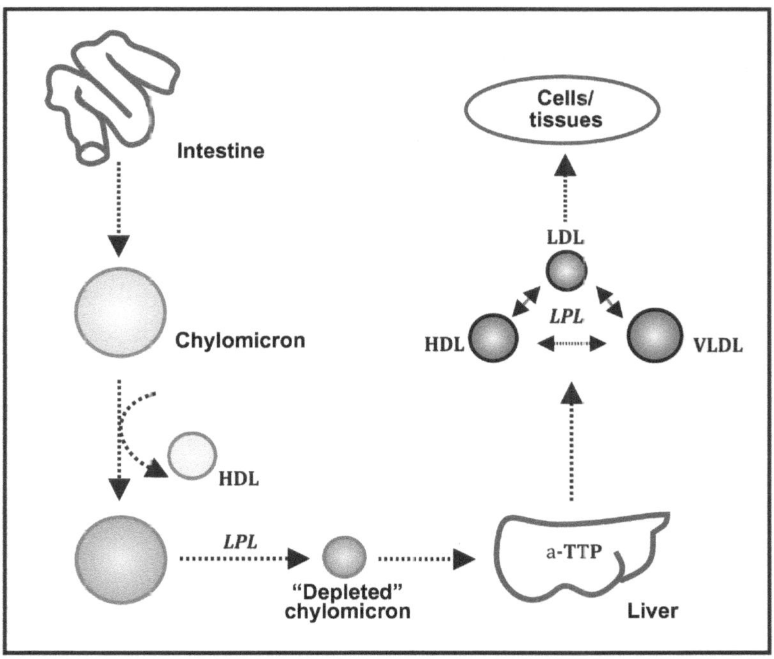

Figure 4.5 Potential clinical application of vitamin E in selected diseases.

α-tocopherol (*RRR*-α-tocopherol) (100%), the relative affinity for other vitamin E homologues is as follows: 38% for β-tocopherol, 9% for γ-tocopherol, 2% for δ-tocopherol, 2% for α-tocopherol acetate, 11% for *SRR*-α-tocopherol, 12% for α-tocotrienol, and 9% for Trolox (water-soluble vitamin E analogue) (Hosomi et al., 1997). In the serum, the levels of remaining vitamin E forms do not exceed 10% of the α-tocopherol level (Nakamura and Omaye, 2009). Those non-α-tocopherol forms are also preferably metabolized by the hepatic cytochrome P450-4F2 and cytochrome P450-3A (Nakamura and Omaye, 2009). The terminal metabolites of vitamin E homologues are the respective 2′-carboxyethyl-6-hydroxychromans, which are excreted via urine and bile (Traber and Atkinson, 2007). It was shown that those metabolites, together with α-tocopherol oxidation products (α-tocopheryloquinone, 5,6-epoxy-α-tocopheryloquinone, and 2,3-epoxy-α-tocopheryloquinone), show biological activity (Grammas et al., 2004; Terentis et al., 2002; Wu and Croft, 2007; Cornwell et al., 2002).

Vitamin E is an essential micronutrient for humans which determines beneficial health outcomes. The recommended dietary allowance (RDA) of vitamin E varies from 3 to 15 mg/day in different countries and depends on the age of a person. In the United States RDA is 15 mg α-tocopherol for adults (22.4 IU of the natural forms or 33.3 IU of synthetic forms) (Galli et al., 2017). In recent years the European Food Safety Authority (EFSA) has recommended replacing RDAs with the Adequate Intake which is as follows: 13 mg/day for men,11 mg/day for women, and 5−13 mg/day for infants/children (depending on age) (Galli et al., 2017). In general, the worldwide intake of vitamin E is low and below the RDA (Galli et al., 2017). The average plasma concentration of vitamin E homologues is about 23.2 μM for α-tocopherol, 2.5 μM for γ-tocopherol, 0.3 μM for δ-tocopherol, and 1 μM for α-tocotrienol (Hensley et al., 2004). The vitamin E tissue distribution and accumulation (adipose tissue, 150 μg/g tissue; the adrenal glands, 132 μg/g; kidney, heart, liver, 7−40 μg/g) point to tissue-specific functions of vitamin E forms (Szymańska et al., 2017).

4.5.2 Biological function of vitamin E

Vitamin E is a natural, strong antioxidant that protects cell components against damage caused by ROS. Tocochromanols inhibit lipid peroxidation that can lead to cell membrane, protein, and DNA alterations

(Traber et al., 2008). Vitamin E homologues are located in cell membranes where they scavenge lipid peroxyl radicals by donating a hydrogen from the phenolic group of the chromanol ring. It was assumed that α-tocopherol has the highest antioxidant activity, followed by β-, γ-, and δ-homologues (Muller et al., 2010). Recent in vitro and in vivo studies suggest that T_3s are more potent antioxidants than tocopherols, mainly due to their higher hydrophobicity and more efficient interaction with the lipid peroxyl radicals in membranes (Gruszka et al., 2008). Different antioxidant activity is also observed between α-, β-, γ-, and δ-homologues. For example, γ-tocopherol is able to trap electrophiles such as RNS, whose generation is enhanced during inflammation. This ability is determined by the homologue structure: γ-tocopherol in contrast to α-homologue has an unsubstituted 5-position in the chromanol ring (Fig. 4.1) (Szymańska et al., 2017).

The effect of vitamin E on fertility and tissue and organ development has been well-documented. Some of these functions have been confirmed in humans, the others need to be evaluated. An emerging role of vitamin E is focused on its antioxidant properties. Oxidative stress underlies many diseases, such as cancer, CVDs, inflammation, and aging. It was shown that vitamin E plays a crucial role in the prevention as well as the treatment of those disorders, not only as an antioxidant, but also as a modulator of signal transduction and a gene expression regulator (Zingg, 2007). The review of literature data has indicated that vitamin E has an impact on numerous diseases (Fig. 4.6). Among them, the most important are:

- *Immune system disorders.* Immune cells, which are endangered by oxidative stress because of a high PUFA content, as well as ROS-mediated antimicrobial response during phagocytosis ("oxidative burst") have a higher content of vitamin E (Mocchegiani et al., 2014). Moreover, it was shown that vitamin E deficiency impairs humoral and cell-mediated immune responses (Peh et al., 2016). It was reported that short vitamin E intake can improve immune responses, including T-cell proliferation, delayed-type hypersensitivity response, interleukin-2 production, and the reduction of prostaglandin E2 synthesis (Meydani et al., 1990). Vitamin E efficiency is dose-dependent. It has to be noted that high-dosage vitamin E supplementation must be considered separately because incautious and high intake may be harmful to the point of mortality (Peh et al., 2016; Szymańska et al., 2017).
- *Cardiovascular diseases.* Numerous in vitro studies have shown the positive effects of vitamin E in reducing the risk of cardiovascular disorders

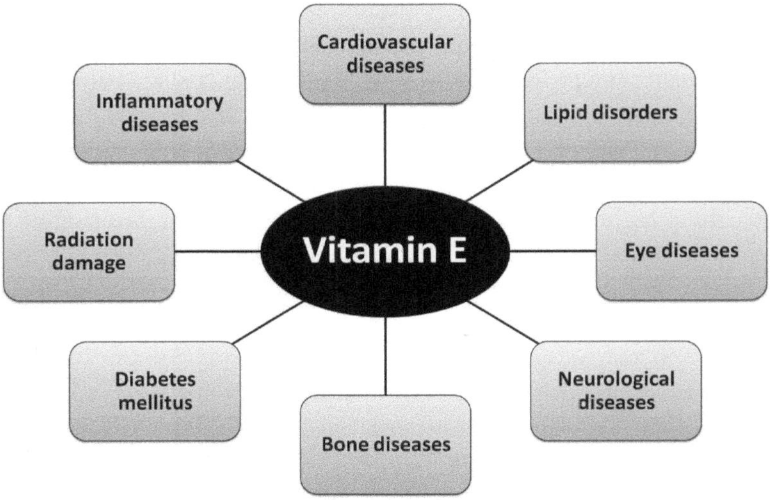

Figure 4.6 Vitamin E transport and distribution within the human body. α-TTP, α-tocopherol transfer protein; HDL, high-density lipoproteins; LDL, low-density lipoproteins; LPL, lipoprotein lipase; VLDL, very-low-density lipoproteins.

mainly by (1) a downregulation of the expression of adhesion molecules, (2) the suppression of monocyte/macrophage activation, and (3) the inhibition of smooth muscle proliferation (Galli et al., 2017; Mocchegiani et al., 2014). High tocotrienol diet is effective in cholesterol lowering in humans with hypercholesterolemia—a risk factor for CVD (Szymańska et al., 2017).

- *Cancer*. The mechanisms of anticancer vitamin E action encompass (1) the stimulation of the *p53* tumor suppressor gene, (2) the activation of heat shock proteins, and (3) the inhibition of transforming growth factor alpha (Szymańska et al., 2017). *In vitro* experiments have shown higher inhibition of cancer growth by γ-tocopherol than by the α-form. γ-Tocopherol was more potent in inducing apoptosis and cell-death pathways, as well as in the reduction of new blood vessel formation (Yan et al., 2015). Nowadays, anticancer properties of tocotrienols are being paid more attention. Studies on human, animal models, and cell lines have shown better antitumor activity by tocotrienols than tocopherols (Mocchegiani et al., 2014). In contrast to *in vitro* and *in vivo* findings on vitamin E anticancer activity, the results obtained from clinical programs are controversial. Several clinical trials have shown no beneficial effects of vitamin E (HOPE-The Ongoing

Outcomes, WHS trials Alpha-Tocopherol and Beta-Carotene Cancer Prevention, and SELECT study) (Szymańska et al., 2017).

- *Neurodegenerative disorders*. It has been observed that vitamin E deficiency increases the risk of dementia and other neurological disorders, such as Alzheimer disease. Moreover, the supplementation of vitamin E could reverse the neurologic dysfunction (Aslam et al., 2004; Peh et al., 2016). In humans the results are contradictory. Some data strongly indicate that vitamin E protects against neurodegeneration (Aslam et al., 2004). In contrast several clinical trials showed that vitamin E has no effect on Alzheimer disease (Szymańska et al., 2017).

References

Asensi-Fabado, M.A., Munné-Bosch, S., 2010. Vitamins in plants: occurrence, biosynthesis and antioxidant function. Trends. Plant. Sci. 15, 582–592.

Aslam, A., Misbah, S.A., Talbot, K., Chapel, H., 2004. Vitamin E deficiency induced neurological disease in common variable immunodeficiency: two cases and a review of the literature of vitamin E deficiency. Clin. Immunol. 112, 24–29.

Bouvier, F., Rahier, A., Camara, B., 2005. Biogenesis, molecular regulation and function of plant isoprenoids. Prog. Lipid. Res. 44, 357–429.

Cahoon, E.B., Hall, S.E., Ripp, K.G., Ganzke, T.S., Hitz, W.D., Coughlan, S.J., 2003. Metabolic redesign of vitamin E biosynthesis in plants for tocotrienol production and increased antioxidant content. Nat. Biotechnol. 21, 1082–1087.

Chun, J., Lee, J., Ye, L., Exler, J., Eitenmiller, R.R., 2006. Tocopherol and tocotrienol contents of raw and processed fruits and vegetables in the United States diet. J. Food Compos. Anal. 19, 196–204.

Cornwell, D.G., Williams, M.V., Wani, A.A., Shen, E., Jones, K.H., 2002. Mutagenicity of tocopherylquinones: evolutionary advantage of selective accumulation of dietary alpha-tocopherol. Nutr. Cancer 43, 111–118.

Delgado, M.A.R., Borges, J.H., 2006. Analytical methodologies for vitamin E analysis. In: Braunstein, M. (Ed.), Focus on Vitamin E Research. Nova Science Publishers, Inc, New York, pp. 141–180.

DellaPenna, D., 2005. Progress in the dissection and manipulation of vitamin E synthesis. Trends. Plant. Sci. 10, 574–579.

Desai, I.D., 1984. Vitamin E analysis methods for animal tissues. Methods Enzymol. 105, 138–147.

Dörmann, P., 2007. Functional diversity of tocochromanols in plants. Planta 225, 269–276.

Dunphy, P.J., Whittle, K.J., Pennock, J.F., Morton, R.A., 1965. Identification and estimation of tocotrienols in *Hevea* latex. Nature 207, 521–522.

Evans, H., Bishop, K.S., 1922. Fetal resorption. Science 55, 650.

Galli, F., Azzi, A., Birringer, M., Cook-Mills, J.M., Eggersdorfer, M., Frank, J., et al., 2017. Vitamin E: emerging aspects and new directions. Free Rad. Biol. Med. 102, 16–36.

Gianello, R., Libinaki, R., Azzi, A., Gavin, P.D., Negis, Y., Zingg, J.M., et al., 2005. α-Tocopheryl phosphate: a novel, natural form of vitamin E. Free Rad. Biol. Med. 39, 970–976.

Gimeno, E., Castellote, A.I., Lamuela-Raventós, R.M., de la Torre, M.C., López-Sabater, M.C., 2000. Rapid determination of vitamin E in vegetable oils by reversed phase high-performance liquid chromatography. J. Chromatogr. A 881, 251–254.

Górnaś, P., Siger, A., Czubinski, J., Dwiecki, K., Seglina, D., Nogala-Kałucka, M., 2014. An alternative RP-HPLC method for the separation and determination of tocopherol and tocotrienol homologues as butter authenticity markers: a comparative study between two European countries. Eur. J. Lipid Sci. Technol. 116, 895–903.

Grammas, P., Hamdheydari, L., Benaksas, E.J., Mou, S., Pye, Q.N., Wechter, W.J., et al., 2004. Anti-inflammatory effects of tocopherol metabolites. Biochem. Biophys. Res. Commun. 319, 1047–1052.

Gruszka, J., Kruk, J., 2007. RP-LC for determination of plastochromanol, tocotrienols and tocopherols in plant oils. Chromatographia 66, 909–913.

Gruszka, J., Pawlak, A., Kruk, J., 2008. Tocochromanols, plastoquinol, and other biological prenyllipids as singlet oxygen quenchers determination of singlet oxygen quenching rate constants and oxidation products. Free Rad. Biol. Med. 45, 920–928.

Hensley, K., Benaksas, E.J., Bolli, R., Comp, P., Grammas, P., Hamdheydari, L., et al., 2004. New perspectives on vitamin E: γ-tocopherol and carboxyelthylhydroxychroman metabolites in biology and medicine. Free Rad. Biol. Med. 36, 1–15.

Herting, D.C., Drury, A.-J.E., 1963. Vitamin E content of vegetable oils and fats. J. Nutr. 81, 335–342.

Hosomi, A., Arita, M., Sato, Y., Kiyose, C., Ueda, T., Igarashi, O., et al., 1997. Affinity for α-tocopherol transfer protein as a determinant of the biological activities of vitamin E analogs. FEBS Lett. 409, 105–108.

Irakli, M.N., Samanidou, V.F., Papadoyannis, I.N., 2011. Development and validation of an HPLC method for the simultaneous determination of tocopherols, tocotrienols and carotenoids in cereals after solid-phase extraction. J. Sep. Sci. 34, 1375–1382.

Kamal-Eldin, A., Appelqvist, L.Å., 1996. The chemistry and antioxidant properties of tocopherols and tocotrienols. Lipids 31 (7), 671–701.

Kamal-Eldin, A., Görgen, S., Pettersson, J., Lampi, A.M., 2000. Normal-phase high-performance liquid chromatography of tocopherols and tocotrienols. J. Chromatogr. A. 881 (1–2), 217–227.

Kruk, J., Pisarski, A., Szymańska, R., 2011. Novel vitamin E forms in leaves of *Kalanchoe daigremontiana* and *Phaseolus coccineus*. J. Plant. Physiol. 168, 2021–2027.

Kruk, J., Szymańska, R., Cela, J., Munné-Bosch, S., 2014. Plastochromanol-8: fifty years of research. Phytochemistry 108, 9–16.

Kruk, J., Szymańska, R., Nowicka, B., Dłużewska, J., 2016. Function of isoprenoid quinones and chromanols during oxidative stress in plants. New Biotechnol. 33, 636–643.

Kusmic, C., Barsacchi, R., Barsanti, L., Gualtieri, P., Passarelli, V., 1999. *Euglena gracilis* as source of the antioxidant vitamin E. Effects of culture conditions in the wild strain and in the natural mutant WZSL. J. Appl. Phycol. 10, 555–559.

Lushchak, V.I., Semchuk, N.M., 2012. Tocopherol biosynthesis: chemistry, regulation and effects of environmental factors. Acta Physiol. Plant. 34, 1607–1628.

Machlin, L.J., Brin, M., 1980. Vitamin E. In: Alfin-Slater, R.B., Kritchevsky, D. (Eds.), Nutrition and the Adult. Springer, Boston, MA, pp. 245–266.

Maeda, H., Sage, T.L., Isaac, G., Welti, R., DellaPenna, D., 2008. Tocopherols modulate extraplastidic polyunsaturated fatty acid metabolism in *Arabidopsis* at low temperature. Plant Cell 20, 452–470.

Mène-Saffrané, L., DellaPenna, D., 2010. Biosynthesis, regulation and functions of tocochromanols in plants. Plant. Physiol. Biochem. 48, 301–309.

Meydani, S.N., Barklund, M.P., Liu, S., Meydani, M., Miller, R.A., Cannon, J.G., et al., 1990. Vitamin E supplementation enhances cell-mediated immunity in healthy elderly subjects. Am. J. Clin. Nutr. 52, 557–563.
Mocchegiani, E., Costarelli, L., Giacconi, R., Malavolta, M., Basso, A., Piacenza, F., et al., 2014. Vitamin E–gene interactions in aging and inflammatory age-related diseases: implications for treatment. A systematic review. Ageing Res. Rev. 14, 81–101.
Moreau, R.A., Lampi, A., 2012. Analysis methods for tocopherols and tocotrienols. In: Xu, Z., Howard, L.R. (Eds.), Analysis of Antioxidant-Rich Phytochemicals. John Wiley & Sons, Inc, UK, pp. 353–386.
Muller, L., Theile, K., Bohm, V., 2010. *In vitro* antioxidant activity of tocopherols and tocotrienols and comparison of vitamin E concentration and lipophilic anti-oxidant capacity in human plasma. Mol. Nutr. Food Res. 54 (5), 731–742.
Munné-Bosch, S., 2005. The role of α-tocopherol in plant stress tolerance. J. Plant. Physiol. 162, 743–748.
Munné-Bosch, S., Alegre, L., 2002. The function of tocopherols and tocotrienols in plants. CRC. Crit. Rev. Plant. Sci. 21, 31–57.
Nakamura, Y.K., Omaye, S.T., 2009. Vitamin E-modulated gene expression associated with ROS generation. J. Funct. Foods 1, 241–252.
Nesaretnam, K., Meganathan, P., Devi Veerasenan, S.D., Selvaduray, K.R., 2012. Tocotrienols and breast cancer: the evidence to date. Genes Nutr. 7, 3–9.
Peh, H.Y., Tan, W.S.D., Liao, W., Wong, W.S.F., 2016. Vitamin E therapy beyond cancer: tocopherol versus tocotrienol. Pharmacol. Ther. 162, 152–169.
Pellaud, S., Mène-Saffrané, L., 2017. Metabolic origins and transport of vitamin E biosynthetic precursors. Front. Plant Sci. 8, 1959.
Pellaud, S., Bory, A., Chabert, V., Romanens, J., Chaisse-Leal, L., Doan, A.V., et al., 2018. WRINKLED1 and ACYL-COA: DIACYLGLYCEROL ACYLTRANSFERASE1 regulate tocochromanol metabolism in Arabidopsis. New Phytol. 217, 245–260.
Piironen, V., Syvaoja, E.L., Varo, P., Salminen, K., Koivistoinen, P., 1986. Tocopherols and tocotrienols in Finnish foods: vegetables, fruits, and berries. J. Agric. Food Chem. 34, 742–746.
Quek, S.-Y., Chu, B.-S., Baharin, B.S., 2007. Commercial extraction of vitamin E from food sources. In: Preedy, V.R., Watson, R.R. (Eds.), The Encyclopedia of Vitamin E. CAB International, UK, pp. 731–739.
Qureshi, A.A., Mo, H.B., Packer, L., Peterson, D.M., 2000. Isolation and identification of novel tocotrienols from rice bran with hypocholesterolemic, antioxidant, and antitumor properties. J. Agric. Food Chem. 48, 3130–3140.
Rowland, R.L., 1958. Flue-cured tobacco. III. Solanochromene and α-tocopherol. J. Am. Chem. Soc. 80, 6130–6133.
Rupérez, F., Martín, D., Herrera, E., Barbas, C., 2001. Chromatographic analysis of α-tocopherol and related compounds in various matrices. J. Chromatogr. A 935 (1–2), 45–469.
Ryan, E., Galvin, K., O'connor, T.P., Maguire, A.R., O'brien, N.M., 2007. Phytosterol, squalene, tocopherol content and fatty acid profile of selected seeds, grains, and legumes. Plant Foods Hum. Nutr. 62, 85–91.
Ryynänen, M., Lampi, A.-M., Salo-Väänänen, P., Ollilainen, V., Piironen, V., 2004. A small-scale sample preparation method with HPLC analysis for determination of tocopherols and tocotrienols in cereals. J. Food Compos. Anal. 17, 749–765.
Saini, R.K., Keum, Y.S., 2016. Tocopherols and tocotrienols in plants and their products: a review on methods of extraction, chromatographic separation, and detection. Food Res. Int. 82, 59–70.
Sen, C.K., Khanna, S., Roy, S., 2006. Tocotrienols: vitamin E beyond tocopherols. Life. Sci. 78, 2088–2098.

Shahidi, F., de Camargo, A.C., 2016. Tocopherols and tocotrienols in common and emerging dietary sources: occurrence, applications, and health benefits. Int. J. Mol. Sci. 17, 1745.
Sjoholm, A., Berggren, P.O., Cooney, R.V., 2000. γ-Tocopherol partially protects insulin-secreting cells against functional inhibition by nitric oxide. Biochem. Biophys. Res. Commun. 277, 334–340.
Szymańska, R., Kruk, J., 2008. Tocopherol content and isomers' composition in selected plant species. Plant Physiol. Biochem. 46, 29–33.
Szymańska, R., Kruk, J., 2010a. Plastoquinol is the main prenyllipid synthesized during acclimation to high light conditions in Arabidopsis and is converted to plastochromanol by tocopherol cyclase. Plant Cell Physiol. 51, 537–545.
Szymańska, R., Kruk, J., 2010b. Identification of hydroxy-plastochromanol in Arabidopsis leaves. Acta Biochim. Pol. 57, 105–108.
Szymańska, R., Kruk, J., 2018. Novel and rare prenyllipids – occurrence and biological activity. Plant. Physiol. Biochem. 122, 1–9.
Szymańska, R., Nowicka, B., Kruk, J., 2017. Vitamin E-occurrence, biosynthesis by plants and functions in human nutrition. Mini-Rev. Med. Chem. 17, 1039–1052.
Terashima, K., Shimamura, T., Tanabayashi, M., Aqil, M., Akinniyi, J.A., Niwa, M., 1997. Constituents of the seeds of Garcinia kola: two new antioxidants, garcinoic acid and garcinal. Heterocycles 45, 1559–1566.
Terentis, A.C., Homas, S.R., Burr, J.A., Liebler, D.C., Stocker, R., 2002. Vitamin E oxidation in human atherosclerotic lesions. Circ. Res. 90, 333–339.
Traber, M.G., Atkinson, J., 2007. Vitamin E, antioxidant and nothing more. Free Rad. Biol. Med. 43, 4–15.
Traber, M.G., Frei, B., Beckman, J.S., 2008. Vitamin E revisited: do new data validate benefits for chronic disease prevention? Curr. Opin. Lipidol. 19, 30–38.
Tsochatzis, E.D., Tzimou-Tsitouridou, R., 2015. Validated RP-HPLC method for simultaneous determination of tocopherols and tocotrienols in whole grain barley using matrix solid-phase dispersion. Food Analyt. Methods 8, 392–400.
Wani, S.H., Sah, S.K., Sági, L., Solymosi, K., 2015. Transplastomic plants for innovations in agriculture. A review. Agron. Sustain. Dev. 35, 1391–1430.
Whittle, K.J., Dunphy, P.J., Pennock, J.F., 1965. Plastochromanol in the leaves of *Hevea brasiliensis*. Biochem. J. 96, 17c–19c.
Wu, J.H., Croft, K.D., 2007. Vitamin E metabolism. Mol. Aspects Med. 28, 437–452.
Xu, Z., 2008. Comparison of extraction methods for quantifying vitamin E from animal tissues. Bioresour. Technol. 99 (18), 8705–8709.
Yamamoto, Y., Fujisawa, A., Hara, A., Dunlap, W.C., 2001. An unusual vitamin E constituent (α-tocomonoenol) provides enhanced antioxidant protection in marine organisms adapted to cold-water environments. Proc. Natl Acad. Sci. USA 98, 13144–13148.
Yan, R.B., Chuang, H.C., Kapuriya, N., Chou, C.C., Lai, P.T., Chang, H.W., et al., 2015. Exploitation of the ability of gamma-tocopherol to facilitate membrane colocalization of Akt and PHLPP1 to develop PHLPP1-targeted Akt inhibitors. J. Med. Chem. 58, 2290–2298.
Zaspel, B.J., Csallany, A.S., 1983. Determination of alpha-tocopherol in tissues and plasma by high-performance liquid chromatography. Anal. Biochem. 130, 146–150.
Zbierzak, A.M., Kanwischer, M., Wille, C., Vidi, P.-A., Giavalisco, P., Lohmann, A., et al., 2010. Intersection of the tocopherol and plastoquinol metabolic pathways at the plastoglobule. Biochem. J. 425, 389–399.
Zingg, J.M., 2007. Vitamin E: an overview of major research directions. Mol. Aspects Med. 28, 400–422.
Zingg, J.M., Azzi, A., 2004. Non-antioxidant activities of vitamin E. Curr. Med. Chem. 11 (9), 1113–1133.

CHAPTER 5

Riboflavin-enriched fermented soy milk for redox-mediated gut modulation: in the search of novel prebiotics

Kiran Thakur[1], Zhao-Jun Wei[2] and Sudhir Kumar Tomar[3]
[1]Associate Professor, School of Food Science and Engineering, Hefei University of Technology, Hefei, People's Republic of China
[2]Professor, School of Food Science and Engineering, Hefei University of Technology, Hefei, People's Republic of China
[3]Principal Scientist, Dairy Microbiology, ICAR-National Dairy Research Institute, Karnal, Haryana, India

Contents

5.1 Introduction

Increasing evidence shows that the trillions of microorganisms (gut microbiota) present in the gastrointestinal tract (GIT) of humans and other mammals play a critical role in both the maintenance of human health and the pathogenesis of many diseases (Steinert et al., 2016). The gut microbiota balance the symbiotic relationship with their host species, aid in biological processes, and aid the host metabolism (Bindels et al., 2017). The insight to modulate the gut microbiota was proposed more than a thousand years ago, giving rise to a spectrum of therapeutic tools and the provision of growth substrates for resident microorganisms (the concept of prebiotics). Until today, any nondigestible food ingredients or substances were considered as prebiotics, originally defined in 1995 by Gibson and

Molecular Nutrition
DOI: https://doi.org/10.1016/B978-0-12-811907-5.00004-X

Roberfroid, which could stimulate the growth and/or activity of these gut residents.

There is, however, an ongoing debate about the strict regulation of food ingredients which qualify as "true" prebiotics. Prebiotic food research has also been limited in recent years, following a ruling from the European regulatory bodies that the labeling of food products with prebiotics and their inherent health claims is not recommended. The use of noncarbohydrate food ingredients to be qualified for prebiotics determines their application as well as their modulatory effects. The effect of certain substances in the manner of ameliorating the certain degree of substances can be utilized. What differentiates the prebiotics from the nonprebiotics is that prebiotics are selectively utilized by host microorganisms and are not just any substance which can affect the microbiome (Gibson et al., 2017).

Besides the existing data which prove all nondigestible carbohydrates to be "true" prebiotics, several noncarbohydrate structures such as polyphenols (Duenas et al., 2015; Queipo-Ortuno et al., 2012), minerals (Chaplin et al., 2016), or vitamins (Steinert et al., 2016; Khan et al., 2012a,b) that can affect the gut microbiota may qualify as prebiotics. The compounds such as vitamins, antibiotics, minerals, and bacteriophages could alter the host microorganisms composition but their acceptability as prebiotics is still under debate.

The relation between diet and health has resulted in the evolution of the idea of "functional foods" which is receiving an increased interest due to many health benefits of certain foods (Thakur et al., 2017a,b,c; Molina et al., 2012; Pophaly et al., 2018; Bansal et al., 2015). Lately, consumers are becoming more inclined toward foods that are beyond basic nutrition. Despite the presence of dairy-based functional foods, the recent inclination toward dairy alternatives has opened up new avenues for cereals-based matrices research and development. Particularly in Asian countries, among the cereal-based foods, soy can be of utmost importance not only because of its low-cost, high-protein content, and polyunsaturated fatty acids, but also it can satisfy the lactose-intolerant individuals and can be considered a good substitute for dairy products (Min et al., 2018). In recent years it has emerged from its reputation as a "poor man's meat" to a value-added food with a promising future in the native food markets (Molina et al., 2012). Besides the popularity of highly nutritious soy milk in Asia, it is recognized as an indispensible part of the diet in China's health program. Despite the rich history of consumption and the

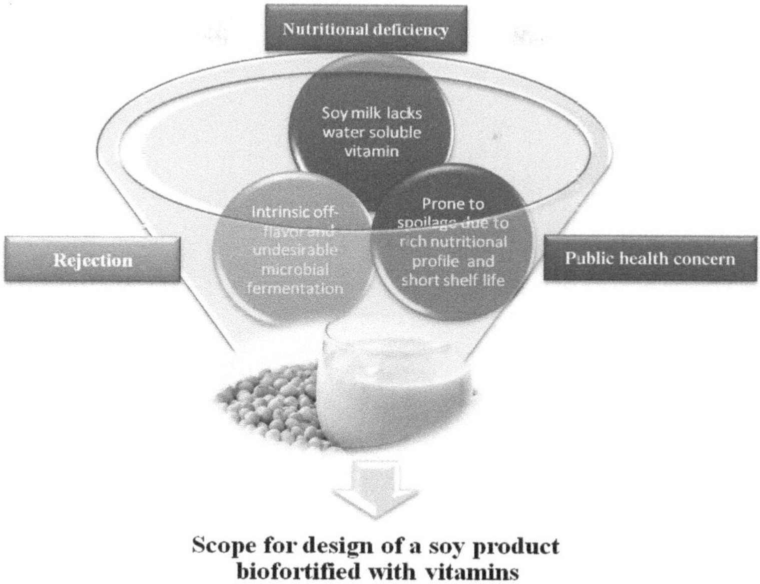

Figure 5.1 Scope for improvement of soy milk with the supplementation of microbial cell factories.

increasing annual production in China, soybeans until recently suffered a severe image problem in many Asian and Western countries (Fig. 5.1). Soybeans lack the presence of many water-soluble vitamins and off-flavors are generated due to oxidative rancidity and undesirable microbial fermentation. Moreover, its highly nutritious nature may be suitable for pathogenic bacteria which may lead to a short shelf (Ma et al., 2017). Although food scientists have tried to resolve these problems by creating some new lines of soybeans, it would be of great interest if improved soy milks could be developed from traditional lines without affecting the composition and which could meet consumers' satisfaction. In the light of existing limitations, the improvement of soy milk-based foods is a hotspot for in vitro fermentation, fortification, and optimization of physicochemical and sensory attributes worldwide (Fig. 5.2). Owing to soy milk's off-flavors, studies have been initiated on the inhibitory role of gut fermentation of soybean carbohydrates in order to suppress the formation of putrefactive compounds (Nakata et al., 2017). The off-flavor compounds have high affinities to soy protein. Therefore the breakdown of the proteins by fermentation can be the possible alternative. With regards to fermentation, it has a long history in Asia and the existing traditional

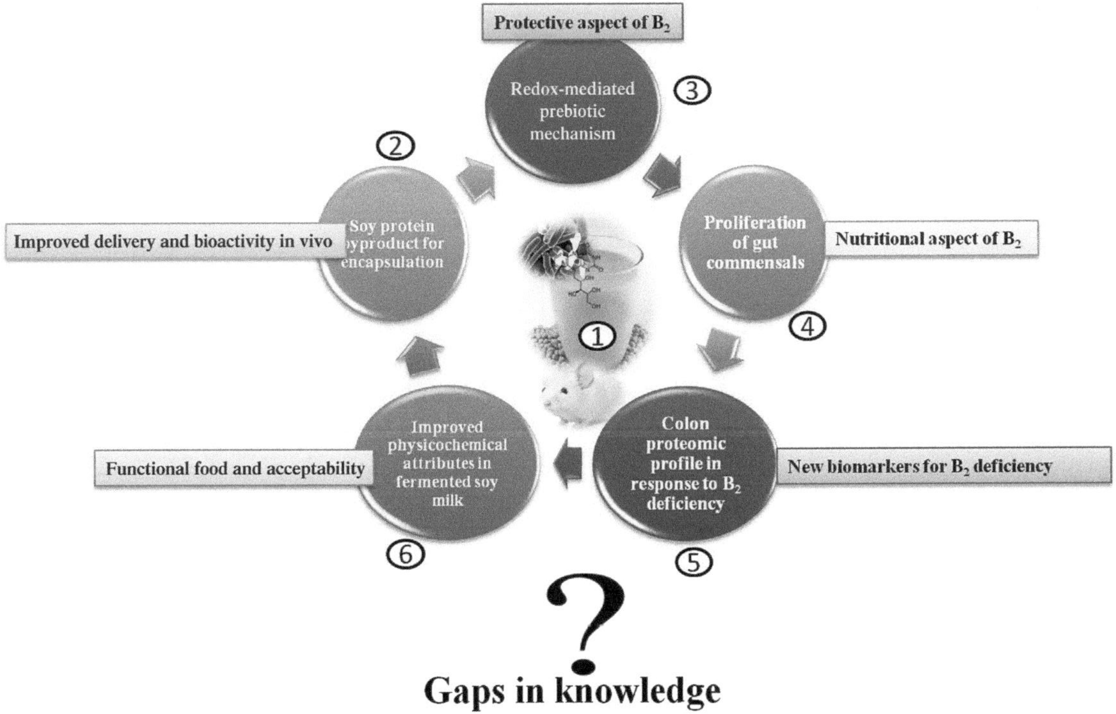

Figure 5.2 The main research issues in the development of vitamin B_2-enriched fermented soy milk.

information can be applied for functional health benefits with a blend of improvised scientific knowledge. Advanced soy fermentation with food grade microbial cell factories (producing various metabolites) could result in better digestibility of soy in the human body by improving the nutritional, consumer, and public health aspects. The versatility of lactic acid bacteria (LAB) has encouraged researchers to obtain new insights in the search for novel compounds for the ever-growing competitive functional food market (Thakur et al., 2016, 2017b; Thakur and Tomar, 2016; Kumar et al., 2018). LAB serve as microbial cell factories for supplying (water-soluble) vitamins to human hosts which make them a good choice for bioprospecting for potent vitamin-producing bacteria (Thakur et al., 2016, 2017b; Thakur and Tomar, 2016). Additionally, LAB have been extensively used in fermentation processes since time immemorial. Therefore these strains have evolved their biosynthetic capability and metabolic versatility for the in situ production of metabolites in dairy and nondairy foods.

5.2 Riboflavin as an essential vitamin

Each B-group vitamin is responsible for regulating the body's homeostasis. Vitamin B_2 is required in numerous enzymatic reactions and for electron transfer in biological oxidation–reduction reactions (Thakur et al., 2017c). Due to various health effects, B_2 is recognized as an indispensable component of cellular metabolism. Additionally, one pioneering report claimed that it can act as a potent prebiotic candidate as well as a remarkable antioxidant vehicle (Steinert et al., 2016). Most of the vitamins and lipids get absorbed in the upper small intestine. What is so far unknown is whether these vitamins can affect the host physiology via the modulation of the gut microbiome. Vitamin B_2, a water-soluble vitamin, is readily taken up in the small intestine. It can therefore be assumed that it is more likely to reach the colon when taken in high doses. The microbial production of B_2 offers a more natural method of increasing vitamin concentrations in foods based on the de novo biosynthetic capacity of certain strains (Thakur et al., 2016).

5.3 Riboflavin as a novel prebiotic ingredient?

To date, studies have recognized prebiotics as substrates for the enhancement of probiotic or gut bacteria. "A nondigestible compound that, through its metabolism by microorganisms in the gut, modulates the composition and/or activity of the gut microbiota, thus conferring a beneficial physiological effect on the host (Steinert et al., 2016)." According to Steinert et al. (2017), several plant components, such as polyphenols, minerals, or vitamins, that can exert beneficial effects through the modulation of the gut microbiota, may qualify as prebiotics in addition to the acceptance of all nondigestible carbohydrates as "true" prebiotics. The recent definition of prebiotics proposed by experts of International Society for Probiotics and Prebiotics emphasized the selective utilization of the substrate for the stimulation of gut microbiota conferring a health benefit (Gibson et al., 2017). The vast understanding of host microbiota and their manifestations has allowed the progress of prebiotic research to stretch beyond the traditional norms. There have been numerous discussions in recent years to order to improve the understanding of the evolution of prebiotics compounds and their microbiome-modulating properties (Fata et al., 2017; Steinert et al., 2016; Bindels et al., 2017; Khan et al., 2012a,b). Therefore the noncarbohydrate compounds can be placed into a category in which, although they may not be selectively utilized by host microbiota, they are accepted as microbiome-modulating substances (Fig. 5.3) (Gibson et al., 2017).

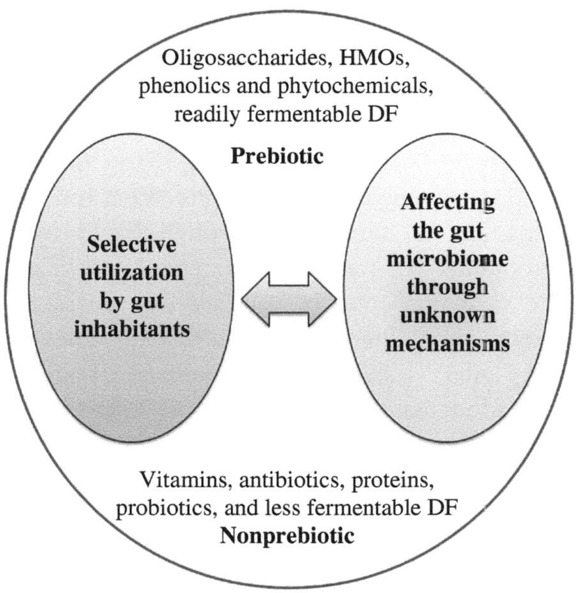

Figure 5.3 What separates probiotics and nonprebiotics?

5.4 Redox-mediated gut modulation by vitamin B_2

Vitamin B_2 was first placed in the prebiotics category because of the amelioration of the growth of a strict anaerobic beneficial bacterium *Faecalibacterium prausnitzii* which comprises 5%–15% of the total number of bacteria in the human gut (Hold et al., 2003). This particular bacterium is extremely sensitive to oxidative stress in the colon. Studies have shown that *F. prausnitzii* has a special ability to use riboflavin as an extracellular electron transporter that allows it to tolerate limited amounts of oxygen (Khan et al., 2012a,b). To emphasize, vitamin B2 intervention not only increased the levels of *F. prausnitzii* but the it also affected the other anaerobes by increasing the *Roseburia* species, and decreasing *Escherichia coli*, indicating an improvement in the redox state which leads to a more favorable gut environment for host microorganisms (Steinert et al., 2016).

In addition to nondigestible carbohydrates, several noncarbohydrate structures, such as polyphenols, minerals, or vitamins have also been found to have a beneficial effect on the modulation of gut microbiota. Besides the existing data which proves all nondigestible carbohydrates to be "true" prebiotics, several noncarbohydrate structures, such as polyphenols (Duenas et al., 2015; Queipo-Ortuno et al., 2012), minerals (Chaplin et al., 2016), vitamins (Steinert et al., 2016; Khan et al., 2012a,b), omega-3 polyunsaturated fatty acids (Watson et al., 2017), and yeast fermentate (Pinheiro et al., 2017), may also qualify as prebiotics. The latter study reported the initial claims of the prebiotic properties of yeast metabolites from *Saccharomyces cerevisiae*. From these above reports, it is clear that in the future, more and more advancements in prebiotic research and gut modulation will help the researchers to understand the exact underlying mechanisms and how they support their prebiotic roles.

To summarize, vitamin B_2 exerts its antioxidant mechanism on the host microbiome by acting as an essential electron transfer shuttle, thereby reducing the oxygen tension inside the gut and making it suitable for the growth of gut anaerobes. This mechanism has been proven by a previous study where vitamin B_2 could mediate the electron transfer to oxygen, thus helping to lower the redox potential (Fig. 5.4). Bacteria do not use vitamin B_2 as a direct substrate for microbial fermentation, however, it should be noted that vitamin B_2 is an essential growth factor for gut inhabitants, in addition to its impact on the gut microbiota by changing the GIT redox state. Even though there is scarce information available on its increased role in nutritional intervention by supporting human health in

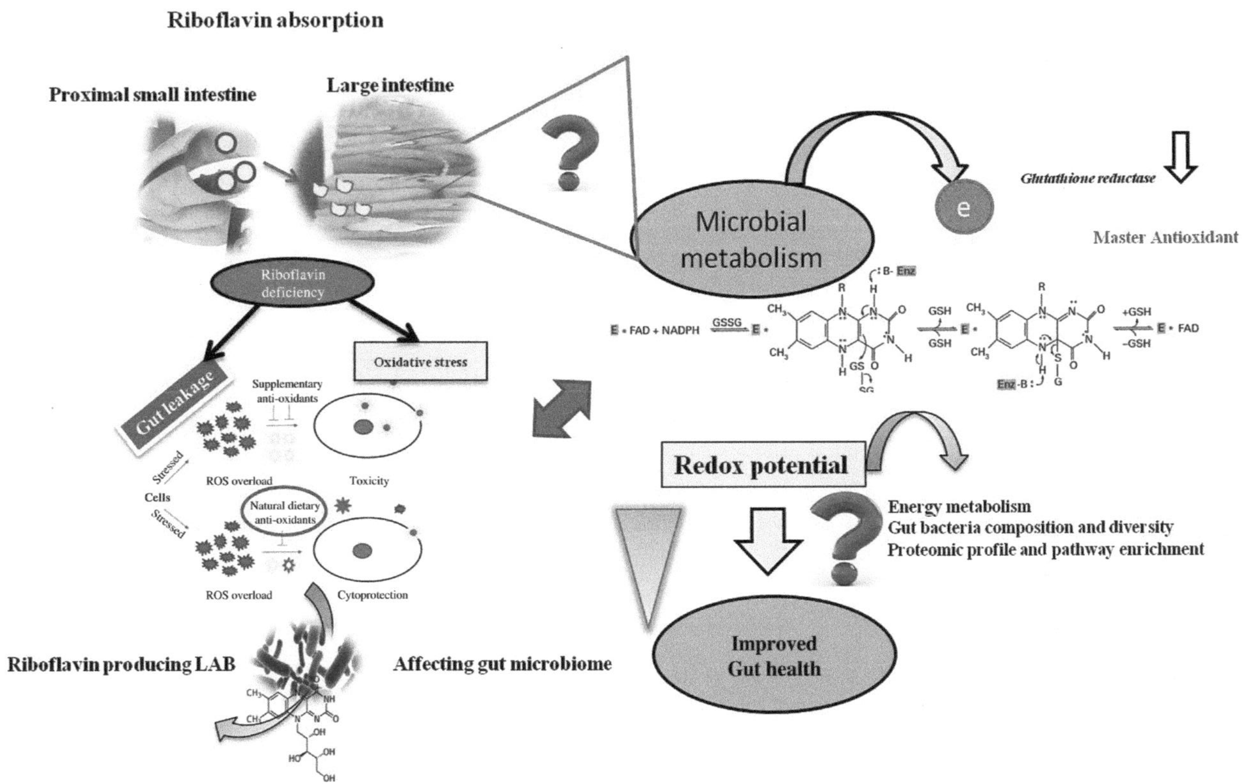

Figure 5.4 Conversion of reduced vitamin B_2 to its oxidized form: a possible mechanism for its antioxidant nature.

relation to *F. prausnitzii*, this finding may lead to further findings supporting the prebiotic potential of vitamin B_2 in the future.

5.5 Soya as an ideal substrate for lactic acid bacteria fermentation

In the Asian countries, various soy products are readily available in the market, for example, soya milk, tofu, and soy paneer, etc., but there are few studies on the development of fermented soya milk. Soya milk is the most commonly used soya-based product consumed in the world, not only because of its potential health benefits but also because it is an alternative for lactose-intolerant individuals, and thus can be considered as a good substitute for dairy products (Fig. 5.5). Particularly in China, the consumers' preference for nondairy fermented drinks (soya milk) over dairy products is increasing day by day. It is widely accepted that fermentation leads to the better digestibility of soya in the human body by reducing the phytate, spoilage bacteria, and antinutritive levels, leading to the better utilization of bioactive compounds by our gut microbes. Moreover, the putrefactive compounds released from soya proteins can be reduced due to the conversion of proteins into peptides by starter lactobacilli during the fermentation process. Considering the beneficial effects of fermentation on soya milk, it is believed that the development of vitamin

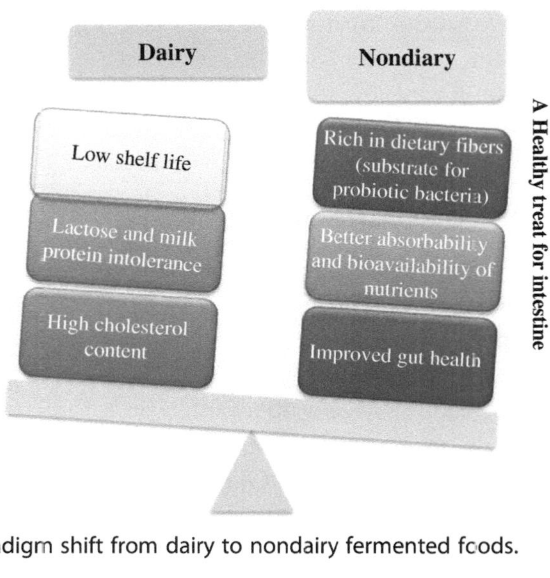

Figure 5.5 Paradigm shift from dairy to nondairy fermented foods.

B_2-enriched fermented soya milk could be the most economical and convenient strategy to reduce the cost of in situ fortification programs. The vitamin B_2-enriched fermented soy milk will contribute to the modification of dietary habits and the diversification of the indigenous foods. Moreover, the high content of nondigestible oligosaccharides in soyabean seeds can provide an ideal substrate for LAB fermentation. In order to develop a healthy food product, the main research issues are the appropriate matrix, the composition and dispensation of substrate, the growth potential of starters and their stability during processing/storage, and the sensory and the nutritional values of the final product. From our previous studies, it is confirmed that riboflavin production is strain specific and not all the bacteria harbor the biosynthesis genes. There is only one report which has demonstrated that soy milk fermented with vitamin B_2-producing *Lactobacillus plantarum* CRL 2130 can revert and prevent ariboflavinosis in murine models (Valle et al., 2016). There is much scope to study this particular vitamin in relation to gut modulation.

Due to various health benefits, fermented soya milk can be considered as potential matrices for vitamin B_2 fortification, yet the stability of in situ-produced riboflavin during the fermentation process is not known. As known previously, nondairy foods contain heterogeneous food matrices, which are the major constraints for the survival of probiotic bacteria. We anticipate that in situ-produced vitamin B_2 can also enhance the fermentation process in soya milk and restore the levels of gut inhabitants which are apparently lowered due to dysbiosis (Fig. 5.6). The putrefactive compounds from soy proteins often lead to off-flavors and affect the overall acceptability. In the future, the effect of vitamin B_2 on the sensory aspect of soya milk should also be taken into consideration.

5.6 Conclusion and future outlook

The correlation of vitamin B_2 with *F. prausnitzii* has helped researchers to explore the potential novel function of this vitamin. It should be taken into consideration further in relation to other gut inhabitants and should be validated in mice models from a mechanistic point of view. Vitamin B_2, although it does not provide a direct substrate for microbial fermentation, may beneficially modulate the composition of the gut microbiota by being metabolized and changing the GIT redox state. To summarize, the physicochemical, technological, nutritional, and functional properties of fermented soy milk, as well as the viability of LAB producing various

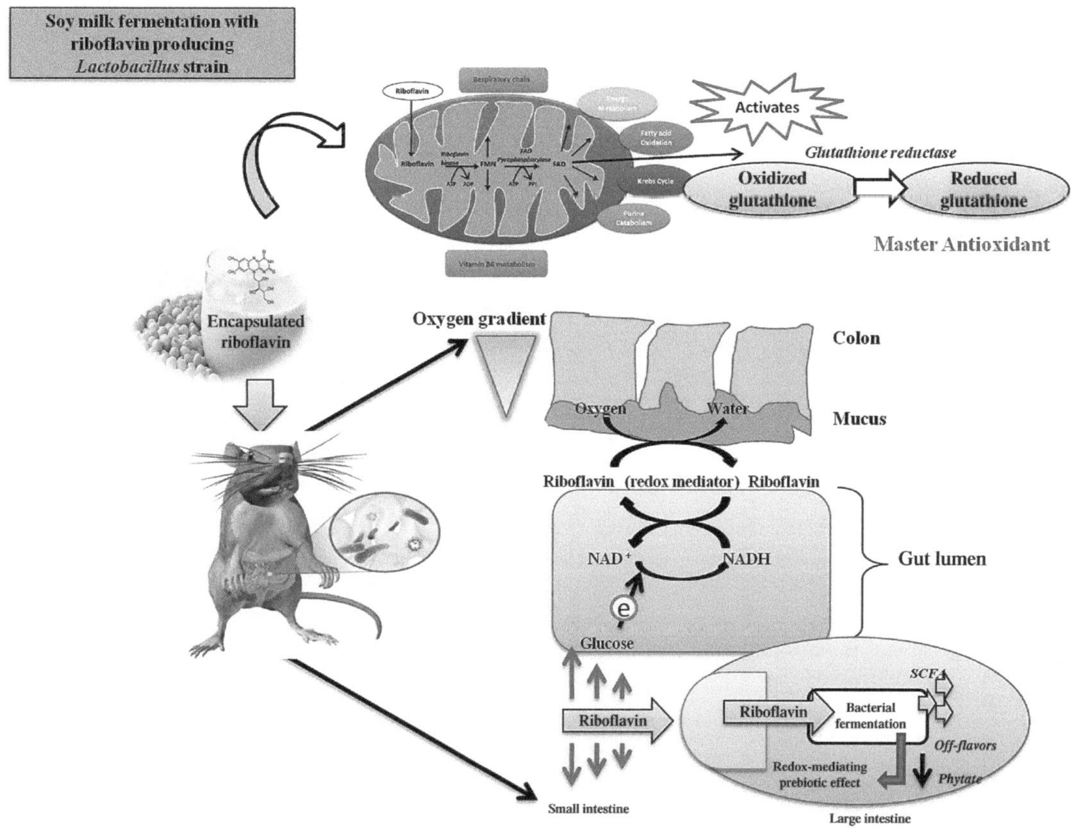

Figure 5.6 Manifestation of redox-mediated modulation of the host microbiome through vitamin B_2-enriched soya milk intervention.

metabolites in fermented products of nondairy origin, are extremely important in order to gain a competitive advantage in the world food market. As long as the relationship between the microbiota composition and the metabolite production has been fully established, the concept of prebiotics will continue to advance. With this mindset, the most recent findings of noncarbohydrate compounds that are yet to be considered as prebiotics would be helpful as future mandates to improve the conception for novel prebiotic food ingredients which if missed now can lead to bigger gaps in prebiotic research in the future. The prebiotic criteria should not only revolve around plant-based fibers; there are already reports emerging about other substances that also confer prebiotic benefits. This way we can take not only limit the manifestation of prebiotic compounds digestive health alone but also understanding their role for metabolism, brain function, and heart health.

References

Bansal, S., Mangal, M., Sharma, S.K., Gupta, R.K., 2015. Non-dairy based probiotics: a healthy treat for intestine. Crit. Rev. Food Sci. Nutr. Available from: https://doi.org/10.1080/10408398.2013.790780.

Bindels, L.B., Delzenne, N.M., Cani, P.D., Walter, J., 2017. Towards a more comprehensive concept for prebiotics. Nat. Rev. Gastroenterol. Hepatol. Available from: https://doi.org/10.1038/nrgastro.2015.47.

Chaplin, A., Parra, P., Laraichi, S., Serra, F., Palou, A., 2016. Calcium supplementation modulates gut microbiota in a prebiotic manner in dietary obese mice. Mol. Nutr. Food Res. 60, 468–480.

Duenas, M., Munoz-Gonzalez, I., Cueva, C., Jimenez-Giron, A., Sanchez-Patan, F., Santos-Buelga, C., et al., 2015. A survey of modulation of gut microbiota by dietary polyphenols. Biomed. Res. Int. 2015. Available from: https://doi.org/10.1155/2015/850902.

Fata, G.L., Rastall, R.A., Lacroix, C., Harmsen, H.J.M., Mohajeri, M.H., Weber, P., et al., 2017. Recent development of prebiotic research—statement from an expert workshop. Nutrients 9, 1376. Available from: https://doi.org/10.3390/nu9121376.

Gibson, G.R., Hutkins, R., Sanders, M.E., Prescott, S.L., Reimer, R.A., Salminen, S.J., et al., 2017. The International Scientific Association for Probiotics and Prebiotics (ISAPP) consensus statement on the definition and scope of prebiotics. Gastroenterol. Hepatol. 14, 491. Available from: https://doi.org/10.1038/nrgastro.2017.75.

Hold, G.L., Schwiertz, A., Aminov, R.I., Blaut, M., Flint, H.J., 2003. Oligonucleotide probes that detect quantitatively significant groups of butyrate-producing bacteria in human feces. Appl. Environ. Microbiol. 69, 4320–4324.

Khan, M.T., Duncan, S.H., Stams, A.J.M., van Dijl, J.M., Flint, H.J., Harmsen, H.J.M., 2012a. The gut anaerobe *Faecalibacterium prausnitzii* uses an extracellular electron shuttle to grow at oxic–anoxic interphases. ISME J. 6, 1578–1585.

Khan, M.T., Browne, W.R., van Dijl, J.M., Harmsen, H.J., 2012b. How can *Faecalibacterium prausnitzii* employ riboflavin for extracellular electron transfer? Antioxid. Redox Signal. 17, 1433–1440.

Kumar, N., Kumari, V., Ram, C., Thakur, K., Tomar, S.K., 2018. Bio-prospectus of lactic acid by bacteria cadmium bioadsorption to mitigate health and environmental impacts. Appl. Microbiol. Biotechnol. 12, 1–17.

Ma, X.H., Hu, X.H., Liu, L., Li, X.P., Ma, Z., Chen, J.H., et al., 2017. The quality changes and microflora analysis of commercial instant soya milk. Food Sci. Nutr. 5, 123–130.

Min, M., Bunt, C.R., Mason, S.L., Hussain, M.A., 2018. Non-dairy probiotic food products: an emerging group of functional foods. Crit. Rev. Food. Sci. Nutr. Available from: https://doi.org/10.1080/10408398.2018.1462760.

Molina, V., Medici, M., de Valdez, G.F., Taranto, M.P., 2012. Soybean-based functional food with vitamin B_{12}-producing lactic acid bacteria. J. Funct. Foods 4, 831–836.

Nakata, T., Kyoui, D., Takahashi, H., Kimura, B., Kuda, T., 2017. Inhibitory effects of soybean oligosaccharides and water-soluble soybean fiber on formation of putrefactive compounds from soyprotein by gut microbiota. Int. J. Biol. Macromol. 97, 173–180.

Pinheiro, I., Robinson, L., Verhelst, A., Marzorati, M., Winkens, B., den Abbeele, P.V., et al., 2017. A yeast fermentate improves gastrointestinal discomfort and constipation by modulation of the gut microbiome: results from a randomized double-blind placebo-controlled pilot trial. BMC Complement Altern. Med. 17, 441. Available from: https://doi.org/10.1186/s12906-017-1948-0.

Pophaly, S., Chauhan, M., Lule, V., Sarang, P., Tarak, J., Thakur, K., et al., 2018. Functional starter cultures for fermented dairy products. In: Öztürkoğlu Budak, Ş., Akal, H.C. (Eds.), Microbial Cultures and Enzymes in Dairy Technology. IGI Global, Hershey, PA, pp. 1–335. Available from: https://doi.org/10.4018/978-1-5225-5363-2.

Queipo-Ortuno, M.I., Boto-Ordonez, M., Murri, M., Gomez-Zumaquero, J.M., Clemente-Postigo, M., Estruch, R., et al., 2012. Influence of red wine polyphenols and ethanol on the gut microbiota ecology and biochemical biomarkers. Am. J. Clin. Nutr. 95, 1323–1334.

Steinert, R.E., Sadabad, M.S., Harmsen, H.J.M., Weber, P., 2016. The prebiotic concept and human health: a changing landscape with riboflavin as a novel prebiotic candidate? Eur. J. Clin. Nutr. 70, 1348–1353.

Thakur, K., Tomar, S.K., 2016. In vitro study of riboflavin producing lactobacilli as potential probiotic. LWT Food Sci. Technol. 68, 570–578.

Thakur, K., Tomar, S.K., De, S., 2016. Lactic acid bacteria as a cell factory for riboflavin production. Microb. Biotechnol. 9, 441–451.

Thakur, K., Zhang, J.G., Wei, Z.J., Kumar, N., Tomar, S.K., Pophaly, S.D., 2017a. Cross talk between functional foods and gut health. In: Nutraceuticals and Innovative Food Products for Healthy Living and Preventive Care. Medical Information Science Reference. ISBN: 1522529705, 9781522529705.

Thakur, K., Tomar, S.K., Wei, Z.J., 2017b. Comparison of relative mRNA expression profiles of riboflavin biosynthesis genes in lactobacilli isolated from human faeces and fermented bamboo shoots. Front. Microbiol. 8, 427. Available from: https://doi.org/10.3389/fmicb.2017.00427.

Thakur, K., Tomar, S.K., Singh, A.K., Mandal, S., Arora, S., 2017c. Riboflavin and health: a review of recent human research. Crit. Rev. Food. Sci. Nutr. 57, 3650–3660.

Valle, M.J., Laiño, J.E., de Moreno de LeBlanc, A., Savoy de Giori, G., LeBlanc, J.G., 2016. Soyamilk fermented with riboflavin-producing *Lactobacillus plantarum* CRL 2130 reverts and prevents ariboflavinosis in murine models. Br. J. Nutr. 116, 1229–1235.

Watson, H., Mitra, S., Croden, F.C., Taylor, M., Wood, H.M., Perry, S.L., et al., 2017. A randomised trial of the effect of omega-3 polyunsaturated fatty acid supplements on the human intestinal microbiota. Gut 67 (11), 1974–1983.

CHAPTER 6

A review of vitamin B12

Gianluca Rizzo[1] and Antonio Simone Laganà[2]
[1]Independent Researcher, Messina, Italy
[2]Department of Obstetrics and Gynecology, "Filippo Del Ponte" Hospital, University of Insubria, Varese, Italy

Contents

Key facts of vitamin B12

- Even if there are different isoforms of cobalamin (Cbl), cofactor forms must follow the endocellular process to be engaged by specific enzymes.
- There is no upper intake level for vitamin B12 because its absorption and retention is limited. Usually the excess vitamin is excreted with urine.
- Only a few microbes can synthesize vitamin B12 but humans can obtain this vitamin through food, due to the bioaccumulation process.
- With senescence, the elevation of gastric pH reduces the ability to digest food efficiently. However, the absorption of the crystalline form of vitamin B12 is not affected.
- Pernicious anemia (PA) is an autoimmune disease that disrupts the gastric mucosa and leads to the incapacity of vitamin B12 absorption.
- Even if vitamin B12 shortage was identified with anemia symptoms, neurological ones can occur without anemia and in an irreversible manner.
- The complexity of the carrier system is well elucidated by modern molecular and cellular techniques; however, there are actually inborn defects that are still unknown.

Molecular Nutrition
DOI: https://doi.org/10.1016/B978-0-12-811907-5.00005-1

Summary points

- Mammals, and so humans, cannot synthesize Cbl.
- Only animal foodstuffs are adequate sources of Cbl.
- If Cbl intake is not sufficient, supplementation is needed.
- Some disease and dysfunction can decrease Cbl absorption.
- Oral Cbl supplementation at a high dosage is as effective as intramuscular injection, as well as in the presence of PA.
- Cbl is crucial for energetic metabolism and in cell replication processes.
- There are only two enzymes that need Cbl for their reactions.
- There is not a gold standard essay for body Cbl status.
- The use of multiple markers can better define Cbl sufficiency than just blood Cbl concentration.
- A wide pool of transporters and endocellular chaperones ensure efficient absorption and utilization of Cbl, minimizing the absorption of useless molecules with no vitamin properties.
- A diffuse Cbl deficiency among the population is a source of concern, in particular among children and pregnant women.
- Among vegetarian people an adequate intake of Cbl can be easily obtained from supplements.

Definitions of words and terms

Corrin: A corrin is a chemical compound formed by a heterocyclic structure. It forms the central ring of vitamin B12 where a cobalt atom is coordinated by four nitrogen atoms, a lateral chain, and a sixth variable ligand for different isoforms.

Cellular trafficking: Endocellular management of molecules through a chaperone system that engages specific elements and escorts them to their cellular fate.

Microbiota: The microbiota is a pool of microorganisms with symbiotic and commensal relationships among strains. Usually the digestive tracts of mammals have specific microbiota associated with various districts with a plethora of functions in food digestion and immunological mechanisms. Sometimes an alteration of these relationships among strains and between host and microbiota can develop negative outcomes.

Bioavailability: The bioavailability of a substance takes into account not only the concentration of it but also some phenomena that alter physiological capabilities to absorb it. This may depend on the presence of other substances or the presence of different mechanisms of transport.

Pernicious anemia: This is an autoimmune disease that disrupts gastric parietal cells due to the production of specific antibodies. This phenomenon alters the secretion of gastric substances, such as the intrinsic factor, a carrier that mediates the absorption of Cbl.

Food-bound malabsorption: The low gastric pH is required for the release of some vitamins from foodstuffs. With senescence the reduction of gastric barriers with the rise of pH reduces the ability to cleave Cbl from food, with a consequent risk of vitamin shortage.

Enterocyte: Enterocyte is a cytotype of the brush border of absorptive gut epithelia. It is a polarized cell characterized by different membrane organization between the apical side, that mediates absorption from gut lumen, and the basolateral side, that mediates the release of substances to the vessel lumen.

Proton pump inhibitors: They are drugs that target the gastric proton pump. They are used to reduce the acidity of the stomach to protect gastric cells in the case of iatrogenic erosion of parietal tissue or in gastroesophageal reflux disease.

Small intestinal bacterial overgrowth: This is a pathological translocation of some strains from large bowel microbiota to the small intestine with the alteration of physiological digestive functions.

Inflammatory bowel disease: This is a group of correlated degenerative diseases that affect bowel tissues with digestive and systemic dysfunctions.

Enterohepatic circulation: The enterohepatic circulation consists of a process of reuptake of some substances that have been excreted with bile. This phenomenon is very important for the efficient use of some vitamins like Cbl.

Microcytemia: This is a disruption of normal hematopoiesis that leads to a low volume of erythrocytes. It depends on an inadequate availability of iron during the process.

Abbreviations

AdoCbl	Adenosylcobalamin
AMN	Amnionless protein
Cbl	Cobalamin
CNCbl	Cyanocobalamin
CNS	Central nervous system

DMB	5,6-Dimethylbenzimidazole
DRI	Dietary reference intake
HC	Haptocorrin
HCY	Homocysteine
HTCII	Holotranscobalamin II
IF	Intrinsic factor
MCM	Methylmalonyl-CoA mutase
MCV	Mean corpuscular volume
MetCbl	Methylcobalamin
MMA	Methylmalonic acid
MMAA	Methylmalonic aciduria type A
MMAB	Methylmalonic aciduria type B
MMACHC	Methylmalonic aciduria type C and homocystinuria
MMADHC	Methylmalonic aciduria type D and homocystinuria
MRP1	Multidrug resistance protein 1
MS	Methionine synthase
MSR	Methionine synthase reductase
OHCbl	Hydroxocobalamin
PA	Pernicious anemia
TCII	Transcobalamin II

6.1 Introduction

Vitamin B12, also called cobalamin (Cbl), is an indispensable molecule with a very complex structure and an intricate pathway of absorption and cellular trafficking that requires molecular escort proteins in body fluids and intracellular chaperones. After the discovery of this vitamin, a lot of mechanisms were clarified, although to date there are still some aspects that need to be elucidated.

The biosynthetic pathway of Cbl numbers about 30 steps, but only some prokaryotes have the required enzyme pool (Martens et al., 2002). Interestingly this complex biosynthetic capacity is limited to some phyla that are not necessarily interrelated (Zhang et al., 2009).

Mammals, humans included, are not able to synthesize Cbl but a highly modulated absorption ability and transport through body fluids prevents any possible shortage even after many years of no intake (Carmel, 2008). Nevertheless, Cbl deficiency can have devastating and sometimes irreversible complications. So the correct sufficiency must be taken in account, especially with a reduced intake or compromised absorption.

Cbl is an organometallic factor composed of a tetrapyrrolic corrinic ring with a cobalt atom coordinated to four equatorial nitrogen atoms. The molecular scaffold is related to well-known prosthetic groups like the protoporphylinic ring of eme group of hemoglobin or cytochromes p450 of the electron transport chain, using the redox state of the metallic atom to produce conformational changes. The central cobalt atom is bound at the lower side with a 5,6-dimethylbenzimidazole base (DMB), with α-axial conformation. DMB is already linked to a lateral chain of the corrinic structure and its conformation seems to be crucial for the interaction with chaperones and final enzymes that use Cbl as a cofactor. At the upper side of the cobalt atom, there is the sixth ligand of the cobalt atom in the β-axial position. There is a variability of this chemical group with relevant significance in catalytic functions. A methyl group on the β-axial position forms a methylcobalamin variant of vitamin B12 (MetCbl), while a 5-deoxyadenosyl group bound to the cobalt atom forms the adenosylcobalamin isoform (AdoCbl). These two alkylcobalamin isoforms have the cofactorial function but there are also other isoforms such as hydroxocobalamin (OHCbl) with a hydroxyl group or cyanocobalamin (CNCbl) with a β-axial cyano group. The Cbl structure with more common β-axial ligands is displayed in Fig. 6.1.

CNCbl was the first isoform characterized by crystallographic techniques and it is currently called vitamin B12. Nowadays we know that it was an artifact of the extraction procedures, but CNCbl functions in the bloodstream are still far from being fully elucidated: maybe it is a

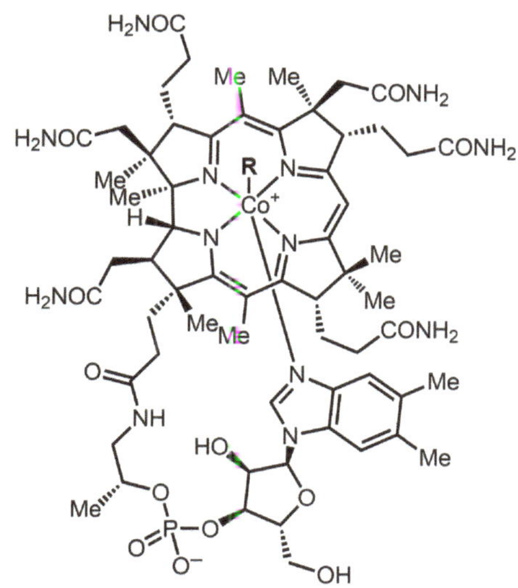

R	Cobalamin isoform
–OH	Hydroxocobalamin
–CN	Cyanocobalamin
$-CH_4$	Methylcobalamin
$-C_{10}H_{13}N_5O_3$	Deoxyadenosylcobalamin

Figure 6.1 Cobalamin structure and isoforms.
The structure of Cb with characteristic corrinic ring and with the most common β-axial ligands that characterize Cbl isoforms.

by-product of scavenger functions for cyanide. Moreover, it was widely described a cellular decyanase activity that enabled the utilization of CNCbl as a vitamin (Kim et al., 2008).

The need for Cbl arose from its ability of reverting hematological signs of pernicious anemia (PA). Nowadays we know that other B vitamins also have related interconnected functions and they take part in the metabolic pathways needed for the cellular replication and the energy production.

6.2 Cobalamin content in food

Because the biosynthetic ability is restricted to a few microorganisms, mostly anaerobes, humans usually need to take advantage of accumulation through the trophic chain in order to obtain a sufficient amount of Cbl from the diet. Ruminants benefit from the microbic biosynthesis of Cbl during vegetable fermentation by gastric microbiota. Thus ruminants accumulate more of the vitamin in their tissues than monogastric animals, such as poultry and pigs (Watanabe, 2007). Moreover, the bioaccumulation of Cbl in tissues is time-dependent so older cattle display higher concentrations of the vitamin (Williams, 2007). In addition, different cuts show variable concentrations depending on their oxidative or glycolytic metabolism tendency, as can be seen in Table 6.1. Red fibers type I (slow) have more mitochondria in the cytosol with a greater oxidative predisposition: on the one hand, cuts with a prevalence of white fibers type II (fast) have low concentrations of Cbl because of the glycolytic metabolism; on the other hand, lean meat has higher vitamin concentrations, due to the water solubility of Cbl (Ortigues-Marty et al., 2005). Table 6.2 summarizes the variability of Cbl concentrations among different species.

Cbl in food is usually photo- and thermolabile, so cooking oxidizes vitamins with the process enhanced in the presence of vitamin C, sulfites, and iron (Gille and Schmid, 2015).

The bioavailability of Cbl in milk seems to be higher compared to other animal food sources, despite its reduced concentration (Tucker et al., 2000). This phenomenon could depend on the vitamin fraction being bound to specific carriers that enhance absorption. Similarly to other food sources, thermal processing and storage in an oxidative environment decrease vitamin retention in milk (Gille and Schmid, 2015). During fermentation food processing some strains that are used for yogurt production (*Streptococcus thermophilus* and *Lactobacillus bulgaricus*) compete with Cbl utilization, thus reducing the final content (Arkbåge et al.,

Table 6.1 Variability of cobalamin (Cbl) (μg) concentration among cuts in different species.

Beef		Lamb	
Brisket	2.25	Foreshank	2.34
Rib eye steak	1.73	Leg	2.50
Shoulder top blade steak	4.33	Loin	2.04
Sirloin cap steak	2.64	Rib	2.09
Tenderloin	3.47	Shoulder	2.53
Pork		**Turkey**	
Leg (ham)	0.63	Breast	0.42
Shoulder	0.74	Leg	0.39
Sirloin	0.56	Wing	0.39
Spareribs	0.38		
Tenderloin	0.52		
Chicken		**Veal**	
Back	0.25	Leg (top round)	1.04
Breast	0.34	Loin	2.46
Drumstick	0.53	Rib	1.29
Leg	0.56	Shank	1.89
Thigh	0.62	Shoulder	1.67
Wing	0.25	Sirloin	1.27

Variability of Cbl concentrations in meat depends on species and cuts. Selected cuts (raw) from different species form US Department of Agriculture database are displayed.

Table 6.2 Mean and range of cobalamin (Cbl) concentration (μg) from different foods.

	Beef	Pork	Chicken	Lamb	Turkey	Veal
Mean	2.66	0.56	0.42	2.3	0.4	1.6
Range	1.73–4.33	0.38–0.74	0.25–0.62	2.04–2.53	0.39–0.42	1.04–2.46

The table summarizes means and range of Cbl concentrations of items from Table 6.1.

2003). However, some strains could be used in biotechnological production to improve Cbl retention in fermented products, and also plant-based products (Gu et al., 2015). In cheese production, the removal of the aqueous phase of whey decreases Cbl content in the final products (Arkbåge et al., 2003).

The highest source of Cbl is the liver, followed by the red meat of ruminants (Gille and Schmid, 2015). However, there is a reverse correlation between the concentration in food and bioavailability (Matte et al., 2012). The best way to absorb the highest fraction of Cbl is to spread discrete intakes of vitamin through the day to avoid the saturation of the absorption system (Allen, 2010).

Although there are official tables about Cbl contents in foods, there could be a wide variability among samples and among detection techniques used to quantify Cbl concentration. Different techniques have variable sensibilities to active and inactive vitamin forms (microbiological, HPLC, or radioisotope) (Gille and Schmid, 2015). Moreover, detailed US Department of Agriculture tables refer to Retail Cuts that could vary from European ones.

Microalgae are inadequate sources of Cbl because of the presence of recurrent inactive analogues (Watanabe, 2007). Inactive corrinoids are not useful for vitamin function and could also block chaperones that transport Cbl, so they cannot be available for active vitamin transport. Some plant foods could show small amounts of Cbl, due to an associated biofilm such as occurs for seaweed or fermented food like tempeh (Watanabe, 2007). Nevertheless, they cannot be considered reliable sources of Cbl because of a missed standardization of products; microorganisms able to perform the biosynthesis of the vitamin could not be represented in the starter pool. Currently, the dietary reference intake (DRI) for Cbl for the general population is 2.4 μg/day (Institute of Medicine, 1998). This requires a normal physiological absorption ability. Moreover, this quantity does not take into account the need of a single ingestion intake, such as in the case of supplementation in the vegetarian diet in the absence of other sources of Cbl or fortified foods. In a single ingestion, the limit of absorption depends on the saturation of transport system, which is capable of binding only 1.5–2 μg (Allen, 2010).

6.3 Absorption and transport through the body

A complex system of carriers escorts Cbl through extracellular fluids from the oral cavity to the final cellular site of utilization. These carriers have high affinity for Cbl but with different specificities that represent the pivotal characteristics of the transport system. Indeed it allows a selection of active molecules, avoiding the absorption of inadequate ones that could show antivitaminic effects.

Except when Cbl is taken as a supplement or by fortified foods (called the crystalline form), it can be found in the cofactorial (MetCbl and AdoCbl) form bound to food proteins or in the dissociated form after cooking or other processing (OHCbl).

The oral mucosa secretes the first carrier R-protein (transcobalamin I). This molecule binds Cbl after gastric dissociation from food. This protein protects Cbl from gastric acidity thanks to a glycosylated structure that is resistant to low pH (Hygum et al., 2011). This carrier has been found in various body fluids such as breast milk and plasma (Morkbak et al., 2007). With the progression to the duodenum, pancreatic proteases promote R-protein degradation with the release of Cbl that is promptly bonded to the second carrier secreted by gastric parietal cells: intrinsic factor (IF) or Castle factor. Also this protein protects the vitamin from enzymatic digestion, a theory that it is supported by the presence of a lot of glycosylation sites in the amino acid sequence (Gordon et al., 1991). In this scenario, different carriers have variable specificity: R-binder is a massive ligand with low specificity that binds also inactive nonvitamin corrinoids, such as a cobinamide that has lost a DMB group; despite IF being secreted in limited quantities, it has a high specificity for vitamin forms with intact DMB groups (Quadros, 2010). The rapid turnover of IF allows the regeneration of the most critical carriers to avoid the persistence of blocked forms by inactive corrinoids. In the terminal ileum, the IF–Cbl complex is internalized by the cubam receptor complex with a receptor-mediated endocytosis process, which is very specific for IF–Cbl, on the luminal side of a polarized enterocyte (Birn et al., 1997).

The cubam complex is located on the brush border of enterocytes and it is composed of a transmembrane domain formed by the amnionless protein (AMN) of 48 kDa that drives internalization, and an extrinsic protein of 460 kDa called cubilin that binds the IF–Cbl complex. Both proteins of the cubam complex are expressed also on the apical membrane of the proximal tubule cells of the kidney and on the visceral side of the yolk sac (Sahali et al., 1988).

After endocytosis, IF is degraded in the lysosome and Cbl crosses the intracellular lysosomial membrane with the help of LMBRD1, a transmembrane protein of 61 kDa (Rutsch et al., 2009). A schematic representation of the absorption process of Cbl is displayed in Fig. 6.2.

In the cytoplasm, Cbl follows cellular utilization or the release from the basolateral side of the enterocyte before entering the blood flow. The gateway for Cbl into the body fluids after digestion is thought to be the

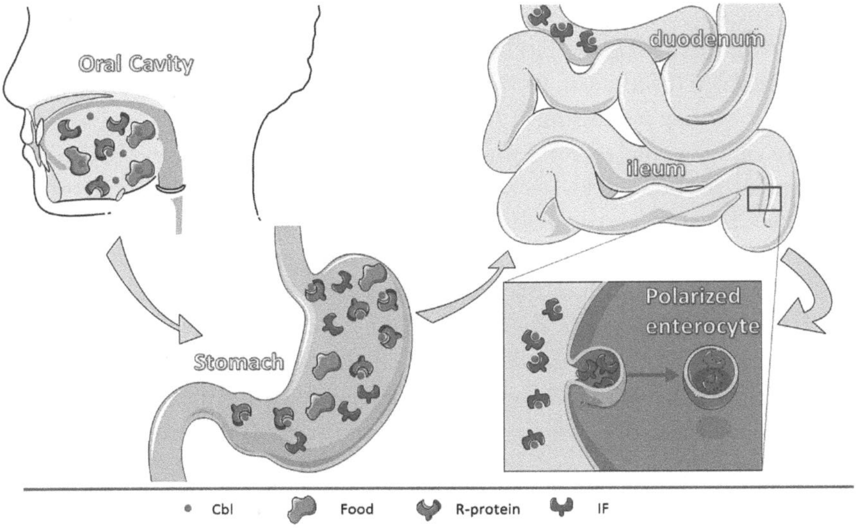

Figure 6.2 Cobalamin uptake.
The absorption process of Cbl from the oral cavity to cellular uptake is displayed. *Modified from Servier Medical Art database by Servier (Creative Commons 3.0).*

multispecific membrane transporter of 190 kDa called multidrug resistance protein 1 (MRP1) (Beedholm-Ebsen et al., 2010). However, the presence of another transporter not yet described or passive diffusion of Cbl in its free form could be possible (Deeley et al., 2006). The mechanism is not well understood, but it is known that Cbl is yielded to the blood carriers transcobalamin II (TCII) and haptocorrin (HC). As occurs for the transporter couple R-binder/IF, these two proteins also have different affinities for the vitamin with a selective significance. TCII is secreted by vascular endothelial cells and binds Cbl with high selectivity to form a complex called holotranscobalamin II (HTCII), which is the circulating bioavailable fraction of the vitamin (Quadros et al., 1989). The remaining Cbl, about 80% of the total blood vitamin, is bound to HC (Seetharam and Yammani, 2003). The function of HC is not well understood, but in light of its low selectivity compared to TCII, it is proposed to have a role in the removal of damaged vitamin molecules or has a vitamin reservoir function (Kanazawa et al., 1983). In fact a reverse transport to the liver is thought because HC receptors are characterized only on hepatocytes' membranes (Mørkbak et al., 2006). However, active molecules captured by reverse transport could be recovered by enterohepatic circulation.

Some microbe strains of gut microbiota are able to biosynthesize Cbl. However, in human feces Cbl is found mostly in the inactive form. Even if the active vitamin could be present in the gut after biosynthesis by symbiotic bacteria, the terminal tract of the bowel is far from the site of IF-mediated absorption. This means that the excess Cbl not bound to IF is lost with the progression to the distal tract of the gut and this phenomenon minimizes acute toxicity events in the case of a higher intake through food or supplements.

Cbl is a water-soluble vitamin, so the excess absorbed is then excreted with urine. There is a reuptake system in the proximal tubule of the kidney that recovers the vitamin through a 600 kDa protein called megalin or low-density lipoprotein receptor-related protein 2. Cbl can follow the cellular storage or bloodstream restitution. It was proposed that there is an interaction with the cubam complex coexpressed in this kidney cytotype. Megalin has high specificity for HTCII that justifies its role in the selection of active forms from urine (Nielsen et al., 2012).

The sophisticated uptake—reuptake process of Cbl allows an efficient economy of vitamin, so if there is a low intake the clinical signs of deficiency need many years to become overt. However, in the case of rapid utilization (such as in infancy or pregnancy) or when absorptive capacity is limited, the manifestation of the shortage speeds up.

The method of delivery to the central nervous system (CNS) is largely unknown, even if the neurological effects of Cbl deficiency have been widely explored.

6.4 Cellular trafficking and metabolism

Cbl enters peripheral cells via a receptor-mediated endocytosis process that involves a 58 kDa protein called CD320 or TCb1R, which belongs to the same receptor family as megalin and the LDL receptor (Quadros and Sequeira, 2013). CD320 is modulated by cellular proliferative signals that suggest the importance of Cbl in cellular replication (Amagasaki et al., 1990). In the lysosome, TCII is degraded and the receptor is recycled to the membrane to make it available again to bind a new Cbl molecule. Leaving the intracellular organelle, Cbl enters the cytoplasm to follow the cellular trafficking that adopts an articulated system of chaperones to deliver activated vitamin cofactor to the final molecular targets. In recent decades the understanding of this pathway has had progressed rapidly due to new molecular techniques that use cell cultures of fibroblasts. Rare inborn mutations of genetic loci encoding for cellular chaperones of Cbl gave the opportunity to understand the multistep pathway from internalization to utilization.

The passage through the lysosomal membrane is mediated by LMBRD1 and ABCD4 proteins, products of genetic loci cblF and cblJ, respectively (Coelho et al., 2012). Within the cytoplasm, Cbl is promptly engaged by the first cytosolic chaperone MMACHC (methylmalonic aciduria type C and homocystinuria), a product of the cblC locus. This molecule is capable of carrying out the dealkylation of alkylcobalamins MetCbl and AdoCbl, mediating also the decyanation of CNCbl. This wide specificity of MMACHC for Cbl with different β-axial ligands highlights the pivotal role of this chaperone molecule (Kim et al., 2008). In detail, this protein uses a glutathione molecule for the dealkylation reaction while it needs a reduced flavin molecule for decyanation (Kim et al., 2008, 2009). Cbl in its provitaminic form (without an upper ligand) can follow the cytosolic pathway acquiring a methyl group, or the mitochondrial pathway where it will be transformed into AdoCbl. In the cytoplasm the OHCbl is engaged by MMADHC (methylmalonic aciduria type D and homocystinuria), a product of the cblD locus. This protein escorts the provitamin to methionine synthase reductase (MSR), a product of the cblE locus, which is the enzyme responsible for MetCbl formation (Coelho et al., 2008). MSR interacts with methionine synthase (MS), a product of the cblG locus, which catalyzes the transfer of a methyl group from N5-methyltetrahydrofolate to a homocysteine (HCY) molecule. MS is one of the two final molecular targets for the Cbl utilization currently known in mammals (Matthews et al., 2008). The catalytic reaction consists of two steps, during which methionine and Cbl(CoI) are generated as reaction intermediates. In a second step, the MetCbl is regenerated with the transformation of N5-methyltetrahydrofolate to tetrahydrofolate. Cbl (CoI) is one of the most reactive compounds currently known and this is why it is called a "supernucleophile" (Schrauzer and Deutsch, 1969). The role of MSR is to intercept molecules of Cbl occasionally oxidated to Cbl (CoII) in order to catalyze their reactivation through reductive methylation, using *S*-adenosylmethionine as a methyl group donor and NADPH as an electron donor. The methyl transfer is an exothermic reaction and drives the unfavorable coupled reduction (Banerjee et al., 1990).

The access to the mitochondrion could be mediated by a not yet characterized transporter, although passive diffusion from cytoplasm to mitochondrial trafficking machinery is not excluded. In the mitochondrial matrix, the provitamin without an upper ligand is engaged by MMAB (methylmalonic aciduria type B), the ATP-dependent Cbl adenosyltransferase that is the product of the cblB locus, and that catalyzes the formation of AdoCbl (Leal et al., 2003). MMAB transfers AdoCbl to methylmalonyl-CoA mutase (MCM), the protein product of the *mut* locus, that is the final mitochondrial molecular target of coenzyme Cbl, one of the only two Cbl utilizer proteins known, together with the aforementioned cytosolic MS.

There is another mitochondrial protein involved in the Cbl pathway. Methylmalonic aciduria type A (MMAA) is the product of the cblA locus and has the role of maintaining Cbl in the AdoCbl active form for the catalytic cycle (Froese and Gravel, 2010). MMAA is a GTPase with the function of expelling Cbl(CoII) from the active site of MCM. This happens when occasionally 5′-deoxyadenosine groups escape from Cbl during the catalytic cycle, by blocking the enzyme (Padovani and Banerjee, 2009). Schematic cellular trafficking of Cbl is displayed in Fig. 6.3. Table 6.3 summarizes proteins involved in Cbl transport, trafficking, and metabolism.

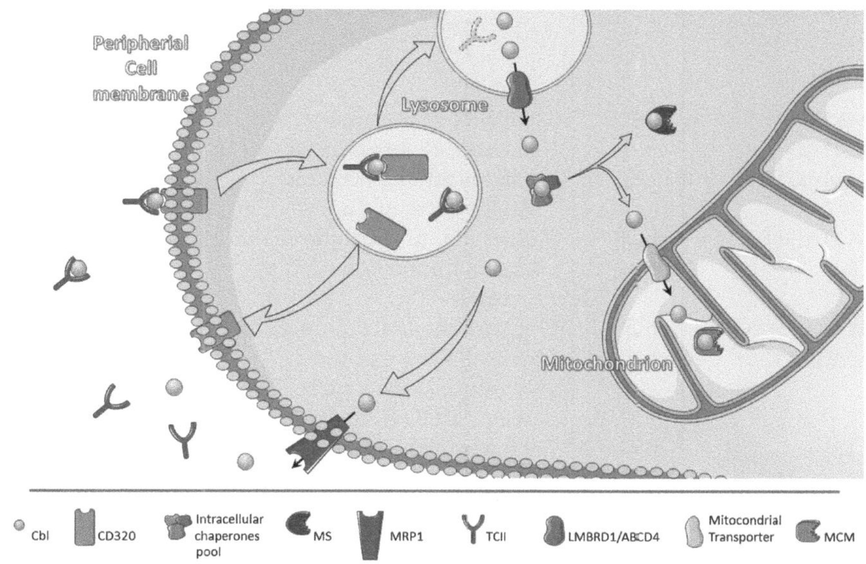

Figure 6.3 Cellular trafficking.
After the cellular uptake of Cbl, a complex pool of chaperones escorts the vitamin to the final enzymes. During these pathways, Cbl is deprived form β-axial ligand and equipped with specific residue to obtain vitamin isoforms. *Modified from Servier Medical Art database by Servier (Creative Commons 3.0).*

Table 6.3 Proteins (and their loci) involved in cobalamin (Cbl) homeostasis and trafficking.

Protein	Locus	Function	Location
R-protein		Binds free Cbl	Oral cavity and stomach
Intrinsic factor		Binds Cbl released from food	Small intestine
AMN	*AMN*	Mediates Cbl-IF internalization (cubam complex)	Enterocyte of the terminal ileum, apical side
Cubilin	*CUMN*	Binds Cbl-IF for the internalization (cubam complex)	Enterocyte of the terminal ileum, apical side
MRP1		Mediates the enter into blood flow	Enterocyte, basolateral side
Transcobalamin II		Transports Cbl through blood flow	Blood
Haptocorrin		Binds Cbl in blood, maybe for an inverse transport to liver	Blood
CD320		Binds Cbl-TCII and mediates its internalization	Peripheral cell membrane
Megalin		Mediates kidney reabsorption	Cell of renal proximal tubule, apical side
MMAA	cblA	Mediates adenosilation of Cbl	Mitochondrion
MMAB	cblB	Catalyzes adenosilation of Cbl	Mitochondrion
MMACHC	cblC	Catalyzes the decyaniation or dealkylation of Cbl	Cytosol
MMADHC	cblD	Routes Cbl to the intracellular destiny (mitochondrion or cytosol)	Cytosol
MSR	cblE	Catalyzes methylation of Cbl	Cytosol
LMBRD1	cblF	Escorts Cbl for exit the lysosome (in a complex with ABCD4)	Lysosomal membrane
MS	cblG	Catalyzes methylation of homocysteine using Cbl as cofactor	Cytosol
ABCD4	cblJ	Escorts Cbl for exit the lysosome (in a complex with LMBRD1)	Lysosomal membrane
MCM	*mut*	Synthesizes succinyl-CoA form methylmalonyl-CoA using Cbl as cofactor	Mitochondrion

Function and tissue location of factors involved in absorption, trafficking, and metabolism of Cbl. Complementation loci are also displayed.

MS has a pivotal role in methyl transfer reactions so it is crucial for nucleic acids synthesis. If one of the cofactors of the enzyme pool (including Cbl) is missing, the metabolic cycle is blocked by the accumulation of by-products of reactions such as HCY.

MCM is an enzyme of odd-chain fatty acids degradation. It is involved also in metabolic pathways of branched-chain amino acids and cholesterol. It catalyzes the conversion of methylmalonyl-CoA into succinyl-CoA, which can enter the Krebs cycle for catabolic utilization. The Krebs cycle accepts only two-carbon molecules so odd-chain fatty acids could not be completely catabolized without this pathway involving the Cbl cofactor. In the absence of AdoCbl, there is an accumulation of methylmalonic acid (MMA) as a by-product.

The central cobalt atom of Cbl structure can exist in three oxidative states (III), (II), and (I), that allow different coordination ligands: six, five, and four, respectively. The conformational state of Cbl is crucial for engagement to chaperones and for adequate intracellular trafficking. In fact in physiological conditions, the DMB group is coordinated to cobalt. This conformation is called "base-on" and protects the molecule from spurious reactivity. The protonation of DMB at low pH allows a change in conformation from "base-on" to "base-off." However, there is another conformational state in which Cbl is bound to a target protein with a "base-off/his-on" in which a histidine residue of the client protein (MS or MCM) is linked to a cobalt atom. This conformation enables the ready utilization of the cofactor in a catalytic process by controlling at the same time its reactivity (Banerjee, 2006). The lability of the β-axial coordination bond is pivotal for cofactor reactivity and the upper ligand shows different bond dissociation energies (Gherasim et al., 2013). IF and TCII bind Cbl only in the base-on conformation, while intracellular carriers MMAB and MMACHC bind vitamin in the base-off conformation, probably because of a higher reactivity of the β-axial position (Gherasim et al., 2013).

6.5 Cobalamin shortage and deficiency processes

If there are animal foods in the diet, the Cbl requirement is easily granted by physiological mechanisms (Allen, 2008). Unfortunately DRI does not take into account the variability in bioavailability of the vitamin in different foods, impairments in absorption capability, increased needs in shortage situations, and the net absorption in the case of a single-dose intake (Allen, 2009). Intakes far above the DRI show improvements in blood markers with better outcomes among older adults (Dullemeijer et al., 2013). Apart from the shortages in the case of inborn defects on loci encoding transporters and chaperone proteins, there is a diffused deficiency state among the population that depends on malnutrition or a vegetarian diet without correct planning and supplementation. Cbl deficiency is typical of low-income countries and among elderly people worldwide because of absorption disturbances (Dali-Youcef and Andrès, 2009; McLean et al., 2008). There are also some clues that a global vitamin insufficiency has an impact on childhood and among women at reproductive age (Allen, 2009). During pregnancy and breastfeeding the transfer of Cbl to the fetus and the infant is crucial, and when the offspring is female it could establish a transgenerational deficiency which self-implements over time. The massive utilization of Cbl for cellular replication processes rapidly decreases vitamin deposits in the case of an inadequate intake (Green et al., 2017). Vitamin requirements are still important in infancy and adolescence and the shortage in these ages is a source of concern (de Benoist, 2008).

Even if PA, a historical pathology of Cbl deficiency, manifests with hematological and neurological signs, often the former could be absent and only CNS dysfunctions could appear during severe shortage (Lindenbaum et al., 1988). Neurological mechanisms need to be better understood but the role of Cbl is suggested by hyperhomocysteinemia involvement in neurotoxic pathways (Fuso and Scarpa, 2011).

The coexistence of Cbl deficiency and dementia with high frequency in senescence suggests multiple mechanisms of correlation between these two phenomena. The most harmful neurological effect of vitamin shortage is characterized by the demyelination of central and peripheral nerves, mostly irreversibly (Stabler, 2013).

Even if there are commercial isoforms of Cbl with different upper axial ligands, the most used form for fortification and supplement formulation is the crystal one (CNCbl), because of its safety and cheapness. Moreover, this provitaminic isoform has a good stability compared to the thermal- and photolability of alkylcobalamins that easily lose the DMB group because of the weak cobalt—carbon bond (Waddington and Finke, 1993). There is no advantage in using alkylcobalamins in place of CNCbl because, as already described above, the decyanation reaction is efficiently carried out by intracellular enzymatic machinery. The CblC complementation group of inborn errors is responsive only to OHCbl because of the inability of decyanation or dealkylation of the Cbl consumed (Andersson and Shapira, 1998).

The shortage of Cbl is more frequent in low-income countries, mostly due to insufficient nutrition or microbial infections (Yajnik et al., 2006). Vegetarians who do not take Cbl supplements or consume fortified foods show deficiency states with variable severity (Rizzo et al., 2016).

The American Institute of Medicine suggests supplementation with crystal Cbl in older people, because of an impaired absorptive functionality typical of this age, and define a vitamin bioavailability of about 50% in supplements (Institute of Medicine, 1998). Usually, these absorption issues depend on low gastric acidity that causes a food-bound malabsorption with the inability to dissociate Cbl from food proteins but without involving an IF dysfunction. The preserved IF activity allows a responsiveness to a physiological dosage of Cbl in a crystal form via the oral route.

Over 80 years old, the prevalence of Cbl deficiency can reach 23%–25% (Johnson et al., 2010).

In the case of PA, Cbl hypovitaminosis is caused by anti-IF or antiparietal antibodies that disrupt receptor-mediated endocytosis. This pathology can affect all ages but it is more frequent after 65 years old (Carmel, 1996). This clinical picture is coherent with the inability of the physiological oral intake of Cbl to grant the vitamin requirement.

Megadoses of oral Cbl can be still absorbed even with PA, due to passive diffusion of Cbl at very high dosage that concerns 1% of total amount taken in a single dose (Berlin et al., 1968). Oral treatment has advantages for compliance for patients and for logistical aspects compared to treatment with injections that often requires the involvement of professional care. Currently, there is no defined tolerable upper intake level for Cbl (Tucker et al., 2000).

Small intestinal bacterial overgrowth or other infections (*Helicobacter pylori, Giardia lamblia*, malaria, or tuberculosis) could promote deficiency through competition with vitamin absorption by microbes. Usually treatments for infection eradication resolve the shortage (Premkumar et al., 2012).

Ileal or gastric resections favor the establishment of clinically evident Cbl deficiency with a spectrum resembling food-bound malabsorption to PA because of reduced absorption, secretive alteration, or disturbance of enterohepatic circulation.

Celiac disease and inflammatory bowel disease can influence absorption processes, especially in the acute phase. Also alcoholism and prolonged pharmacological treatments could interfere with various steps of Cbl absorption. Proton pump inhibitors attenuate the gastric acidity needed for the release of the vitamin from food and the following engagement by IF, while metformin interferes with Cbl internalization by sequestering calcium that is needed for endocytic cubam receptor process (Bauman et al., 2000). Cholestyramine, colchicine, and some antibiotics can block IF (Green et al., 2017).

Currently, there is no consensus or gold standard for adequate markers of Cbl deficiency. Taking into account that total blood Cbl concentration cannot discriminate between the active and inactive vitamin (bound to HC for reverse transport), low–normal blood concentrations are not preventive for Cbl shortage. Moreover, some hepatic and myeloproliferative diseases can raise blood HC (Arendt and Nexo, 2013). So in the process of evaluation for Cbl adequacy it could be helpful to verify normal hepatic functionality. Occasionally blood concentrations of Cbl show normal levels in diagnosed PA (Carmel and Agrawal, 2012). To better understand the vitamin status, it could be useful to measure HTCII, the only available form for cellular uptake (Nexo and Hoffmann-Lücke, 2011). However, total Cbl and HTCII are not adequate as markers for follow-up improvements during treatments because of their rapid rise after Cbl injection (Carmel, 2008). There are also functional markers, namely HCY and MMA, that are useful to verify cellular sufficiency (Green, 1995). Both markers can rise in the case of renal insufficiency, so an interpretation of their blood levels could be puzzling in older age (Loikas et al., 2007). Moreover, HCY increases also in the case of the shortage of other B vitamins, such as folate (vitamin B9) and pyridoxine (vitamin B6). Conversely, in the case of small intestinal bacterial overgrowth there is an increase of MMA in blood flow that can confuse the diagnosis. The increase in MMA may depend on bacterial propionate production captured by a portal system that acts as an MMA precursor (Leonard, 1997). Translocation of microbes to the upper intestinal tract can compete with Cbl utilization and produce inactive corrinoids that could distort blood Cbl detection by hiding a shortage below a normal apparent concentration (Degnan et al., 2014). Cbl heterotrophic utilization can take place in blind loop syndrome after the creation of surgical anastomosis. An increase of propionate also could derive from odd-chain fatty acids degradation from milk, thus affecting the utility of this marker in nursling infants (Monsen et al., 2003).

Even if not so specific there are other useful hematic markers in the case of Cbl shortage, because of the influence of this vitamin in cell replication. Mean corpuscular volume (MCV) is one of the signs of macrocytic anemia in the case of hematopoiesis disturbance (Stabler, 2013). However, iron deficiency anemia causes microcytemia so it can mask this marker utility. Cbl deficiency can also disturb hematopoiesis of leukocytes by causing hypersegmented neutrophils. The progression of the shortage causes pancytopenia.

Using various blood markers may have enhanced the comprehension of metabolic pathways that use Cbl for a better prevention of a deficit by identifying the transition from subclinical to shortage conditions (Green et al., 2017). Nevertheless, from another point of view, these tools can cause overdiagnosis and overprescription, in some cases without any clinical relevance (Carmel and Sarrai, 2006).

Herbert proposed the use of multiple markers to define a staging of Cbl deficiency in vegetarians (Herbert, 1994). Even if there are different cutoff values depending on diagnostic method used or clinical reference method, Herrmann proposed a particularly higher threshold for total blood Cbl to define deficiency among vegetarians (Herrmann and Geisel, 2002).

Underestimating deficiency without an adequate program of treatment can lead to serious dysfunctions such as megaloblastic anemia and neurological disorders that can cause death.

There is a good characterization of inherited genetic defects of cellular trafficking but there is still 15%–20% of malabsorption caused by unknown recessive inborn errors that needs to be clarified by the characterization of other pivotal proteins (Shah et al., 2011).

6.6 How other vitamins are affected or behave

The B vitamins are a group of water-soluble vitamins not necessarily linked by structure homology but with interconnected metabolic functions in catabolic and anabolic pathways, in particular regarding one-carbon metabolism (Kennedy, 2016).

Even if the involvement of Cbl, folate, and pyridoxine in the HCY cycle is widely known and explored, the contribution of other B vitamins is often underestimated. For example, riboflavin (vitamin B2) is the coenzyme of methyltetrahydrofolate reductase, while niacin (vitamin B3) is converted to NAD and used as a cofactor for dihydrofolate reductase and *S*-adenosylhomocysteine hydrolase. Moreover, while interconnection among Cbl and folate in dementia has been highlighted (Reynolds, 2006), niacin also seems to have a role in Parkinson disease (Wakade et al., 2015).

Treatments with a pool of B vitamins seem to better improve HCY status than the use of just a single vitamin (Haskell et al., 2010).

The interplay between Cbl and folate is still debated. The folate trap is a phenomenon in which an elevation of serum folate depends on an HCY blockage because of Cbl shortage. Folate accumulates in the methyltetrahydrofolate form without the chance of a methyl transfer (Reynolds, 2006). In this case the high blood folate does not ensure repletion of peripheral cell deposits.

The rise of HCY in high-income countries often reflects a low folate status (Monsen et al., 2003). In countries with mandatory fortification program of flours with folate, HCY better reflects Cbl status (Green and Miller, 2005).

Cbl and folate have other interactions that are still unknown, such as the effect of folate supplementation when there is a Cbl deficiency. There is a higher risk of anemia and cognitive impairment in patients with low blood concentration of Cbl and high concentration of folate than in patients with low Cbl but normal folate (Morris et al., 2007). Moreover, a high intake of folate can mask early hematic signs of a Cbl shortage (MCV and hypersegmented neutrophils), delaying the diagnosis and increasing the risk of neurological damage and therefore of possible irreversible damage (Campbell, 1996). There are some clues suggested with the worsening neurological status in patients with a Cbl shortage after the intake of folate supplements, even with hematological improvement (Brito et al., 2016). These aspects need to be clarified carefully, taking into account that some countries have a fortification policy to prevent congenital malformation but that can cause uncontrolled vitamin intakes. This phenomenon could confuse the differential diagnosis and even worsen some medical aspects. Epidemiological and clinical trial studies focused on a subgroup of B vitamins are still needed, but some clues suggest a wider interdependence among B vitamins and there is the possibility that a more concerted approach to vitamin deficiency could be useful (Kennedy, 2016).

References

Allen, L.H., 2008. Causes of vitamin B12 and folate deficiency. Food Nutr. Bull. 29, . Available from: https://doi.org/10.1177/15648265080292S105S20-34-37.

Allen, L.H., 2009. How common is vitamin B-12 deficiency? Am. J. Clin. Nutr. 89, 693S–696SS. Available from: https://doi.org/10.3945/ajcn.2008.26947A.

Allen, L.H., 2010. Bioavailability of vitamin B12. Int. J. Vitam. Nutr. Res. 80, 330–335. Available from: https://doi.org/10.1024/0300-9831/a000041.

Amagasaki, T., Green, R., Jacobsen, D.W., 1990. Expression of transcobalamin II receptors by human leukemia K562 and HL-60 cells. Blood 76, 1380–1386.
Andersson, H.C., Shapira, E., 1998. Biochemical and clinical response to hydroxocobalamin versus cyanocobalamin treatment in patients with methylmalonic acidemia and homocystinuria (cblC). J. Pediatr. 132, 121–124.
Arendt, J.F.B., Nexo, E., 2013. Unexpected high plasma cobalamin : proposal for a diagnostic strategy. Clin. Chem. Lab. Med. 51, 489–496. Available from: https://doi.org/10.1515/cclm-2012-0545.
Arkbåge, K., Witthöft, C., Fondén, R., Jägerstad, M., 2003. Retention of vitamin B12 during manufacture of six fermented dairy products using a validated radio protein-binding assay. Int. Dairy J. 13, 101–109. Available from: https://doi.org/10.1016/S0958-6946(02)00146-2.
Banerjee, R., 2006. B12 trafficking in mammals: a for coenzyme escort service. ACS Chem. Biol. 1, 149–159. Available from: https://doi.org/10.1021/cb6001174.
Banerjee, R.V., Harder, S.R., Ragsdale, S.W., Matthews, R.G., 1990. Mechanism of reductive activation of cobalamin-dependent methionine synthase: an electron paramagnetic resonance spectroelectrochemical study. Biochemistry (Mosc) 29, 1129–1135.
Bauman, W.A., Shaw, S., Jayatilleke, E., Spungen, A.M., Herbert, V., 2000. Increased intake of calcium reverses vitamin B12 malabsorption induced by metformin. Diabetes Care 23, 1227–1231.
Beedholm-Ebsen, R., van de Wetering, K., Hardlei, T., Nexø, E., Borst, P., Moestrup, S.K., 2010. Identification of multidrug resistance protein 1 (MRP1/ABCC1) as a molecular gate for cellular export of cobalamin. Blood 115, 1632–1639. Available from: https://doi.org/10.1182/blood-2009-07-232587.
Berlin, H., Berlin, R., Brante, G., 1968. Oral treatment of pernicious anemia with high doses of vitamin B12 without intrinsic factor. Acta Med. Scand. 184, 247–258.
Birn, H., Verroust, P.J., Nexo, E., Hager, H., Jacobsen, C., Christensen, E.I., et al., 1997. Characterization of an epithelial approximately 460-kDa protein that facilitates endocytosis of intrinsic factor-vitamin B12 and binds receptor-associated protein. J. Biol. Chem. 272, 26497–26504.
Brito, A., Verdugo, R., Hertrampf, E., Miller, J.W., Green, R., Fedosov, S.N., et al., 2016. Vitamin B-12 treatment of asymptomatic, deficient, elderly Chileans improves conductivity in myelinated peripheral nerves, but high serum folate impairs vitamin B-12 status response assessed by the combined indicator of vitamin B-12 status. Am. J. Clin. Nutr. 103, 250–257. Available from: https://doi.org/10.3945/ajcn.115.116509.
Campbell, N.R., 1996. How safe are folic acid supplements? Arch. Intern. Med. 156, 1638–1644.
Carmel, R., 1996. Prevalence of undiagnosed pernicious anemia in the elderly. Arch. Intern. Med. 156, 1097–1100.
Carmel, R., 2008. How I treat cobalamin (vitamin B12) deficiency. Blood 112, 2214–2221. Available from: https://doi.org/10.1182/blood-2008-03-040253.
Carmel, R., Agrawal, Y.P., 2012. Failures of cobalamin assays in pernicious anemia. N. Engl. J. Med. 367, 385–386. Available from: https://doi.org/10.1056/NEJMc1204070.
Carmel, R., Sarrai, M., 2006. Diagnosis and management of clinical and subclinical cobalamin deficiency: advances and controversies. Curr. Hematol. Rep. 5, 23–33.
Coelho, D., Suormala, T., Stucki, M., Lerner-Ellis, J.P., Rosenblatt, D.S., Newbold, R. F., et al., 2008. Gene identification for the cblD defect of vitamin B12 metabolism. N. Engl. J. Med. 358, 1454–1464. Available from: https://doi.org/10.1056/NEJMoa072200.
Coelho, D., Kim, J.C., Miousse, I.R., Fung, S., du Moulin, M., Buers, I., et al., 2012. Mutations in ABCD4 cause a new inborn error of vitamin B12 metabolism. Nat. Genet. 44, 1152–1155. Available from: https://doi.org/10.1038/ng.2386.

Dali-Youcef, N., Andrès, E., 2009. An update on cobalamin deficiency in adults. QJM 102, 17–28. Available from: https://doi.org/10.1093/qjmed/hcn138.
de Benoist, B., 2008. Conclusions of a WHO Technical Consultation on folate and vitamin B12 deficiencies. Food Nutr. Bull. 29, S238–S244. Available from: https://doi.org/10.1177/15648265080292S129.
Deeley, R.G., Westlake, C., Cole, S.P.C., 2006. Transmembrane transport of endo- and xenobiotics by mammalian ATP-binding cassette multidrug resistance proteins. Physiol. Rev. 86, 849–899. Available from: https://doi.org/10.1152/physrev.00035.2005.
Degnan, P.H., Taga, M.E., Goodman, A.L., 2014. Vitamin B12 as a modulator of gut microbial ecology. Cell Metab. 20, 769–778. Available from: https://doi.org/10.1016/j.cmet.2014.10.002.
Dullemeijer, C., Souverein, O.W., Doets, E.L., van der Voet, H., van Wijngaarden, J.P., de Boer, W.J., et al., 2013. Systematic review with dose-response meta-analyses between vitamin B-12 intake and European Micronutrient Recommendations Aligned's prioritized biomarkers of vitamin B-12 including randomized controlled trials and observational studies in adults and elderly persons. Am. J. Clin. Nutr. 97, 390–402. Available from: https://doi.org/10.3945/ajcn.112.033951.
Froese, D.S., Gravel, R.A., 2010. Genetic disorders of vitamin B_{12} metabolism: eight complementation groups—eight genes. Expert Rev. Mol. Med. 12, e37. Available from: https://doi.org/10.1017/S1462399410001651.
Fuso, A., Scarpa, S., 2011. One-carbon metabolism and Alzheimer's disease: is it all a methylation matter? Neurobiol. Aging 32, 1192–1195. Available from: https://doi.org/10.1016/j.neurobiolaging.2011.01.012.
Gherasim, C., Lofgren, M., Banerjee, R., 2013. Navigating the B(12) road: assimilation, delivery, and disorders of cobalamin. J. Biol. Chem. 288, 13186–13193. Available from: https://doi.org/10.1074/jbc.R113.458810.
Gille, D., Schmid, A., 2015. Vitamin B12 in meat and dairy products. Nutr. Rev. 73, 106–115. Available from: https://doi.org/10.1093/nutrit/nuu011.
Gordon, M.M., Hu, C., Chokshi, H., Hewitt, J.E., Alpers, D.H., 1991. Glycosylation is not required for ligand or receptor binding by expressed rat intrinsic factor. Am. J. Physiol. 260, G736–G742. Available from: https://doi.org/10.1152/ajpgi.1991.260.5.G736.
Green, R., 1995. Metabolite assays in cobalamin and folate deficiency. Baillieres Clin. Haematol. 8, 533–566.
Green, R., Miller, J.W., 2005. Vitamin B12 deficiency is the dominant nutritional cause of hyperhomocysteinemia in a folic acid-fortified population. Clin. Chem. Lab. Med. 43, 1048–1051. Available from: https://doi.org/10.1515/CCLM.2005.183.
Green, R., Allen, L.H., Bjørke-Monsen, A.-L., Brito, A., Guéant, J.-L., Miller, J.W., et al., 2017. Vitamin B12 deficiency. Nat. Rev. Dis. Primer 3, 17040. Available from: https://doi.org/10.1038/nrdp.2017.40.
Gu, Q., Zhang, C., Song, D., Li, P., Zhu, X., 2015. Enhancing vitamin B12 content in soy-yogurt by *Lactobacillus reuteri*. Int. J. Food Microbiol. 206, 56–59. Available from: https://doi.org/10.1016/j.ijfoodmicro.2015.04.033.
Haskell, C.F., Robertson, B., Jones, E., Forster, J., Jones, R., Wilde, A., et al., 2010. Effects of a multi-vitamin/mineral supplement on cognitive function and fatigue during extended multi-tasking. Hum. Psychopharmacol. 25, 448–461. Available from: https://doi.org/10.1002/hup.1144.
Herbert, V., 1994. Staging vitamin B-12 (cobalamin) status in vegetarians. Am. J. Clin. Nutr. 59, 1213S–1222S. Available from: https://doi.org/10.1093/ajcn/59.5.1213S.
Herrmann, W., Geisel, J., 2002. Vegetarian lifestyle and monitoring of vitamin B-12 status. Clin. Chim. Acta Int. J. Clin. Chem. 326, 47–59.
Hygum, K., Lildballe, D.L., Greibe, E.H., Morkbak, A.L., Poulsen, S.S., Sorensen, B.S., et al., 2011. Mouse transcobalamin has features resembling both human

transcobalamin and haptocorrin. PLoS One 6, e20638. Available from: https://doi.org/10.1371/journal.pone.0020638.
Institute of Medicine, 1998. Dietary Reference Intakes for Thiamin, Riboflavin, Niacin, Vitamin B6, Folate, Vitamin B12, Pantothenic Acid, Biotin, and Choline, The National Academies Collection: Reports funded by National Institutes of Health. National Academies Press, Washington, DC.
Johnson, M.A., Hausman, D.B., Davey, A., Poon, L.W., Allen, R.H., Stabler, S.P., et al., 2010. Vitamin B12 deficiency in African American and white octogenarians and centenarians in Georgia. J. Nutr. Health Aging 14, 339–345.
Kanazawa, S., Herbert, V., Herzlich, B., Drivas, G., Manusselis, C., 1983. Removal of cobalamin analogue in bile by enterohepatic circulation of vitamin B12. Lancet Lond. Engl. 1, 707–708.
Kennedy, D.O., 2016. B vitamins and the brain: mechanisms, dose and efficacy—a review. Nutrients 8, 68. Available from: https://doi.org/10.3390/nu8020068.
Kim, J., Gherasim, C., Banerjee, R., 2008. Decyanation of vitamin B12 by a trafficking chaperone. Proc. Natl. Acad. Sci. U.S.A. 105, 14551–14554. Available from: https://doi.org/10.1073/pnas.0805989105.
Kim, J., Hannibal, L., Gherasim, C., Jacobsen, D.W., Banerjee, R., 2009. A human vitamin B12 trafficking protein uses glutathione transferase activity for processing alkylcobalamins. J. Biol. Chem. 284, 33418–33424. Available from: https://doi.org/10.1074/jbc.M109.057877.
Leal, N.A., Park, S.D., Kima, P.E., Bobik, T.A., 2003. Identification of the human and bovine ATP:Cob(I)alamin adenosyltransferase cDNAs based on complementation of a bacterial mutant. J. Biol. Chem. 278, 9227–9234. Available from: https://doi.org/10.1074/jbc.M212739200.
Leonard, J.V., 1997. Stable isotope studies in propionic and methylmalonic acidaemia. Eur. J. Pediatr. 156 (Suppl. 1), S67–S69.
Lindenbaum, J., Healton, E.B., Savage, D.G., Brust, J.C., Garrett, T.J., Podell, E.R., et al., 1988. Neuropsychiatric disorders caused by cobalamin deficiency in the absence of anemia or macrocytosis. N. Engl. J. Med. 318, 1720–1728. Available from: https://doi.org/10.1056/NEJM198806303182604.
Loikas, S., Koskinen, P., Irjala, K., Löppönen, M., Isoaho, R., Kivelä, S.-L., et al., 2007. Renal impairment compromises the use of total homocysteine and methylmalonic acid but not total vitamin B12 and holotranscobalamin in screening for vitamin B12 deficiency in the aged. Clin. Chem. Lab. Med. 45, 197–201. Available from: https://doi.org/10.1515/CCLM.2007.028.
Martens, J.H., Barg, H., Warren, M.J., Jahn, D., 2002. Microbial production of vitamin B12. Appl. Microbiol. Biotechnol. 58, 275–285. Available from: https://doi.org/10.1007/s00253-001-0902-7.
Matte, J.J., Guay, F., Girard, C.L., 2012. Bioavailability of vitamin B_{12} in cows' milk. Br. J. Nutr. 107, 61–66. Available from: https://doi.org/10.1017/S0007114511002364.
Matthews, R.G., Koutmos, M., Datta, S., 2008. Cobalamin-dependent and cobamide-dependent methyltransferases. Curr. Opin. Struct. Biol. 18, 658–666. Available from: https://doi.org/10.1016/j.sbi.2008.11.005.
McLean, E., de Benoist, B., Allen, L.H., 2008. Review of the magnitude of folate and vitamin B12 deficiencies worldwide. Food Nutr. Bull. 29, S38–S51. Available from: https://doi.org/10.1177/15648265080292S107.
Monsen, A.-L.B., Refsum, H., Markestad, T., Ueland, P.M., 2003. Cobalamin status and its biochemical markers methylmalonic acid and homocysteine in different age groups from 4 days to 19 years. Clin. Chem. 49, 2067–2075. Available from: https://doi.org/10.1373/clinchem.2003.019869.

Mørkbak, A.L., Hvas, A.-M., Lloyd-Wright, Z., Sanders, T.A.B., Bleie, O., Refsum, H., et al., 2006. Effect of vitamin B12 treatment on haptocorrin. Clin. Chem. 52, 1104–1111. Available from: https://doi.org/10.1373/clinchem.2005.061549.

Morkbak, A.L., Poulsen, S.S., Nexo, E., 2007. Haptocorrin in humans. Clin. Chem. Lab. Med. 45, 1751–1759. Available from: https://doi.org/10.1515/CCLM.2007.343.

Morris, M.S., Jacques, P.F., Rosenberg, I.H., Selhub, J., 2007. Folate and vitamin B-12 status in relation to anemia, macrocytosis, and cognitive impairment in older Americans in the age of folic acid fortification. Am. J. Clin. Nutr. 85, 193–200. Available from: https://doi.org/10.1093/ajcn/85.1.193.

Nexo, E., Hoffmann-Lücke, E., 2011. Holotranscobalamin, a marker of vitamin B-12 status: analytical aspects and clinical utility. Am. J. Clin. Nutr. 94, 359S–365S. Available from: https://doi.org/10.3945/ajcn.111.013458.

Nielsen, M.J., Rasmussen, M.R., Andersen, C.B.F., Nexø, E., Moestrup, S.K., 2012. Vitamin B12 transport from food to the body's cells—a sophisticated, multistep pathway. Nat. Rev. Gastroenterol. Hepatol. 9, 345–354. Available from: https://doi.org/10.1038/nrgastro.2012.76.

Ortigues-Marty, I., Micol, D., Prache, S., Dozias, D., Girard, C.L., 2005. Nutritional value of meat: the influence of nutrition and physical activity on vitamin B12 concentrations in ruminant tissues. Reprod. Nutr. Dev. 45, 453–467. Available from: https://doi.org/10.1051/rnd:2005038.

Padovani, D., Banerjee, R., 2009. A G-protein editor gates coenzyme B12 loading and is corrupted in methylmalonic aciduria. Proc. Natl. Acad. Sci. U.S.A. 106, 21567–21572. Available from: https://doi.org/10.1073/pnas.0908106106.

Premkumar, M., Gupta, N., Singh, T., Velpandian, T., 2012. Cobalamin and folic acid status in relation to the etiopathogenesis of pancytopenia in adults at a tertiary care centre in north India. Anemia 2012, 707402. Available from: https://doi.org/10.1155/2012/707402.

Quadros, E.V., 2010. Advances in the understanding of cobalamin assimilation and metabolism. Br. J. Haematol. 148, 195–204. Available from: https://doi.org/10.1111/j.1365-2141.2009.07937.x.

Quadros, E.V., Sequeira, J.M., 2013. Cellular uptake of cobalamin: transcobalamin and the TCblR/CD320 receptor. Biochimie 95, 1008–1018. Available from: https://doi.org/10.1016/j.biochi.2013.02.004.

Quadros, E.V., Rothenberg, S.P., Jaffe, E.A., 1989. Endothelial cells from human umbilical vein secrete functional transcobalamin II. Am. J. Physiol. 256, C296–C303. Available from: https://doi.org/10.1152/ajpcell.1989.256.2.C296.

Reynolds, E., 2006. Vitamin B12, folic acid, and the nervous system. Lancet Neurol. 5, 949–960. Available from: https://doi.org/10.1016/S1474-4422(06)70598-1.

Rizzo, G., Laganà, A.S., Rapisarda, A.M.C., La Ferrera, G.M.G., Buscema, M., Rossetti, P., et al., 2016. Vitamin B12 among vegetarians: status, assessment and supplementation. Nutrients 8. Available from: https://doi.org/10.3390/nu8120767.

Rutsch, F., Gailus, S., Miousse, I.R., Suormala, T., Sagné, C., Toliat, M.R., et al., 2009. Identification of a putative lysosomal cobalamin exporter altered in the cblF defect of vitamin B12 metabolism. Nat. Genet. 41, 234–239. Available from: https://doi.org/10.1038/ng.294.

Sahali, D., Mulliez, N., Chatelet, F., Dupuis, R., Ronco, P., Verroust, P., 1988. Characterization of a 280-kD protein restricted to the coated pits of the renal brush border and the epithelial cells of the yolk sac. Teratogenic effect of the specific monoclonal antibodies. J. Exp. Med. 167, 213–218.

Schrauzer, G.N., Deutsch, E., 1969. Reactions of cobalt(I) supernucleophiles. The alkylation of vitamin B12s cobaloximes(I), and related compounds. J. Am. Chem. Soc. 91, 3341–3350.

Seetharam, B., Yammani, R.R., 2003. Cobalamin transport proteins and their cell-surface receptors. Expert. Rev. Mol. Med. 5, 1–18. Available from: https://doi.org/10.1017/S1462399403006422.

Shah, N.P., Beech, C.M., Sturm, A.C., Tanner, S.M., 2011. Investigation of the ABC transporter MRP1 in selected patients with presumed defects in vitamin B12 absorption. Blood 117, 4397–4398. Available from: https://doi.org/10.1182/blood-2010-12-322750.

Stabler, S.P., 2013. Clinical practice. Vitamin B12 deficiency. N. Engl. J. Med. 368, 149–160. Available from: https://doi.org/10.1056/NEJMcp1113996.

Tucker, K.L., Rich, S., Rosenberg, I., Jacques, P., Dallal, G., Wilson, P.W., et al., 2000. Plasma vitamin B-12 concentrations relate to intake source in the Framingham Offspring study. Am. J. Clin. Nutr. 71, 514–522. Available from: https://doi.org/10.1093/ajcn/71.2.514.

Waddington, M.D., Finke, R.G., 1993. Neopentylcobalamin (neopentylB12) cobalt-carbon bond thermolysis products, kinetics, activation parameters, and bond dissociation energy: a chemical model exhibiting 106 of the 1012 enzymic activation of coenzyme B12's cobalt-carbon bond. J. Am. Chem. Soc. 115, 4629–4640. Available from: https://doi.org/10.1021/ja00064a026.

Wakade, C., Chong, R., Bradley, E., Morgan, J.C., 2015. Low-dose niacin supplementation modulates GPR109A, niacin index and ameliorates Parkinson's disease symptoms without side effects. Clin. Case Rep. 3, 635–637. Available from: https://doi.org/10.1002/ccr3.232.

Watanabe, F., 2007. Vitamin B12 sources and bioavailability. Exp. Biol. Med. (Maywood, NJ) 232, 1266–1274. Available from: https://doi.org/10.3181/0703-MR-67.

Williams, P., 2007. Nutritional composition of red meat. Nutr. Diet 64, S113–S119. Available from: https://doi.org/10.1111/j.1747-0080.2007.00197.x.

Yajnik, C.S., Deshpande, S.S., Lubree, H.G., Naik, S.S., Bhat, D.S., Uradey, B.S., et al., 2006. Vitamin B12 deficiency and hyperhomocysteinemia in rural and urban Indians. J. Assoc. Phys. India 54, 775–782.

Zhang, Y., Rodionov, D.A., Gelfand, M.S., Gladyshev, V.N., 2009. Comparative genomic analyses of nickel, cobalt and vitamin B12 utilization. BMC Genomics 10, 78. Available from: https://doi.org/10.1186/1471-2164-10-78.

CHAPTER 7

Nutrigenomic aspects of dietary pyridoxine (vitamin B_6) and selenium interaction and their implications in reproduction

Danyel Bueno Dalto[1] and Jean-Jacques Matte[1]
[1]Sherbrooke Research and Development Centre, Agriculture and Agri-Food Canada, Sherbrooke, QC, Canada

Contents

Key facts of transmethylation and transsulfuration in embryos and the impact of vitamin B_6 to the interplay between them

- Vitamin B_6 (B_6) participates as a cofactor in a series of essential enzymes for amino acids metabolism.
- Methionine is a remarkable amino acid contributing to protein mass and the synthesis of homocysteine.
- Homocysteine connects two major metabolisms, the one-carbon metabolism and the antioxidative system.

DOI: https://doi.org/10.1016/B978-0-12-811907-5.00015-4

- The remethylation of homocysteine generates *S*-adenosyl methionine, an important contributor for the one-carbon metabolism and that performs crucial functions in genetic stability.
- Mammals metabolize sulfur and selenomethionine interchangeably. Consequently B_6-dependent enzymes catalyze the transsulfuration of selenohomocysteine to selenocysteine and further into selenoproteins.
- Selenoproteins have remarkable actions on antioxidant defense during embryo development.
- The influence of dietary B_6 on those metabolisms is especially important in early gestation because the transsulfuration pathway is not fully functional in embryos.
- The immature embryonic transsulfuration pathway implies the possible existence of alternative routes for the transfer of maternal selenium to preimplantation embryos for the synthesis of selenoproteins.
- Redox alterations brought by the placentation process makes this scenario even more complex.

Summary points

- Vitamin B_6 (B_6) is essential in reproduction, and acts on redox reactions through the synthesis of antioxidants.
- In mammals, the metabolism of sulfur- and selenoamino acids metabolism is similar.
- B_6 modulates the fate of sulfur- and selenohomocysteine between transsulfuration and transmethylation pathways, especially under high oxidative states.
- Ovulation generates oxidative molecules that may impair ovarian functions and early embryo development.
- After placentation the greater embryo oxygen tension may increase oxidative pressure and embryo losses.
- Excessive metabolic oxidation stimulates transsulfuration in preference to remethylation, but in embryos this pathway is not fully functional.
- Understanding the interactions between these two pathways is essential to improve embryo development.

Abbreviations

B_6 vitamin B_6
CBS cystathionine β-synthase

CGL	cystathionine γ-lyase
GSH	glutathione
MTR	methionine synthase
SAM	*S*-adenosylmethionine
SCLY	selenocysteine lyase
Se	selenium
THF	tetrahydrofolate

7.1 Introduction

Vitamin B_6 (B_6) participates as a cofactor in a series of enzymes catalyzing transamination, decarboxylation, and elimination/replacement reactions and therefore is essential for the metabolism of amino acids. Among the various amino acids the metabolism of methionine is remarkably important because, besides contributing to the protein mass, it is the substrate for the synthesis of the key metabolite homocysteine, which connects two major metabolic systems, the one-carbon metabolism and the antioxidative system (Dalto and Matte, 2017).

Methionine is first activated by adenosine triphosphate synthesizing the methyl donor *S*-adenosylmethionine (SAM) (Mudd and Cantoni, 1958). After donating its methyl group, SAM produces *S*-adenosylhomocysteine and further homocysteine (Ulrey et al., 2005). Homocysteine has two fates, either remethylation to methionine or transsulfuration to cysteine. Remethylation may be indirectly impacted by B_6 through reactions involving B_6-dependent enzymes for the synthesis of one-carbon carrier folates (Perry et al., 2007) that, together with SAM, are major contributors for the one-carbon metabolism. By linking amino acids and nucleotides, this fundamental metabolism performs crucial functions in genetic stability (Selhub, 1999).

Mammals metabolize sulfur- and selenoamino acids interchangeably (Schrauzer, 2003). Consequently in the case of selenomethionine, the B_6-dependent enzymes of the transsulfuration pathway catalyze the synthesis of selenocysteine from selenohomocysteine. Selenocysteine is further reduced by selenocysteine lyase (SCLY; a B_6-dependent enzyme) to form selenide that in a series of B_6-dependent reactions is incorporated into selenoproteins (Johansson et al., 2005), such as glutathione peroxidases, thioredoxin reductases, iodothyronine deiodinases, among others. Peroxidases play major roles in maintaining the cellular redox state with remarkable actions on antioxidant defense during spermiogenesis, maturation of spermatozoa, and embryo development (Ursini, 2000).

The influence of dietary B_6 on the above metabolisms and its interactions with selenium (Se) are especially important in early gestation because the transsulfuration pathway is not fully functional in embryos (Levonen et al., 2000), suggesting the existence of alternative routes for the transfer of maternal Se to preimplantation embryos for the synthesis of selenoproteins. Additionally, redox alterations due to the exposure to oxygen brought by the placentation process (Jauniaux et al., 2000) make this scenario even more complex.

This chapter discusses the impact of B_6 on the interplay between transmethylation and transsulfuration pathways under different redox states, focusing on the interaction between dietary B_6 and Se in embryos at 5 and 30 days of gestation in a pig model.

7.2 Pyridoxine sources, recommendations, and bioavailability

Vitamin B_6 is a water-soluble compound necessary for normal growth, development, and biological functions. Most animals lack the ability to synthesizse B_6 and rely upon an external supply, such as natural foods (whole grain cereals, nuts, lean meat, fish, and vegetables). Yeast extract, wheat bran, and liver contain the highest concentrations of the vitamin (FSA, 2002).

The metabolically active forms of B_6 (pyridoxine, pyridoxal, and pyridoxamine, and their phosphorylated forms) vary among foods of plant and animal origin. Roth-Maier et al. (2002) reported that in foods of plant origin, pyridoxine and pyridoxamine are the main forms, except for maize (50% of the vitamin is pyridoxal). In raw animal tissue, the major form is pyridoxal phosphate (Ball, 2006). Using a rat model, Benedikt et al. (1996) showed that the content of B_6 in milk consisted of 80.0% pyridoxal, 15.0% pyridoxamine, and 5.0% pyridoxine. Pyridoxine hydrochloride is used in multivitamin supplements and food fortification (Dove and Cook, 2001). Although bacterial B_6 synthesis at the colon may also contribute to the total intestinal input of the vitamin (Allgood and Cidlowski, 1991), it cannot be locally absorbed and therefore only coprophagous animals would obtain benefits from this source of B_6 (Combs Jr., 2012).

According to Driskell (1994) the minimum daily B_6 requirement of humans appears to range from 0.65 to 1.25 mg. These daily values are greater (2.1–7.6 mg) in pregnant and lactating women. Dietary proteins (level, source, and quality) have been shown to impact the metabolic needs of B_6. This may be related to the fact that cellular levels of all nonessential amino acids are influenced by reactions catalyzed by pyridoxal-5-phosphate. In fact, greater serine (Aboaysha and Kratzer, 1980) or methionine supplementation (Kazemi and Daghir, 1971) increases B_6 requirements for growth. Primary B_6 deficiency and toxicity are uncommon. However, at high doses (150 mg/kg of body weight) it has been shown to induce sensory neuropathy in dogs (Hoover et al., 1981).

Depending on food origin, the bioavailability of B_6 may range between 40%–80% for all metabolically active forms (Ball, 2006). The absorption site of B_6 is mainly the jejunum. Dephosphorylated forms are capable of crossing cell membranes, whereas phosphorylated forms are not, causing metabolic trapping (Gregory, 1997). Dephosphorylated forms (pyridoxine, pyridoxal, and pyridoxamine) are rapidly absorbed by passive diffusion (Gregory, 1997), and once within the enterocyte they are converted into their corresponding phosphates by the catalytic action of cytoplasmic pyridoxal kinase. These phosphorylated vitamers are eventually dephosphorylated, facilitating the easy diffusion of B_6 compounds across the basolateral membrane (Middleton, 1985). Much of the ingested pyridoxine is released into the portal circulation as pyridoxal and further taken up by the liver. In the liver the inactive forms of vitamin B_6 are phosphorylated by pyridoxal kinase, yielding pyridoxal-5-phosphate (physiologically active form of B_6), pyridoxine phosphate, and pyridoxamine phosphate. These two inactive phosphorylated forms are eventually oxidized to ultimately yield pyridoxal-5-phosphate (Wada and Snell, 1961). Free pyridoxal-5-phosphate is hydrolyzed to pyridoxal, is released, and then circulates bound to albumin (Anderson et al., 1974) and/or hemoglobin (Mehansho and Henderson, 1980). Once pyridoxal crosses the cell membrane pyridoxal-5-phosphate is regenerated through the action of pyridoxal kinase. Free pyridoxal not leaving the cell goes through oxidation to yield 4-pyridoxic acid (Gregory, 1997), which is further excreted in the urine.

7.3 Selenium sources, recommendations, and bioavailability

Dietary Se may be obtained from both organic and inorganic sources (Dumont et al., 2006). Inorganic Se (sodium selenite) has been the main source of Se added to nutritional supplements and is naturally present in phytoplankton (Whanger, 2002). Organic Se is normally ingested from plants and animal-derived food products in the form of selenomethionine (Combs and Combs, 1986).

For human nutrition, selenomethionine is currently considered the most appropriate source of Se (Schrauzer, 2003) due to the higher bioavailability and greater body tissue accumulation, as well as lower toxicity potential and environmental pollution compared to sodium selenite (Swanson, 1991; Vendeland et al., 1994). However, its metabolic fate is dependent upon the pyridoxine status (Pavlata et al., 2011). In fact, low pyridoxine levels in the body may impair the utilization of organic Se and, consequently, increase Se requirements (Yin, 1992).

Recommended Dietary Allowances have been proposed by the Food and Nutrition Board of the Institute of Medicine (United States). The daily intake ranges from 55 μg (recommended) to 400 μg (tolerable upper intake) of Se for adults (Institute of Medicine, 2000). However, studies in pregnant and lactating rats (Smith and Picciano, 1986) and pigs (Mahan and Peters, 2004; Dalto et al., 2016) have reported that Se requirement increases during pregnancy and lactation due to a higher demand for maternal transfer to conceptuses and newborns. This greater demand for Se may also be required in situations of high metabolic oxidative stress (Dalto et al. 2015a, 2016). Therefore studies involving the effects of supranutritional Se supplementation in humans have aroused great interest.

The bioavailability and mechanisms of absorption of Se are dependent upon the chemical forms in which it is absorbed and metabolized, but both sources are preferentially absorbed in the ileum (McDowell, 2003). In general, organic Se is more bioavailable than inorganic Se (Rider et al., 2010). Measurements of Se crossing portal-drained viscera (blood plasma porto-arterial differences) indicated a bioavailability of approximately 43% for selenite and 65% for organic Se (yeast) (Matte, unpublished data). Selenite is passively absorbed by simple diffusion (Wolfram, 1989), quickly transformed into hydrogen selenide, and further into selenophosphates, the substrate to the synthesis of functional selenoproteins (Windisch, 2002), with little tissue accumulation of Se. Differently, organic Se is actively absorbed through amino acid (methionine) transport mechanisms (McDowell, 2003) and follows the methionine metabolism or is metabolized to synthesize selenoproteins (Sunde, 1984). Because the methionine-tRNA cannot discriminate between methionine and selenomethionine, using both interchangeably in protein synthesis, organic Se is effective in building Se reserves in tissues (Schrauzer, 2003).

7.4 Transmethylation and transsulfuration pathways

Demethylation and remethylation reactions consist of metabolic reactions involving the transfer of methyl groups. These two reactions are generally known as transmethylation. A good example of transmethylation reactions is the methionine cycle. By the action of adenosine triphosphate, the methyl group of methionine is activated and forms SAM (Mudd and Cantoni, 1958), one of the most important metabolic donors of methyl groups. After donating its methyl group, SAM is transformed into *S*-adenosylhomocysteine that is promptly hydrolyzed to homocysteine (Ulrey et al., 2005). Homocysteine may follow two pathways: remethylation to methionine or transsulfuration to cysteine (Fig. 7.1). Remethylation may occur by two pathways that are differentiated by the donor of one-carbon molecules (betaine or folate) (Födinger et al., 2000). Independently of its redox states, folates in the form of tetrahydrofolate (THF) serve as donors of single carbons (Tibbetts and Appling, 2010). The one-carbon donor 5-methyl-THF catalyzes the conversion of homocysteine to methionine. In brief, the methyl donor 5-methyl-THF is transformed into THF while the methyl recipient homocysteine forms methionine (Berg et al., 2002) in a reaction catalyzed by methionine synthase (MTR), a vitamin B_{12}-dependent enzyme (Li et al., 1996). Under folate and/or vitamin B_{12} deficiency, MTR reactions are severely impaired.

Although not directly demonstrated (Martinez et al., 2000; Perry et al., 2007), the impact of B_6 status on the remethylation of methyl groups can be inferred by the influence of B_6-dependent enzymes on the synthesis of 5,10-methylene-THF in a reaction involving the methylene group of serine along with THF. Serine and THF are considered as the major carriers of one-carbon groups; however, SAM is the most important one-carbon donor (Selhub, 1999) due to its more energetically favorable reactions. The transfer of these volatile and easy-binding single carbons from folate and SAM are major contributors to the one-carbon metabolism. The one-carbon metabolism links amino acid and nucleotide metabolisms, performing critical roles in DNA synthesis, repair, and replication (Selhub, 1999).

Transsulfuration is a metabolic pathway involving the conversion of homocysteine into cysteine through the intermediate metabolite cystathionine. Briefly, in a reaction catalyzed by the B_6-dependent enzyme cystathionine β-synthase (CBS), the acetyl or succinyl group of homoserine replaces the thiol group of homocysteine to form

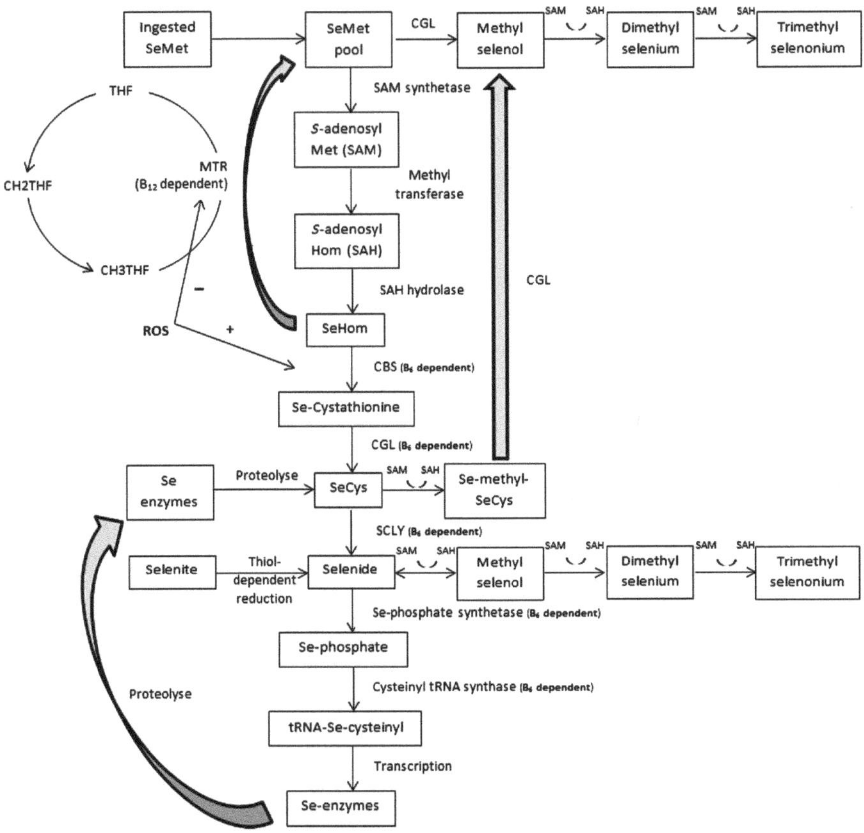

Figure 7.1 Transmethylation and transsulfuration pathways of selenium (similar for sulfur counterparts) in adults. The substrate-specific enzyme selenocysteine lyase (SCLY) represents the landmark step between sulfur and selenium metabolisms. *Se*, Selenium; *SeMet*, selenomethionine; *SeHom*, selenohomocysteine; *SeCys*, selenocysteine; *THF*, tetrahydrofolate; *CH2THF*, 5,10-methylene-THF; *CH3THF*, 5-methyl-THF; *MTR*, methionine synthase; *CBS*, cystathionine β synthase; *CGL*, cystathionine γ-lyase; *SCLY*, selenocysteine lyase; *ROS*, reactive oxygen species. *Adapted from Dalto, D.B., Matte, J.J., 2017. Pyridoxine (vitamin B6) and the glutathione peroxidase system; a link between one-carbon metabolism and antioxidation. Nutrients 9, 189.*

cystathionine (Aitken et al., 2011). This critical action at the homocysteine junction indicates that CBS performs key roles in both the maintenance of the methionine pool and the synthesis of cysteine (Dalto and Matte, 2017) but also suggests that this enzyme would be, in turn, strictly regulated. Indeed, CBS is regulated by a feedback mechanism in which low concentrations of SAM stimulates the remethylation of homocysteine, whereas high concentrations of SAM favor the transsulfuration pathway (Ereno-Orbea et al., 2014). After cystathionine synthesis from homocysteine, this molecule is cleaved by the B_6-dependent enzyme cystathionine γ-lyase (CGL) to form cysteine (Flavin and Slaughter, 1964) that, in a series of reactions catalyzed by γ-glutamylcysteine synthetase and glutathione (GSH) synthetase, will form GSH. In this sense, the transsulfuration pathway directly connects homocysteine and GSH, the major redox buffer in mammalian cells. Therefore it is likely that enzymes regulating this metabolic pathway might be sensitive to redox changes. Indeed, oxidizing conditions increase transsulfuration through higher CBS activity (Taoka et al., 1998), whereas MTR activity is reduced resulting in less remethylation (Chen et al., 1995).

7.5 Pyridoxine and selenium interaction for the synthesis of selenoproteins

Considering that mammals metabolize selenoamino acids in the same way as their sulfur counterparts (Schrauzer, 2003), the same B_6-dependent enzymes are expected to catalyze reactions of the transsulfuration pathway for selenomethionine but using Se-homocysteine to form selenocysteine. Similar to cysteine, selenocysteine may be used as substrate for the synthesis of GSH, but this is likely insignificant compared to the much greater pool of GSH synthesized from (sulfur)cysteine (Osawa et al., 1992). The most important reaction of selenocysteine is its reduction to selenide via SCLY (B_6-dependent enzyme). Considering that SCLY is substrate specific, this step is the landmark between sulfur and Se metabolisms (Dalto and Matte, 2017). Further, selenophosphates are synthesized by selenophosphate synthetase, a B_6-dependent enzyme. Finally, in another B_6-dependent reaction, selenophosphates donate Se molecules that will be incorporated into the phosphate moiety of Ser-tRNA, generating a selenocysteine-specific tRNA[Ser]Sec. This unique tRNA that contains the selenocysteine insertion sequence (SECIS) combines with a selenocysteine-tRNA-specific elongation factor and a specific SECIS binding protein to incorporate selenocysteine into selenoproteins (Johansson et al., 2005).

It is noteworthy to mention that, as for methionine/homocysteine, in the metabolism of their seleno equivalents high oxidative states not only reduce the remethylation of Se-homocysteine to selenomethionine, but also stimulate the transsulfuration pathway. This control does not occur for inorganic Se because selenite obtained from the diet is directly reduced to selenide, shortcutting the transsulfuration pathway for the synthesis of selenoproteins (Mosharov et al., 2000), which could allow an eventual accumulation of toxic levels of selenide. Although organic Se also generates selenide, the saturability of the enzyme SCLY prevents the accumulation of excessive selenide.

These effects of oxidative status on the transsulfuration pathway and the importance of B_6 for those reactions were further supported by recent studies of this laboratory on the effects of Se sources and levels combined or not with B_6 on reproductive traits and redox balance in pigs. According to Dalto et al. (2015a, 2016), B_6 supplementation (10 mg/kg) does not impact on blood or tissue accumulation of inorganic or organic Se from estrus 1 to estrus 5 or during the periestrus period (an oxidative stress condition) (Figs. 7.2 and 7.3). This is expected for inorganic Se because absorbed selenite is immediately reduced to selenide, independently of redox or B_6 status, for the synthesis of selenoproteins or excretion (methylation) rather than building body reserves (Windisch, 2002).

In contrast, organic Se metabolism is highly impacted by both oxidative stress conditions and B_6 status. Under basal oxidative stress conditions, the remethylation of Se-homocysteine back to selenomethionine is likely the preferential pathway due to the lack of positive feedback by oxidative molecules on CBS. Davis (2006) and Lima (2006) suggested that B_6 may not be a significant aspect influencing the transsulfuration of homocysteine, which is likely primarily controlled by oxidative molecules and SAM levels. In fact, Dalto et al. (2016) showed no effect of B_6 on SCLY gene expression and selenoproteins gene expression and activity in gilts at 30 day of gestation, a physiological state shown to be of limited oxidative stress in sows. Conversely, under the redox conditions brought by the periestrus period, Dalto et al. (2015a) reported high gene expressions of SCLY and glutathione peroxidase 1 (GPX1) in the liver (Fig. 7.4) and kidneys of organic Se + B_6 supplemented animals, which is in line with the positive feedback of oxidative molecules on CBS. In that study, however, no B_6 effects were found on GPX activity (liver, kidneys, and whole blood) during the same periestrus period. In this regard, Lubos et al. (2011) reported that because GPX has multi regulation factors (transcriptional, posttranscriptional, translational, or posttranslational), changes in gene expression may not parallel its enzymatic activity.

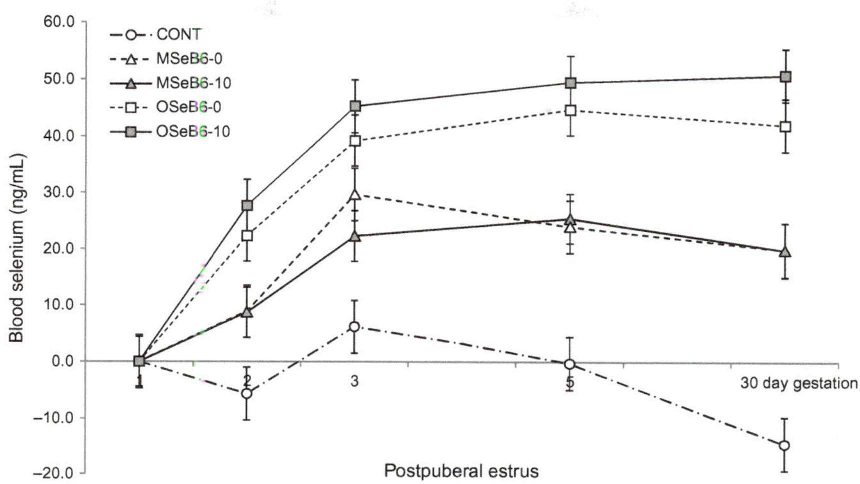

Figure 7.2 Blood selenium concentration (ng/mL) of gilts on each estrus, expressed as increases relative to pretreatment values at estrus 1, presented as LS means ± SEM. *CONT*, Basal diet containing 0.3 mg/kg and 2.4 mg/kg of natural Se and pyridoxine respectively; *MSe*, basal diet supplemented with 0.3 mg/kg of sodium selenite; *$MSeB_6$10*, basal diet supplemented with 0.3 mg/kg of sodium selenite and 10 mg/kg of hydrochloride pyridoxine; *OSe*, basal diet supplemented with 0.3 mg/kg of Se-enriched yeast; *$OSeB_6$10*, basal diet supplemented with 0.3 mg/kg of Se-enriched yeast and 10 mg/kg of hydrochloride pyridoxine. *Adapted from Dalto, D. B., Audet, I., Lapointe, J., Matte, J.J., 2016. The importance of pyridoxine for the impact of the dietary selenium sources on redox balance, embryo development, and reproductive performance in gilts. J. Trace Elem. Med. Biol. 34, 79–89.*

7.6 Dietary pyridoxine and selenium on embryo development: studies using a pig model

7.6.1 Five-day porcine expanded blastocysts

Recent studies of this laboratory using a microarray technology provided unique and interesting insights on B_6 and Se interactions and their effects on the interplay between remethylation and transsulfuration pathways during early porcine embryo development.

Dalto et al. (2015b) reported no difference in B_6 levels in uterine flushings between inorganic or organic Se combined with B_6. These authors also reported that Se was undetectable in those same samples, indicating that the uptake of Se from this source by the preimplantation embryo is insignificant. However, maternal supplementation with organic Se combined (or not) with B_6 supplies embryos with more Se compared to maternal inorganic Se combined (or not) with B_6 supplementation

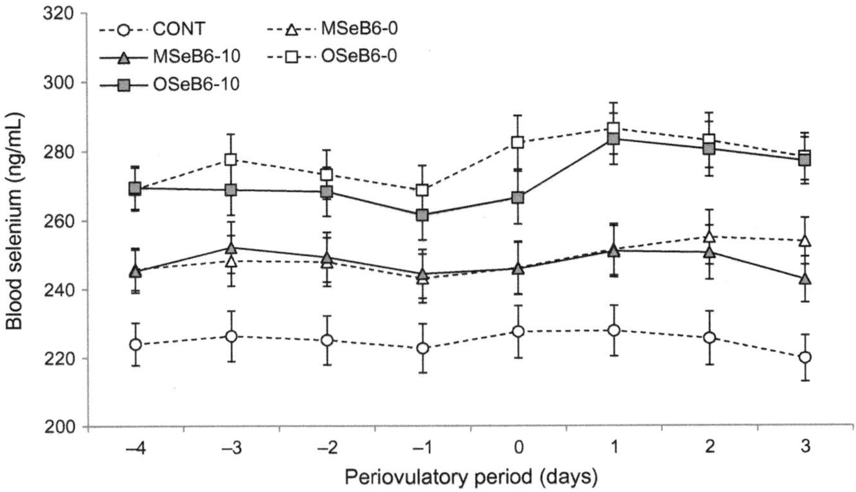

Figure 7.3 Blood selenium concentration (ng/mL of blood) of gilts at fourth estrus, shown as LS means ± SEM. Physiological estrus indicated as d0. *CONT,* Basal diet containing 0.2 and 1.7 mg/kg of natural Se and pyridoxine respectively; *MSe,* basal diet supplemented with 0.3 mg/kg of sodium selenite; *$MSeB_6$10,* basal diet supplemented with 0.3 mg/kg of sodium selenite and 10 mg/kg of hydrochloride pyridoxine; *OSe,* basal diet supplemented with 0.3 mg/kg of Se-enriched yeast; *$OSeB_6$10,* basal diet supplemented with 0.3 mg/kg of Se-enriched yeast and 10 mg/kg of hydrochloride pyridoxine. *Adapted from Dalto, D.B., Roy, M., Audet, I., Palin, M.-F., Guay, F., Lapointe, J., et al., 2015a. Interaction between vitamin B6 and source of selenium on the response of the selenium-dependent glutathione peroxidase system to oxidative stress induced by oestrus in pubertal pig. J. Trace Elem. Med. Biol. 32, 21–29.*

(Fortier et al., 2012; Ma et al., 2014; Dalto et al., 2016). Considering that organic Se is deposited in tissues more efficiently than is inorganic Se (Mahan et al., 1999), the most likely source of this mineral would be the preovulatory oocyte because it might be impacted by systemic maternal Se levels through the follicular fluid. In this sense, Dalto et al. (2015b) reported that maternal supplementation with organic Se combined with B_6 stimulated about 30 times more genes in porcine expanded blastocysts compared to inorganic Se combined with B_6. These results suggest that embryos from organic Se + B_6 supplemented dams would have greater Se reserves, likely selenomethionine, and are more suitable to go through demethylation to Se-homocysteine.

A relevant aspect to consider is the fact that from conception to neonatal age, embryos, fetuses, and newborns are not capable of converting selenomethionine into selenocysteine via the transsulfuration pathway

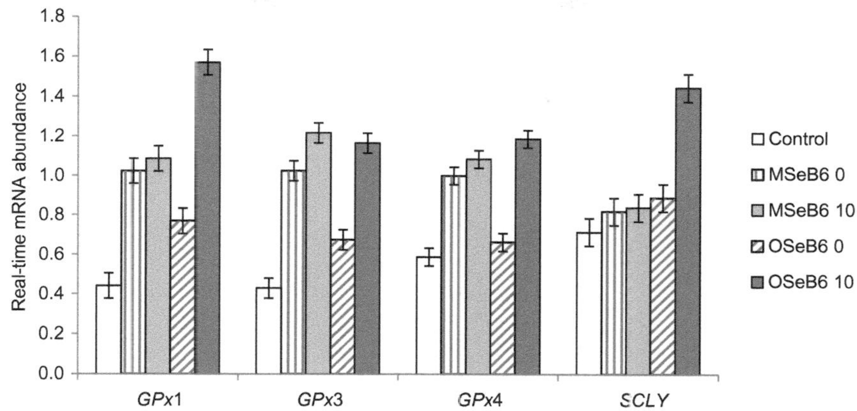

Figure 7.4 Gene expression of *GPX1*, *GPX3*, *GPX4*, and *SCLY* in liver of gilts 3 days after fourth oestrus, shown as least square means ± SEM. CONT = basal diet containing 0.3 mg/kg and 2.4 mg/kg of natural Se and pyridoxine respectively, MSe = basal diet supplemented with 0.3 mg/kg of sodium selenite, $MSeB_610$ = basal diet supplemented with 0.3 mg/kg of sodium selenite and 10 mg/kg of hydro-chloride pyridoxine, OSe = basal diet supplemented with 0.3 mg/kgof Se-enriched yeast, $OSeB_610$ = basal diet supplemented with 0.3 mg/kg of Se-enriched yeast and 10 mg/kg of hydro-chloride pyridoxine. *Adapted from Dalto, D.B., Roy, M., Audet, I., Palin, M.-F., Guay, F., Lapointe, J., et al., 2015a. Interaction between vitamin B6 and source of selenium on the response of the selenium-dependent glutathione peroxidase system to oxidative stress induced by oestrus in pubertal pig. J. Trace Elem. Med. Biol. 32, 21–29.*

because they lack CGL activity, despite detectable mRNA expression (Gardiner and Reed, 1995; Levonen et al., 2000) (Fig. 7.5). This implies that selenomethionine would be either incorporated into unspecific protein or demethylated to Se-homocysteine followed by remethylation to selenomethionine. Dalto et al. (2015b), studying specific gene expression according to Se source (common genes between sources were excluded from analysis), reported no differentially expressed genes in the demethylation or remethylation pathway in 5-day embryos from gilts supplemented with organic or inorganic Se combined with B_6. However, several genes related to elongation factors, translation, and mitotic cell cycle were impacted by maternal organic Se supplementation. Those authors concluded that protein deposition is the preferential route for selenomethionine in 5-day porcine embryos. Nevertheless, a recent study from this laboratory (Dalto et al., 2018), using the database generated by Dalto et al. (2015b) but considering common genes between sources of Se in the analysis (global gene expression), suggests that maternal organic Se supplementation combined with B_6 may affect DNA methylation through

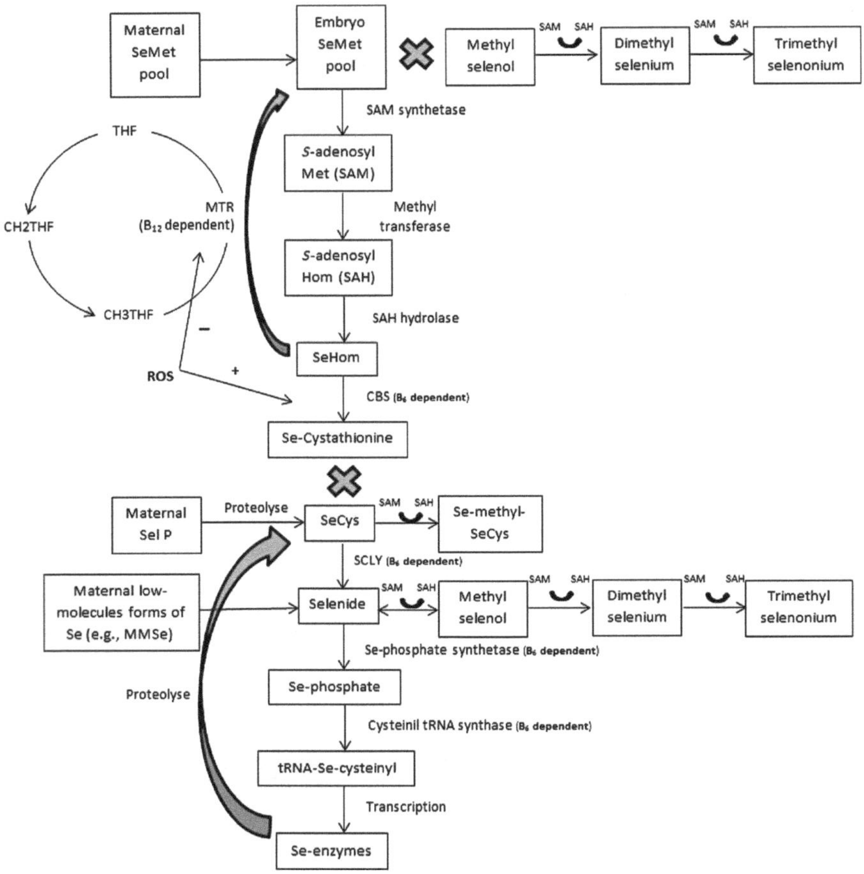

Figure 7.5 Embryo transmethylation and transsulfuration pathways of selenium (similar for sulfur counterparts) and possible maternal selenium transfer routes.
Se, Selenium; *SeMet*, selenomethionine; *SeHom*, selenohomocysteine; *SeCys*, selenocysteine; *THF*, tetrahydrofolate; *CH2THF*, 5,10-methylene-THF; *CH3THF*, 5-methyl-THF; *MTR*, methionine synthase; *CBS*, cystathionine β synthase; *CGL*, cystathionine γ-lyase; *SCLY*, selenocysteine lyase; *ROS*, reactive oxygen species. *Adapted from Dalto, D.B., Matte, J.J., 2017. Pyridoxine (vitamin B6) and the glutathione peroxidase system; a link between one-carbon metabolism and antioxidation. Nutrients 9, 189.*

methyltransferases and SAM carrier genes (generation of methyl groups) and eventually epigenetic events. In this sense, although protein deposition may be the preferential route for selenomethionine in 5-day porcine embryos, the importance of transmethylation reactions should not be overlooked. It is noteworthy to mention that in Dalto et al. (2015b) the greatest number of viable embryos (although not statistically significant)

Table 7.1 Average recovery rate and number of porcine embryos according to viability and stages of development collected at 5 days of gestation.

Measurements	CONT	MSeB$_6$10	OSeB$_6$10
Embryo recovery rate (%)	76.92	85.61	92.74
Viable embryos (*n*)	14.17	13.50	18.17
Degenerated embryos (*n*)	0.50	2.00	0.00
Early stage embryos (*n*)	3.33	4.30	3.67
Advanced stage embryos (*n*)	10.83	9.17	14.50
Total embryos (*n*)	14.67	15.50	18.17

CONT, Basal diet containing 0.3 mg/kg and 1.7 mg/kg of natural Se and pyridoxine respectively; *MSeB610*, basal diet supplemented with 0.3 mg/kg of sodium selenite and 10 mg/kg of hydrochloride pyridoxine; *OSeB610*, basal diet supplemented with 0.3 mg/kg of Se-enriched yeast and 10 mg/kg of hydrochloride pyridoxine.
Source: Adapted from Dalto, D.B., Tsoi, S., Audet, I., Dyck, M.K., Foxcroft, G.R., Matte, J.J., 2015b. Gene expression of porcine blastocysts from gilts fed organic or inorganic selenium and pyridoxine. Reproduction 149, 31–42.

was collected from gilts supplemented with organic Se combined with B_6 and this was in the absence of degenerated embryos (Table 7.1). Dalto et al. (2015b) also reported several genes related to the synthesis of selenoenzymes in 5-day embryos, suggesting the potential to synthesize these enzymes at this early stage of development. As transsulfuration is not fully functional in embryos, the most likely sources of Se to the preimplantation embryo for the synthesis of selenoenzymes would be maternal selenocysteine, methylselenol, and/or selenoproteins (after proteolysis in the embryo) originating from the preovulatory oocyte. Consequently, independently of maternal dietary Se (inorganic and organic), the preimplantation embryo Se content would derive from an organic metabolite (oocyte selenomethionine pool and/or oocyte selenoproteins). In this sense, the synthesis of selenoproteins would unlikely be regulated by the previously mentioned feedback mechanism promoted by oxidative molecules but controlled by the B_6-dependent enzyme SCLY, which limits the synthesis of selenide (Fig. 7.5). Considering the key roles of methyl donors and the one-carbon metabolism, this metabolically imposed transfer of organic Se to preimplantation embryos may be considered a mechanism to protect DNA processing and genetic stability.

7.6.2 Thirty-day porcine embryos

Although the transsulfuration pathway is not fully functional in 30-day embryos (similar to 5-day embryos) the placentation process which begins at approximately 25 days of gestation in pigs may change the dynamic between transmethylation and transsulfuration.

Increasing levels of oxidative molecules are expected in the embryo as a result of the greater transport of oxygen by the placenta raising embryonic oxygen tension. According to Jauniaux et al. (2000), in early pregnancy in humans these levels are higher than at mid- or end-pregnancy likely because of the underdeveloped embryonic antioxidant system. As discussed above, high oxidative stress conditions stimulate CBS activity and transsulfuration, whereas they reduce MTR activity and remethylation. Besides the negative effects on embryo/fetal development caused by disturbances to the metabolism of one-carbon (Kalhan, 2016), an unusual accumulation of Se-cystathionine may be expected in Se-enriched embryos due to the inactive enzyme CGL. Under these circumstances, careful consideration should be made regarding B_6 supplementation because it stimulates CBS activity. In pigs, Dalto et al. (2016) observed evidence of disturbed embryo development (greater within-litter weight variation) after maternal supplementation with 12.4 mg/kg compared to 2.4 mg/kg feed of B_6. Under similar experimental conditions and pig genetic lines, Fortier et al. (2012) reported no negative effect of maternal supplementation in gilts fed 3 mg/kg of feed of B_6 combined with different sources of Se (inorganic vs organic Se) at 0.5 mg/kg of feed. In fact those authors observed better morphological and metabolic indicators (embryo weight and length, and protein and DNA content) in supplemented animals than in the control group at similar levels of B_6 but at 0.2 mg/kg of feed of Se.

The above mentioned greater organic Se incorporation compared to inorganic Se in adult individuals, which is independent of B_6 status, is also observed in 30-day porcine embryos (Fortier et al., 2012; Dalto et al., 2016). This higher load of Se-methionine in embryos derived from dams supplemented with organic Se may not be used for the synthesis of selenoenzymes (immature transsulfuration pathway) but will be possibly incorporated into general proteins and/or transmethylated, producing methyl groups that supply the one-carbon metabolism. Similarly to 5-day embryos, dams supplemented with inorganic Se supply this mineral in the organic form to their embryos, not as Se-methionine but as selenocysteine, after the catabolism of selenoproteins in the placenta (Burk et al., 2013). According to Soda et al. (1999), although SCLY has low activity in vivo, it is expected that selenocysteine would be metabolized to a great extent because the tissue concentration as well as the K_M (Michaelis constant) value of the enzyme is greater than that of the substrate. Considering that no effects of maternal Se (levels or sources) were observed on the activity of Se-GPX in 30-day porcine embryos (Fortier et al., 2012; Dalto et al., 2016), it appears that at this stage of development the flow of Se through SCLY is not primarily substrate driven. Consequently it is reasonable to suppose that, after the lyse of selenoproteins in the placenta supplying selenocysteine to the embryo, this metabolite would be directed preferentially to protein deposition and secondarily to catabolism by SCLY (not influenced by redox status) for the synthesis of selenide and further selenoenzymes. This alternative metabolism of selenoproteins synthesis may protect embryos from wasting one-carbon groups (methylation of excess selenide) and, as for 5-day embryos, promote genetic stability.

7.7 Conclusions

Vitamin B_6 is important for the equilibrium between the synthesis of methyl groups and antioxidants. This vitamin helps to control the enzymatic activity at the homocysteine junction between transmethylation and transsulfuration pathways and, consequently, the flow of methyl molecules between the one-carbon and selenoproteins metabolisms. However, the impact of oxidative stress conditions and metabolic maturity cannot be disregarded.

Although at high levels B_6 may possibly disturb embryo development when combined with organic Se at adequate levels, this interaction modulates important metabolic mechanisms impacting embryo development at both morphological and metabolic levels.

References

Aboaysha, A.M., Kratzer, F.H., 1980. Serine utilization in the chick as influenced by dietary pyridoxine. Proc. Soc. Exp. Biol. Med. 163, 490–495.

Aitken, S.M., Lodha, P.H., Morneau, D.J.K., 2011. The enzymes of the transsulfuration pathways:aActive-site characterizations. BBA Proteins Proteom. 1814, 1511–1517.

Allgood, V.E., Cidlowski, J.A., 1991. Novel role for vitamin B6 in steroid hormone action: a link between nutrition and the endocrine system. J. Nutr. Biochem. 2, 523–534.

Anderson, B.B., Newmark, P.A., Rawlins, M., Green, R., 1974. Plasma binding of vitamin B6 compounds. Nature 250, 502–504.

Ball, G.F.M., 2006. Vitamins in Foods: Analysis, Bioavailability, and Stability. CRC Press, Boca Raton.

Benedikt, J., Roth-Maier, D.A., Kirchgessner, M., 1996. Influence of dietary vitamin B6 supply during gravidity and lactation on total vitamin B6 concentration (pyridoxine, pyridoxal and pyridoxamine) on blood and milk. Int. J. Vitam. Nutr. Res. 66, 146–150.

Berg, J.M., Tymoczko, J.L., Stryer, L., 2002. Biochemistry, fifth ed. W.H. Freeman and Company, New York.

Burk, R.F., Olson, G.E., Hill, K.E., Winfrey, V.P., Motley, A.K., Kurokawa, S., 2013. Maternal-fetal transfer of selenium in the mouse. FASEB J. 27, 3249–3256.

Chen, Z., Chakraborty, S., Banerjee, R., 1995. Demonstration that mammalian methionine synthases are predominantly cobalamin-loaded. J. Biol. Chem. 270, 19246–19249.

Combs Jr., G.F., 2012. The Vitamins—Fundamental Aspects in Nutrition and Health. Academic Press, San Diego.

Combs Jr, G.F., Combs, S.B., 1986. The Role of Selenium in Nutrition. Academic Press, New York.

Dalto, D.B., Roy, M., Audet, I., Palin, M.-F., Guay, F., Lapointe, J., et al., 2015a. Interaction between vitamin B6 and source of selenium on the response of the selenium-dependent glutathione peroxidase system to oxidative stress induced by oestrus in pubertal pig. J. Trace Elem. Med. Biol. 32, 21–29.

Dalto, D.B., Tsoi, S., Audet, I., Dyck, M.K., Foxcroft, G.R., Matte, J.J., 2015b. Gene expression of porcine blastocysts from gilts fed organic or inorganic selenium and pyridoxine. Reproduction 149, 31–42.

Dalto, D.B., Audet, I., Lapointe, J., Matte, J.J., 2016. The importance of pyridoxine for the impact of the dietary selenium sources on redox balance, embryo development, and reproductive performance in gilts. J. Trace Elem. Med. Biol. 34, 79–89.

Dalto, D.B., Matte, J.J., 2017. Pyridoxine (vitamin B6) and the glutathione peroxidase system; a link between one-carbon metabolism and antioxidation. Nutrients 9, 189.

Dalto, D.B., Tsoi, S., Dyck, M.K., Matte, J.J., 2018. Gene ontology analysis of expanded porcine blastocysts from gilts fed organic or inorganic selenium combined with pyridoxine. BMC Genomics 19, 836–846.

Davis, S.R., Quinlivan, E.P., Stacpoole, P.W., Gregory 3rd, J.F., 2006. Plasma glutathione and cystathionine concentrations are elevated but cysteine flux is unchanged by dietary vitamin B-6 restriction in young men and women. J. Nutr. 136, 373–378.

Dove, C.R., Cook, D.A., 2001. Water-Soluble Vitamins in Swine Nutrition Swine Nutrition, second ed. CRC Press, Boca Raton.

Driskell, J.A., 1994. Vitamin B-6 requirements of humans. Nutr. Res. 14, 293–324.

Dumont, E., Vanhaecke, F., Cornels, R., 2006. Selenium speciation from food source to metabolites: a critical review. Anal. Bioanal. Chem. 385, 1304–1323.

Ereno-Orbea, J., Majtan, T., Oyenarte, I., Kraus, J.P., Martinez-Cruz, L.A., 2014. Structural insight into the molecular mechanism of allosteric activation of human cystathionine beta-synthase by *S*-adenosylmethionine. Proc. Natl. Acad. Sci. U.S.A. 111, E3845–E3852.

Flavin, M., Slaughter, C., 1964. Cystathionine cleavage enzymes of neurospora. J. Biol. Chem. 239, 2212–2219.

Födinger, M., Hörl, W., Sunder-Plassmann, G., 2000. Molecular biology of 5,10-methylenetetrahydrofolate reductase. J. Nephrol. 13, 20–33.

Fortier, M.-E., Audet, I., Giguère, A., Laforest, J.-P., Bilodeau, J.-F., Quesnel, H., et al., 2012. Effect of dietary organic and inorganic selenium on antioxidant status, embryo development, and reproductive performance in hyperovulatory first-parity gilts. J. Anim. Sci. 90, 231–240.

FSA, 2002. The Composition of Foods, sixth ed. Royal Society of Chemistry, Cambridge.

Gardiner, C.S., Reed, D.J., 1995. Glutathione redox cycle-driven recovery of reduced glutathione after oxidation by tertiary-butyl hydroperoxide in preimplantation mouse embryos. Arch. Biochem. Biophys. 321, 6–12.
Gregory, J.F., 1997. Bioavailability of vitamin B-6. Eur. J. Clin. Nutr. 51, 43–48.
Hoover, D.M., Carltoannd, W., Henrikso, C.K., 1981. Ultrastructural lesions of pyridoxine toxicity in beagle dogs. Vet. Pathol. 18, 769–777.
Institute of Medicine, 2000. Dietary Reference Intakes for Vitamin C, Vitamin E, Selenium, and Carotenoids. The National Academies Press, Washington.
Jauniaux, E., Watson, A.L., Hempstock, J., Bao, Y.P., Skepper, J.N., Burton, G.J., 2000. Onset of maternal arterial blood flow and placental oxidative stress. A possible factor in human early pregnancy failure. Am. J. Pathol. 157, 2111–2122.
Johansson, L.G., Gafvelin, G., Arner, E.S.J., 2005. Selenocysteine in proteins—properties and biotechnological use. BBA Gen. Subj. 1726, 1–13.
Kalhan, S.C., 2016. One carbon metabolism in pregnancy: Impact on maternal, fetal and neonatal health. Mol. Cell. Endocrinol. 435, 48–60.
Kazemi, R., Daghir, N.J., 1971. Interrelationships between methionine and vitamin B6 in chick diets. Poult. Sci. 50, 1296–1302.
Levonen, A.L., Lapatto, R., Saksela, M., Raivio, K.O., 2000. Human cystathionine gamma-lyase: developmental and in vitro expression of two isoforms. Biochem. J. 347, 291–295.
Li, Y.N., Gulati, S., Baker, P.J., Brody, L.C., Banerjee, R., Kruger, W.D., 1996. Cloning, mapping and RNA analysis of the human methionine synthase gene. Hum. Mol. Genet. 5, 1851–1858.
Lima, C.P., Davis, S.R., Mackey, A.D., Scheer, J.B., Williamson, J., Gregory 3rd, J.F., 2006. Vitamin B-6 deficiency suppresses the hepatic transsulfuration pathway but increases glutathione concentration in rats fed AIN-76A or AIN-93G diets. J. Nutr. 136, 2141–2147.
Lubos, E., Loscalzo, J., Handy, D.E., 2011. Glutathione peroxidase-1 in health and disease: from molecular mechanisms to therapeutic opportunities. Antioxid. Redox Signal. 5, 1957–1997.
Ma, Y.L., Lindemann, M.D., Pierce, J.L., Unrine, J.M., Cromwell, G.L., 2014. Effect of inorganic or organic selenium supplementation on reproductive performance and tissue trace mineral concentrations in gravid first-parity gilts, fetuses, and nursing piglets. J. Anim. Sci. 92, 5540–5550.
Mahan, D.C., Peters, J.C., 2004. Long-term effects of dietary organic and inorganic selenium sources and levels on reproducing sows and their progeny. J. Anim. Sci. 82, 1343–1358.
Mahan, D.C., Cline, T.R., Richert, B., 1999. Effects of dietary levels ofselenium-enriched yeast and sodium selenite as selenium sources fed togrowing-finishing pigs on performance, tissue selenium, serum glutathione peroxidase activity, carcass characteristics, and loin quality. J. Anim. Sci. 77, 2172–2179.
Martinez, M., Cuskelly, G.J., Williamson, J., Toth, J.P., Gregory, J.F., 2000. Vitamin B6 deficiency in rats reduces hepatic serine hydroxymethyltransferase and cystathionine beta-synthase activities and rates of in vivo protein turnover, homocysteine remethylation and transsulfuration. J. Nutr. 130, 1115–1123.
McDowell, L.R., 2003. Minerals in Animal and Human Nutrition, second ed. Elsevier Science, Amsterdam.
Mehansho, H., Henderson, L.M., 1980. Transport and accumulation of pyridoxine and pyridoxal by erythrocytes. J. Biol. Chem. 255, 11901–11907.
Middleton, H.M., 1985. Uptake of pyridoxine by in vivo perfused segments of rat small intestine: a possible role for intracellular vitamin metabolism. J. Nutr. 115, 1079–1088.

Mosharov, E., Cranford, M.R., Banerjee, R., 2000. The quantitatively important relationship between homocysteine metabolism and glutathione synthesis by the transsulfuration pathway and its regulation by redox changes. Biochemistry 39, 13005–13011.
Mudd, S.H., Cantoni, G.L., 1958. Activation of methionine for transmethylation. III. The methionine-activating enzyme of bakers' yeast. J. Biol. Chem. 231, 481–492.
Osawa, S., Jukes, T.H., Watanabe, K., Muto, A., 1992. Recent evidence for evolution of the genetic code. Microbiol. Rev. 56, 229–264.
Pavlata, L., Misurova, L., Pechova, A., Dvorak, R., 2011. The effect of inorganic and organically bound forms of selenium on glutathione peroxidase activity in the blood of goats. Vet. Med. Czech. 56, 75–81.
Perry, C., Yu, S., Chen, J., Matharu, K., Stover, P., 2007. Effect of vitamin B6 availability on serine hydroxymethyltransferase in MCF-7 cells. Arch. Biochem. Biophys. 462, 21–27.
Rider, S.A., Davies, S.J., Jha, A.N., Clough, R., Sweetman, J.W., 2010. Bioavailability of co-supplemented organic and inorganic zinc and selenium sources in a white fishmeal-based rainbow trout (*Oncorhynchus mykiss*) diet. J. Anim. Physiol. Anim. Nutr. 94, 99–110.
Roth-Maier, D.A., Kettler, S.I., Kirchgessner, M., 2002. Availability of vitamin B6 from different food sources. Int. J. Food Sci. Nutr. 53, 171–179.
Schrauzer, G.N., 2003. The nutritional significance, metabolism and toxicology of selenomethionine. Adv. Food Nutr. Res. 47, 73–112.
Selhub, J., 1999. Homocysteine metabolism. Annu. Rev. Nutr. 19, 217–246.
Smith, A.M., Picciano, M.F., 1986. Evidence for increased selenium requirement for the rat during pregnancy and lactation. J. Nutr. 116, 1068–1079.
Soda, K., Oikawa, T., Esaki, N., 1999. Vitamin B6 enzymes participating in selenium amino acid metabolism. BioFactors 10, 257–262.
Sunde, R.A., 1984. The biochemistry of selenoproteins. J. Am. Oil Chem. Soc. 61, 1891–1900.
Swanson, C.A., 1991. Human (74Se)selenomethionine metabolism: a kinetic model. Am. J. Clin. Nutr. 54, 917–926.
Taoka, S., Ohja, S., Shan, X., Kruger, W.D., Banerjee, R., 1998. Evidence for heme-mediated redox regulation of human cystathionine β-synthase activity. J. Biol. Chem. 273, 25179–25184.
Tibbetts, A.S., Appling, D.R., 2010. Compartmentalization of mammalian folate-mediated one-carbon metabolism. Annu. Rev. Nutr. 30, 57–81.
Ulrey, C.L., Liu, L., Andrews, L.G., Tollefsbol, T.O., 2005. The impact of metabolism on DNA methylation. Hum. Mol. Genet. 14, R139–R147.
Ursini, F., 2000. The world of glutathione peroxidases. J. Trace Elem. Med. Biol. 14, 116–121.
Vendeland, S.C., Deagen, J.T., Butler, J.A., Whanger, P.D., 1994. Uptake of selenite, selenomethionine and selenate by brush border membrane vesicles isolated from rat small intestine. Biometals 7, 305–312.
Wada, H., Snell, E.E., 1961. The enzymatic oxidation of pyridoxine and pyridoxamine phosphates. J. Biol. Chem. 236, 2089–2095.
Whanger, P.D., 2002. Selenocompounds in plants and animals and their biological significance. J. Am. Coll. Nutr. 21, 223–232.
Windisch, W., 2002. Interaction of chemical species with biological regulation of the metabolism of essential trace elements. Anal. Bioanal. Chem. 372, 421–425.
Wolfram, S., Berger, B., Grenacher, B., Scharrer, E., 1989. Transport of seleno amino acids and their sulphur analogues across the intestinal brush border membrane. J. Nutr. 119, 706–712.

Yin, S.A., Sato, I., Yamagushi, K., 1992. Comparison of selenium level and glutathione peroxidase activity in tissues of vitamin B6 deficient rats fed sodium selenite or Dl selenomethionine. J. Nutr. Biochem. 3, 633–639.

Further reading

Davis, S., Scheer, J., Quinlivan, E., Coats, B., Stacpoole, P., Gregory, J., 2005. Dietary vitamin B6 restriction does not alter rates of homocysteine remethylation or synthesis in healthy young women and men. Am. J. Clin. Nutr. 81, 648–655.

CHAPTER 8

Vitamin K2 is a key regulator of clinically relevant molecular processes

Maria Fusaro[1,2], Mario Plebani[3], Giovanni Tripepi[4], Giorgio Iervasi[1], John Cunningham[5], Francesco Locatelli[6], Martina Zaninotto[3], Andrea Aghi[7], Maria Cristina Mereu[8] and Maurizio Gallieni[9]

[1]National Research Council (CNR) – Institute of Clinical Physiology (IFC), Pisa, Italy
[2]Department of Medicine, University of Padova, Padova, Italy
[3]Department of Medicine, University of Padova, Laboratory Medicine Unit, Padova, Italy
[4]Clinical Epidemiology and Physiopathology of Renal Diseases and Hypertension, CNR, Institute of Clinical Physiology, Reggio Calabria, Italy
[5]University College London, London, United Kingdom
[6]Division of Nephrology and Dialysis, A. Manzoni Hospital, Lecco, Italy
[7]Department of Medicine, Clinica Medica 1, University of Padova, Padova, Italy
[8]Nephrologist Independent Researcher, Cagliari, Italy
[9]Nephrology and Dialysis Unit, Department of Clinical and Biomedical Sciences 'Luigi Sacco', University of Milan, Milan, Italy

Contents

Summary points

- This chapter is about vitamin K [K1 or phylloquinone (PK), and K2 or menaquinone (MKn)].

Molecular Nutrition
DOI: https://doi.org/10.1016/B978-0-12-811907-5.00029-4

- PK is found in vegetables, MKn is produced by bacteria in the intestine and in fermented foods.
- The main role of vitamin K is as the coenzyme for gamma-glutamyl carboxylase (GGCX), forming gamma-carboxyglutamic acid (Gla) residues on target proteins.
- Vitamin K also acts as a ligand for the steroid and xenobiotic receptor (SXR) in the nucleus.
- Gla residues are essential for the activity of vitamin K–dependent proteins (VKDPs), such as coagulation factors (prothrombin, factor VII, IX,X, and proteins C, M, S, Z), bone Gla protein (BGP, or osteocalcin), matrix Gla protein (MGP), Gas6 (growth arrest-specific 6 protein), GRP (Gla-rich protein), and periostin.
- Recommended intakes for vitamin K are not well-established and significantly different indications can be found in the literature.
- An adequate vitamin K intake in the general population and in patients affected by bone and mineral disorders (e.g., osteoporosis) and cardiovascular calcifications can lead to benefits.
- Its use as a dietary supplement and as a pharmacological treatment for bone and mineral abnormalities should be further explored.

Abbreviations

AI	adequate intake
Apo	apolipoprotein
BGP	bone Gla protein (or osteocalcin)
BMP-2	bone morphogenetic protein-2
CKD	chronic kidney disease
cMGP	carboxylated MGP
dp-cMGP	dephosphorylated-carboxylated MGP
dp-ucMGP	dephosphorylated-undercarboxylated MGP
Gas6	growth arrest-specific 6 protein
GGCX	gamma-glutamyl carboxylase
Gla	gamma-carboxyglutamic acid
GRP	Gla-rich protein
MGP	matrix Gla protein
MKn	menaquinones
p-cMGP:	phosphorylated-carboxylated MGP
PK	phylloquinone
p-ucMGP	phosphorylated-undercarboxylated MGP
PXR	pregnane X receptor
RDA	recommended dietary allowance
SXR	steroid and xenobiotic receptor

uc-BGP undercarboxylated BGP
ucMGP undercarboxylated MGP
VKDP vitamin K–dependent protein
VSMCs vascular smooth muscle cells

8.1 Introduction

The first descriptions of vitamin K in the literature date back to the 1930s (Dam, 1935; Schønheyder, 1936; MacCorquodale et al., 1939). The discovery of vitamin K marked a seminal achievement in the field of coagulation and thrombosis, so important that less than a decade later, in 1943, Henrik Carl Peter Dam and Edward Adelbert Doisy won the Nobel Prize in Physiology or Medicine for their work on the characterization of vitamin K and its effects on the coagulation system. However, in the following years no significant further developments were observed, until recently when other vitamin K–dependent proteins (VKDPs)were identified, and a role of vitamin K was proposed for bone and mineral metabolism. Vitamin K deficiency may be associated with bone fractures and vascular calcifications and therefore is important for bone and cardiovascular health. More clinically relevant areas are being explored, including cancer, which has been linked to vitamin K deficiency (Dahlberg et al., 2017).

Vitamin K acts as a cofactor for the posttranslational modification of specific proteins, denominated VKDPs, through carboxylation of glutamate residues. A 2-methyl-1,4-naphthoquinone nucleus characterizes the K vitamers, which exist in two forms based on the different side-chains at the 3-position: vitamin K1 (or phylloquinone, PK, with a phytyl side chain) and K2 (or menaquinone, MKn, with a variable number of condensed isoprenic units). Another K vitamer without a side chain is a synthetic form called menadione or K3 (Fig. 8.1) (Fusaro et al., 2011).

The sources of vitamin K are different according to the type of vitamer considered. In particular, PK can be found mostly in green leafy vegetables, such as cabbage, spinach, cauliflower, and green fruits, such as kiwi and avocado (Booth et al., 2003). In Japan a significant dietary intake of MKn has been associated with the consumption of natto, a soybean-based fermented food (Fujita et al., 2012). In Western diets MKn has been found in fermented foods such as curdled cheese, egg yolk, butter, and beef liver (Schurgers et al., 2007). The intestinal bacterial flora also generate MKn, which is characterized by long lateral chains: MK-10 and MK-11 are synthesized by Bacteroides, MK-8 by Enterobacteria, MK-7

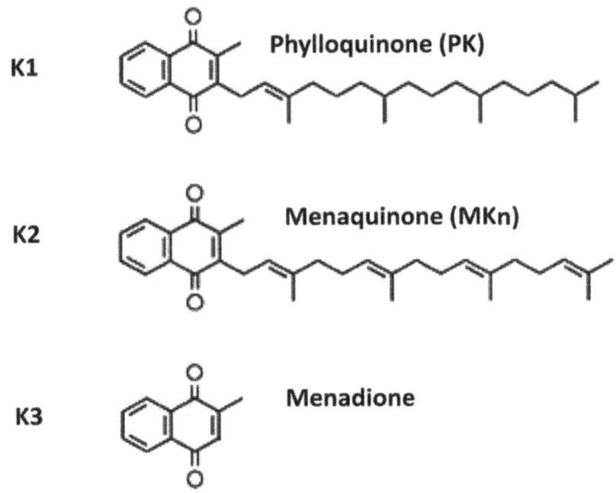

Figure 8.1 The three main forms of vitamin K.
Vitamin K1 (phylloquinone) is found in plants, and it is the main dietary source of vitamin K.
Vitamin K2 can be defined as a group of related compounds, menaquinones (MKs). The side chain of vitamin K2 can be of different length, with a variable number of isoprenoid units (MKn). In humans some of the ingested vitamin K1 is converted to menaquinone-4 (MK-4), the specific mammalian vitamin K2.
Vitamin K3 (menadione), a synthetic form of vitamin K1, has the same naphthoquinone ring as K1 and K2, but lacks a side chain. Menadione may also be converted into MK-4 in the liver.

by Veillonella, and MK-6 by *Eubacterium lentum* (Conly and Stein, 1992; Walther et al., 2013). A peculiar case is represented by MK-4, which is the only one not produced by the intestinal bacterial flora but it is converted from PK through a side chain removal/addition mechanism in specific tissues such as pancreas, testes, and vessel wall, with menadione as the intermediate molecule (Walther et al., 2013). The synthetic form menadione, K3, is also converted into MK-4 in the liver (Sato et al., 2012).

8.2 Metabolism, recycling, and functions of vitamin K

Reflecting the different dietary sources and mechanisms of vitamin K synthesis, intestinal absorption follows different pathways: MKn is absorbed in the colon by a passive diffusion mechanism, while PK is absorbed by the small bowel with a saturable, energy-dependent mechanism (Shearer and Newman, 2008). Normal pancreatic function and the presence of bile salts are necessary conditions for normal absorption of vitamin K (Shearer and Newman, 2008). In the enterocyte vitamin K becomes part of micelle that assembles chylomicrons with apolipoprotein A, apoB-48, ApoC, and ApoE, thus arriving into the circulation (Shearer and Newman, 2008). Chylomicrons are converted into remnants because triglycerides are removed by lipoprotein lipase in the capillaries and they then reach the liver as very-low-density lipoprotein. The latter, together with apolipoprotein B, C, and E, leave the circulation and arrive into bone by an endocytosis mechanism (Shearer and Newman, 2008; Cooper, 1997). Apolipoprotein E polymorphisms influence vitamin K levels (Kohlmeier et al., 1996). Of all the fat-soluble vitamins, vitamin K is the one with the lowest serum levels in humans. Recycling helps to maintain adequate stores of vitamin K (Fig. 8.2) (Stafford, 2005).

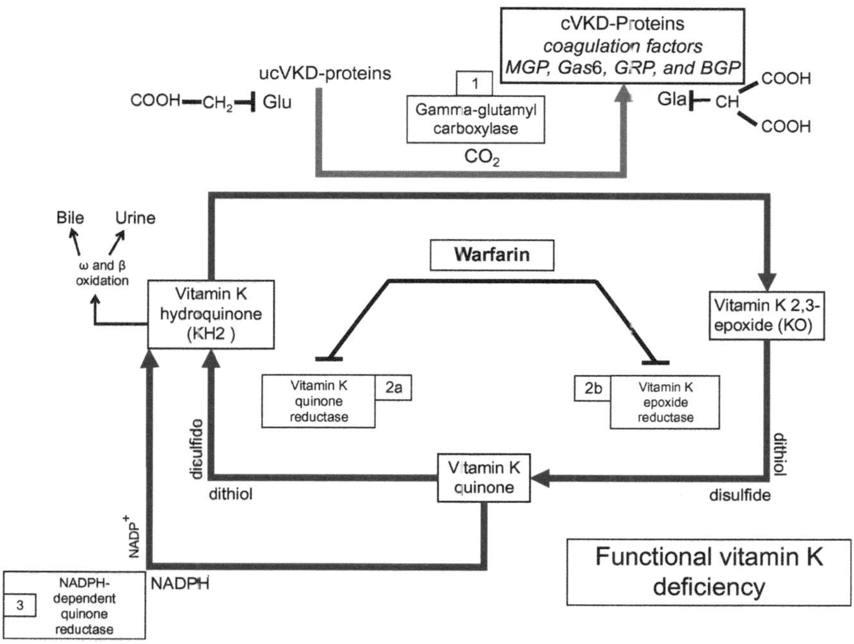

Figure 8.2 The vitamin K cycle.
Vitamin K acts as a coenzyme of gamma-glutamyl carboxylase (GGCX) (1). The reaction is the carboxylation of glutamic acid (Glu), transformed into gamma-carboxyglutamic acid (Gla) residues. Warfarin, an antagonist of vitamin K, blocks two important reactions: vitamin K quinone reductase (2a) and vitamin K epoxide reductase (VKOR) (2b), leading to a functional deficit of vitamin K. Quinone reductase NADPH (3) is insensitive to the inhibitory action of warfarin and can be an escape route for the transformation of vitamin K quinone into vitamin K hydroquinone.

The main role of vitamin K is acting as the coenzyme for the gamma-glutamyl carboxylase (GGCX) enzyme (Fig. 8.2), leading to the carboxylation of glutamic acid residues (Glu), which are transformed into gamma-carboxyglutamic acid (Gla) (Fusaro et al., 2011, 2017a; Gallieni and Fusaro, 2014). Gla residues are essential for the activity of VKDPs, such as coagulation factors (prothrombin, factor VII, IX,X, and proteins C, M, S, Z), bone Gla protein (BGP, or osteocalcin), matrix Gla protein (MGP), Gas6 (growth arrest-specific 6 protein), GRP (Gla-rich protein), and periostin (Oldenburg et al., 2006; Vermeer, 1990, 2012; Merle and Garnero, 2012; Wen et al., 2018).

Less studied is another vitamin K action as a ligand of the steroid and xenobiotic receptor (SXR) in the nucleus (Fusaro et al., 2017b; Horie-Inoue and Inoue, 2008). SXR is also known as the murine homolog pregnane X receptor, PXR. SXR/PXR is mainly expressed in the liver and intestine (Sultana et al., 2018). Vitamin K2 appears to modulate, through this nuclear receptor, the expression of genes involved in bile acid synthesis and glucose homeostasis in mice (Sultana et al., 2018). SXR/PXR has also been found in osteoblastic cell lines, which are activated by vitamin K (Horie-Inoue and Inoue, 2008). In fact SXR/PXR seems to regulate bone homeostasis by promoting bone formation and suppressing bone resorption (Fusaro et al., 2017b). Furthermore, transcriptional control of SXR/PXR target genes by vitamin K induces bone protective effects through the regulation of collagen proteins, osteoclastogenesis, and osteoblastogenesis (Fusaro et al., 2017b; Azuma et al., 2014).

8.3 Vitamin K status and vitamin K–dependent proteins

Recommended intakes for vitamin K are not well-established and significantly different recommendations can be found in the literature. The Food and Nutrition Board (FNB) at the Institute of Medicine of the National Academies (Institute of Medicine, 2001) postulates a dietary reference intake defined by four sets of reference values, which may vary by age and gender. They include the recommended dietary allowance (RDA), defined as the average daily level of intake sufficient to meet the nutrient requirements of nearly all (up to 98%) healthy individuals. The adequate intake (AI) refers to the amount ensuring nutritional adequacy and it is established when evidence is insufficient to develop an RDA. The estimated average requirement is the average daily level of intake estimated to meet the requirements of 50% of healthy individuals. Finally, the tolerable upper intake level (UL) is the maximum daily intake unlikely to cause adverse health effects. Due to insufficient available data, Institute of Medicine (2001) suggests for vitamin K an AI of 120 mcg/day in adult males and 90 mcg/day in adult females, with no distinction between vitamin K1 and K2. These values have been endorsed by the National Institutes of Health (National Institutes of Health, 2018). In Europe the European Food Safety Authority recommends 70 mcg/day of PK for all adults including pregnant and lactating women (EFSA Panel on Dietetic Products, Nutrition and Allergies, 2017). Furthermore, authorities of individual European countries recommend higher intakes of vitamin K; according to the Italian Nutritional Guideline the AI for vitamin K for adults is 140 mcg/day under 60 years of age and 170 mcg/day in individuals older than 60 years (Società Italiana di Nutrizione Umana, 2014). The Belgian authorities also raised the maximum intake of vitamin K to 210 mcg/day (Conseil Supérieur de la Santé, 2016). There is no known toxicity associated with high doses of vitamin K1 or K2, which is why no tolerable UL of intake has been established for vitamin K1 or K2 (Institute of Medicine, 2001).

Vitamin K is essential for the function of VKDPs but it is not precisely known what levels of vitamin K1 and/or K2 are required for an adequate activity of a range of VKDPs involved in the regulation of physiologic functions, such as coagulation, bone and cartilage mineralization, inhibition of vascular calcifications, anticancer mechanisms, etc. (Shiozawa et al., 2010; Naito et al., 2012; Rafael et al., 2014) (Table 8.1). Specific claims for recommending a higher intake of vitamin K2 have been published (Bruno, 2016), suggesting 180 mcg/day for adults.

Among the liposoluble vitamins, vitamin K has the lowest circulating levels in healthy humans (Sadowski et al., 1989), which translates into difficulties when trying to assess vitamin K status. Furthermore, the variation of serum levels of vitamin K vitamers also depends on serum triglyceride concentrations and apoE genotype: these two factors accounted for 64% of the interindividual variation (Fusaro et al., 2011). Thus the measurement standardization of vitamin K levels is to date undefined and vitamin K status is mainly assessed by evaluating the carboxylation level of VKDPs (Fusaro et al., 2017c). Sadowski et al. (1989) assessed vitamin K levels in the general population and found that the normal concentration of plasma PK ranged between 0.29 and 2.64 nmol/L, with a median value of 0.86 nmol/L. Elderly subjects had slightly higher PK levels than the young subjects (means = 1.05 vs 0.94 nmol/L), but when plasma PK

Table 8.1 Physiologic function of vitamin K–dependent proteins (VKDP), effects of vitamin K deficiency in the general population and in chronic kidney disease (CKD) patients on VKDPs, and the use of VKDPs as biomarkers.

Vitamin K–dependent proteins	Physiologic function	Vitamin K deficiency in the general population	Vitamin K deficiency in CKD patients	Use as biomarker
Matrix Gla protein (MGP)	• Inhibition of osteogenic factors (blocking the growth of mineralized crystals) and consequently vascular and soft tissue calcification.	Vascular calcifications, mortality	Vascular calcifications, mortality	Total MGP is not currently used as an indicator of vitamin K deficiency
Dephosphorylated-undercarboxylated MGP (dp-uc MGP)	• A reduced number of carboxyl residues is a consequence of vitamin K deficiency, reducing VKDP activity • Dp-uc MGP is a posttranslational molecule, probably physiologically inactive	Renal dysfunction, cardiovascular calcification	Cardiovascular calcification	Low serum levels may be a marker of cardiovascular disease. High serum levels may be a marker of vitamin K deficiency, renal dysfunction, cardiovascular, and soft tissue calcification.
Bone Gla protein (BGP, osteocalcin)	• Involved in bone mineralization: attract and bind calcium ions for the translocation of calcium ions to the bone matrix	Bone fragility, vascular calcifications, abnormal glucose metabolism, and mortality	Bone fragility, vascular calcifications, and mortality	Bone anabolic marker
Undercarboxylated BGP (uc-BGP)	• uc-BGP has been implicated in the hormonal regulation of glucose homeostasis.	Abnormal glucose metabolism	Unknown consequences	uc-BGP is a biomarker of vitamin K deficiency and osteoarthritis.

Growth arrest-specific 6 (GAS6). expressed in endothelial cells, vascular smooth muscle cells, and bone marrow	• Mediated by TAM receptors activation • Effects on primary hemostasis, vascular remodeling, and coagulation • Produced by platelets and blood vessel walls • Antiinflammatory effect, depending on cell type • Protect endothelial cells and VSMCs against apoptosis	Unknown consequences Putative: effects on hemostasis, inflammation, and cancer growth	Unknown consequences	Uncertain
Gla-rich protein (GRP)	• Inhibitor of osteoblast differentiation and maturation • Inhibitor of calcification in vascular and articular tissue • Novel antiinflammatory agent, with potential beneficial effects on osteoarthritis progression • Decreases the activity of alkaline phosphate	Unknown consequences	Unknown consequences	Association between osteoarthritis and carboxylation deficiency
Periostin and periostin-like-factor (PLF)	• Promotes the differentiation, aggregation, adhesion, and proliferation of osteoblasts • Involvement in collagen folding (bone strength)	Increase risk of fibrosis in heart, myocardial hypertrophy, and dysfunction of heart	Increase risk of fibrosis in heart, myocardial hypertrophy, and dysfunction of heart	High periostin levels as marker high pressure of bone tissue PLF: indicator of adaptive bone remodeling

Gla-rich protein (GRP), Gas6, and MGP are likely to exhibit a synergistic effect on the inhibition of cardiovascular calcification. TAM receptors (Tyro3, Axl, and Mer) comprise a unique family of receptor tyrosine kinases.

concentrations were expressed as nanomoles of PL per millimole of triglyceride, the elderly subjects showed decreased levels for PK compared with the young subjects. Neogi et al. (2006) found a lower prevalence of osteoarthritis of the hand and knee with increasing plasma PK levels. Based on this study, a plasma PK level below 1 nmol/L may carry an increased risk for the development of osteoarthritis, while levels above this threshold were not associated with further decreases in osteoarthritis prevalence (Neogi et al., 2006). Among the individuals included in this study, the median plasma PK concentration was 1.03 nmol/L, suggesting that half of them had insufficient levels for adequate osteoarticular metabolism. Plasma PK levels adjusted for triglycerides have also been found to be inversely associated with femur neck bone mineral density (BMD) in men and with vertebral BMD in postmenopausal women not using estrogen replacements (Booth et al., 2004). In contrast, there were no significant associations between biochemical measures of vitamin K and BMD in either premenopausal women or postmenopausal women using estrogen replacements.

In the population-based Rotterdam Study, the dietary intake of MK was related to aortic calcification and coronary heart disease (Geleijnse et al., 2004). The relative risk of coronary heart disease mortality was significantly reduced in the mid (0.73) and upper (0.43) tertiles of dietary MK compared to the lower tertile. Furthermore, the upper tertile of MK intake was also significantly and inversely related to all-cause mortality (RR 0.74) and severe aortic calcification (odds ratio 0.48), suggesting that an adequate MK intake may be instrumental in the prevention of cardiovascular diseases and the related morbidity and mortality. Interestingly PK intake was not related to any of the outcomes (Geleijnse et al., 2004).

As indicated in Table 8.1 vitamin K regulates several VKDPs, with relevant physiologic functions. A total of 17 different VKDPs have been identified to date (Wen et al., 2018). A short review of the most relevant and well-studied follows here.

8.3.1 Bone Gla protein (osteocalcin)

Osteocalcin, or BGP, is a protein of 49 amino acids, containing three Gla residues. BGP synthesis is modulated by vitamin D, acting as a promoter for its gene synthesized by the activating transcription factor 4, which regulates terminal osteoblast differentiation and virtually all functions of the osteoblast related to the control of bone mass (Yoshizawa et al., 2009). Unexpectedly, it was found that $1,25(OH)_2D_3$ increases BGP expression in humans (Kerner et al., 1989) and rats, while it decreases its expression in mice. BGP is produced by osteoblasts, odontoblasts, cartilage cells, and osteoblast-like vascular smooth muscle cells (VSMCs) as proprotein in a first step of the synthesis and after removal of the signal peptide it is transformed into its undercarboxylated form (uc-BGP) (Wen et al., 2018). Uc-BGP is then converted to its active form, carboxylated (cBGP), by GGCX, with an enzymatic reaction requiring the presence of vitamin K. BGP binds calcium ions and incorporates them in the hydroxyapatite crystals forming the bone matrix (Fusaro et al., 2011; Wen et al., 2018). While in animals all three BGP vitamin K–dependent Gla sites are fully carboxylated, in humans the BGP molecules found in bone and serum are incompletely carboxylated (undercarboxylated BGP). Carboxylation is also influenced by the osteotesticular protein tyrosine phosphatase (OST-PTP), whose gene name is ESP (Wen et al., 2018). OST-PTP contributes to maintaining the carboxylated state of BGP and experimental studies showed that a deletion of the epithiospecifier protein (ESP) gene in mice ($Esp^{-/-}$) is associated with alterations of glucose metabolism (Kim et al., 2010) and with a reduced BGP production in organs of the male reproductive system (Karsenty and Oury, 2014). Thus the activity of BGP is diversified and complex. Carboxylated BGP locally inhibits osteoclast-mediated bone resorption and it binds to calcium deposits in the bone matrix. BGP can also be found in the blood circulation, but whether it promotes or inhibits the calcification of blood vessels has not been elucidated (Wen et al., 2018).

8.3.2 Matrix Gla protein

MGP is a protein of 84 amino acids, produced by cells of bone and the cardiovascular system, namely osteoclasts, chondrocytes, vascular endothelial cells, macrophages, and the VSMCs. It contains five Gla residues and it has a high affinity for calcium and hydroxyapatite (Schurgers et al., 2008). Its biological activity depends on the vitamin K–dependent physiologic regulation of the Gla residues. In addition, the protein can be phosphorylated on three serine residues at positions 3, 6, and 9. Thus MGP can be found in the circulation in different forms, depending on the carboxylation and phosphorylation status: dephosphorylated-undercarboxylated MGP (dp-ucMGP); dephosphorylated-carboxylated MGP (dp-cMGP); and phosphorylated-carboxylated MGP (p-cMGP) (Schurgers et al., 2008). After the synthesis of dp-ucMGP, GGCX and its coenzyme vitamin K carboxylate the five Glu residues into Gla molecules and transform the protein into dp-cMGP. Subsequently, the latter become phosphorylated to generate p-cMGP, which is the active molecule.

In the case of vitamin K deficiency due to a low oral intake or to warfarin treatment, there will be an increase in the inactive ucMGP and in particular the p-ucMGP will bind to calcium without inhibiting calcification. MGP prevents blood vessel calcification forming a molecular compound made of fetuin-A (80%), Gla (2%), and calcium-phosphorous ions (18%). This complex inhibits the promotion and growth of potential calcification foci. In addition, MGP activates phagocytosis of apoptotic bodies, blocking their potential contribution to ectopic calcifications. During warfarin treatment, or inadequate vitamin K intake, matrix vesicles are formed and apoptotic bodies appear in VSMCs, favoring the formation of calcification foci on the vascular wall. VSMCs may also differentiate into osteoblast-like cells (Wen et al., 2018). P-cMGP inhibits the production of bone morphogenetic protein-2 (BMP-2), a powerful osteoinductive protein which in turn regulates another VKDP, GRPA lack of GRP promotes the osteogenic differentiation of VSMCs. In several chronic diseases, such as chronic kidney disease (CKD), diabetes, and inflammatory conditions, an increased local synthesis of MGP by VSMC at the level of the arterial tunica media is observed in order to try to inhibit the vascular calcifications which characterize these conditions (Schurgers et al., 2008; Murshed et al., 2004). Keutel Syndrome, a rare recessive autosomal genetic disease clinically characterized by diffuse, severe cartilage and vascular calcification, is caused by a mutation in the gene encoding MGP (Munroe et al., 1999). A similar phenotype has been obtained in mice with MGP gene knockout, developing early in their life pathological fractures due to severe osteoporosis and severe medial vascular calcifications, resulting in aortic rupture and death (Luo et al., 1997).

8.3.3 Growth arrest-specific 6 protein

Gas6 is a vitamin K–dependent, Gla-containing (11–12 residues) protein involved in the stimulation of cell proliferation (Hafizi and Dahlbäck, 2006). It has 44% homology with plasma anticoagulant protein S (Mark et al., 1996). Their action is mediated by the binding to and activation of the receptor tyrosine kinases Axl, Sky, and Mer. Gas6 regulates cell survival, proliferation, migration, adhesion, and phagocytosis. In addition,

Gas6 and protein S connect their nonreceptor-binding regions to the negatively charged membranes of apoptotic cells. Gas6 protein expression is common in the lung, endometrium, and 24 other tissues and cells, including the osteoblasts (Shiozawa et al., 2010). It was found to be overexpressed in many cancers and has been implicated as an adverse prognostic marker, but Gas6 also inhibits vascular calcification by interfering with VSMC apoptosis (Hasanbasic et al., 2005).

8.3.4 Gla-rich protein

GRP is characterized by a large number of Gla residues, in humans up to 15, conferring the highest ratio between number of Gla residues and size of the protein among VKDPs (Viegas et al., 2009). Such abundance of Gla residues and therefore its marked affinity for mineral binding suggests that GRP may directly influence mineral formation, thereby protecting from soft tissue mineralization. Consistent with this, its distribution is primarily in the bone, cartilage, skin, and vasculature, where it serves an important role in inhibiting vascular calcification. GRP is also a circulating protein, activated following γ-carboxylation. Its expression may be inhibited by BMP-2, a protein associated with bone. In turn GRP may inhibit the differentiation and maturation of osteoblasts, activity of alkaline phosphatase, and expression of osteogenic genes, thus acting as a negative regulator of osteogenic differentiation (Wen et al., 2018). Importantly GRP may be involved in the mechanisms of calcification of articular tissues associated with inflammation in osteoarthritis (Cavaco et al., 2016).

8.3.5 Periostin

Periostin is a large VKDP, with a molecular weight of ~90 kDa. Also known as osteoblast-specific factor 2, it is an extracellular matrix protein (Wen et al., 2018). Periostin is expressed during ontogenesis and in adult connective tissues submitted to mechanical strains, most notably in periosteum, periodontal ligaments, tendons, heart valves, and skin (Merle and Garnero, 2012). It is also expressed in neoplastic tissues, cardiovascular and fibrotic diseases, and during wound repair. Isoforms of periostin have been identified (Litvin et al., 2004), differing in their C-terminal sequences. Periostin isoforms are expressed in vivo and in vitro during the stages of osteoblast differentiation and maturation. Because antisense oligonucleotides and antibodies directed against and blocking the activity of periostin isoforms induced a marked reduction of osteoblast-specific-differentiation markers, a role for these proteins in osteoblast differentiation has been proposed (Litvin et al., 2004). By binding to cell surface receptors, periostin stimulates the differentiation, aggregation, adhesion, and proliferation of osteoblasts. In addition, its action on collagen folding, favoring matrix assembly, may be relevant for improving bone strength (Merle and Garnero, 2012). Of four different subtypes (Pn-1 to -4), Pn-1 but not Pn-2 inhibited the adhesion of cardiac fibroblasts and cardiac muscle cells and also promoted cardiac fibrosis and remodeling following myocardial infarction. Furthermore, Pn-2 has been associated with angiogenesis, but Pn-1 was not. Overall, periostin may increase myocardial hypertrophy, myocardial fibrosis, and dysfunction of the heart.

8.4 Clinical use of menaquinones

The nine different but related compounds known as MKn are generally classified into the short-chain MKn (with MK-4 as the most relevant) and the long-chain MKn (of which MK-7 is the most studied). It occurs naturally in some animal-derived and fermented foods, most notably the traditional Japanese breakfast food natto (Marles et al., 2017). MK-7 has greater bioavailability than other forms of vitamin K, which has led to a comparatively large use of this product as an ingredient of dietary supplements.

Natto is the product of fermentation of a traditional Japanese soybean, due to the presence of *Bacillus subtilis natto* (Booth, 2012). The fermented food contains large amounts of MK-7 and traces of MK-6; 100 g of natto may contain as much as 950 mcg of MK-7. The use of natto in Japan has been known since 1600 by Samurai warriors, who used it to increase their strength and speed of reactions. Furthermore, ancient Japanese physician registers contained recommendations to pregnant women to take a daily dose of natto in order to obtain healthy offspring. Natto provides a natural form of MK-7, commonly used by the general population in Japan and globally as a supplement by physicians to prevent bone and cardiovascular diseases (Gallieni and Fusaro, 2014; Fusaro et al., 2011, 2017a,b; Marles et al., 2017). We would point out that the bioactivity and toxicity of MK-7 depends on the bacillus used for the fermentation process. In particular, the use of microorganisms different from *B. subtilis natto* may have possible side effects (Haydushka et al., 2012; Salkinoja-Salonen et al., 1999).

Data available in the literature regarding the potential toxicity of vitamin K intake conclude that MK-7 is safe and adverse events are extremely rare, except for gastrointestinal disorders such as diarrhea. On the other hand, special attention should be given to patients treated with warfarin or similar oral vitamin K antagonist anticoagulants, because there is a risk of interaction with vitamin K and interference with the activity of VKDPs (Marles et al., 2017).

Furthermore, MK-7 also exists in a synthetic form, *all-trans*, which seems be bioequivalent to the natural *cis* isomer (Møller et al., 2016). Among the side effects of the synthetic MK-7, dry mouth and diarrhea have been reported (Møller et al., 2016).

Menatetrenone or MK-4 was approved as a drug for the treatment for osteoporosis in Japan in 1960. Indeed interventional studies with MK-4 (45 mg/day orally) demonstrated improvements of BMD and a reduction of the incidence of bone fractures (Shiraki et al., 2000; Inoue et al., 2009; Fang et al., 2012). Moreover, other studies have highlighted an association between high dietary MKn intake, but not PK, and reduced cardiovascular calcifications (Beulens et al., 2009; Fusaro et al., 2012). A recent meta-analysis of cohort or nested case-control studies investigated the relationship between dietary vitamin K intake and the risk of fractures (Hao et al., 2017). Four cohort studies and one nested case-control study, with a total of 1114 fractures cases and 80,982 participants were included in the meta-analysis. In all studies only the intake of PK (vitamin K1), was calculated. A statistically significant inverse association between dietary vitamin K intake and risk of fractures (highest vs. the lowest intake, RR = 0.78) was detected. When stratified by follow-up duration, the RR of fracture for dietary vitamin K intake was 0.76 in studies with more than 10 years of follow-up, suggesting that higher dietary vitamin K intake may moderately decrease the risk of fractures. Iwamoto (2014) reviewed the results of eight randomized controlled trials (RCTs) that investigated the effect of menatetrenone on BMD, measured by dual-energy X-ray absorptiometry and the incidence of fractures in postmenopausal women with osteoporosis. Small RCTs showed that MK-4 (menatetrenone) monotherapy decreased serum uc-BGP concentrations, modestly increased lumbar spine BMD, and reduced the incidence of fractures (mainly vertebral fracture). In addition, combined alendronate and menatetrenone therapy enhanced the decrease in serum uc-BGP concentrations and further increased femoral neck BMD.

Regarding vascular calcifications, observational studies have found higher dietary MKn, but not PK, to be associated with less calcification (Shea and Holden, 2012). Because vascular calcification is highly prevalent in certain populations, such as patients with CKD, it is important to establish whether vitamin K may reduce vascular calcification in patients at higher risk. Overall, the available observational population-based evidence, based on dietary intake measures, suggests that MKn intake may be more likely to protect against vascular calcification than PK intake. However, the available intervention studies suggest that PK supplementation slows the progression of vascular calcification (Braam et al., 2004; Shea et al., 2009).

MKn have not been fully tested. A small Japanese study (Ikari et al., 2016) failed to demonstrate a clear benefit. Despite high dose MK-4 administration (45 mg/day for 1 year), coronary artery calcification increased + 14% annually and brachial ankle pulse wave velocity did not change significantly. The benefits of MK-4 supplementation were only observed in patients with vitamin K insufficiencies correlated with high PIVKA-2 baseline levels, reducing pulse wave velocity but not vascular calcifications. A larger, ongoing randomized controlled study, the VitaK-CAC trial, will analyze the effects of MK-7 supplementation on the progression of coronary artery calcifications. The trial is a double-blind, randomized, placebo-controlled trial including patients with coronary artery disease (Vossen et al., 2015).

8.5 Conclusion

Consideration of the issue of adequate vitamin K intake in the general population and in patients affected by bone and mineral abnormalities, specifically osteoporosis and cardiovascular calcification, has often underestimated the distinction between PK (vitamin K1) and MKn (vitamin K2). Although the two forms of vitamin K have similar activity in sustaining the vitamin K cycle and the carboxylation of VKDPs, their role may be markedly different and therefore their use for the prevention and treatment of bone and mineral abnormalities could follow different pathways and require different doses. We have outlined in this article evidence that vitamin K2 is a key regulator of clinically relevant molecular processes. Its use as a dietary supplement and as a pharmacological treatment for bone and mineral abnormalities should be further explored.

References

Azuma, K., Ouchi, Y., Inoue, S., 2014. Vitamin K: Novel molecular mechanisms of action and its roles in osteoporosis. Geriatr. Gerontol. Int. 14, 1–7.

Beulens, J.W., Bots, M.L., Atsma, F., Bartelink, M.L., Prokop, M., Geleijnse, J.M., et al., 2009. High dietary menaquinone intake is associated with reduced coronary calcification. Atherosclerosis 203, 489–493.

Booth, S.L., 2012. Vitamin K: food composition and dietary intakes. Food Nutr. Res. 2012, 56.

Booth, S.L., Martini, L., Peterson, J.W., Saltzman, E., Dallal, G.E., Wood, R.J., 2003. Dietary phylloquinone depletion and repletion in older women. J. Nutr. 133, 2565–2569.

Booth, S.L., Broe, K.E., Peterson, J.W., Cheng, D.M., Dawson-Hughes, B., Gundberg, C.M., et al., 2004. Associations between vitamin K biochemical measures and bone mineral density in men and women. J. Clin. Endocrinol. Metab. 89, 4904–4909.

Braam, L.A., Hoeks, A.P., Brouns, F., Hamulyak, K., Gerichhausen, M.J., Vermeer, C., 2004. Beneficial effects of vitamins D and K on the elastic properties of the vessel wall in postmenopausal women: a follow-up study. Thromb. Haemost. 91, 373–380.

Bruno, E.J., 2016. The prevalence of vitamin K deficiency/insufficiency, and recommendations for increased intake. J. Hum. Nutr. Food Sci. 4, 1077.

Cavaco, S., Viegas, C.S., Rafael, M.S., Ramos, A., Magalhães, J., Blanco, F.J., et al., 2016. Gla-rich protein is involved in the cross-talk between calcification and inflammation in osteoarthritis. Cell Mol. Life Sci. 73, 1051–1065.

Conly, J.M., Stein, K., 1992. The production of menaquinones (vitamin K2) by intestinal bacteria and their role in maintaining coagulation homeostasis. Prog. Food Nutr. Sci. 16, 307–343.

Conseil Supérieur de la Santé, 2016. Recommandations nutritionnelles pour la Belgique — 2016 CSS n. 9285. Available from: <https://www.health.belgium.be/sites/default/files/uploads/fields/fpshealth_theme_file/css_9285_avis_rec_nutr.pdf>.

Cooper, A.D., 1997. Hepatic uptake of chylomicron remnants. J. Lipid Res. 38, 2173–2192.

Dahlberg, S., Ede, J., Schött, U., 2017. Vitamin K and cancer. Scand. J. Clin. Lab. Invest. 77, 555–567.

Dam, C.P.H., 1935. The antihaemorrhagic vitamin of the chick: occurrence and chemical nature. Nature 135, 652–653.

EFSA Panel on Dietetic Products, Nutrition and Allergies, 2017. Dietary reference values for vitamin K. EFSA J. 15, 4780.

Fang, Y., Hu, C., Tao, X., Wan, Y., Tao, F., 2012. Effect of vitamin K on bone mineral density: a meta-analysis of randomized controlled trials. J. Bone Miner. Metab. 30, 60–68.

Fujita, Y., Iki, M., Tamaki, J., et al., 2012. Association between vitamin K intake from fermented soybeans, natto, and bone mineral density in elderly Japanese men: the Fujiwara-kyo Osteoporosis Risk in Men (FORMEN) study. Osteoporos. Int. 23, 705–714.

Fusaro, M., Crepaldi, G., Maggi, S., et al., 2011. Vitamin K, bone fractures, and vascular calcifications in chronic kidney disease: an important but poorly studied relationship. J. Endocrinol. Invest. 34, 317–323.

Fusaro, M., Noale, V., Viola, V., et al., 2012. Vitamin K, vertebral fractures, vascular calcifications, and mortality: vitamin K Italian (VIKI) dialysis study. J. Bone Miner. Res. 27, 2271–2278.

Fusaro, M., Gallieni, M., Rizzo, M.A., Stucchi, A., Delanaye, P., Cavalier, E., et al., 2017a. Vitamin K plasma levels determination in human health. Clin. Chem. Lab. Med. 55, 789–799.

Fusaro, M., Mereu, M.C., Aghi, A., Iervasi, G., Gallieni, M., 2017b. Vitamin K and bone. Clin. Cases Miner. Bone Metab. 14, 200–206.

Fusaro, M., Plebani, M., Iervasi, G., Gallieni, M., 2017c. Vitamin K deficiency in chronic kidney disease: evidence is building up. Am. J. Nephrol. 45, 1–3.

Gallieni, M., Fusaro, M., 2014. Vitamin K and cardiovascular calcification in CKD: is patient supplementation on the horizon? Kidney Int. 86, 232–234.

Geleijnse, J.M., Vermeer, C., Grobbee, D.E., Schurgers, L.J., Knapen, M.H., van der Meer, I.M., et al., 2004. Dietary intake of menaquinone is associated with a reduced risk of coronary heart disease: the Rotterdam Study. J. Nutr. 134, 3100–3105.

Hafizi, S., Dahlbäck, B., 2006. Gas6 and protein S. Vitamin K-dependent ligands for the Axl receptor tyrosine kinase subfamily. FEBS J. 273, 5231–5244.

Hao, G., Zhang, B., Gu, M., Chen, C., Zhang, Q., Zhang, G., et al., 2017. Vitamin K intake and the risk of fractures: a meta-analysis. Medicine (Baltimore) 96, e6725.

Hasanbasic, I., Rajotte, I., Blostein, M., 2005. The role of gamma-carboxylation in the anti-apoptotic function of Gas6. J. Thromb. Haemost. 3, 2790–2797.

Haydushka, I.A., Markova, N., Kirina, V., Atanassova, M., 2012. Recurrent sepsis due to bacillus licheniformis. J. Glob. Infect. Dis. 4, 82–83.

Horie-Inoue, K., Inoue, S., 2008. Steroid and xenobiotic receptor mediates a novel vitamin K2 signaling pathway in osteoblastic cells. J. Bone Miner. Metab. 26, 9–12.

Ikari, Y., Torii, S., Shioi, A., Okano, T., 2016. Impact of menaquinone-4 supplementation on coronary artery calcification and arterial stiffness: an open label single arm study. Nutr. J. 15, 53.

Inoue, T., Fujita, T., Kishimoto, H., Makino, T., Nakamura, T., Nakamura, T., et al., 2009. Randomized controlled study on the prevention of osteoporotic fractures (OF study): a phase IV clinical study of 15-mg menatetrenone capsules. J. Bone Miner. Metab. 27, 66–75.

Institute of Medicine, 2001. Dietary Reference Intakes for Vitamin A, Vitamin K, Arsenic, Boron, Chromium, Copper, Iodine, Iron, Manganese, Molybdenum, Nickel, Silicon, Vanadium, and Zinc. National Academy Press, Washington, DC.

Iwamoto, J., 2014. Vitamin K2 therapy for postmenopausal osteoporosis. Nutrients 6, 1971–1980.

Karsenty, G., Oury, F., 2014. Regulation of male fertility by the bone-derived hormone osteocalcin. Mol. Cell. Endocrinol. 382, 521–526.

Kerner, S.A., Scott, R.A., Pike, J.W., 1989. Sequence elements in the human osteocalcin gene confer basal activation and inducible response to hormonal vitamin D3. Proc. Natl Acad. Sci. USA 86, 4455–4459.

Kim, Y.S., Paik, I.Y., Rhie, Y.J., Suh, S.H., 2010. Integrative physiology: defined novel metabolic roles of osteocalcin. J. Korean Med. Sci. 25, 985–991.

Kohlmeier, M., Salomon, A., Saupe, J., Shearer, M.J., 1996. Transport of vitamin K to bone in humans. J. Nutr. 126, 1192S–1196S.

Litvin, J., Selim, A.H., Montgomery, M.O., Lehmann, K., Rico, M.C., Devlin, H., et al., 2004. Expression and function of periostin-isoforms in bone. J. Cell. Biochem. 92, 1044–1061.

Luo, G., Ducy, P., McKee, M.D., Pinero, G.J., Loyer, E., Behringer, R.R., et al., 1997. Spontaneous calcification of arteries and cartilage in mice lacking matrix GLA protein. Nature 386, 78–81.

MacCorquodale, D.W., Binkley, S.B., Thayer, S.A., Doisy, E.A., 1939. On the constitution of Vitamin K1. J. Am. Chem. Soc. 61, 1928–1929.

Mark, M.R., Chen, J., Hammonds, R.G., Sadick, M., Godowsk, P.J., 1996. Characterization of Gas6, a member of the superfamily of G domain-containing proteins, as a ligand for Rse and Axl. J. Biol. Chem. 271, 9785–9789.

Marles, R.J., Roe, A.L., Oketch-Rabah, H.A., 2017. US pharmacopeial convention safety evaluation of menaquinone-7, a form of vitamin K. Nutr. Rev. 75, 553–578.

Merle, B., Garnero, P., 2012. The multiple facets of periostin in bone metabolism. Osteoporos. Int. 23, 1199–1212.

Møller, M., Gjelstad, I.M., Baksaas, I., Grande, T., Aukrust, I.R., Drevon, C.A., 2016. Bioavailability and chemical/functional aspects of synthetic MK-7 vs fermentation-derived MK-7 in randomised controlled trials. Int. J. Vitam. Nutr. Res. 2016, 1–15.

Munroe, P.B., Olgunturk, R.O., Fryns, J.P., Van Maldergem, L., Ziereisen, F., Yuksel, B., et al., 1999. Mutations in the gene encoding the human matrix Gla protein cause Keutel syndrome. Nat. Genet. 21, 142–144.
Murshed, M., Schinke, T., McKee, M.D., Karsenty, G., 2004. Extracellular matrix mineralization is regulated locally; different roles of two Gla-containing proteins. J. Cell. Biol. 165, 625–630.
Naito, K., Watari, T., Obayashi, O., Katsube, S., Nagaoka, I., Kaneko, K., 2012. Relationship between serum undercarboxylated osteocalcin and hyaluronan levels in patients with bilateral knee osteoarthritis. Int. J. Mol. Med. 29, 756–760.
National Institutes of Health, Updated 2018. Vitamin K. Fact sheet for health professionals. <https://ods.od.nih.gov/factsheets/VitaminK-HealthProfessional/> (accessed 28.02.19.).
Neogi, T., Booth, S.L., Zhang, Y.Q., Jacques, P.F., Terkeltaub, R., Aliabadi, P., et al., 2006. Low vitamin K status is associated with osteoarthritis in the hand and knee. Arthritis Rheum. 54, 1255–1261.
Oldenburg, J., Bevans, C.G., Muller, C.R., Watzka, M., 2006. Vitamin K epoxide reductase complex subunit 1 (VKORC1): the key protein of the vitamin K cycle. Antioxid. Redox. Signal. 8, 347–353.
Rafael, M.S., Cavaco, S., Viegas, C.S., Santos, S., Ramos, A., Willems, B.A., et al., 2014. Insights into the association of Gla-rich protein and osteoarthritis, novel splice variants and γ-carboxylation status. Mol. Nutr. Food Res. 58, 1636–1646.
Sadowski, J.A., Hood, S.J., Dallal, G.E., Garry, P.J., 1989. Phylloquinone in plasma from elderly and young adults: factors influencing its concentration. Am. J. Clin. Nutr. 50, 100–108.
Salkinoja-Salonen, M.S., Vuorio, R., Andersson, M.A., Kämpfer, P., Andersson, M.C., Honkanen-Buzalski, T., et al., 1999. Toxigenic strains of *Bacillus licheniformis* related to food poisoning. Appl. Environ. Microbiol. 65, 4637–4645.
Sato, T., Schurgers, L.J., Uenishi, K., 2012. Comparison of menaquinone-4 and menaquinone-7 bioavailability in healthy women. Nutr. J. 11, 93.
Schønheyder, F., 1936. The quantitative determination of vitamin K. Biochem. J. 30, 890–896.
Schurgers, L.J., Teunissen, K.J., Hamulyak, K., et al., 2007. Vitamin K-containing dietary supplements: comparison of synthetic vitamin K1 and natto-derived menaquinone-7. Blood 109, 3279–3283.
Schurgers, L.J., Cranenburg, E.C., Vermeer, C., 2008. Matrix Gla-protein: the calcification inhibitor in need of vitamin K. Thromb. Haemost. 100, 593–603.
Shea, M.K., Holden, R.M., 2012. Vitamin K status and vascular calcification: evidence from observational and clinical studies. Adv. Nutr. 3, 158–165.
Shea, M.K., O'Donnell, C.J., Hoffmann, U., Dallal, G.E., Dawson-Hughes, B., Ordovas, J.M., et al., 2009. Vitamin K supplementation and progression of coronary artery calcium in older men and women. Am. J. Clin. Nutr. 89, 1799–1807.
Shearer, M.J., Newman, P., 2008. Metabolism and cell biology of vitamin K. Thromb. Haemost. 100, 530–547.
Shiozawa, Y., Pedersen, E.A., Patel, L.R., Ziegler, A.M., Havens, A.M., Jung, Y., et al., 2010. GAS6/AXL axis regulates prostate cancer invasion, proliferation, and survival in the bone marrow niche. Neoplasia 12, 116–127.
Shiraki, M., Shiraki, Y., Aoki, C., Miura, M., 2000. Vitamin K2 (menatetrenone) effectively prevents fractures and sustains lumbar bone mineral density in osteoporosis. J. Bone Miner. Res. 15, 515–521.
Società Italiana di Nutrizione Umana, 2014. Assunzione raccomandata per la popolazione (PRI) e assunzione adeguata (AI). LARN—Livelli di assunzione di riferimento per la popolazione italiana: Vitamine. Available from: <http://www.sinu.it/html/pag/09-VITAMINE.asp>.

Stafford, D.W., 2005. The vitamin K cycle. J. Thromb. Haemost. 3, 1873–1878.
Sultana, H., Watanabe, K., Rana, M.M., Takashima, R., Ohashi, A., Komai, M., et al., 2018. Effects of vitamin K_2 on the expression of genes involved in bile acid synthesis and glucose homeostasis in mice with humanized PXR. Nutrients 10, 8.
Vermeer, C., 1990. Gamma-carboxyglutamate-containing proteins and the vitamin K-dependent carboxylase. Biochem. J. 266, 625–636.
Vermeer, C., 2012. Vitamin K: the effect on health beyond coagulation—an overview. Food Nutr. Res. 2012, 56.
Viegas, C.S., Cavaco, S., Neves, P.L., Ferreira, A., João, A., Williamson, M.K., et al., 2009. Gla-rich protein is a novel vitamin K-dependent protein present in serum that accumulates at sites of pathological calcifications. Am. J. Pathol. 175, 2288–2298.
Vossen, L.M., Schurgers, L.J., van Varik, B.J., Kietselaer, B.L., Vermeer, C., Meeder, J.G., et al., 2015. Menaquinone-7 supplementation to reduce vascular calcification in patients with coronary artery disease: rationale and study protocol (VitaK-CAC Trial). Nutrients 7, 8905–8915.
Walther, B., Karl, J.P., Booth, S.L., Boyaval, P., 2013. Menaquinones, bacteria, and the food supply: the relevance of dairy and fermented food products to vitamin K requirements. Adv. Nutr. 4, 463–473.
Wen, L., Chen, J., Duan, L., Li, S., 2018. Vitamin K-dependent proteins involved in bone and cardiovascular health. Mol. Med. Rep. 18, 3–15.
Yoshizawa, T., Hinoi, E., Jung, D.Y., Kajimura, D., Ferron, M., Seo, J., et al., 2009. The transcription factor ATF4 regulates glucose metabolism in mice through its expression in osteoblasts. J. Clin. Invest. 119, 2807–2817.

CHAPTER 9

Biotin status screening

Shin-ichiro Hagiwara
Department of Pediatric Gastroenterology, Nutrition and Endocrinology, Osaka Medical Center and Research Institute for Maternal and Child Health, Osaka, Japan

Contents

Summary points

- Biotin is a water-soluble vitamin, also known as vitamin H.
- Biotin is an essential micronutrient for the metabolism and survival of all organisms due to its function as a cofactor of enzymes, known as biotin-dependent carboxylases.
- Biotin deficiency presents various clinical manifestations such as hair loss, red rash, neurologic symptoms, and susceptibility to infection.
- The main causes of biotin deficiency include: (1) total parenteral nutrition without biotin supplementation, (2) excessive consumption of raw egg white, (3) intake of infant formulas with inadequate biotin, (4) long-term use of anticonvulsants and antibiotics, (5) smoking and chronic alcoholism, (6) inflammatory bowel disease, (7) inborn metabolic disorders, and (8) pregnancy.

Molecular Nutrition
DOI: https://doi.org/10.1016/B978-0-12-811907-5.00026-9

- Markers of biotin deficiency include: (1) plasma concentration of 3-hydroxyisovaleric acid measured by liquid chromatography—tandem mass spectroscopy, (2) increased 3-hydroxyisovaleric acid (3HIA) and 3-hydroxyisovaleryl carnitine (3HIA-carnitine) level in urine, and (3) gel densitometry analysis of biotinylated 3-methylcrotonyl-CoA carboxylase and propionyl-CoA carboxylase in peripheral blood lymphocytes.
- Urinary 3HIA and 3HIA-carnitine markers have been proved valid in healthy adults. However the markers may not accurately reflect the biotin status in pregnant women or lactating women.

Definitions of words and terms

ACC ACC is an abbreviation for acetyl-CoA carboxylase, comprised of ACC-α and ACC-β. Acetyl CoA is converted to malonyl CoA by ACC-α which is a key enzyme in lipid synthesis. ACC-β catalyzes an identical reaction in the mitochondria and is associated with fatty acid oxidation.

Carboxylase An enzyme that catalyzes carboxylation or decarboxylation. Carboxylation is a reaction in which carboxylic acid group is introduced to a substrate.

Inflammatory bowel disease Inflammatory bowel diseases (IBDs), including Crohn's disease and ulcerative colitis, are chronic inflammatory disorders of the intestine. The incidence of IBD is increasing worldwide.

LC—MS/MS LC—MS/MS is an abbreviation for liquid chromatography—tandem mass spectroscopy. This tandem method is used for the analysis of small molecules.

MCC MCC is an abbreviation for 3-methylcrotonyl-CoA carboxylase. 3-Methylcrotonyl-CoA carboxylase is an essential enzyme for the catabolism of the branched-chain amino acid, leucine.

PC PC is an abbreviation for pyruvate carboxylase. Pyruvate carboxylase catalyzes the conversion of pyruvate to oxaloacetate, which is associated with gluconeogenesis and lipogenesis.

PCC PCC is abbreviation for propionyl-CoA carboxylase. Propionyl-CoA carboxylase catalyzes the conversion of propionyl CoA to methylmalonyl CoA. Methylmalonyl CoA is converted to succinyl CoA and enters the tricarboxylic acid cycle.

9.1 Introduction

Biotin was first found from yeast as a growth factor in the early 20th century and was later identified as biotin (Boas, 1927). Biotin, a water-soluble vitamin, acts as a cofactor for carboxylase in fatty acid synthesis, amino acid metabolism and gluconeogenesis. Emerging evidence has revealed that biotin deficiency affects inflammation (Cowan et al., 1979; Elahi et al., 2018; Fernandez-Banares et al., 1989). Elahi et al. (2018)

demonstrated that "biotin deficiency enhances the inflammatory responses in $CD4^+$ T cells, which may contribute to inflammation associated with biotin deficiency". Since the diagnosis of biotin deficiency can be difficult due to various symptoms, screening methods for biotin deficiency are required in clinical practice. This chapter discusses the screening methods used for biotin deficiency as well its symptoms and causes.

9.2 What is biotin?

Biotin, a water-soluble family of vitamins, is composed of a ureido ring fused with a tetrahydrothiophene ring (Fig. 9.1). This micronutrient acts as a covalently bound coenzyme for five carboxylases—acetyl-CoA carboxylase α (ACC-α), acetyl-CoA carboxylase β (ACC-β), pyruvate carboxylase (PC), propionyl-CoA carboxylase (PCC), and 3-methylcrotonyl-CoA carboxylase (MCC)—in fatty acid synthesis, amino acid metabolism, and gluconeogenesis (Lanska, 2012; Zempleni and Mock, 1999). First, biotin-dependent carboxylases are formed as "enzymatically inactive apocarboxylase proteins" (Mock, 2017). After the covalent attachment of biotin by the enzyme holocarboxylase synthetase (HLCS), inactive apocarboxylase can convert to active holocarboxylases (Mock, 2017). Biotin also regulates the expression of various genes (e.g., transcriptional regulation of the glucokinase gene and reduction of mRNA levels of lipogenic genes) (Chauhan and Dakshinamurti, 1991; Dakshinamurti, 2013; Larrieta et al., 2010).

9.3 Biotin physiology

Biotin is available from various food sources. It mostly exists in food in protein-bound forms that are digested by gastrointestinal peptidases and

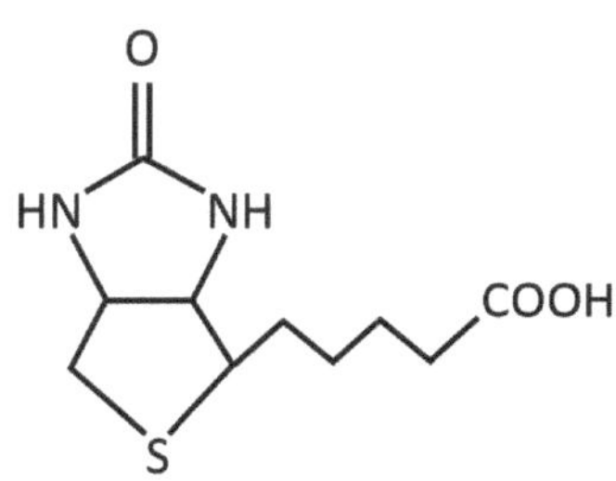

Figure 9.1 Skeletal formula of biotin. Bicyclic molecule composed of an ureido ring fused with a tetrahydrothiophene ring.

proteases to form biotinyl peptide and biocytin. Biotin and lysine in biotinyl peptides and biocytin are hydrolyzed by intestinal biotinidase (BTD) to release biotin. Subsequently, free biotin is absorbed in the small intestine, predominantly the jejunum. On the other hand, bacterially derived biotin exists in its unbound form and is absorbed in the colon (Said, 2012). Once absorbed, biotin is used for various biotinylation processes. Biotin binds to each of the five apocarboxylases, leading to the formation of their corresponding holocarboxylase (ACC-α, ACC-β, PC, PCC, and MCC) via the action of HLCS (Fig. 9.2). Biotin deficiency causes increases plasma concentration of 3-hydroxyisovaleryl carnitine (3HIA-carnitine) and urinary excretion of 3-hydroxyisovaleric acid (3HIA) and 3HIA-carnitine because of reduced activity of MCC (Mock et al., 2011) (Table 9.1).

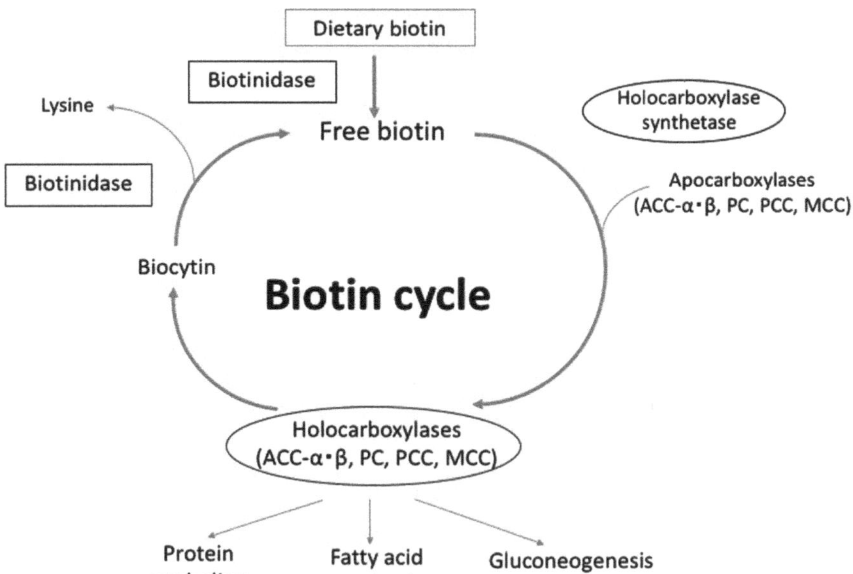

Figure 9.2 Schematic representation of the biotin cycle. Free biotin obtained from food or the cleavage of biocytin via the action of biotinidase (BTD) is covalently attached to the five apocarboxylases, ACC-α, ACC-β, PC, PCC, and MCC via the action of biotin holocarboxylase synthetase (HLCS), thereby forming active holocarboxylases. The holocarboxylases are subsequently proteolyzed to biocytin, which is then further cleaved by BTD. As a result, free biotin reenters the cycle. *ACC*, Acetyl-CoA carboxylase; *PC* pyruvate carboxylase; *PCC*, propionyl-CoA carboxylase; *MCC*, 3-methylcrotonyl-CoA carboxylase.

Table 9.1 Key facts about biotin, including the function of biotin, and the causes and symptoms of biotin deficiency.

- Biotin plays an important role in fatty acid synthesis, gluconeogenesis, and branched – chain amino acid catabolism.
- Emerging evidence has shown that biotin is associated with the immune response.
- Biotin deficiency is caused by various conditions, such as inadequate nutrition therapy, prolonged use of anticonvulsants and antibiotics, pregnancy, and inherited metabolic disorders.
- Symptoms of biotin deficiency vary. (e.g., hair loss and a scaly red rash around the eyes, nose, mouth, and genitals).
- Adult neurological symptoms include depression, hallucinations, lethargy, ataxia, numbness and tingling of the extremities, and seizures.
- Inborn metabolic disorders such as biotinidase deficiency and holocarboxylase synthetase deficiency often show similar symptoms to biotin deficiency and increased susceptibility to bacterial and fungal infections.

9.4 Causes of biotin deficiency

Various causes of biotin deficiency have been reported, including:

1. *Total parenteral nutrition without biotin*. Patients who receive long-term total parenteral nutrition therapy without biotin supplementation, develop biotin deficiency (Khalidi et al., 1984).
2. *Excessive consumption of raw egg whites*. Avidin, contained in raw egg white, has a high binding affinity to biotin, making it unavailable for absorption. Prolonged consumption of raw egg, not cooked egg, was reported to be a predisposing factor for biotin deficiency (Adhisivam et al., 2007).
3. *Intake of infant formulas with insufficient biotin*. Biotin deficiency has been reported in infants with milk allergy, receiving hypoallergenic formulas containing low levels of biotin (Hagiwara et al., 2017; Hayashi et al., 2014).
4. *Long-term anticonvulsant therapy*. Long-term administration of anticonvulsants, such as phenytoin, phenobarbital, carbamazepine, and primidone, may cause biotin deficiency. Possible mechanisms include inhibition of intestinal biotin uptake, accelerated biotin catabolism, and impaired renal tubular reabsorption of biotin (Mock and Dyken, 1997; Said, 2012).
5. *Long-term oral antibiotic therapy*. Long-term administration of oral antibiotics has been linked to biotin deficiency because of disturbance of

the intestinal microbiome induced by antibiotics. In mice antibiotic-induced overgrowth of bacteria, *Lactobacillus murinus*, was shown to increase biotin consumption (Hayashi et al., 2017).

6. *Smoking and chronic alcoholism.* Smoking accelerates biotin metabolism, especially in women (Sealey et al., 2004). Animal studies showed that chronic alcohol exposure has negative impact on biotin uptake in pancreatic acinar cells and renal biotin reabsorption (Srinivasan et al., 2014; Subramanian et al., 2011).
7. *Inflammatory bowel disease (IBD).* IBD is a group of chronic inflammatory disorders of the intestine, including Crohn's disease and ulcerative colitis. A clinical study showed that biotin levels in IBD patients were significantly lower than in controls (Fernandez-Banares et al., 1989). However, biotin deficiency has not been conclusively demonstrated in IBD, and reports are inconsistent (Ghishan and Kiela, 2017).
8. *Pregnancy and lactation.* Emerging studies have shown decreased biotin levels in a significant proportion of pregnant and lactating women (Mock, 2009, 2017). Some experts recommend a higher intake of biotin for pregnant women because marginal biotin deficiency during pregnancy might be teratogenic (Mock, 2017; Mock et al., 2003).
9. *Inborn errors of metabolism: BTD deficiency and HLCS deficiency.* Biotin deficiency can arise due to rare inborn errors of metabolism, including deficiencies of BTD (MIM 253260) and HLCS (MIM 253270).

9.4.1 Biotinidase deficiency

Mutations in the *BTD* gene that encodes BTD. BTD functions to remove biotin bound to proteins in food, leaving biotin in its free form. Free biotin is required by five biotin-dependent carboxylases, necessary for fatty acid synthesis, amino acid metabolism, and gluconeogenesis. BTD deficiency is a hereditary disorder in which the body is unable to recycle biotin, with subsequent impairments of the main biotin-dependent carboxylases and accumulation of potentially toxic substance in the human body (Mastrangelo, 2018).

9.4.2 Holocarboxylase synthetase deficiency

Mutations in the *HLCS* gene. HLCS is the enzyme that catalyzes the binding of biotin to carboxylases and histones (Suormala et al., 1998). Defects in this gene cause failure to attach biotin, leading to reduced activity of the biotin-dependent carboxylases. This process results in multiple carboxylase deficiency (Donti et al., 2016).

9.5 Symptoms

Biotin deficiency leads to an array of pathological conditions, including alopecia, conjunctivitis, skin rash and neurological symptoms, such as depression, lethargy, hallucination, and hypotonia. Patients with hereditary disorders of biotin deficiency also develop immune dysfunction, including increased susceptibility to bacterial and fungal infections (Elahi et al., 2018; Krol and Krafchik, 2006; Seymons et al., 2004; Trueb, 2016).

9.6 Biotin status screening

While a universal biotin status screening has not yet been established, several screening methods have been proposed.

9.6.1 Plasma concentration of 3-hydroxyisovaleryl carnitine

As mentioned previously, biotin acts as a covalently bound coenzyme for five carboxylases (ACC-α, ACC-β, PC, PCC, and MCC). Plasma 3HIA-carnitine concentrations are increased in isolated genetic deficiency of MCC (Roschinger et al., 1995) and deficiency of multiple carboxylases because of BTD or HLCS deficiency (Raha and Udani, 2011; Van Hove et al., 2008; Stratton et al., 2010). Stratton et al. (2010) reported that plasma 3HIA-carnitine concentration is an early and sensitive biomarker of marginal biotin deficiency in humans. They measured plasma concentration of 3HIA-carnitine using liquid chromatography—tandem mass spectroscopy (LC—MS/MS).

The usefulness of LC—MS/MS using dry blood spots (DBSs) in pediatrics has been reported (Hagiwara et al., 2017). Previous studies showed that LC—MS/MS using DBSs, used for new-born mass screening of metabolic inherited disorders, is available for the detection of biotin deficiencies in infants because an increase of 3HIA-carnitine (C5-OH) measured by LC—MS/MS reflects biotin deficiency (Tokuriki et al., 2013). Hagiwara et al. (2017) reported that C5-OH measured by LC—MS/MS from DBSs was >1.00 nmol/L in a pediatric patients who developed biotin deficiency. In inherited metabolic disorders, such as BTD and HLCS deficiency, conditions are screened for using new-born screening tandem mass spectroscopy to detect elevated C5-OH levels in DBSs.

9.6.2 Urinary concentrations of 3-hydroxyisovaleric acid and 3-hydroxyisovaleryl carnitine

Stratton et al. (2011) reported that urinary 3HIA and 3HIA-carnitine levels, measured by LC–MS/MS, are sensitive biomarkers of marginal biotin deficiency in experimentally induced biotin-deficient adults. However, Perry et al. (2014) reported that urinary 3HIA-carnitine was lower among pregnant women than among nonpregnant control women, indicating that urinary 3HIA-carnitine is not a reliable biomarker of marginal biotin deficiency in pregnancy (Mock, 2017). In children, an increase of urinary 3HIA level beyond the normal range (3.4–12.5 μg/mg creatinine) is considered a biomarker of biotin deficiency (Hayashi et al., 2014).

9.6.3 Abundance of biotinylated 3-methylcrotonyl-CoA carboxylase and propionyl-CoA carboxylase

Eng et al. (2013) showed that an "abundance of holo-MCC and holo-PCC allowed for distinguishing biotin-deficient and biotin-sufficient individuals". According to their study, an abundance of holo-MCC and holo-PCC in peripheral blood lymphocytes determined by gel densitometry and fluorescent-labeled streptavidin were reliable indicators of marginal biotin deficiency (Eng et al., 2013). In theory, "activity of PCC and MCC (two of the five biotin-dependent carboxylases) in peripheral blood lymphocytes should be as sensitive and specific as the abundance of holo-PCC and holo-MCC" (Mock et al., 2002; Mock, 2017). This novel "assay quantitates the catalysis by PCC or MCC of ^{14}C-bicarbonate incorporation into acid-precipitable material" (Mock et al., 2002; Mock, 2017). However, this method is not suitable for screening biotin deficiency because it is technically difficult, as blood samples require special handling and storage.

References

Adhisivam, B., Mahto, D., Mahadevan, S., 2007. Biotin responsive limb weakness. Indian Pediatr. 44, 228–230.

Boas, M.A., 1927. The effect of desiccation upon the nutritive properties of egg-white. Biochem. J. 21, 712–724.

Chauhan, J., Dakshinamurti, K., 1991. Transcriptional regulation of the glucokinase gene by biotin in starved rats. J. Biol. Chem. 266, 10035–10038.

Cowan, M.J., Wara, D.W., Packman, S., Ammann, A.J., Yoshino, M., Sweetman, L., et al., 1979. Multiple biotin-dependent carboxylase deficiencies associated with defects in T-cell and B-cell immunity. Lancet 2, 115–118.
Dakshinamurti, K., 2013. Regulation of gene expression by biotin, vitamin B6 and vitamin C. Molecular Nutrition. CABI Publishing, Wallingford, pp. 151–166.
Donti, T.R., Blackburn, P.R., Atwal, P.S., 2016. Holocarboxylase synthetase deficiency pre and post newborn screening. Mol. Genet. Metab. Rep. 7, 40–44.
Elahi, A., Sabui, S., Narasappa, N.N., Agrawal, S., Lambrecht, N.W., Agrawal, A., et al., 2018. Biotin deficiency induces Th1- and Th17-mediated proinflammatory responses in human CD4(+) T lymphocytes via activation of the mTOR signaling pathway. J. Immunol. 200, 2563–2570.
Eng, W.K., Giraud, D., Schlegel, V.L., Wang, D., Lee, B.H., Zempleni, J., 2013. Identification and assessment of markers of biotin status in healthy adults. Br. J. Nutr. 110, 321–329.
Fernandez-Banares, F., Abad-Lacruz, A., Xiol, X., Gine, J.J., Dolz, C., Cabre, E., et al., 1989. Vitamin status in patients with inflammatory bowel disease. Am. J. Gastroenterol. 84, 744–748.
Ghishan, F.K., Kiela, P.R., 2017. Vitamins and minerals in inflammatory bowel disease. Gastroenterol. Clin. N. Am. 46, 797–808.
Hagiwara, S.I., Kubota, M., Nambu, R., Kagimoto, S., 2017. Screening of carnitine and biotin deficiencies on tandem mass spectrometry. Pediatr. Int. 59, 458–461.
Hayashi, H., Tokuriki, S., Okuno, T., Shigematsu, Y., Yasushi, A., Matsuyama, G., et al., 2014. Biotin and carnitine deficiency due to hypoallergenic formula nutrition in infants with milk allergy. Pediatr. Int. 56, 286–288.
Hayashi, A., Mikami, Y., Miyamoto, K., Kamada, N., Sato, T., Mizuno, S., et al., 2017. Intestinal dysbiosis and biotin deprivation induce alopecia through overgrowth of *Lactobacillus murinus* in mice. Cell Rep. 20, 1513–1524.
Khalidi, N., Wesley, J.R., Thoene, J.G., Whitehouse Jr., W.M., Baker, W.L., 1984. Biotin deficiency in a patient with short bowel syndrome during home parenteral nutrition. J. Parenter. Enteral Nutr. (JPEN) 8, 311–314.
Krol, A., Krafchik, B., 2006. The differential diagnosis of atopic dermatitis in childhood. Dermatol. Ther. 19, 73–82.
Lanska, D.J., 2012. The discovery of niacin, biotin, and pantothenic acid. Ann. Nutr. Metab. 61, 246–253.
Larrieta, E., Velasco, F., Vital, P., Lopez-Aceves, T., Lazo-de-la-Vega-Monroy, M.L., Rojas, A., et al., 2010. Pharmacological concentrations of biotin reduce serum triglycerides and the expression of lipogenic genes. Eur. J. Pharmacol. 644, 263–268.
Mastrangelo, M., 2018. Actual insights into treatable inborn errors of metabolism causing epilepsy. J. Pediatr. Neurosci. 13, 13–23.
Mock, D.M., 2009. Marginal biotin deficiency is common in normal human pregnancy and is highly teratogenic in mice. J. Nutr. 139, 154–157.
Mock, D.M., 2017. Biotin: from nutrition to therapeutics. J. Nutr. 147, 1487–1492.
Mock, D.M., Dyken, M.E., 1997. Biotin catabolism is accelerated in adults receiving long-term therapy with anticonvulsants. Neurology 49, 1444–1447.
Mock, D., Henrich, C., Carnell, N., Mock, N., Swift, L., 2002. Lymphocyte propionyl-CoA carboxylase and accumulation of odd-chain fatty acid in plasma and erythrocytes are useful indicators of marginal biotin deficiency small star, filled. J. Nutr. Biochem. 13, 462.
Mock, D.M., Mock, N.I., Stewart, C.W., LaBorde, J.B., Hansen, D.K., 2003. Marginal biotin deficiency is teratogenic in ICR mice. J. Nutr. 133, 2519–2525.
Mock, D.M., Stratton, S.L., Horvath, T.D., Bogusiewicz, A., Matthews, N.I., Henrich, C.L., et al., 2011. Urinary excretion of 3-hydroxyisovaleric acid and 3-hydroxyisovaleryl

carnitine increases in response to a leucine challenge in marginally biotin-deficient humans. J. Nutr. 141, 1925–1930.
Perry, C.A., West, A.A., Gayle, A., Lucas, L.K., Yan, J., Jiang, X., et al., 2014. Pregnancy and lactation alter biomarkers of biotin metabolism in women consuming a controlled diet. J. Nutr. 144, 1977–1984.
Raha, S., Udani, V., 2011. Biotinidase deficiency presenting as recurrent myelopathy in a 7-year-old boy and a review of the literature. Pediatr. Neurol. 45, 261–264.
Roschinger, W., Millington, D.S., Gage, D.A., Huang, Z.H., Iwamoto, T., Yano, S., et al., 1995. 3-Hydroxyisovalerylcarnitine in patients with deficiency of 3-methylcrotonyl CoA carboxylase. Clin. Chim. Acta 240, 35–51.
Said, H.M., 2012. Biotin: biochemical, physiological and clinical aspects. Subcell Biochem. 56, 1–19.
Sealey, W.M., Teague, A.M., Stratton, S.L., Mock, D.M., 2004. Smoking accelerates biotin catabolism in women. Am. J. Clin. Nutr. 80, 932–935.
Seymons, K., De Moor, A., De Raeve, H., Lambert, J., 2004. Dermatologic signs of biotin deficiency leading to the diagnosis of multiple carboxylase deficiency. Pediatr. Dermatol. 21, 231–235.
Srinivasan, P., Kapadia, R., Biswas, A., Said, H.M., 2014. Chronic alcohol exposure inhibits biotin uptake by pancreatic acinar cells: possible involvement of epigenetic mechanisms. Am. J. Physiol. Gastrointest. Liver Physiol. 307, G941–G949.
Stratton, S.L., Horvath, T.D., Bogusiewicz, A., Matthews, N.I., Henrich, C.L., Spencer, H.J., et al., 2010. Plasma concentration of 3-hydroxyisovaleryl carnitine is an early and sensitive indicator of marginal biotin deficiency in humans. Am. J. Clin. Nutr. 92, 1399–1405.
Stratton, S.L., Horvath, T.D., Bogusiewicz, A., Matthews, N.I., Henrich, C.L., Spencer, H.J., et al., 2011. Urinary excretion of 3-hydroxyisovaleryl carnitine is an early and sensitive indicator of marginal biotin deficiency in humans. J. Nutr. 141, 353–358.
Subramanian, V.S., Subramanya, S.B., Said, H.M., 2011. Chronic alcohol exposure negatively impacts the physiological and molecular parameters of the renal biotin reabsorption process. Am. J. Physiol. Renal Physiol. 300, F611–F617.
Suormala, T., Fowler, B., Jakobs, C., Duran, M., Lehnert, W., Raab, K., et al., 1998. Late-onset holocarboxylase synthetase-deficiency: pre- and post-natal diagnosis and evaluation of effectiveness of antenatal biotin therapy. Eur. J. Pediatr. 157, 570–575.
Tokuriki, S., Hayashi, H., Okuno, T., Yoshioka, K., Okazaki, S., Kawakita, A., et al., 2013. Biotin and carnitine profiles in preterm infants in Japan. Pediatr. Int. 55, 342–345.
Trueb, R.M., 2016. Serum biotin levels in women complaining of hair loss. Int. J. Trichol. 8, 73–77.
Van Hove, J.L., Josefsberg, S., Freehauf, C., Thomas, J.A., Thuy le, P., Barshop, B.A., et al., 2008. Management of a patient with holocarboxylase synthetase deficiency. Mol. Genet. Metab. 95, 201–205.
Zempleni, J., Mock, D.M., 1999. Biotin biochemistry and human requirements. J. Nutr. Biochem. 10, 128–138.

PART II

Molecular Biology of the Cell

CHAPTER 10

Vitamin B_1 and the pyruvate dehydrogenase complex

Yuliya Parkhomenko[1], Andriy Vovk[2] and Zoya Protasova[1]
[1]Department of Vitamins and Coenzymes Biochemistry, A.V. Palladin Institute of Biochemistry of the National Academy of Sciences of Ukraine, Kyiv, Ukraine
[2]Department of Bioorganic Mechanisms, V.P. Kukhar Institute of Bioorganic Chemistry and Petrochemistry of the National Academy of Sciences of Ukraine, Kyiv, Ukraine

Contents

Key facts of vitamin B_1

- A deep deficiency of thiamine leads to a disease that was long known as "beriberi," which is accompanied by convulsions, paralysis, and without treatment ends with death.
- According to Japanese authors, the first descriptions of a beriberi clinic occurring were in 808, but it is officially recognized that the presence in natural foods of a compound that treats this disease was discovered

Molecular Nutrition
DOI: https://doi.org/10.1016/B978-0-12-811907-5.00012-9

by the observations of Eijkman during 1898–1906 which he spent in a prison hospital on the island of Java.

- The substance that cured polyneuritis was first isolated and crystallized in 1926 by Jansen and Donath.
- Eijkman and Hopkins in 1929 received the Nobel Prize in the field of physiology and medicine for research leading to the discovery of vitamins.
- Classic forms of vitamin B_1 deficiency are currently extremely rare, but hypovitaminosis (low provision of the vitamin) is quite common in people even in developed countries due to an unhealthy diet (lack of vitamin B_1 intake) and/or effects on the body of adverse factors of exogenous (environmental pollution) and endogenous (e.g., increased consumption of alcohol and drugs) origin.
- A universal criterion for estimation of the body's thiamine status is the measurement of the content of thiamine diphosphate in erythrocytes.
- Vitamin B_1 is supplied to organisms by foods such as whole grains, pork, beef, legumes, egg yolk, nuts, and others.

Summary points

- This chapter is devoted to the analysis of the relationship between two factors: the supply of the body with vitamin B_1 (thiamine) and the activity of the pyruvate dehydrogenase complex (PDC), the coenzyme of which is a phosphorylated form of thiamine, thiamine diphosphate (ThDP).
- The PDC is a multienzyme structure consisting of three enzymes: pyruvate dehydrogenase itself [E1, pyruvate dehydrogenase (PDH)], dihydrolipoamide acetyltransferase (E2), and dihydrolipoamide dehydrogenase (E3). This complex catalyzes the oxidative decarboxylation of pyruvate with the formation of acetyl-CoA as a final product.
- PDC in animal tissues is subject to multifactorial regulation mediated mainly by PDH kinase and PDH phosphatase, which carry out phosphorylation (inactivation) and dephosphorylation (activation) of the first component of the complex (E1, PDH), respectively.
- Thus under certain physiological conditions, part of the PDC can be in an inactive form and the ratio of the active and inactive forms of the PDC is determined by the activities of PDH kinase and PDH phosphatase.
- Despite the fact that ThDP is a coenzyme of PDH, there is no strong relationship between the content of ThDP in tissues and the activity of E1. This can be attributed to a noncoenzymic function of ThDP in PDC regulation.

- ThDP and thiamine triphosphate (ThTP) are involved in the regulation of PDC by acting on regulatory enzymes. ThDP inhibits PDH kinase, which leads to activation of the PDC, and ThTP inhibits PDH phosphatase, resulting in inactivation of the multienzyme complex.
- The relative flow of glucose carbon atoms through metabolic pathways such as the tricarboxylic acid cycle, gluconeogenesis, and fatty acids biosynthesis is distributed at the level of the PDC.
- In nerve cells, vitamin B_1 is involved in the regulation of acetylcholine synthesis from pyruvate, mediated by the effects of its phosphates on PDC activity.
- PDC and its regulatory enzymes can be considered as potential therapeutic targets for thiamine and its derivatives in the treatment of obesity, diabetes, and neurological disorders.

Definitions of words and terms

- *Acetylcholine*: Acetylcholine is a chemical transmitter (mediator) of nervous excitation, which is synthesized in nerve cells; the ends of the nerve fibers for which it serves as a mediator are called cholinergic.
- *Apoenzyme*: Apoenzyme is a protein part of an enzyme that binds a coenzyme to exhibit the catalytic activity.
- *Homeostasis*: Homeostasis is a state of relative balance (equilibrium) of the metabolic processes in separate living system.
- *Coenzyme*: Coenzyme is a low-molecular organic compound located at the active site of an enzyme and is indispensable for the catalytic transformation of the enzyme substrate.
- *Lipogenesis*: Lipogenesis is the process of fatty acids synthesis with subsequent formation of triglycerides involving several biochemical reactions.
- *Metabolism*: Metabolism is considered to be the summation of biochemical reactions that take place in a living organism during its vital activity.
- *Metabolite*: Metabolite is an intermediate or final product of the metabolism.
- *Mitochondria*: Mitochondria are subcellular structures in eukaryotic cells providing energy and metabolic intermediates in aerobic biochemical processes. The ketoacid dehydrogenase complexes are also located in mitochondria
- *PDC*: PDC is an abbreviation for pyruvate dehydrogenase complex.
- *PDH_a*: It means the active form of pyruvate dehydrogenase (PDH, E1 enzyme of PDC).

- *PDH_{total}*: It means the amount of active and inactive (phosphorylated) forms of PDC.
- *Pyruvate*: Pyruvate is an anionic form of pyruvic acid (2-oxopropionic acid), which is formed in the body during the breakdown of carbohydrates. Pyruvate is a key metabolite of energy metabolism, including the conversion of carbohydrates, proteins, and lipids.
- *Vitamins*: Vitamins are biologically active low-molecular compounds that participate in biochemical pathways, which are also important as regulatory agents. These organic compounds of different classes are not synthesized in humans and animals and must come from the outside.
- *Synaptosomes*: Synaptosomes are isolated nerve endings that retain all the properties of a nerve cell.

Abbreviations

Ach	Acetylcholine
AThTP	Adenylated thiamine triphosphate
ATP	Adenosine triphosphate
CoA	Coenzyme A
FAD	Flavin adenine dinucleotide
HCD	High-carbohydrate diet
NAD	Nicotinamide adenine dinucleotide
OTh	Oxythiamine
OThDP	Oxythiamine diphosphate
PDC	Pyruvate dehydrogenase complex
PDH	Pyruvate dehydrogenase
ThDP	Thiamine diphosphate
ThMP	Thiamine monophosphate
ThTP	Thiamine triphosphate

Vitamin B_1 (thiamine) is one of the essential micronutrients involved in many physiological processes in humans such as energy metabolism and functions of the nervous system. This nitrogen-containing and water-soluble compound was named by Funk as "vitamine," which was applied to the whole group of other structurally diverse compounds in food called vitamins (Rosenfeld, 1997). Since the discovery of thiamine, it was understood that the lack of this low-molecular compound can be responsible for developing polyneuropathy known as the disease "beriberi." This disease is characterized by severe nerve paralysis, apathy, lack of activity, memory impairment, depression, as well as symptoms of hysteria and heart disorders (Muralt, 1947; Carpenter, 2012).

The works of Peters and his school in Oxford laid the foundation for studying the role of vitamin B_1 in cell metabolism. Summarizing his experiments, Peters wrote that "the view can now be advanced that the action of vitamin B_1 is related specifically to pyruvate oxidase in its aerobic reaction" (Peters, 1936). Further studies led to the opinion that thiamine's effect was not due to this compound itself, but to a derivative that was synthesized from the natural vitamin (Jansen, 1949). These were the first steps on the path to the elucidation of the role of thiamine diphosphate (ThDP) in biochemical transformations of pyruvate.

An important stage in the study of the biochemistry of vitamin B_1 was the identification of its basic biologically active form, ThDP, which, as is now known, is a coenzyme of several enzymes that catalyzes the forming and breaking of carbon—carbon bonds and is involved in key metabolic pathways. Among them, the pyruvate dehydrogenase complex (PDC) catalyzes the transformation of pyruvate into acetyl-CoA, a substrate for the tricarboxylic acid cycle and acetylcholine (ACh) synthesis. One of the early hypotheses concerning a neurotropic action of thiamine was proposed by Peters (1967). This hypothesis suggested that a pathological change in nervous tissue at thiamine deficiency can be attributed to a disturbance in the synthesis of acetyl-CoA, which is the precursor for the biosynthesis of neurotransmitter ACh. A reduction in the acetyl-CoA synthesis under thiamine deficiency was explained by the decrease in the activity of PDC due to a deficiency of its coenzyme ThDP. However, the relationship between tissue supply with thiamine, the ThDP content, and the PDC activity turned out to be more complex than previously assumed (Parkhomenko et al., 1996). The study of this issue is important because the experimental data obtained to date strongly suggest that functional impairment of thiamine-dependent processes in the human organism may be one of the important pathogenetic factors in the development of most metabolic and neurodegenerative diseases (Bunik et al., 2013; Parkhomenko et al., 2016).

In this chapter, we consider the results of research, including our own ones, which might expand our understanding of the effects of thiamine provision to tissues on PDC activity.

10.1 Biologically active derivatives of vitamin B_1 in living tissues

It is now established that in the cells of all living organisms vitamin B_1 is represented by its nonphosphorylated form and phosphoric esters

(Bettendorff and Wins, 2009; Gangolf et al., 2010a). The oxidized thiamine derivatives, such as thiochrome and disulfide, also occur in minor amounts (Parkhomenko et al., 2012). The biological effects of these compounds being catabolites of thiamine are still an open question.

Thiamine molecules penetrate into the cells in a free nonphosphorylated form and are phosphorylated immediately to ThDP by the cytosolic enzyme thiamine pyrophosphokinase (EC 2.7.6.2), which catalyzes the transfer of a pyrophosphate group from ATP to thiamine (Manzetti et al., 2014). In living tissues, the phosphorylated derivatives of vitamin B_1 are shared between ThDP, thiamine monophosphate (ThMP), and thiamine triphosphate (ThTP). Recently a new natural thiamine derivative, adenylated thiamine triphosphate (AThTP) (Fig. 10.1), has been identified (Bettendorff et al., 2007). ThDP is considered to be the most studied of

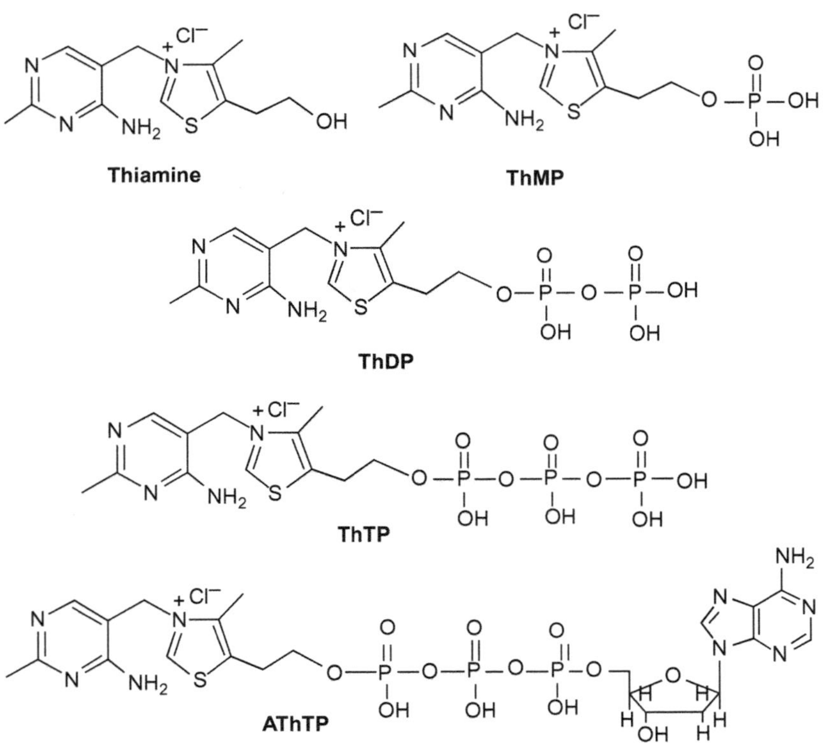

Figure 10.1 ***Thiamine and its phosphorylated derivatives.*** *AThTP*, Adenylated thiamine triphosphate; *ThDP*, thiamine diphosphate; *ThMP*, thiamine monophosphate; *ThTP*, thiamine triphosphate.

the phosphorylated thiamine derivatives. This compound functions as a coenzyme for the enzymes playing key roles in energy generation in mitochondria, among which the most significant could be pyruvate dehydrogenase (PDH) and α-ketoglutarate dehydrogenase as well as branched-chain ketoacid dehydrogenases (Bunik et al., 2013). As a cofactor, ThDP enables the activity of other enzymes, including transketolase, which participates in the pentose phosphate pathway.

ThMP and ThTP do not show coenzyme functions, and their roles still have not been determined. ThTP, which was discovered more than 60 years ago in liver tissue (Rossi-Fanelli et al., 1952), remains the most mysterious compound among the thiamine phosphates. Evidence for a specific role of this thiamine ester in the neural tissue was obtained later (Cooper et al., 1963). To date the following information about ThTP can be undeniable. ThTP is found to be synthesized in all living cells (Chagovec and Rybina, 1959; Berman and Fishman, 1975; Miyoshi et al., 1990), both in the cytosol and in the mitochondria (Gangolf et al., 2010b). There are enzymes that are able to hydrolyze ThTP in all cells (Makarchikov et al, 2003; Sidorova et al., 2009). ThTP could be a phosphate donor for protein phosphorylation, which has been shown to occur in postsynaptic membranes containing endogenous kinase, for 43K rapsyn, a protein required for the clustering of ACh receptors at the neuromuscular junction (Nghiêm et al., 2000). It should be noted that some fragmentary knowledge on the metabolism of ThTP and its involvement in cellular processes, accumulated to date, still does not allow the completion of the overall picture on the role of this compound in living cells.

10.2 Pyruvate dehydrogenase complex

10.2.1 Structure and function of pyruvate dehydrogenase complex

The PDC catalyzes the oxidative decarboxylation of pyruvate with the formation of acetyl-CoA. Three different enzymes are involved in this transformation of pyruvate (Patel et al., 2014). The first one, pyruvate dehydrogenase (E1, PDH), along with enzyme-bound ThDP, catalyzes the decarboxylation of pyruvate and acetylation of the lipoamide group of dihydrolipoamide acetyltransferase (E2) forming S-acetyldihydrolipoyl-E2. Then the enzyme E2 carries the acetyl group to coenzyme A providing acetyl-CoA to the tricarboxylic acid cycle. The reduced lipoamide fragment of E2 is oxidized by a flavoprotein, dihydrolipoamide dehydrogenase (E3).

I. Pyruvate + ThDP-E1 → CO_2 + Hydroxyethyl-ThDp-E1
II. Hydroxyethyl-ThDP-E1 + Lip$(S)_2$-E2 → ThDP-E1 + Lip(SH)(S-acetyl)-E2
III. Lip(SH)(S-acetyl)]-E2 +CoA → acetyl-CoA + Lip$(SH)_2$-E2
IV. Lip$(SH)_2$-E2 + FAD-E3 → Lip$(S)_2$-E2 + FAD_{red}-E3
V. FAD_{red}-E3 + NAD^+ → FAD-E3 + NADH + H^+

Figure 10.2 ***Stepwise reactions of pyruvate dehydrogenase complex.*** Lip(S_2), Lip(SH)(S-acetyl), and Lip$(SH)_2$ are lipoate, acetylhydrolipoate, and dihydrolipoate, respectively. *FAD_{red}*, Reduced FAD.

Two electrons are transferred to NAD^+ via flavin adenine dinucleotide (FAD) of the E3 subunit, and NADH and a proton are produced by this reaction (Fig. 10.2). Among the coenzymes participating in the reactions catalyzed by PDC, ThDP is associated with E1 noncovalently, lipoamide is covalently bound to the lysine residue of E2, and FAD is strongly associated with E3.

Under certain conditions, for example, with deficiency of CoA and NAD^+, E2 and E3 activities may be reduced as compared with the activity of the ThDP-dependent pyruvate decarboxylate subunit. In this case, the formation of by-products, mainly acetoin, was observed (Alkonyi et al., 1976). This unusual product of E1 activity is generated at a higher level in tumors (Baggetto and Lehninger, 1987).

The molecular mechanism of catalysis by E1 of PDC explains how the decarboxylation is coupled with acetyl transfer. The enzyme-bound ThDP exists in a V-conformation which can provide the reactive C2 deprotonated form of ThDP. This ylide attacks the α-carbon atom of pyruvate to form the C2α-lactyl-ThDP intermediate which yields C2α-carbanion (enamine) after decarboxylation. The enamine intermediate acylates the lipoyl group of E2 releasing S-acetyldihydrolipoate and the initial thiazolium ylide. It should be noted that the first stages of this mechanism can by supplemented by protonation and tautomerization of the 4′-aminopyrimidine ring of ThDP (Nemeria et al., 2009). In the later stages of the reaction the acylation of lipoamide can occur through the mechanism of the formation of 2-acetyl-ThDP intermediates (Gruys et al., 1989).

Many years of effort by scientists to elucidate the structural intracellular organization and interaction of the enzymes in the PDC led to the understanding of PDC as a great macromolecular machine consisting of many interacting enzymes "that are connected and regulated by highly flexible domains, also called swinging arms" (Hezaveh et al., 2018). However, the complete structure and function of these domains have not been clarified in detail until today.

The discovery of the mechanism of PDC activity regulation by phosphorylation—dephosphorylation of its E1 component (Linn et al., 1969) was a turning point for understanding and further studying the PDC physiological role.

10.2.2 General views on the key role of PDC in cellular metabolism and its regulation

PDC occupies a central position in the metabolism of carbohydrates in animal cells, being responsible for the pyruvate oxidative decarboxylation to acetyl-CoA in mitochondria. The acetyl-CoA is further used in the tricarboxylic acid cycle, but it can also be involved in fatty acids synthesis (Choi et al., 2010). Thus at the PDC level the flow of glucose carbon between these metabolic pathways is distributed. This is possible due to a mechanism of PDC regulation by phosphorylation—dephosphorylation of its E1 component, which is PDH.

The strict regulation of PDC is known to be very important for maintaining glucose homeostasis, since chronic disorders in glucose homeostasis lead to the development of many metabolic diseases, such as obesity, type 2 diabetes, and even cancer (Gray et al., 2014; Jeoung, 2015). PDH phosphorylation and dephosphorylation can proceed with the participation of specific regulatory enzymes, PDH kinase and PDH phosphatase, respectively. PDH kinase is strongly associated with dihydrolipoamide acetyltransferase and remains bound after purification of the complex, whereas PDH phosphatase binds to the complex via the Ca^{2+} ion (Pettit et al., 1972; Denton et al., 1972) and readily dissociates during purification.

Impaired glucose homeostasis is one of the main risk factors for metabolic diseases, in particular obesity. Since PDC plays a key role in glucose metabolism, this complex can be considered as a possible therapeutic target for the prevention and treatment of such diseases. ThDP is a starting coenzyme of PDC and it was logical to assume that the activity of the complex would directly depend on the vitamin B_1 content and its metabolism in the tissues. In this case, modulators of PDC activity could also be searched for among the thiamine derivatives. We were guided by these considerations to elucidate the effects of thiamine on PDC activity under different physiological conditions. These studies were carried out in the experiments on rats in vivo, on the isolated mitochondria as well as partially purified PDC and PDH phosphatase from rat liver.

10.3 Thiamine, pyruvate dehydrogenase complex, and obesity

10.3.1 Effect of thiamine on the pyruvate dehydrogenase complex activity in lipogenesis in vivo

The experiments were performed on rats of four groups with different models of lipid metabolism, namely: I—control animals, which were kept on a balanced diet; II—3 days of starvation (lipolysis activation); III—a high-carbohydrate diet (HCD) for 3 days after 3 days of starvation (a model for lipogenesis activation); and IV—after 3 days of starvation, the animals were given an HCD and 250 μg thiamine per 100 g of body weight daily for 3 days (Parkhomenko et al., 1983a,b, 1986).

Samples of liver from rats of the above four groups were taken for further study. The activity of PDC, PDH, the content of thiamine and its phosphates, the concentration of pyruvate, and the content of free fatty acids in the liver samples were determined (Parkhomenko et al., 1983a,b).

According to the data given in Table 10.1, the activities of PDC and PDH were critically reduced in rat liver after 3 days of fasting and raised above the same level in the control group after 3 days of keeping the animals on HCD. Changes in the values of concentrations of pyruvate and free fatty acids in the liver indicated the trend of the alteration in the metabolic processes. Thus under the fasting conditions, the activation of lipolysis in rat liver (increased level of free fatty acids) and gluconeogenesis (decreased concentration of pyruvate at decreased PDC activity) was observed. However, when animals were given HCD, there was a tendency for lipogenesis activation (increased concentration of free fatty acids).

It should be noted that the decrease in PDC and PDH activity in rat liver in the state of "Starvation" and "Starvation + HCD + B_1" was accompanied by a significant increase in the ability of the tissue to synthesize acetoin, which confirms a change in the functional state of the PDC (Table 10.1.).

The decrease in the activities of PDC and PDH in the liver of rats in the "Starvation + HCD + B_1" group was unexpected. This effect was confirmed by a significant increase in the concentration of pyruvate and a decrease in free fatty acids. Under the same conditions, the content of thiamine and thiamine phosphates in the liver, including ThDP and ThTP, increased significantly as can be seen from Table 10.1.

We continued our research to make sure that changes in the activity of PDC and PDH were caused by alterations in concentrations of phosphorylated thiamine derivatives. Thiamine at a dose of 250 μg per 100 g of body weight was administered to rats, which after 3 days of fasting were kept for

Table 10.1 Biochemical indices characterizing the functional state of pyruvate dehydrogenase complex (PDC) in the liver of rats with different feeding regimes, namely, PDC and pyruvate dehydrogenase (PDH) activity, the synthesis of acetoin, concentrations of pyruvate and free fatty acids, and content of thiamine phosphates.

Parameters	Animal groups			
	Control	Starvation	Starvation + HCD	Starvation + HCD + B_1
PDC activity, *nmoles of NADH formed per 1 g of wet tissue/min* ($n = 7$)	243.9 ± 62.4	60.5 ± 13.7^{a,b}	349.3 ± 42.9	220.5 ± 37.1^{b}
PDH activity, *nmoles reduced* $K_3Fe(CN)_6$ *per 1 g of wet tissue/min* ($n = 7$)	237.8 ± 19.4	63.3 ± 14.3^{a,b}	270.4 ± 49.0	104.10 ± 21.4^{a,b}
PDH activity, *nmoles of* $^{14}CO_2$ *output per 1 g of wet tissue/min* ($n = 5$)	49.72 ± 10.18	24.62 ± 7.62^{b}	55.67 ± 12.51	23.76 ± 2.02^{a,b}
Acetoin synthesis, *nmoles per 1 g of wet tissue/min* ($n = 3$)	193.3 ± 4.0	933.3 ± 280.0^{a,b}	266.7 ± 33.3	486.7 ± 113.3^{a,b}
Pyruvate concentration, *nmoles per 1 g of wet tissue* ($n = 5–7$)	57.50 ± 3.19	35.43 ± 6.15^{a,b}	64.30 ± 5.95	92.92 ± 9.32^{a}
Free fatty acid content, *microequivalent per 1 g of wet tissue* ($n = 7$)	5.90 ± 0.33	6.96 ± 0.37^{a}	6.36 ± 0.35	5.47 ± 0.40^{b}
ThDP content, *nmoles per 1 g wet tissue* ($n = 3$)	10.0 ± 1.5	11.8 ± 1.1	10.6 ± 0.8	17.0 ± 1.3^{a,b}
ThTP content, *nmoles per 1 g wet tissue* ($n = 3$)	2.9 ± 0.5	3.6 ± 0.4^{b}	2.6 ± 0.3	4.3 ± 0.6^{a,b}

Each value represents the mean ± SEM.
$^{a}P < .05$, compared with the control.
$^{b}P < .05$, compared with "Starvation + HCD + B_1" group. (Old data in Parkhomenko et al., 1983a—Tables 1 and 3; 1983b—Tables 1 and 2). The methods used to analyze the above indices were described in detail earlier (Parkhomenko et al., 1979, 1983a,b).

3 days on HCD. The activity of PDH, active and total (the last was measured after endogenous PDH phosphatase activation), and the content of thiamine derivatives were analyzed in dynamics 1, 2, 6, and 12 hours after thiamine injection (Parkhomenko et al., 1983b). The inverse changes in PDH_a activity (Fig. 10.3A) and in the content of thiamine phosphates,

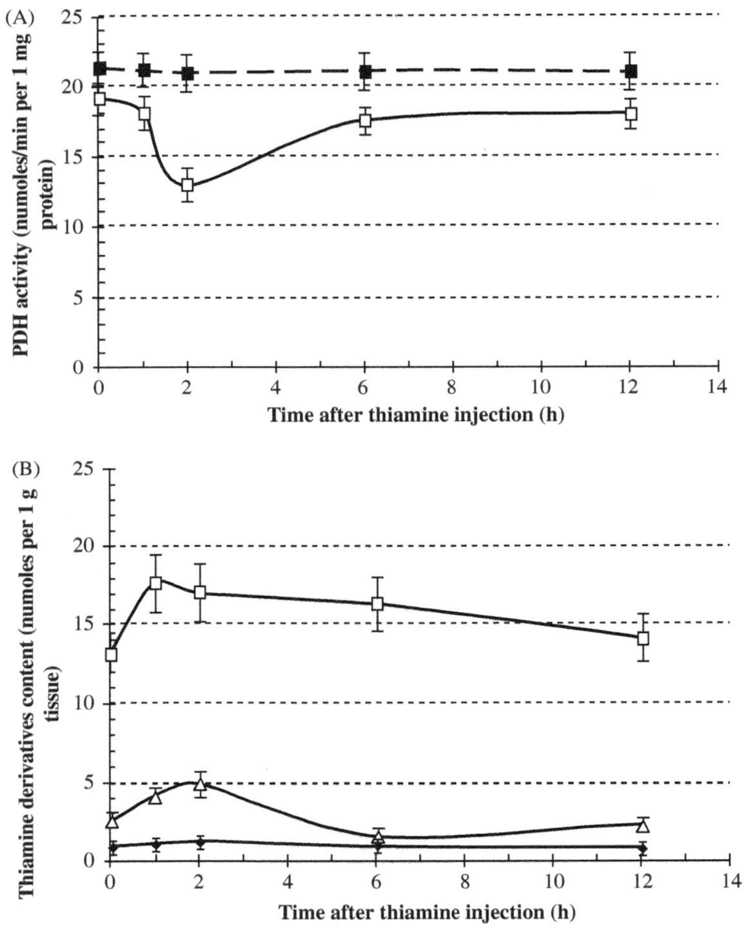

Figure 10.3 PDH activity and the content of thiamine derivatives in the liver of rats of "Starvation + HCD" group at start and 1 h, 2 h, 6 h, and 12 h after injection of 250 μg thiamine per 100 g of weight.
Values are mean ± SEM ($n = 3-6$). (A) activities of PDH_a (active PDH, –□–) and PDH_{total} (–■–); (B) content of thiamine derivatives: total thiamine (–□–), free thiamine (–◆–), and thiamine triphosphate (–△–) (old data in Parkhomenko et al., 1983b, Figs. 10.1–10.3.) The methods used for the analysis of activities of PDH_a and PDH_{total}, and thiamine phosphates were described in detail earlier (Parkhomenko et al., 1979, 1983b).

primarily ThTP (Fig. 10.3B), were observed in the rat liver homogenates. No changes in the PDH_{total} activity were observed under these conditions.

Thus the obtained data confirmed that the PDH activity decreased in liver of rats with activated lipogenesis for the first hours after vitamin B_1 administration. It might be initiated by the variation in concentration of thiamine derivatives in living tissue providing the increased concentration of ThTP. To verify this conclusion, the isolated mitochondria and partially purified enzymes were used in further experiments.

10.3.2 Thiamine diphosphate and thiamine triphosphate involvement in pyruvate dehydrogenase complex regulation: studies on isolated mitochondria and partially purified enzymes

The experiments were performed on mitochondria isolated from the liver of rats of four groups, namely, control animals, starved animals, and animals receiving HCD or HCD and vitamin B_1 after 3-day fasting (Parkhomenko et al., 1986). It was shown that the increasing ThDP concentration in the medium during the incubation of liver mitochondria of all rat groups did not result in increased PDC activity, indicating a low probability of the existence of the operative mechanism of the PDC regulation by association–dissociation ThDP with apoenzyme PDH in animal cells. On the other hand, the incubation of mitochondria with ThTP as well as with ATP significantly decreased the PDC activity. The studies with partially purified complex indicated that ThTP cannot replace ATP in the PDH kinase reaction but is able to inhibit reactivation of the complex by exogenous PDH phosphatase.

Further experiments on the isolated enzyme preparations, PDC and PDH phosphatase, confirmed that ThTP inhibited phosphatase competitively with respect to its substrate, phosphorylated PDH (Parkhomenko et al., 1987). Both the thiamine phosphates inhibited the activity of PDH kinase at concentrations exceeding 1 μM. The inhibitory effect of ThTP on the PDH phosphatase activity was confirmed experimentally using two methodological approaches: (1) measuring the reactivation rate of the phosphorylated PDC with exogenous PDH phosphatase, in the presence of various ThTP concentrations; and (2) under the same conditions measuring the ^{32}P release. In the second case, PDC used as a substrate was inactivated by $[\gamma\text{-}^{32}P]ATP$ (Parkhomenko et al, 1987). As seen in Fig. 10.4 the dependence of inhibition of PDH phosphatase activity on

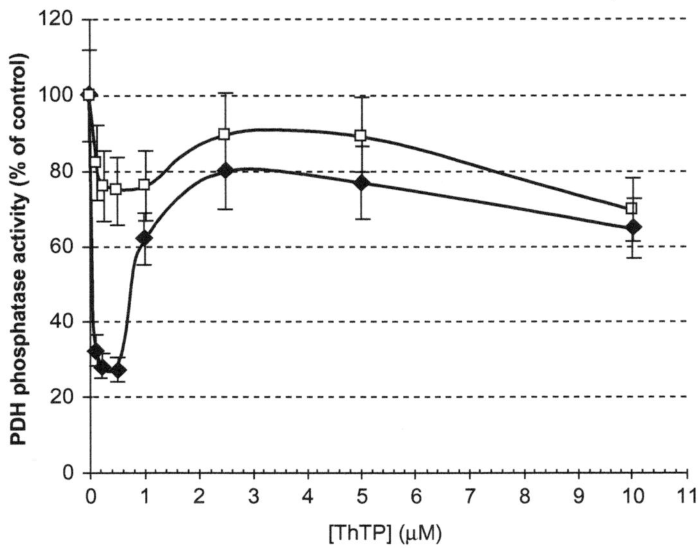

Figure 10.4 ***Effect of thiamine triphosphate (ThTP) on the pyruvate dehydrogenase (PDH) phosphatase activity.*** Values, expressed as % of the control values (synaptosomes were incubated without any additions), are the mean ± SEM ($n = 3–4$). PDH phosphatase activity was measured by the rate of reactivation of complex (–◆–) and by the release rate of ^{32}P (–□–). (Old data in Parkhomenko et al., 1987, Fig. 10.3). The experimentation and the methods used for the analysis of PDH phosphatase activity were described in detail earlier (Parkhomenko et al., 1987).

ThTP concentration has a nonlinear character. The maximum of the inhibition is observed in the low-micromolar range of ThTP concentrations.

Thus according to the data obtained ThDP and ThTP exhibited almost the same inhibitory activity toward PDH kinase. Only one of the thiamine phosphates, ThTP at concentrations close to its physiological levels, had an inhibitory effect on the activity of PDH phosphatase. With respect to in vivo activity the ThTP synthesized after the injection of vitamin B_1 is suggested to be responsible for the temporary decrease in PDC activity in liver of rats in lipogenesis.

Activation of lipogenesis in liver of rats on a HCD was accompanied by an increase in PDC activity due to the conversion of its inactive form to the active one catalyzed by PDH phosphatase. To provide PDC dephosphorylation, PDH phosphatase binds to the complex via a calcium ion (Hansford, 1981). A possible mechanism may be that ThTP interferes with the binding of PDH phosphatase to the complex, interacting with one of the protein molecules or with a calcium ion.

However, it is impossible to be sure that the determined ThTP concentrations correspond to the physiological ones at the end of the experiments. There is a wide range in the values of ThTP content in animal tissues, as given by various authors (Rindi and De Giuseppe, 1961; Kawasaki, 1986; Parkhomenko et al., 1979; Gangolf et al., 2010a). The ThTP seems to be a transit labile macroergic compound. Quantity determination of ThTP may depend on the physiological state of the animal, the method of its killing, the way of extraction from tissues, and a number of other factors. Thus the noncoenzyme regulation of glucose metabolism on the PDC level by thiamine derivatives can be a subject for further study in order to understand the molecular mechanisms of some metabolic disorders.

10.3.3 Physiological significance of noncoenzyme action of vitamin B_1 derivatives on pyruvate dehydrogenase complex

10.3.3.1 Metabolic diseases, pyruvate dehydrogenase complex, and thiamine

Obesity, which has become widespread in our time, is considered to play an important role in the etiology of severe metabolic diseases, such as hepatic steatosis, insulin resistance, and type 2 diabetes mellitus (Zhang et al., 2018). The disorders in the homeostasis of glucose and free fatty acids can also cause cancer, cardiovascular, and neurodegenerative diseases (Schummer et al., 2008; Patel et al., 2014; Lee, 2014; Jeoung, 2015). The ThDP-dependent multienzyme PDC plays a key role in maintaining glucose homeostasis in cells and abnormalities in its functioning may cause metabolic disorders (Schummer et al., 2008; Choi et al., 2010; Gray et al., 2014; Eyassu and Angione, 2017; Maguire et al., 2018).

The PDC activity under different physiological conditions is determined by the change in the ratio of its active (dephosphorylated) and inactive (phosphorylated) forms (Linn et al., 1969). Four isoenzymes of PDH kinase (PDH kinase 1, 2, 3, and 4) and two isoenzymes of PDH phosphatase are involved in PDC regulation (Lee, 2014). The isoenzymes of PDH kinase in mammals exhibit tissue specificity (Bowker-Kinley et al., 1998; Jeoung and Harris, 2008). The regulatory enzyme PDH kinase, like the basic enzymes of PDC, undergo multidimensional regulation both at the level of protein expression and at the level of metabolic interaction with regulatory molecules (Kerbey et al., 1984; Caterson et al., 1987; Lee, 2014; Patel et al., 2014; Jeoung, 2015;

Mahmood et al., 2016). An increase in the activity of this enzyme in patients with diabetes, cancer, and some other metabolic pathologies leads to an excessive undesirable decrease in PDC activity which may be corrected by inhibitors of PDH kinase as possible therapeutic agents. The search for the effective and selective inhibitors of PDH kinase is particularly topical at this time (Lee, 2014; Zhang et al., 2015, 2018; Jeoung, 2015; Wu et al., 2018).

Thiamine deficiency in people with obesity and diabetes has been repeatedly reported in the literature (Carrodeguas et al., 2005; Pácal et al., 2014; Kerns et al., 2015; Nath et al., 2017). Analysis of literature data and the results of our own studies indicate that vitamin B_1 and its derivatives could also be promising for the treatment of the metabolic disorders. We used an animal model of lipogenesis activation and showed that thiamine administration inhibits the PDC reactivation in the liver of rats transferred after fasting to high-carbon diets, and, accordingly, inhibits the lipogenesis. It was suggested that the mechanism of this thiamine action might have reference to noncoenzyme effects of thiamine derivatives, primarily thiamine phosphates. This action of vitamin B_1 was confirmed in experiments on rats with the model of obesity and metabolic disorders (Tanaka et al, 2010). The addition of 0.2% thiamine to the drinking water of such rats prevented obesity. The positive effect was also obtained by the addition of thiamine to a drug for the treatment of obesity caused by diabetes in mice (Muroyama et al., 2003). In view of the foregoing, we consider it to be promising to create drugs for the treatment of metabolic diseases on the basis of thiamine derivatives.

10.3.3.2 Vitamin B_1, pyruvate dehydrogenase complex, and modulation of acetylcholine synthesis

Numerous research has shown that glucose-derived pyruvate through the PDC reaction is a main source of acetyl-CoA for ACh synthesis in nerve cells (Lefresne et al., 1978; Perry et al., 1980; Szutowicz et al., 2013). Although the regulation of PDC from rat brain is similar to that of the enzyme complex derived from other tissues, some features of the regulation of the brain PDH in vivo should be pointed out (Schaffer and Olson, 1980; Aiuchi et al., 1984). In particular, it has been shown that the regulation of PDC through the phosphorylation–dephosphorylation mechanism is tightly coupled with the functioning of an excitable membrane in nerve cells (Browning et al., 1981; Schaffer and Olson, 1980).

The early studies aimed at elucidating the role of vitamin B_1 in the functioning of nerve cells showed that at stimulation of the nerve fiber, thiamine was released together with ACh into the environment, which indicates the interrelation of the metabolism of these substances (Muralt, 1947). Taking into account all the above and our data on the participation of ThDP and ThTP in the regulation of PDC from liver tissue, we suggested that such regulation can take place in nerve cells. The initial studies with synaptosomes demonstrated a nonlinear dependence of label incorporation from [2-^{14}C]pyruvate into ACh at incubation of the synaptosomes with increasing thiamine concentration (Parkhomenko et al., 1991). Under these conditions the PDC activity analyzed by the formation of acetyl-CoA were changed synchronously with the change in the degree of the label incorporation into ACh.

To be sure that the effect of thiamine and its phosphorylated derivatives on the ACh synthesis in nerve cells was caused by their noncoenzyme action on PDC activity, we used the methodological approach described by Parkhomenko et al. (1991), with synaptosomes from the brain of normal and B_1-deficient rats, and thiamine or oxythiamine (OTh) was added to the incubation mixture. Both thiamine and OTh can form mono-, di-, and triphosphates in a cell, and oxythiamine diphosphate is known to be the antagonist of ThDP.

It was assumed that if thiamine affected the synthesis of ACh only because of an increase in concentration of TDP as coenzyme of PDC, the thiamine antagonist oxythiamine in form of diphosphate would not contribute to PDC activity. But if the effect of phosphorylated thiamine derivatives on the synthesis of ACh under these conditions was due to the regulation of PDC, OTh through its phosphorylated derivatives would be affected in a similar way as thiamine.

As seen in Fig. 10.5, both thiamine and OTh exhibit similar effects on the activity of PDH (Fig. 10.5A) and on the incorporation of a label from [2-^{14}C]pyruvate into Ach (Fig. 10.5B) in synaptosomes isolated from normal and B_1-deficient rats, which confirms the hypothesis of a noncoenzyme mechanism of vitamin B_1 action. Thus during thiamine interaction with excitable membranes the signal is transferred to the systems providing synthesis of ACh (including PDC). It is probable that thiamine phosphates and certain proteins, including cytoskeleton ones, are involved in the transfer of this signal (Parkhomenko et al., 2016).

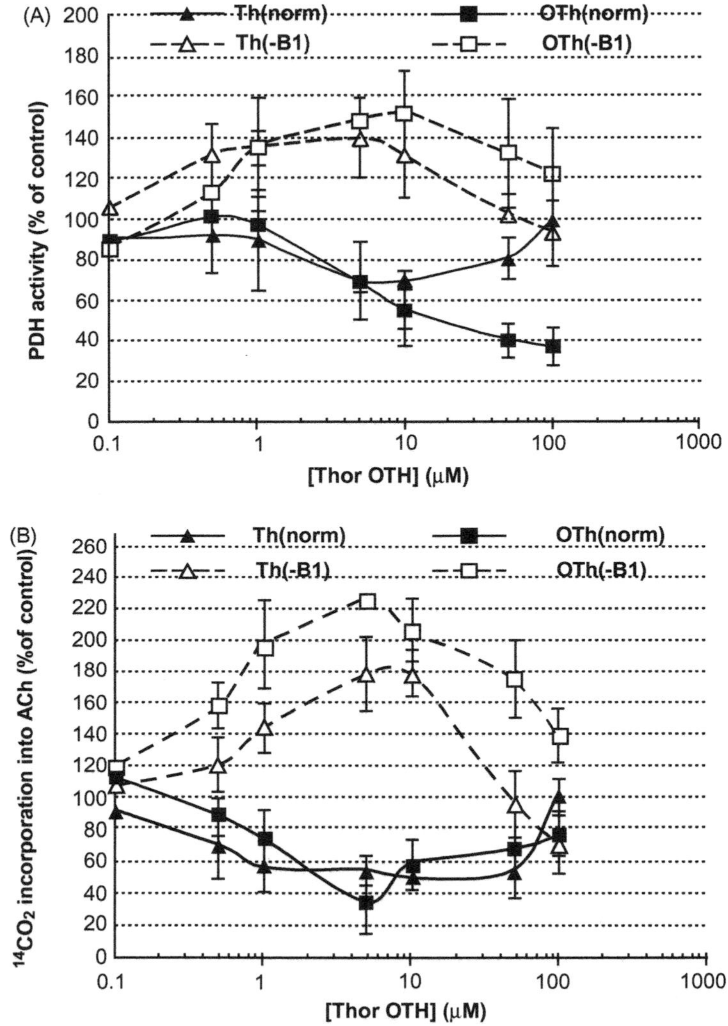

Figure 10.5 The effect of thiamine and oxythiamine on PDH activity (A) and the incorporation of a label from [2-^{14}C]pyruvate into ACh (B) in synaptosomes isolated from the brain of normal and thiamine-deficient rats.
Values are mean ± SEM ($n = 3–6$). The experimentation and the methods used in that study for the analysis of PDH activity, and ACh radioactivity were described in detail earlier (Parkhomenko et al., 1983a, 1991).

Summarizing the information presented above, it can be concluded that not only a sufficient content of vitamin B_1 in tissues but also a regime of thiamine intake into cells and its active metabolism are important in maintaining the normal level of metabolic processes.

References

Aiuchi, T., Matsunaga, M., Daimatsu, T., Nakaya, K., Nakamura, Y., 1984. Effect of glucose and pyruvate metabolism on membrane potential in synaptosomes. Biochim. Biophys. Acta 771, 228–234.

Alkonyi, I., Bolygy, E., Gyycsi, L., Szaby, D., 1976. Studies on the formation of acetoin from acetaldehyde by the pyruvate dehydrogenase complex and its regulation. Eur. J. Biochem. 66, 551–557.

Baggetto, L.G., Lehninger, A.L., 1987. Isolated tumoral pyruvate dehydrogenase can synthesize acetoin which inhibits pyruvate oxidation as well as other aldehydes. Biochem. Biophys. Res. Commun. 145, 153–159.

Berman, K., Fishman, R.A., 1975. Thiamine phosphate metabolism and possible coenzyme-independent functions of thiamine in brain. J. Neurochem. 24, 457–465.

Bettendorff, L., Wins, P., 2009. Thiamin diphosphate in biological chemistry: new aspects of thiamin metabolism, especially triphosphate derivatives acting other than as cofactors. FEBS. J. 276, 2917–2925.

Bettendorff, L., Wirtzfeld, B., Makarchikov, A.F., Mazzucchelli, G., Frédérich, M., Gigliobianco, T., et al., 2007. Discovery of a natural thiamine adenine nucleotide. Nat. Chem. Biol. 3, 211–212.

Bowker-Kinley, M.M., Davis, W.I., Wu, P., Harris, R.A., Popov, K.M., 1998. Evidence for existence of tissue-specific regulation of the mammalian pyruvate dehydrogenase complex. Biochem. J. 329, 191–196.

Browning, M., Bennett, W.F., Kelly, P., Lynch, G., 1981. Evidence that the 40,000 Mr phosphoprotein influenced by high frequency synaptic stimulation is the alpha subunit of pyruvate dehydrogenase. Brain Res. 218, 255–266.

Bunik, V.I., Tylicki, A., Lukashev, N.V., 2013. Thiamin diphosphate-dependent enzymes: from enzymology to metabolic regulation, drug design and disease models. FEBS. J. 280, 6412–6442.

Carpenter, K.J., 2012. The discovery of thiamin. Ann. Nutr. Metab. 61, 219–223.

Carrodeguas, L., Kaidar-Person, O., Szomstein, S., Antozzi, P., Rosenthal, R., 2005. Preoperative thiamine deficiency in obese population undergoing laparoscopic bariatric surgery. Surg. Obes. Relat. Dis. 1, 517–522.

Caterson, I.D., Astbury, L.D., Williams, P.F., Vanner, M.A., Cooney, G.J., Turtle, J.R., 1987. The activity of the pyruvate dehydrogenase complex in heart and liver from mice during the development of obesity and insulin resistance. Biochem. J. 243, 549–553 (Printed in Great Britain).

Chagovec, R.V., Rybina, A.A., 1959. Investigation on the forms and metabolism of thiamine in tissues of the animal organism by means of thiamine-^{35}S. in: international Symposium on B vitamins, Poznan, 21–24, IX, pp. 324–338.

Choi, C.S., Ghoshal, P., Srinivasan, M., Kim, S., Cline, G., Patel, M.S., 2010. Liver-specific pyruvate dehydrogenase complex deficiency upregulates lipogenesis in adipose tissue and improves peripheral insulin sensitivity. Lipids 45, 987–995.

Cooper, J.R., Roth, R.H., Kini, M.M., 1963. Biochemical and physiological function of thiamine in nervous tissue. Nature 199, 609–610.

Denton, R.M., Randle, P.J., Martin, B.R., 1972. Stimulation by calcium ions of pyruvate dehydrogenase phosphate phosphatase. Biochem. J. 128, 161–163.

Eyassu, F., Angione, C., 2017. Modelling pyruvate dehydrogenase under hypoxia and its role in cancer metabolism. R. Soc. Open Sci. 4, 170360.

Gangolf, M., Czerniecki, J., Radermecker, M., Detry, O., Nisolle, M., Jouan, C., et al., 2010a. Thiamine status in human and content of phosphorylated thiamine derivatives in biopsies and cultured cells. PLoS One 5, e13616.

Gangolf, M., Wins, P., Thiry, M., El Moualij, B., Bettendorff, L., 2010b. Thiamine triphosphate synthesis in rat brain occurs in mitochondria and is coupled to the respiratory chain. J. Biol. Chem. 285, 583–594.
Gray, L.R., Tompkins, S.C., Taylor, E.B., 2014. Regulation of pyruvate metabolism and human disease. Cell Mol. Life Sci. 71, 2577–2604.
Gruys, K.J., Datta, A., Frey, P.A., 1989. 2-Acetylthiamin pyrophosphate (acetyl-TPP) pH-rate for hydrolysis of acetyl-TPP and isolation of acetyl-TPP as a transient species in pyruvate dehydrogenase catalyzed reactions. Biochemistry 28, 9071–9080.
Hansford, R.G., 1981. Effect of micromolar concentration of free Ca^{2+} ions on pyruvate dehydrogenase interconvertion in intact rat heart mitochondria. Biochem. J. 194, 721–732.
Hezaveh, S., Zeng, A.P., Jandt, U., 2018. Full enzyme complex simulation: interactions in human pyruvate dehydrogenase complex. J. Chem. Inf. Model. 58, 362–369.
Jansen, B.C.P., 1949. The physiology thiamine. Vitam. Horm. VII, 84–106.
Jeoung, N.H., 2015. Pyruvate dehydrogenase kinases: therapeutic targets for iabetes and cancers. Diabetes Metab. J. 39, 1881–1897.
Jeoung, N.H., Harris, R.A., 2008. Pyruvate dehydrogenase kinase-4 deficiency lowers blood glucose and improves glucose tolerance in diet-induced obese mice. Am. J. Physiol. Endocrinol. Metab. 295, 46–54.
Kawasaki, T., 1986. Determination of thiamin and its phosphate esters by high-performance liquid chromatography, Methods Enzymology, vol. 122. Academic Press, New York, pp. 15–20.
Kerbey, A.L., Caterson, I.D., Williams, P.F., Turtle, J.R., 1984. Proportion of active dephosphorylated pyruvate dehydrogenase complex in heart and isolated heart mitochondria is decreased in obese hyperinsulinaemic mice. Biochem. J. 217, 117–121.
Kerns, J.C., Arundel, C., Chawla, L.S., 2015. Thiamin deficiency in people with obesity. Adv. Nutr. 6, 147–153.
Lee, I.K., 2014. The role of pyruvate dehydrogenase kinase in diabetes and obesity. Diabetes Metab. J. 38 (3), 181–186.
Lefresne, P., Beaujouan, J.C., Glowinski, J., 1978. Origin of the acetyl moiety of acetylcholine in rat striatal synaptosomes: a specific pyruvate dehydrogenase involved in ACh synthesis? Biochimie 60, 479–487.
Linn, T.C., Pettit, F.H., Hucho, F., Reed, L.J., 1969. Alpha-keto acid dehydrogenase complexes. XI. Comparative studies of regulatory properties of the pyruvate dehydrogenase complexes from kidney, heart, and liver mitochondria. Proc. Natl. Acad. Sci. U.S.A. 64, 227–234.
Maguire, D., Talwar, D., Shiels, P.G., McMillan, D., 2018. The role of thiamine dependent enzymes in obesity and obesity related chronic disease states: a systematic review. Clin. Nutr. ESPEN 25, 8–17.
Mahmood, S., Birkaya, B., Rideout, T.C., Patel, M.S., 2016. Lack of mitochondria-generated acetyl-CoA by pyruvate dehydrogenase complex downregulates gene expression in the hepatic de novo lipogenic pathway. Am. J. Physiol. Endocrinol. Metab. 311, 117–127.
Makarchikov, A.F., Lakaye, B., Gulyai, I.E., Czerniecki, J., Coumans, B., Wins, P., et al., 2003. Thiamine triphosphate and thiamine triphosphatase activities: from bacteria to mammals. Cell Mol. Life Sci. 60, 1477–1488.
Manzetti, S., Zhang, J., Spoel, D., 2014. Thiamin function, metabolism, uptake, and transport. Biochemistry 53, 821–835.
Miyoshi, K., Egi, Y., Shioda, T., Kawasaki, T., 1990. Evidence for in vivo synthesis of thiamin triphosphate by cytosolic adenylate kinase in chicken skeletal muscle. J. Biochem. 108, 267–270.

Muralt, A., 1947. Thiamine and peripheral neurophysiology. In: Harris, R.S., Thimann, K.,V. (Eds.), Vitamins and Hormones, vol. V. Academic Press Inc, New York, pp. 93–118.
Muroyama, K., Murosaki, S., Yamamoto, Y., Odaka, H., Chung, H.C., Miyoshi, M., 2003. Anti-obesity effects of a mixture of thiamin, arginine, caffeine, and citric acid in non-insulin dependent diabetic KK mice. J. Nutr. Sci. Vitaminol. (Tokyo) 49, 56–63.
Nath, A., Tran, T., Shope, T.R., Koch, T.R., 2017. Prevalence of clinical thiamine deficiency in individuals with medically complicated obesity. Nutr. Res. 37, 29–36.
Nemeria, N.S., Chakraborty, S., Balakrishnan, A., Jordan, F., 2009. Reaction mechanisms of thiamin diphosphate enzymes: defining states of ionization and tautomerization of the cofactor at individual steps. FEBS J. 276, 2432–2446.
Nghiêm, H.O., Bettendorff, L., Changeux, J.P., 2000. Specific phosphorylation of torpedo 43K rapsyn by endogenous kinase(s) with thiamine triphosphate as the phosphate donor. FASEB J. 14, 543–554.
Pácal, L., Kuricová, K., Kaňková, K., 2014. Evidence for altered thiamine metabolism in diabetes: is there a potential to oppose gluco-and lipotoxicity by rational supplementation? World J. Diabetes 5, 288–295.
Parkhomenko, J.M., Rybina, A.A., Khalmuradov, A.G., 1979. Separation of thiamine phosphoric esters on sephadex cation exchanger, Methods Enzymology, vol. 62. Academic Press, New York, pp. 59–62.
Parkhomenko, Iu.M., Vovk, A.I., Protasova, Z.S., Chernysh, I.Iu, Khalmuradov, A.G., 1983a. Effect of thiamine on the activity of the pyruvate dehydrogenase complex in rat liver following stimulation of lipogenesis. Ukr. Biokhim. Zh. 55, 408–414 (in Russian).
Parkhomenko, Iu.M., Rybina, A.A., Klimchuk, S.A., Khalmuradov, A.G., 1983b. Interrelation between the content of thiamine phosphates and pyruvate dehydrogenase activity in the liver of rats with intensified lipogenesis. Ukr. Biokhim. Zh. 55, 517–522 (in Russian).
Parkhomenko, Iu.M., Protasova, Z.S., Khalmuradov, A.G., 1986. Thiamine phosphates and regulation of the pyruvate dehydrogenase complex activity in rat liver mitochondria. Ukr. Biokhim. Zh. 58 (6), 35–41 (in Russian).
Parkhomenko, Iu.M., Chernysh, I.Iu, Churilova, T.Ia, Khalmuradov, A.G., 1987. Effect of thiamine phosphates on the activity of regulatory enzymes of the pyruvate dehydrogenase complex. Ukr. Biokhim. Zh. 59 (5), 49–54 (in Russian).
Parkhomenko, Yu.M., Protasova, Z.S., Chernysh, I.Yu, Pkhakadze, E.G., 1991. Modulation of acetylcholine synthesis in the rat brain synaptosomes by thiamine and its relation to the regulation of the pyruvate dehydrogease complex activity. In: Bisswanger, H. (Ed.), Biochemistry and Physiology of ThDP-Dependent Enzymes. VCH Verlagsgesellschaft Mbh, New York, pp. 375–381.
Parkhomenko, Iu.M., Donchenko, G.V., Protasova, Z.S., 1996. The neural activity of thiamine: facts and hypotheses. Ukr. Biokhim. Zh. 68 (2), 3–14 (in Russian).
Parkhomenko, Iu.M., Stepuro, I.I., Donchenko, G.V., Stepuro, V.I., 2012. Oxidized derivatives of thiamine: formation, properties, biological role. Ukr. Biokhim. Zh. 84 (5), 5–24 (in Russian).
Parkhomenko, Yu. M., Pavlova, A.S., Mezhenskaya, O.A., 2016. Mechanisms responsible for the high sensitivity of neural cells to vitamin B_1 deficiency. Neurophysiology 48, 429–448.
Patel, M.S., Nemeria, N.S., Furey, W., Jordan, F., 2014. The pyruvate dehydrogenase complexes: structure-based function and regulation. J. Biol. Chem. 289, 16615–16623.
Perry, E.K., Perry, R.H., Tomlinson, B.E., Blessed, G., Gibson, P.H., 1980. Coenzyme A-acetylating enzymes in alzheimer's disease: possible cholinergic 'compartment' of pyruvate dehydrogenase. Neurosci. Lett. 18, 105–110.

Peters, R.A., 1936. Pyruvic acid oxidation in brain.I. vitamin B_1 and the pyruvate oxidase in pigeon brain. Biochem. J. 30, 2206–2218.
Peters, R.A., 1967. The biochemical lasion of thiamine deficiency, Thiamine Deficiency, vol. 28 (6). J. & A. Churchill, Ciba Foundation, Study Group, London, pp. 1–8.
Pettit, F.H., Roche, Th.E., Reed, L.J., 1972. Function of calcium ions in pyruvate dehydrogenase phosphatase activity. Biochem. Biophys. Res. Commun. 49, 563–571.
Rindi, G., De Giuseppe, L., 1961. The content of thiamine and its mono-, di-and triphosphoric esters in different biological materials. Int. Z. Vitaminforsch. 31, 321–326.
Rosenfeld, L., 1997. Vitamine - vitamin. The early years of discovery. Clin. Chem. 43, 680–685.
Rossi-Fanelli, A., Siliprandi, N., Fasella, P., 1952. On the presence of the triphosphothiamine (TPT) in the liver. Science 116, 711–713.
Schaffer, W.T., Olson, M.S., 1980. The regulation of pyruvate oxidation during membrane depolarization of rat brain synaptosomes. Biochem. J. 192, 741–751.
Schummer, C.M., Werner, U., Tennagels, N., Schmoll, D., Haschke, G., Juretschke, H. P., et al., 2008. Dysregulated pyruvate dehydrogenase complex in Zucker diabetic fatty rats. Am. J. Physiol. Endocrinol. Metab. 294, E88–E96.
Sidorova, A.A., Stepanenko, S.P., Parkhomenko, Iu.M., 2009. Characteristics of thiamine triphosphatase from neural cells plasma membranes. Ukr. Biokhim. Zh. 81 (3), 57–65 (in Russian).
Szutowicz, A., Bielarczyk, H., Jankowska-Kulawy, A., Pawełczyk, T., Ronowska, A., 2013. Acetyl-coA the key factor for survival or death of cholinergic neurons in course of neurodegenerative diseases. Neurochem. Res. 38, 1523–1542.
Tanaka, T., Kono, T., Terasaki, F., Yasui, K., Soyama, A., Otsuka, K., et al., 2010. Thiamine prevents obesity and obesity-associated metabolic disorders in OLETF rats. J. Nutr. Sci. Vitaminol. (Tokyo) 56, 335–346.
Wu, C.Y., Satapati, S., Gui, W., Wynn, R.M., Sharma, G., Lou, M., et al., 2018. A novel inhibitor of pyruvate dehydrogenase kinase stimulates myocardial carbohydrate oxidation in diet-induced obesity. J. Biol. Chem. 293, 9604–9613.
Zhang, S.L., Hu, X., Zhang, W., Yao, H., Tam, K.Y., 2015. Development of pyruvate dehydrogenase kinase inhibitors in medicinal chemistry with particular emphasis as anticancer agents. Drug Discov. Today 20, 1112–1119.
Zhang, M., Zhao, Y., Li, Z., Wang, C., 2018. Pyruvate dehydrogenase kinase 4 mediates lipogenesis and contributes to the pathogenesis of nonalcoholic steatohepatitis. Biochem. Biophys. Res. Commun. 495, 582–586.

Further reading

Cooper, R.H., Randle, P.J., Denton, R.M., 1974. Regulation of heart muscle dehydrogenase kinase. Biochem. J. 143, 625–641.
Kawasaki, T., 1992. Thiamin triphosphate synthesis in animals. J. Nutr. Sci. Vitaminol. (Tokyo) Spec No. 383–386.
Patel, M.S., Roche, T.E., 1990. Molecular biology and biochemistry of pyruvate dehydrogenase complexes. FASEB J. 4, 3224–3233.

CHAPTER 11

Thiamine, oxidative stress, and ethanol

Álisson de Carvalho Gonçalves[1], Luiz Ricardo Soldi[1] and Guilherme Vannucchi Portari[2]
[1]Laboratory of Experimental Nutrition, Federal University of Triangulo Mineiro, Uberaba, Brazil
[2]Health Institute, Department of Nutrition, Federal University of Triangulo Mineiro, Uberaba, Brazil

Contents

Key facts of oxidative stress

- Some situations produce high levels of free radicals and/or mitigate antioxidant activity.
- Oxidative stress is an imbalance between prooxidant activity and antioxidant capacity in favor of the former.
- In an oxidative stress framework, free radicals react with other molecules and cause cell damage.
- Thus antioxidant defenses are essential to combat oxidative damage and protect cell function.
- Oxidative stress triggers or mediates several health disturbances, and it is responsible for several harmful effects due to alcohol consumption.
- Some nutrients can act directly against free radicals or can assist impaired antioxidant mechanisms.

Molecular Nutrition
DOI: https://doi.org/10.1016/B978-0-12-811907-5.00018-X

- Molecules, enzymes, and nutrients with antioxidant capacity are responsible for the maintenance of redox balance, especially during events with high production of free radicals.

Summary points

- This chapter focuses on thiamine and its relation with alcohol intake and oxidative stress.
- Vitamin B1 is a generic term utilized to describe the existent forms of thiamine, a micronutrient essential to humans, which mainly plays a role in energy metabolism.
- Thiamine deficiency is correlated to neurological disorders, heart disease, and other pathological conditions.
- Alcohol intake is intimately related to thiamine deficiency, because of inadequate eating habits and failure in thiamine absorption.
- Alcohol metabolism aggravates the production of reactive species and/or reduces antioxidant capacity, while also provoking oxidative stress that can mediate the harmful effects of chronic alcohol intake.
- Several studies have shown the antioxidant role of thiamine, including against the effects of excessive alcohol consumption.
- Thiamine supplementation has shown positive effects against neurodegenerative disorders and liver disease related to ethanol metabolism.
- Therefore there is a consensus that thiamine supplementation must be part of the treatment of alcoholics, mainly during withdrawal periods.

Definition of words/terms

***Alcoholism*:** Excessive and chronic alcoholic beverage intake can trigger neuropathy, cardiopathy, hepatic disease, and others.

***Thiamine deficiency*:** Low thiamine availability to cells caused by poor ingestion or failure in thiamine uptake and/or transport.

***Free radical*:** Atoms or molecules that have unpaired electrons in the last atomic layer. This characteristic causes the free radical to react with other molecules, sharing, donating, or absorbing electrons. Despite promoting some damage in macromolecules, free radicals play an essential role in processes of cellular signaling and control.

***Antioxidant*:** Molecule or mechanism able to scavenge free radicals and/or protect other molecules against free radical reaction.

***Oxidative stress*:** Imbalance between oxidative reactions and antioxidant capacity in favor of oxidation.

***Lipid peroxidation*:** Oxidative damage to lipids. Generally, the main lipids affected by oxidative stress are the phospholipids that comprise the cell membrane.

Abbreviations

ADH	Alcohol dehydrogenase
CAT	Catalase
GPx	Glutathione peroxidase
GR	Glutathione reductase
GSH	Reduced glutathione
GSSG	Oxidized glutathione
NAD	Nicotinamide adenine dinucleotide
PPP	Pentose phosphate pathway
SOD	Superoxide dismutase
TDP	Thiamine diphosphate
TMP	Thiamine monophosphate
TPKase	Thiamin pyrophosphokinase
TTP	Thiamine triphosphate

11.1 Introduction

Thiamine by definition is a micronutrient essential to humans, intimately related to pathologies caused by the consumption of ethanol, mainly due to its deficiency. This deficiency observed in chronic alcoholics can be primary, due to lack of proper food consumption, or secondary, due to disturbances in absorption and metabolic processes (biotransformation, use, and excretion) (Martin, 2001), and has been extensively described in the scientific literature, mainly as Wernicke–Korsakoff Syndrome (Butterworth et al., 1993).

Studies that have evaluated thiamine diet deprivation have shown negative effects on various health issues (Abdou and Hazell, 2015). In fact its deficiency is strongly related to neurodegenerative diseases (Butterworth et al., 1993). On the other hand, supplementation with thiamine analogs have shown promising results. Several studies showed a reversal of pathological conditions, prevention of diseases, and improvement of energy metabolism in response to an increase in thiamine intake (Chou et al., 2018; Masuda et al., 2015; Woelk et al., 1998). Special attention has been given to the relationship between this vitamin and chronic alcoholism, since this condition is closely linked to thiamine deficiency and health disorders (Hoyumpa Jr., 1983).

Although commonly studied due to its metabolic effects on the citric acid cycle, thiamine has gathered attention due to its antioxidant effects, be they due to properties on its chemical structure or its influence in inducing pathways related to oxidative stress. In fact studies have shown some antioxidant effects in response to thiamine supplementation (Bozic et al., 2015; Schmid et al., 2008). Thus it was hoped that thiamine could be part of the treatment against alcoholism-associated disorders, since oxidative stress mediates the harmful effects of ethanol intake. In reality studies have shown positive effects of thiamine treatment in alcoholics, and works are currently being publishing describing mechanisms by which this vitamin can contribute to prevent negative alcoholism effects (Martin et al., 2003; Portari et al., 2016; Vidhya et al., 2013; Yilmaz et al., 2015).

11.2 Structure and function of thiamine

Vitamin B1 is a generic term utilized to describe the existent forms of thiamine (Fig. 11.1A), that is, nonphosphorylated thiamine, mono-, di-, and triphosphates. Chemically, the thiamine molecule is composed of two rings united by a methyl bridge, with one being a pyrimine ring (2,5-dimethyl-6-aminopyrimidine) and the other being a thiazole ring (4-methyl-5-hydroxy ethyl thiazole) (Manzetti et al., 2014).

Following its ingestion, the absorption of thiamine occurs mainly in the proximal regions of the small intestine (jejunum). Although there is a spontaneous diffusion through the wall of the intestine, high levels of thiamine require the participation of specific carriers to cross the biological barriers and reach the bloodstream. In the blood thiamine is mainly concentrated in erythrocytes, although some is present in plasma, platelets, and leucocytes. Thiamine can be found in the human organism in its free or phosphate-esterified forms: thiamine monophosphate (Fig. 11.1B), thiamine diphosphate (TDP) (Fig. 11.1C), thiamine triphosphate (Fig. 11.1D), and adenosine thiamine triphosphate (Fig. 11.1E) (Pácal et al., 2014).

TDP is the biologically active form of thiamine and is formed in the cytosol through the action of the enzyme pyrophosphokinase. The enzymatic complex pyruvate—dehydrogenase utilizes TDP as a cofactor to promote the oxidative decarboxylation of pyruvate and produce acetyl coenzyme-A (acetyl-CoA). The molecule acetyl-CoA participates in the production of citrate, the first component in the citric acid cycle. TDP functions also in the activity of α-ketoglutarate dehydrogenase, the enzymatic complex responsible for the decarboxylation of α-ketoglutarate and the formation of succinate in the citric acid cycle. Furthermore, concerning the metabolism of carbohydrates, TDP is an important cofactor in the normal activity of transketolase, a regulatory enzyme in the pentose phosphate pathway, which produces precursors of nucleic acids and potential antioxidant reduction agents (Manzetti et al., 2014). Aside from these

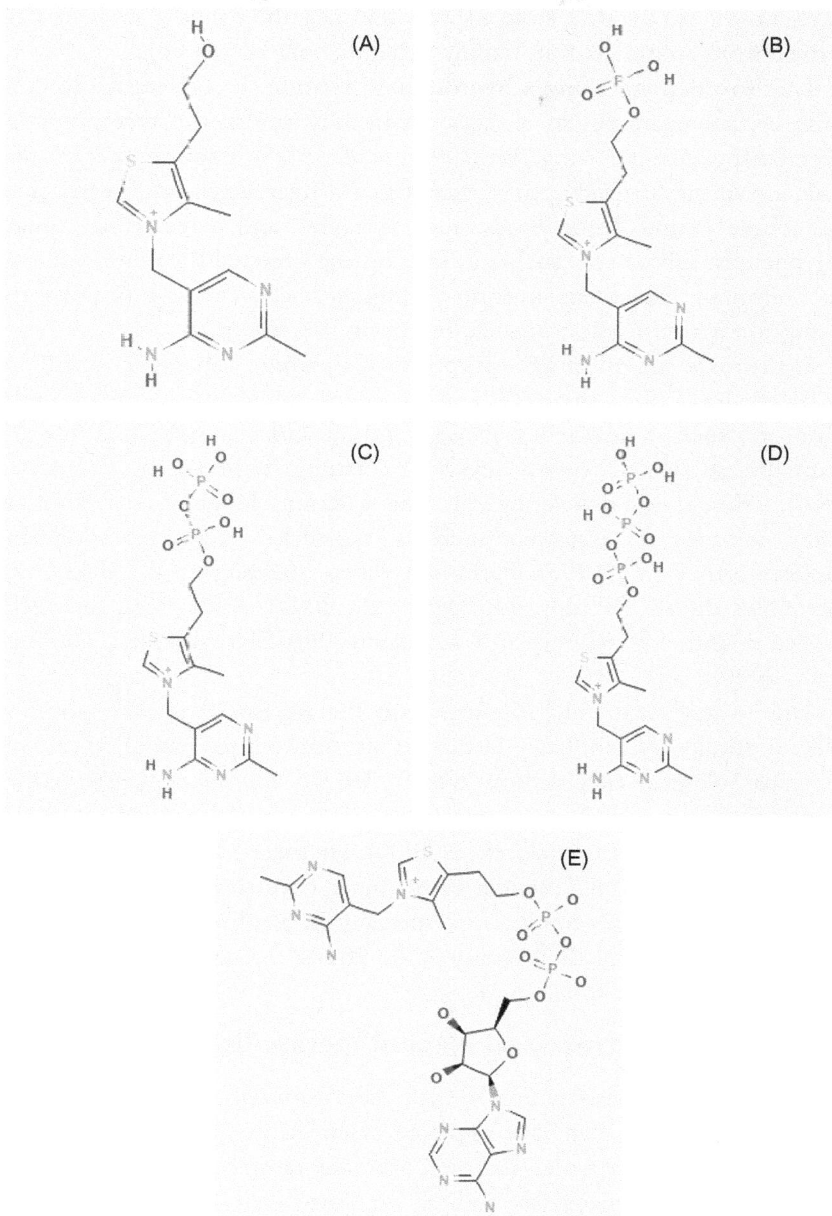

Figure 11.1 Thiamine's chemical structure. (A) Nonphosphorylated thiamine. (B) Thiamine monophosphate (TMP). (C) Thiamine diphosphate (TDP). (D) Thiamine triphosphate (TTP). (E) Adenosine thiamine diphosphate.

mechanisms, TDP is a cofactor in the decarboxylation of ketoacids derived from amino acids in ramified chains (Lonsdale, 2006).

Due to thiamine being a hydrosoluble vitamin, it is necessary to consume certain quantities of it daily. In healthy adults, the recommended dietary allowance is 1.2 mg/day (Otten et al., 2006). Food sources of thiamine are meats (specially pork), wheat germ, liver, eggs, fish, beans, nuts, and whole grains. Some foods, such as coffee and a few teas, contain polyphenols, substances capable of inactivating ingested thiamine. Chronic alcoholism or inadequate nutritional ingestion can also compromise the absorption and utilization of thiamine (Lonsdale, 2006).

Inadequate ingestion or absorption of thiamine can cause deficiency in its levels of both thiamine and its esters, which can cause, acutely, symptoms such as headaches, nausea, and muscular fatigue. The first and main disease related to low levels of thiamine is beri-beri (Carpenter, 2000). However, deficiency of this vitamin is also correlated to other neurological disorders such as Wernicke–Korsakoff syndrome (Butterworth et al., 1993), Parkinson disease (Zhang et al., 2011), and Alzheimer disease (Karuppagounder et al., 2009). Aside from these, the lack of thiamine is possibly also associated with heart disease (Hanninen et al., 2006).

Due to its fundamental role in energy metabolism, it is quite common to find studies which have evaluated its relation to physiological and physiopathological mechanisms which depend on an adequate energy supply and/or metabolism of energetic substrates. (Masuda et al., 2015; Pácal et al., 2014; Pannunzio et al., 2000). However, studies which investigated the antioxidant potential of thiamine have shown positive results, in distinct prooxidant conditions, especially in alcoholism (Portari et al., 2016; Vidhya et al., 2013; Vignisse et al., 2017; Yilmaz et al., 2015).

11.3 Oxidative stress and alcohol metabolism

Several endogen processes involve free radical formation. Free radicals are atoms or molecules that have unpaired electrons in the last atomic layer. However, other molecules that are not free radicals, but are similar in action or can become a free radical, are known as nonradicals. Besides their role in cell signaling and function, both kinds of reactive species can interact with other molecules while aiming to reestablish the electronic balance and change their structure. However, there are molecules and mechanisms that work against the reactive species, known as antioxidants.

In fact antioxidant systems include molecules and enzymes capable of converting the reactive species into stable molecules, mitigating their harmful potential (Halliwell and Gutteridge, 2015).

Aerobic organisms have developed antioxidant systems capable of donating, sharing, or sequestering electrons from unstable molecules and thus preventing a cascade of unwanted oxidation reactions. Thus molecules, enzymes, and nutrients with antioxidant capacity are responsible for the maintenance of redox balance, especially during events of high reactive species production, being able to prevent or reduce the potential damages promoted by such prooxidant species. The enzymes that compose the antioxidant system are superoxide dismutase (SOD), catalase (CAT), glutathione peroxidase (GPx), and glutathione reductase (GR). Nonenzymatic antioxidants are mainly vitamins C and E and the reduced glutathione (GSH) molecules (Pisoschi and Pop, 2015).

An imbalance between oxidative reactions and antioxidant capacity in favor of oxidation, which leads to the destabilization of signaling and control of redox reactions, is defined as oxidative stress (Jones, 2006). Aside from oxidative stress impairing processes of cell signaling, it can also promote damage to macromolecules, especially lipids, proteins, and nucleic acids. Thus oxidative damage can harm the function and signaling of cells, impair other metabolic pathways, promote apoptosis, and trigger diseases (Carocho and Ferreira, 2013).

Studies have shown that oxidative stress is related to several diseases. In the liver oxidative stress plays a role in nonalcoholic liver disease and in triggering a fibrosis framework. A study (Barnham et al., 2004) discussed the reactive species participation in the emergence of several neurodegenerative diseases and there are studies that also related the oxidative stress to diabetic retinopathy (Kowluru, 2001), myopathies (Arbogast et al., 2009), and heart failure (Münzel et al., 2015). Thus the proper functioning of the antioxidant system is essential for the maintenance of the redox homeostasis and, consequently, the adequate health status.

Some conditions or situations aggravate the reactive species production and/or reduce antioxidant capacity, causing an oxidative stress framework. Inflammatory diseases, radiation exposition, smoking, and strenuous exercise are example of situations which cause a redox imbalance (Pisoschi and Pop, 2015). Alcoholic drink is a powerful promoter of oxidative stress, since ethanol metabolism produces a large amount of reactive species. The oxidative stress produced from ethanol metabolism mainly damages the liver and neural tissues, while also affecting several other organs and tissues (Zima et al., 2001).

Not all ingested ethanol is absorbed and reaches the bloodstream, as a small part of alcohol is oxidized in stomach by isoforms of alcohol dehydrogenase (ADH), exhaled by the lungs, or excreted in urine. However, almost 90% of ingested alcohol is absorbed into the gastrointestinal tract and metabolized in liver. Ethanol is completely metabolized in three steps. First, alcohol is converted to acetaldehyde, a toxic molecule. Second, acetaldehyde is oxidized and converted to acetate. Finally, the acetate molecules break down into water and carbon dioxide (Cederbaum, 2012; Zakhari, 2006).

There are three pathways capable of oxidizing ethanol and forming acetaldehyde. ADH is the major enzyme responsible for ethanol oxidation in liver, and it is present mainly in hepatocyte cytosol. Cytochrome P450, a family of heme enzymes, catalyzes the oxidation of ethanol in the microsomal region of endoplasmic reticulum and mitochondria. CAT, an antioxidant enzyme, is capable of oxidizing ethanol, but has little importance in ethanol metabolism in liver. CAT activity is more significant in alcohol oxidation in neural tissue (Cederbaum, 2012; Zakhari, 2006).

The enzyme ADH catalyzes the reversible reaction between ethanol and the oxidized form of nicotinamide adenine dinucleotide (NAD^+). This reaction transfers two hydrogens from ethanol to NAD^+, producing acetaldehyde and the reduced form of nicotinamide adenine dinucleotide, reduced form (NADH) plus a hydrogen ion (H^+) (Cederbaum, 2012).

P450 enzymes are a family of enzymes involved in the oxidation of xenobiotics. In the liver they are mainly in the microsomal fraction of endoplasmic reticulum. While other P450 enzymes also participate in ethanol oxidation, CYP2E1 is the major P450 enzyme that converts ethanol to acetaldehyde. CYP2E1 catalyzes the reaction between acetaldehyde, $NADPH + H^+$ and oxygen, producing $NADP^+$, acetaldehyde, and two molecules of water. CYP2E1 has an important role during chronic ethanol intake. Studies show that chronic ethanol administration increases CYP2E1 as an adaptive response, enhancing ethanol metabolism in the liver (Cederbaum, 2012; Wu and Cederbaum, 2003; Zakhari, 2006).

CAT is an antioxidant enzyme that scavenges hydrogen peroxide (H_2O_2), a reactive species produced in different metabolic steps. In fact CAT causes a reaction between two molecules of H_2O_2 and produces water and oxygen. However, CAT can also react with ethanol and H_2O_2, forming acetaldehyde and water (Cederbaum, 2012). As mentioned, the participation of CAT in alcohol oxidation is lower in the liver than in the brain. Studies have shown that CAT inhibitors reduce ethanol-induced locomotor effects (Sanchis-Segura et al., 2005) and the level of ethanol intake (Aragon and Amit, 1992). Thus if on one hand CAT prevents the oxidative damage caused by H_2O_2, on the other hand it produces the acetaldehyde, a toxic molecule for brain cells. Fortunately, there are mechanisms specialized at blunting acetaldehyde.

Acetaldehyde produced in the first step of ethanol metabolism is converted to acetate by the activity of aldehyde dehydrogenase, which uses the NAD^+ as cofactor, and produces NADH. The acetate produced from acetaldehyde reaches peripheral tissues and it can form acetyl-CoA, which can be a precursor of carbohydrate, lipids, and proteins (Setshedi et al., 2010; Zakhari, 2006). In addition, acetate is an important mediator of ethanol effects, mainly in the central nervous system, such as motor coordination and locomotor activity (Israel et al., 1994).

The toxic potential of acetaldehyde is related to its capacity to interact with other molecules. It can form adducts with proteins and DNA molecules, which can impair cellular function and signaling (Eriksson, 2001). In addition, acetaldehyde production by CYP2E1 can form superoxide anions, hydroxyethyl radicals, and H_2O_2, which can react with metal ions to produce hydroxyl radicals, highly reactive free radicals (Wu and Cederbaum, 2003; Zakhari, 2006). In fact several studies have showed that ethanol intake increases the level of oxidative damage markers and impairs antioxidant systems in different tissues and organs (Müller et al., 2017; Nordmann et al., 1990; Scott et al., 2000).

Ethanol intake increases lipid peroxidation in liver, kidney, lungs, and brain (Nordmann et al., 1990). In addition, Scott et al. (2000) showed that ethanol ingestion reduces SOD activity and GSH concentration in the liver of rats. A study realized with zebra fish showed that repeated exposure to ethanol reduces SOD and CAT activity and nonprotein thiols (represented mainly by GSH) concentration in brain tissue (Müller et al., 2017). In rats chronic ethanol treatment reduced the activity of SOD and GPx and increased oxidative damage to protein and lipids in the cortex and hippocampus (Gong et al., 2017).

Besides accentuating the oxidative stress the ingestion of alcohol is associated with nutritional deficiency. Alcoholics often have low levels of vitamins, due to either the greater degradation, higher excretion, and/or lower intake of these nutrients. The reduced levels of antioxidant vitamins may be related to the increase of the oxidative stress because of the ethanol metabolism (Tanner et al., 1986). However, other vitamins are also present in concentrations lower than the recommended levels in alcoholics. For example, thiamine deficiency has been associated with ethanol intake. In addition, supplementation with thiamine analogs has been shown to be effective against some adverse effects of ethanol intake (Hoyumpa, 1983).

11.4 Thiamine and alcohol metabolism

The major cause of thiamine deficiency in alcoholics is related to eating habits. Erratic eating habits and/or lack of available food contribute to the low intake of thiamine. However, ethanol consumption can influence parameters of absorption, storage, and excretion of thiamine (Hoyumpa, 1983). Alcohol intake affects thiamine absorption directly and indirectly. Ethanol impairs the Na/K-ATPase, which modulates the active thiamine transport. Moreover, ethanol consumption is related to deficiency of other nutrients, which participate in the thiamine absorption process (Hoyumpa, 1983). Studies show that ethanol treatment causes a dose-dependent reduction in thiamine pyrophosphokinase (TPKase) activity in different neural tissues (Rindi et al., 1986). TPKase catalyzes the conversion of thiamine to TDP, the biological active form. Thus ethanol intake impairs also the thiamine metabolism, and may harm several metabolic processes in which TDP plays a role.

TDP is essential to several metabolic process in neural tissue, such as in the synthesis of neurotransmitters, nucleic acids, fatty acids, antioxidants, and steroids. In addition, thiamine plays a role in carbohydrate metabolism and thiamine deficiency causes a disturbance in this pathway (Martin et al., 2003). Evidence suggests that a disturbance in carbohydrate metabolism can lead to damage to mitochondria and increase oxidative stress (Dmitriev and Dugin, 2007). Both events can cause cell damage and cell death (Hazell et al., 2013). Thus thiamine deficiency is strongly related to brain disorders, such as Wernicke–Korsakoff syndrome, Parkinson, and Alzheimer diseases (Abdou and Hazell, 2015). However, thiamine deficiency contributes to other neurodegenerative disorders related to alcohol consumption, including alcohol dementia (Chou et al., 2018).

A study (Pannunzio et al., 2000) that analyzed the effects of thiamine deficiency in vitro exposed cultures of rat cerebellar granule cells to a thiamine-deficient medium and did not find an increase in cell death. However, treatment with a thiamine antagonist (pyrithiamine) reduced the thiamine esters concentration, decreased activities of the thiamine-dependent enzymes, and increased cell death. Interestingly the addition of antioxidant substances (α-tocopherol or butylated hydroxyanisole) to the cultures of cells treated with pyrithiamine showed a neuroprotective effect (Pannunzio et al., 2000). These data indicate that oxidative stress plays an important role in neuronal cell death related to thiamine deficiency.

Since alcohol consumption has been linked to thiamine deficiency, several studies have used thiamine supplementation to treat and prevent health disorders related to ethanol intake. Thiamine supplementation has shown positive effects against neurodegenerative disorders and liver disease related to ethanol metabolism. An experimental study (Woelk et al., 1998) showed that treatment with a thiamine analog improved the symptoms of alcoholic polyneuropathy in humans. A population-based cohort study showed that thiamine therapy could be an efficient strategy to prevent alcoholic dementia (Chou et al., 2018).

The positive effects of thiamine on alcohol-induced health disorders are the consequence of the improvement of several metabolic pathways. As mentioned above, TDP is a cofactor of enzymes involved in macronutrient catabolism. The activity of thiamine-dependent enzymes would be harmed by alcohol intake, since ethanol promotes thiamine deficiency. Thus thiamine supplementation can recover the TDP levels and, consequently, recover or enhance the enzyme's activity. In fact a study (Vidhya et al., 2013) showed that thiamine supplementation increases the transketolase activity in the brain tissue of rats treated with ethanol.

The effects of thiamine supplementation against ethanol-induced damage in the brain may be related to its antioxidant effects (Vignisse et al., 2017). A study (Lukienko et al., 2000) showed the antioxidant effects of thiamine, and proposed that it could react with reactive species, sharing its electrons with them. Benfotiamine showed a direct antioxidant activity against the oxidative damage induced by three different prooxidant agents in a culture of human kidney cells (Schmid et al., 2008). Other studies showed indirect antioxidant effects of thiamine. In a culture of microglial cells, benfotiamine treatment reduced production of reactive species and lipid peroxidation marker and increased gene expression and activity of antioxidant enzymes (Bozic et al., 2015). After exposing rats to ethanol intake for 90 days, a study showed that supplementation with thiamine during a period of abstinence promoted significant increases in the activity of antioxidant enzymes (Vidhya et al., 2013).

The antioxidant effects of thiamine against ethanol-induced oxidative damage in liver is well evidenced. A study (Portari et al., 2016) found lower levels of oxidative damage markers in liver tissue of rats submitted to chronic ethanol intake and supplemented with benfotiamine. In a similar study, supplementation with thiamine pyrophosphate showed to be efficient against liver oxidative damage caused by alcohol intake (Yilmaz et al., 2015).

The improvement of antioxidant enzyme activity may still be related to molecular factors. Increases in TDP levels could inhibit the binding and activity of the p53 protein (McLure et al., 2004), a protein capable of inhibiting the gene expression of enzymes with antioxidant function (Drane et al., 2001). Confirming this, a study (Zhao et al., 2005) showed that the translocation of the p53 gene to mitochondria promoted the inactivation of mitochondrial SOD. Thus the recovery of TDP levels could increase the expression of antioxidant enzymes genes in thiamine-deficient people. In addition, thiamine analog supplementation is effective in enhancing the activity of transketolase, the pentose phosphate pathway regulatory enzyme (Schmid et al., 2008; Vidhya et al., 2013). Increased transketolase activity contributes to increases in NADPH production by pentose phosphate pathway. NADPH is essential for reducing oxidized glutathione in GSH, retaking the antioxidant capacity of the peptide (Lu, 2009). NADPH also preserves the normal functioning of CAT (Kirkman et al., 1987).

The evidence suggests that thiamine supplementation is efficient in mitigating the damage caused by high ethanol intake. Thus there are discussions about the possibility of adding thiamine to alcoholic beverages consumed, but there are technical problems such as vitamin stability, absorption, or beverage taste (Binns et al., 1989). However, there is a consensus that thiamine supplementation must be part of the treatment of alcoholics, mainly during withdrawal periods.

11.5 Alcohol metabolism and other vitamins

Thiamine serves a role as an antioxidant in the organism's defense against harmful oxidative stress toxicity. This role is not unique to thiamine as several other substances also possess a similar protective action, such as ascorbic acid, glutathione, lipoic acid, uric acid, carotenes, α-tocopherol, and ubiquinol. Treatments developed to alleviate the consequential effects of alcohol consumption by use of supplementation with thiamine in conjunction with several other substances have been and are currently undergoing research (Ambadath et al., 2010). The possible synergistic effect of thiamine with other antioxidants stems from the increased antioxidant potential that results from the administration of two or more of these substances. While each individual antioxidant acts in a different manner, the end result is a decrease in and stabilization of reactive oxygen species.

Two of the most referred to nonenzymatic antioxidants are ascorbic acid and α-tocopherol. Vitamin C, ascorbic acid, is a molecule capable of removing oxygen in the cellular environment through the scavenging of reactive oxygen species and also acts by recycling antioxidants such as α-tocopherol leading to a one-electron reduction of lipid hydroperoxyl radicals. The molecule α-tocopherol in itself is found mostly in lipoproteins and the cell membrane, acting as an inhibitor of lipid peroxidation through the capture of peroxyl (Carocho and Ferreira, 2013). Each molecule of α-tocopherol can donate two electrons before it requires recycling. When peroxyl radicals are formed, these react preferably with vitamin E than with fatty acids. The hydroxyl group of α-tocopherol reacts with the radical to form the corresponding lipid hydroperoxide and the tocopheryl radical which oxidizes ascorbic acid and recycles by returning to its reduced state. Thiamine sums to this by inhibiting lipid peroxidation and interacting with free radicals/hydroperoxides alongside these antioxidants which causes it to suffer oxidation becoming thiochrome and thiamine disulfide, limiting the potential for cellular damage. In models of both acute and chronic alcoholism, vitamin C and vitamin E alongside thiamine have been shown to possess a protective role, especially in avoiding membrane-related damage (Reddy et al., 2017). This "antioxidant network" depends upon the supply of antioxidants available in the cellular environment and the organism itself (Traber and Stevens, 2011).

The modern diet in general is capable of providing the necessary quantities of different vitamins, thiamine included. Yet a few situations, such as an excessively high-carb diet (e.g., consumption of polished rice and processed noodles), can lead to a deficiency of thiamine and other vitamins. The deficiency of a single vitamin can lead to a range of consequences, while severe malnutrition can lead to even more advanced disease models and death. Even considering this, the modern physician rarely considers vitamin deficiency as an initial diagnosis. While the use of multivitamins and different supplements can help alleviate the risk, the precarious dietary condition of individuals should be considered as a top candidate in the cause and development of disease (Martin, 2001). In individuals suffering from chronic alcoholism, the lack of a proper diet is critical in the development of the disease leading to a grave deficiency of thiamine and other vitamins. In a healthy individual, the united front of several antioxidants to combat oxidative stress is necessary and even more so in individuals who ingest alcohol on a regular basis as the oxidative stress provoked is greater and requires an even larger quantity of antioxidants capable of counteracting harmful reactive oxygen species. Ergo vitamin deficiency can aggravate an already precarious illness and heighten oxidative stress-related damage.

11.6 Conclusions and perspectives

Thiamine and its many forms have been studied and tested as an antioxidant in several different pathologies including those caused by the use of alcohol.

Although there are several studies focusing on thiamine versus ethanol/alcoholism, there is still a lack of research dedicated to the use of thiamine as an effective antioxidant in the prevention and treatment of diseases associated with alcoholism, which would justify its use in humans.

The exact biochemical and molecular mechanisms should still be targets of investigation as well as clinical trials in humans to ascertain the effectiveness of thiamine against oxidative stress caused by ethanol.

References

Abdou, E., Hazell, A.S., 2015. Thiamine deficiency: an update of pathophysiologic mechanisms and future therapeutic considerations. Neurochem. Res. 40, 353–361.

Ambadath, V., Venu, R.G., Madambath, I., 2010. Comparative study of the efficacy of ascorbic acid, quercetin, and thiamine for reversing ethanol-induced toxicity. J. Med. Food 13, 1485–1489.

Aragon, C., Amit, Z., 1992. The effect of 3-amino-1, 2, 4-triazole on voluntary ethanol consumption: evidence for brain catalase involvement in the mechanism of action. Neuropharmacology 31, 709–712.

Arbogast, S., Beuvin, M., Fraysse, B., Zhou, H., Muntoni, F., Ferreiro, A., 2009. Oxidative stress in SEPN1-related myopathy: from pathophysiology to treatment. Ann. Neurol. Off. J. Am. Neurol. Assoc. Child Neurol. Soc. 65, 677–686.

Barnham, K.J., Masters, C.L., Bush, A.I., 2004. Neurodegenerative diseases and oxidative stress. Nat. Rev. Drug Discov. 3, 205.

Binns, C.W., Carruthers, S.J., Howat, P.A., 1989. Thiamin in beer: a health promotion perspective. Community Health Stud. 13, 301–305.

Bozic, I., Savic, D., Stevanovic, I., Pekovic, S., Nedeljkovic, N., Lavrnja, I., 2015. Benfotiamine upregulates antioxidative system in activated BV-2 microglia cells. Front. Cell Neurosci. 9, 351.

Butterworth, R.F., Kril, J.J., Harper, C.G., 1993. Thiamine-dependent enzyme changes in the brains of alcoholics: relationship to the Wernicke–Korsakoff syndrome. Alcohol. Clin. Exp. Res. 17, 1084–1088.

Carocho, M., Ferreira, I.C., 2013. A review on antioxidants, prooxidants and related controversy: natural and synthetic compounds, screening and analysis methodologies and future perspectives. Food Chem. Toxicol. 51, 15–25.
Carpenter, K.J., 2000. Beriberi, White Rice, and Vitamin B: a Disease, a Cause, and a Cure. University of California Press.
Cederbaum, A.I., 2012. Alcohol metabolism. Clin. Liver Dis. 16, 667–685.
Chou, W.-P., Chang, Yu-Han, Lin, H.-C., Chang, Yi-Hsin, Chen, Y.-Y., Ko, C.-H., 2018. Thiamine for preventing dementia development among patients with alcohol use disorder: a nationwide population-based cohort study. Clin. Nutr. Available from: https://doi.org/10.1016/j.clnu.2018.05.009.
Dmitriev, L., Dugin, S., 2007. Aldehydes and disturbance of carbohydrate metabolism: some consequences and possible approaches to its normalization. Arch. Physiol. Biochem. 113, 87–95.
Drane, P., Bravard, A., Bouvard, V., May, E., 2001. Reciprocal down-regulation of p53 and SOD2 gene expression–implication in p53 mediated apoptosis. Oncogene 20, 430.
Eriksson, C.P., 2001. The role of acetaldehyde in the actions of alcohol (update 2000). Alcohol. Clin. Exp. Res. 25, 15S–32S.
Gong, Y.-S., Hu, K., Yang, L.-Q., Guo, J., Gao, Y., Song, F., et al., 2017. Comparative effects of EtOH consumption and thiamine deficiency on cognitive impairment, oxidative damage, and β-amyloid peptide overproduction in the brain. Free Radic. Biol. Med. 108, 163–173.
Halliwell, B., Gutteridge, J.M., 2015. Free Radicals in Biology and Medicine. Oxford University Press, USA.
Hanninen, S.A., Darling, P.B., Sole, M.J., Barr, A., Keith, M.E., 2006. The prevalence of thiamin deficiency in hospitalized patients with congestive heart failure. J. Am. Coll. Cardiol. 47, 354–361.
Hazell, A.S., Faim, S., Wertheimer, G., Silva, V.R., Marques, C.S., 2013. The impact of oxidative stress in thiamine deficiency: a multifactorial targeting issue. Neurochem. Int. 62, 796–802.
Hoyumpa Jr, A.M., 1983. Alcohol and thiamine metabolism. Alcohol. Clin. Exp. Res. 7, 11–14.
Israel, Y., Orrego, H., Carmichael, F., 1994. Acetate-mediated effects of ethanol. Alcohol. Clin. Exp. Res. 18, 144–148.
Jones, D.P., 2006. Redefining oxidative stress. Antioxid. Redox Signal. 8, 1865–1879.
Karuppagounder, S.S., Xu, H., Shi, Q., Chen, L.H., Pedrini, S., Pechman, D., et al., 2009. Thiamine deficiency induces oxidative stress and exacerbates the plaque pathology in Alzheimer's mouse model. Neurobiol. Aging. 30, 1587–1600.
Kirkman, H.N., Galiano, S., Gaetani, G., 1987. The function of catalase-bound NADPH. J. Biol. Chem. 262, 660–666.
Kowluru, R., 2001. Diabetes-induced elevations in retinal oxidative stress, protein kinase C and nitric oxide are interrelated. Acta Diabetol. 38, 179–185.
Lonsdale, D., 2006. A review of the biochemistry, metabolism and clinical benefits of thiamin (e) and its derivatives. Evid. Based Complement. Alternat. Med. 3, 49–59.
Lu, S.C., 2009. Regulation of glutathione synthesis. Mol. Aspects Med. 30, 42–59.
Lukienko, P., Mel'nichenko, N., Zverinskii, I., Zabrodskaya, S., 2000. Antioxidant properties of thiamine. Bull. Exp. Biol. Med. 130, 874–876.
Manzetti, S., Zhang, J., van der Spoel, D., 2014. Thiamin function, metabolism, uptake, and transport. Biochemistry 53, 821–835.
Martin, P., 2001. Molecular mechanisms of thiamine utilization. Curr. Mol. Med. 1, 197–207.
Martin, P.R., Singleton, C.K., Hiller-Sturmhofel, S., 2003. The role of thiamine deficiency in alcoholic brain disease. Alcohol. Res. Health 27, 134–142.

Masuda, H., Masuda, T., Hatta, H., 2015. Effect of thiamin (vitamin B1) on carbohydrate metabolism at rest and during exercise. J. Phys. Fit. Sports Med. 4, 337−341.
McLure, K.G., Takagi, M., Kastan, M.B., 2004. NAD+ modulates p53 DNA binding specificity and function. Mol. Cell. Biol. 24, 9958−9967.
Müller, T.E., Nunes, S.Z., Silveira, A., Loro, V.L., Rosemberg, D.B., 2017. Repeated ethanol exposure alters social behavior and oxidative stress parameters of zebrafish. Prog. Neuropsychopharmacol. Biol. Psychiatry 79, 105−111.
Münzel, T., Gori, T., Keaney Jr, J.F., Maack, C., Daiber, A., 2015. Pathophysiological role of oxidative stress in systolic and diastolic heart failure and its therapeutic implications. Eur. Heart J. 36, 2555−2564.
Nordmann, R., Ribière, C., Rouach, H., 1990. Ethanol-induced lipid peroxidation and oxidative stress in extrahepatic tissues. Alcohol Alcohol. 25, 231−237.
Otten, J.J., Hellwig, J.P., Meyers, L.D., 2006. Dietary Reference Intakes: the Essential Guide to Nutrient Requirements. National Academies Press.
Pácal, L., Kuricová, K., Kaňková, K., 2014. Evidence for altered thiamine metabolism in diabetes: is there a potential to oppose gluco- and lipotoxicity by rational supplementation? World J. Diabetes 5, 288.
Pannunzio, P., Hazell, A.S., Pannunzio, M., Rao, K.R., Butterworth, R.F., 2000. Thiamine deficiency results in metabolic acidosis and energy failure in cerebellar granule cells: an in vitro model for the study of cell death mechanisms in Wernicke's encephalopathy. J. Neurosci. Res. 62, 286−292.
Pisoschi, A.M., Pop, A., 2015. The role of antioxidants in the chemistry of oxidative stress: a review. Eur. J. Med. Chem. 97, 55−74.
Portari, G.V., Ovidio, P.P., Deminice, R., Jordão Jr, A.A., 2016. Protective effect of treatment with thiamine or benfotiamine on liver oxidative damage in rat model of acute ethanol intoxication. Life Sci. 162, 21−24.
Reddy, V.D., Padmavathi, P., Bulle, S., Hebbani, A.V., Marthadu, S.B., Venugopalacharyulu, N.C., et al., 2017. Association between alcohol-induced oxidative stress and membrane properties in synaptosomes: a protective role of vitamin E. Neurotoxicol. Teratol. 63, 60−65.
Rindi, G., Imarisio, L., Patrini, C., 1986. Effects of acute and chronic ethanol administration on regional thiamin pyrophosphokinase activity of the rat brain. Biochem. Pharmacol. 35, 3903−3908.
Sanchis-Segura, C., Correa, M., Miquel, M., Aragon, C.M., 2005. Catalase inhibition in the Arcuate nucleus blocks ethanol effects on the locomotor activity of rats. Neurosci. Lett. 376, 66−70.
Schmid, U., Stopper, H., Heidland, A., Schupp, N., 2008. Benfotiamine exhibits direct antioxidative capacity and prevents induction of DNA damage in vitro. Diabetes Metab. Res. Rev. 24, 371−377.
Scott, R., Reddy, K., Husain, K., Schlorff, E., Rybak, L., Somani, S., 2000. Dose response of ethanol on antioxidant defense system of liver, lung, and kidney in rat. Pathophysiology 7, 25−32.
Setshedi, M., Wands, J.R., de la Monte, S.M., 2010. Acetaldehyde adducts in alcoholic liver disease. Oxid. Med. Cell. Longev. 3, 178−185.
Tanner, A., Bantock, I., Hinks, L., Lloyd, B., Turner, N., Wright, R., 1986. Depressed selenium and vitamin E levels in an alcoholic population. Dig. Dis. Sci. 31, 1307−1312.
Traber, M.G., Stevens, J.F., 2011. Vitamins C and E: beneficial effects from a mechanistic perspective. Free Radic. Biol. Med. 51, 1000−1013.
Vidhya, A., Renjugopal, V., Indira, M., 2013. Impact of thiamine supplementation in the reversal of ethanol induced toxicity in rats. Indian J. Physiol. Pharmacol. 57, 406−417.

Vignisse, J., Sambon, M., Gorlova, A., Pavlov, D., Caron, N., Malgrange, B., et al., 2017. Thiamine and benfotiamine prevent stress-induced suppression of hippocampal neurogenesis in mice exposed to predation without affecting brain thiamine diphosphate levels. Mol. Cell. Neurosci. 82, 126–136.
Woelk, H., Lehrl, S., Bitsch, R., Köpcke, W., 1998. Benfotiamine in treatment of alcoholic polyneuropathy: an 8-week randomized controlled study (BAP I Study). Alcohol Alcohol. 33, 631–638.
Wu, D., Cederbaum, A.I., 2003. Alcohol, oxidative stress, and free radical damage. Alcohol. Res. Health 27, 277–284.
Yilmaz, I., Demiryilmaz, I., Turan, M., Cetin, N., Gul, M., Suleyman, H., 2015. The effects of thiamine and thiamine pyrophosphate on alcohol-induced hepatic damage biomarkers in rats. Eur. Rev. Med. Pharmacol. Sci. 19, 664–670.
Zakhari, S., 2006. Overview: how is alcohol metabolized by the body? Alcohol Res. 29, 245.
Zhang, Q., Yang, G., Li, W., Fan, Z., Sun, A., Luo, J., et al., 2011. Thiamine deficiency increases β-secretase activity and accumulation of β-amyloid peptides. Neurobiol. Aging 32, 42–53.
Zhao, Y., Chaiswing, L., Velez, J.M., Batinic-Haberle, I., Colburn, N.H., Oberley, T.D., et al., 2005. p53 translocation to mitochondria precedes its nuclear translocation and targets mitochondrial oxidative defense protein-manganese superoxide dismutase. Cancer Res. 65, 3745–3750.
Zima, T., Fialová, L., Mestek, O., Janebová, M., Crkovská, J., Malbohan, I., et al., 2001. Oxidative stress, metabolism of ethanol and alcohol-related diseases. J. Biomed. Sci. 8, 59–70.

CHAPTER 12

Riboflavin (vitamin B2) and mitochondrial energy

Bárbara J. Henriques and Cláudio M. Gomes
Biosystems and Integrative Sciences Institute, Faculdade de Ciências, Universidade de Lisboa, and Departamento de Química e Bioquímica, Faculdade de Ciências, Universidade de Lisboa, Lisboa, Portugal

Contents

Key facts about riboflavin

- Riboflavin belongs to the vitamin B group of water-soluble vitamins.
- Riboflavin is not synthesized in mammalian cells, and is therefore only obtained through diet.
- Major dietary sources of riboflavin include eggs, green vegetables, milk, meat, and cereal products.
- The recommended vitamin B2 dietary intake is about 1.5 mg/day for healthy adults, but several conditions require higher riboflavin doses, such as during pregnancy, practice of demanding physical exercise, chronic alcoholism, or some disease states.
- Riboflavin deficiency due to malnutrition is rare.

Molecular Nutrition
DOI: https://doi.org/10.1016/B978-0-12-811907-5.00011-7

- Riboflavin is the precursor of two extremely versatile cofactors, flavin mononucleotide and flavin adenine dinucleotide.
- Riboflavin supplementation corrects some metabolic defects associated with inherited rare disorders. It has been suggested that the pharmacological effect of this vitamin is due to chemical chaperone effects by flavins, whose elevated cellular levels improve flavoprotein folding, stability, and function.

Key facts about riboflavin-responsive disorders

- Mitochondrial energy production results from a combination of oxidation reactions, such as those occurring in mitochondrial β-oxidation or in oxidative phosphorylation processes. Disease mutations associated with genes that encode proteins involved in these pathways result in defective proteins and in impaired mitochondrial energy production.
- The number of cases of mitochondrial energy deficiencies reported to respond to riboflavin supplementation is limited, although there are two diseases for which this number has recently increased.
- Mitochondrial β-oxidation disorders present a broad range of clinical phenotypes, ranging from lethal to milder forms. In the case of less aggressive forms, some patients have been reported to respond successfully to high doses of riboflavin supplementation.
- Riboflavin-responsive multiple acyl-CoA dehydrogenase deficiency (RR-MADD) relates to a subgroup of patients with a remarkable response to high doses of riboflavin supplementation.
- RR-MADD patients are associated with late-onset multiple acyl-CoA dehydrogenase deficiency, the majority of which present genetic defects in the *ETFDH* gene.
- Acyl-CoA dehydrogenase family member 9 (ACAD9) deficiency was genetically defined in 2010 and is the respiratory chain deficiency with the highest number of cases reported to benefit from vitamin B2 therapeutic intake.
- ACAD9 deficiency patient-derived fibroblasts showed an increase in complex I activity, after riboflavin supplementation, in agreement with the improvement of clinical symptoms.
- Until the present date no major side effects have been reported to be associated with vitamin B2 supplementation; therefore patients diagnosed with a disorder affecting a flavoprotein might be eligible for prompt riboflavin therapy.

- Worldwide newborn screening programs allow early diagnosis of inborn errors of metabolism, and in general prompt riboflavin therapeutic intervention can have a positive effect on disease outcomes.

Summary points

- This chapter focuses on the impact of vitamin B2 (riboflavin) supplementation on mitochondria energy processes.
- Riboflavin is the precursor of flavin cofactors, FAD and FMN, that are essential for the structure and function of several mitochondrial flavoproteins.
- Mitochondrial β-oxidation defects and respiratory chain deficiencies are associated with mitochondrial energy deficiencies; therefore these pathologies will be addressed in this chapter.
- Riboflavin-responsive multiple acyl-CoA dehydrogenase deficiency (RR-MADD) belongs to the group of β-oxidation disorders and presents a remarkable therapeutic response to riboflavin intake.
- Riboflavin supplementation has been recently reported to be effective in ACAD9 deficiency patients.
- Riboflavin supplementation increases cellular FAD content, favoring mitochondrial energy production by promoting the folding, stability, and function of flavoproteins.

Definitions of words and terms

- *Mitochondrial β oxidation*: A biochemical pathway through which activated fatty acids are catabolized, producing an activated fatty acid that is a two-carbon chain shorter, an acetyl-coA, and nicotinamide adenine dinucleotide (NADH) and flavin adenine dinucleotide, reduced form ($FADH_2$) energetic molecules. In mammals, fatty acid β-oxidation provides a major source of adenosine triphosphate (ATP) for the heart and skeletal muscle.
- *Oxidative phosphorylation*: Designates the process in which NADH and $FADH_2$, from a series of electron carriers, reduces molecular oxygen to water, with the formation of ATP. In aerobic organisms this is the major source of ATP.
- *Flavin cofactors*: Two redox active protein cofactors that participate in many biological processes and which can carry out one-electron or two-electron transfer reactions.

- Short-chain acyl-CoA dehydrogenase *deficiency*: A very rare inborn error of fatty acid β-oxidation caused by mutation on the *ACADS* gene. Most patients remain asymptomatic, although in some cases disease manifestations include failure to thrive, hypotonia, seizures, developmental delay, and progressive myopathy.
- Medium-chain acyl-CoA dehydrogenase *deficiency*: An inborn error of fatty acid oxidation (FAO) that affects medium-chain acyl-CoA dehydrogenase. Usually disease onset occurs during infancy or early childhood in previously healthy infants, although there are many affected individuals that remain asymptomatic throughout life. Typically, symptomatic patients present with hypoketotic hypoglycemia, lethargy, vomiting, and seizures.
- Very long-chain acyl-CoA dehydrogenase *deficiency*: An inborn error of long-chain FAO associated with mutations on the *ACADVL* gene. VLADD is clinically very heterogeneous and can be divided into three types: severe infantile with early onset, moderately severe infantile/childhood with a later onset, and a late-onset myopathic (usually after 10 years of age). Clinically manifestations include cardiomyopathy, hypoketotic hypoglycemia, liver disease, exercise intolerance, and rhabdomyolysis.
- *Glutaric aciduria type 1*: Autosomal recessive neurometabolic disorder caused by mutations on the *GCDH* gene involved in L-lysine, L-hydroxylysine, and L-tryptophan catabolism. It is clinically characterized by an encephalopathic crisis resulting in striatal injury and severe movement disorder. Over 200 disease mutations have been reported.
- *Multiple acyl-CoA dehydrogenase deficiency (MADD)*: A disorder of fatty acid and amino acid metabolism, which is clinically very heterogeneous, ranging from a severe neonatal presentation with metabolic acidosis, cardiomyopathy, and liver disease, to a mild childhood/adult disease with episodic metabolic decompensation, muscle weakness, and respiratory failure. MADD is caused by mutations in any of these genes: *ETFA*, *ETFB*, and *ETFDH*.
- *Leigh syndrome*: A severe neurological disorder that usually becomes apparent in the first year of life. Leigh syndrome results from defective mitochondrial energy generation, and the cause can be an alteration of any of the mitochondrial respiratory chain complexes. It is clinically and genetically heterogeneous and can be characterized by progressive loss of mental and movement abilities (psychomotor regression). Typically, it results in death within 2–3 years, usually due to respiratory failure.
- *ACAD9 deficiency*: Rare disorder leading to mitochondrial complex I deficiency, characterized by neurological dysfunction, hepatic failure,

cardiomyopathy, and exercise intolerance. It is caused by mutations in the gene that encodes for ACAD9 protein which has activity as acyl-CoA dehydrogenase and as an assembly factor for complex I.

Abbreviations

AMP	Adenosine monophosphate
ATP	Adenosine triphosphate
FAD	Flavin adenine dinucleotide
$FADH_2$	Flavin adenine dinucleotide, reduced form
FMN	Flavin mononucleotide
NADH	Nicotinamide adenine dinucleotide, reduced form
FAO	Fatty acid oxidation
ACAD	Acyl-CoA dehydrogenase
ETF	Electron transfer flavoprotein
ETF:QO	Electron transfer flavoprotein:ubiquinone oxidoreductase
MADD	Multiple acyl-CoA dehydrogenase deficiency
RR-MADD	Riboflavin responsive-MADD
SCAD	Short-chain acyl-CoA dehydrogenase
MCAD	Medium-chain acyl-CoA dehydrogenase
VLCAD	Very long-chain acyl-CoA dehydrogenase
GCDH	Glutaryl-CoA dehydrogenase

12.1 Riboflavin and mitochondrial energy

Vitamins are biomolecules present in the regular diet which are essential for normal development, growth, reproduction, lactation, physical performance, and general well-being. They participate in many cellular processes, such as biosynthesis of coenzyme Q, mitochondrial respiration and energy production, or antioxidant reactions (Kucharská, 2008). In general, mammalian cells do not synthesize these biomolecules, therefore they depend on dietary intake. This chapter is dedicated to vitamin B2, also known as riboflavin, and to the relation of this water-soluble vitamin with mitochondrial energy-producing enzymes. More specifically, we delve into the importance of riboflavin availability for the onset, development, and progression of mitochondrial energy deficiency pathologies.

Mitochondrial energy production results from a series of oxidation reactions within this organelle, ultimately producing adenosine triphosphate (ATP) molecules which power the processes for cell survival (Bratic and Trifunovic, 2010). Riboflavin is the biological precursor of flavin cofactors which are present in several enzymes involved in many of these reactions, such as the electron transport chain (ETC) or β-oxidation pathways. The two flavin cofactors, flavin mononucleotide (FMN) and flavin adenine dinucleotide (FAD), have high functional diversity, part of which is due to their broad range of physiologically attainable redox potentials (from −210 to +600 mV). Also, flavins have the ability to switch between one or two-electron redox chemistry processes, and can therefore act as catalytic cofactors in multiple enzymes that participate in a wide array of essential biochemical oxidation–reduction reactions (Merrill et al., 1981). Indeed, it is estimated that 1%–3% of the genes in bacteria and eukaryotic genomes encode for flavoproteins (De Colibus and Mattevi, 2006). Fig. 12.1 is a schematic representation of mitochondrial

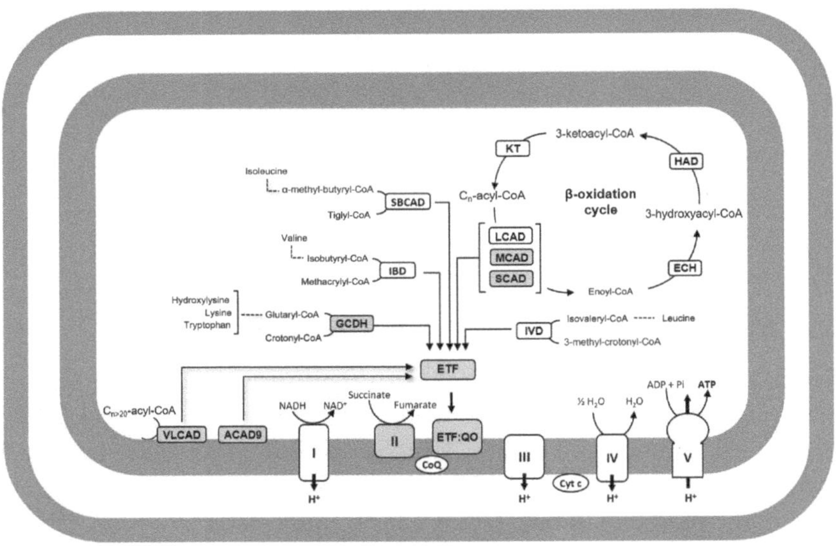

Figure 12.1 ***Schematic representation of pathways involved in mitochondrial energy production.*** Schematic representation of mitochondrial β-oxidation and *ETC*, highlighting the flavoenzymes associated with energy deficiency pathologies that respond to riboflavin supplementation. This simplified scheme of a mitochondrion (crista in the inner membrane are omitted for clarity) depicts reactions and enzymes that are overviewed in this chapter. *LCAD*, Long-chain acyl-CoA dehydrogenase; *MCAD*, medium-chain acyl-CoA dehydrogenase; *SCAD*, short-chain acyl-CoA dehydrogenase; *ECH*, enoyl-CoA hydratase; HAD, 3-L-hydroxyacyl-CoA dehydrogenase; *KT*, β-ketoacyl-CoA thiolase; *IVD*, isovaleryl-CoA dehydrogenase; *SBCAD*, short-branched chain acyl-CoA dehydrogenase; *IBD*, isobutyryl-CoA dehydrogenase; *GCDH*, glutaryl-CoA dehydrogenase; *ETF*, electron transfer flavoprotein; ETF:QO, electron transfer flavoprotein:ubiquinone oxidoreductase; *VLCAD*, very long-chain acyl-CoA dehydrogenase; *ACAD9*, acyl-CoA dehydrogenase family member 9; respiratory chain complexes I–V; *CoQ*, coenzyme Q; *Cyt c*, cytochrome c.

pathways related to energy production highlighting the involved flavoenzymes, thus showing the central importance of vitamin B2 for mitochondrial energy metabolism.

Riboflavin intake is achieved through a regular diet that should include eggs, milk, meat products, yeast, and vegetables, which are the main sources of this vitamin. Under normal conditions, the recommended daily allowance for riboflavin ranges from 0.5 to 0.9 mg/day for children (1−13 years), 1.3 mg/day for male adults, and 1−1.6 mg/day for female adults, depending on several factors such as age (14−18 years, lower value), pregnancy (1.4 mg/day), or during lactation (upper value) (Food and Nutrition Board Washington, D.C, 1998). Vitamin B2 can be found in food in the free form, or already as FAD and FMN in flavoproteins. Briefly, riboflavin is released from its carriers through the action of stomach acid and gastric/intestinal proteases, and is transported into enterocytes through an energy-dependent and sodium-independent riboflavin carrier being then phosphorylated to FMN by a flavokinase and subsequently converted to FAD by a FAD synthetase, with ATP consumption (Barile et al., 2013). In the case of FMN and FAD forms in flavoproteins, they must first be sequentially hydrolyzed to riboflavin in the gastrointestinal tract in order to be absorbed (Depeint et al., 2006). The human body has a very low storage capacity for riboflavin, whose excess is eliminated in urine. In fact, the median plasma concentrations of riboflavin, FMN, and FAD are 10.5, 6.6, and 74 nmol/L, respectively (Hustad et al., 2002).

12.2 Riboflavin deficiency

Adults with a regular diet rarely present symptoms of riboflavin deficiency, although in malnutrition (more frequently in adolescence), pregnancy, chronic alcoholism, or disease states (such as diabetes mellitus or inflammatory bowel disease), vitamin B2 can decrease to suboptimal levels (Grosch, 1999; Powers, 2003). Vitamin supplementation is widely accepted, and this also applies to riboflavin, which has been long used as an approved drug. Vitamin B2 therapeutic doses are dependent on the type of condition, but until now, as no major side effects have been reported, the prescription of this vitamin is straightforward. Although the molecular mechanisms accounting for the benefits associated with vitamin B2 supplementation are not fully clarified, one can anticipate that it will result in an increase in cofactor availability in cells that will favorably impact on flavin-dependent protein levels. Riboflavin therapy is more relevant in cases associated with defects in mitochondrial flavoenzymes (see list in Table 12.1), that depend on flavin cofactors to be functional and/or to improve protein folding and stability (Henriques et al., 2009; Lucas et al., 2011; Saijo and Tanaka, 1995). These diseases are associated

Table 12.1 Flavoenzymes involved in mitochondrial energy production.

Protein	OMIM	Gene	Disorder	Therapeutic riboflavin dosage
Short-chain acyl-CoA dehydrogenase (SCAD)	606885	*ACADS*	SCAD deficiency	10–150 mg/kg/day
Medium-chain acyl-CoA dehydrogenase (MCAD)	607008	*ACADM*	MCAD deficiency	50–150 mg/day
Very long-chain Acyl-CoA dehydrogenase (VLCAD)	609575	*ACADVL*	VLCAD deficiency	50 mg/day
Glutaryl-CoA dehydrogenase (GCDH)	608801	*GCDH*	Glutaric aciduria type 1 (GA-1)	100–150 mg/day
Electron transfer flavoprotein (ETFα and ETFβ subunits)	608053 130410	*ETFA* *ETFB*	Multiple acyl-CoA dehydrogenase deficiency (MADD)	100–400 mg/day
Electron transfer flavoprotein: ubiquinone oxidoreductase (ETF:QO)	231675	*ETFDH*		
Acyl-CoA dehydrogenase family member 9 (ACAD9)	611103	*ACAD9*	Mitochondrial complex I deficiency	150 mg/day
Succinate dehydrogenase, subunit A of complex II, (SDHA)	600857	*SDHA*	Leigh syndrome	40–200 mg/day

Defects in these enzymes are associated with rare metabolic disorders that are potentially responsive to riboflavin supplementation therapy.

with genetic defects in mitochondrial proteins that are somehow involved in mitochondrial energy production (Table 12.1) and will be discussed throughout the following sections. Also important are the reported cases of rare disorders of riboflavin metabolism, such as the Brown–Vialetto–Van Laere syndrome, Fazio–Londe syndrome, or transient multiple acyl-CoA dehydrogenase deficiency (MADD) phenotype. In such cases there is insufficient absorption of the vitamin due to alterations of riboflavin transporters and enzymes of riboflavin metabolism (further details can be found in Henriques et al., 2016).

12.3 Mitochondrial β-oxidation disorders responsive to vitamin B2

The fatty acid β-oxidation pathway is one of the main contributors to energy production in the mitochondria, and each fatty acid degradation cycle results in the formation of flavin adenine dinucleotide, reduced form ($FADH_2$), nicotinamide adenine dinucleotide (NADH), and acetyl-CoA molecules. This pathway is highly dependent on flavoproteins that act on the first steps of fatty acid catabolism. The first oxidation reaction is catalyzed by a group of flavoenzymes named acyl-CoA dehydrogenases (ACADs), with the reducing power from these reactions then funneled into the respiratory chain (RC) via quinone reduction through the hub composed of electron transfer flavoprotein (ETF) and electron transfer flavoprotein:ubiquinone oxidoreductase (ETF:QO) (Alves et al., 2012; Henriques et al., 2011). The ACAD family comprises not only the dehydrogenases for fatty acid β-oxidation [such as the very long-chain acyl-CoA dehydrogenase (VLCAD), long-chain acyl-CoA dehydrogenase (LCAD), medium-chain acyl-CoA dehydrogenase (MCAD), and short-chain acyl-CoA dehydrogenase (SCAD) according to their substrate chain-length specificity], but also dehydrogenases involved in amino acid metabolism [glutaryl-CoA dehydrogenase (GCDH), isovaleryl-CoA dehydrogenase, short-branched chain acyl-CoA dehydrogenase, and isobutyryl-CoA dehydrogenase)] (see Fig. 12.1) (Henriques et al., 2010a). Vitamin B2 intake is extremely important in order to maintain a balanced content of the cofactor in the cell, as all these enzymes depend on flavin to carry out their biological functions and, in many cases, to improve protein folding and stability (Henriques et al., 2009; Lucas et al., 2011; Nagao and Tanaka, 1992; Saijo and Tanaka, 1995).

Genetic defects of these enzymes result in inherited autosomal recessive metabolic disorders, usually referred as fatty acid oxidation (FAO) defects. Severe cases result in neonatal death, but in mild cases, disease symptoms can be triggered by adverse physiological conditions, such as prolonged fasting, exercise, infections, or by a fat-rich diet, and/or decreased dietary intake of riboflavin (Chiong et al., 2007; Harpey et al., 1983). Maintaining or restoring normal flavin levels should in principle improve impaired enzymatic function. Indeed, these beneficial effects associated with riboflavin supplementation have been widely studied (Gianazza et al., 2006; Hoppel et al., 1979; Ross and Hansen, 1992) and we will next present a brief overview of β-oxidation disorders that have been reported to respond to vitamin B2 supplementation.

12.3.1 Riboflavin-responsive multiple acyl-CoA dehydrogenase deficiency

Riboflavin-responsive multiple acyl-CoA dehydrogenase deficiency (RR-MADD) is the β-oxidation disorder for which riboflavin treatment is better established, and a great number of successful cases have been reported. MADD, also termed glutaric aciduria type 2 (GA-2), results from genetic defects in one of three genes: *ETFA* and *ETFB*, which encode the two subunits of ETF, and *ETFDH*, which encodes for ETF:QO (Henriques et al., 2010b). Mutations on any of these genes will affect fatty acid and amino acid metabolism as the two flavoproteins are responsible for receiving electrons from at least 12 mitochondrial dehydrogenases, and for shuttling them to the RC via ubiquinone. The MADD clinical picture is very heterogeneous, ranging from severe forms with neonatal death to late-onset forms with clinical symptoms associated with cellular energy deficiency, such as episodic metabolic decompensation, muscle weakness, and respiratory failure. Generally, patients presenting mild phenotypes are advised to avoid long periods of fasting, and are treated with high doses of riboflavin (Angelini et al., 2006). A special group of MADD patients, known as RR-MADD, show a spectacular response to vitamin B2 supplementation. The first reported case was in the early 1980s, in which a 3-year-old boy with episodic vomiting, lethargy, and hypoglycemia, significantly reduced the excreted amounts of pathologic metabolites and improved disease symptoms after riboflavin therapy at 300 mg/day (Gregersen et al., 1982). Since then, other successful cases have been reported worldwide, with prescribed riboflavin therapies ranging from 100–400 mg/day administered

2–3 times a day (Fan et al., 2018; Goh et al., 2018; Lammer et al., 2011; Lan et al., 2010; Law et al., 2009; Liang et al., 2009; Missaglia et al., 2018; Vergani et al., 1999; Wang et al., 2011; Wen et al., 2010). A recent review reported that 98% of RR-MADD cases are attributed to late-onset MADD, and that the majority of cases are due to mutations in *ETFDH* (93%) rather than mutations in *ETFA* and *ETFB* (Grunert, 2014). This was already proposed by Olsen et al. (2007) back in 2007 in a study on 11 individuals with RR-MADD, where all reported cases had mutations in the *ETFDH* gene. Moreover, seven patients with myopathic forms of coenzyme Q10 deficiency who responded to riboflavin therapy were also shown to have a mutation in *ETFDH* (Gempel et al., 2007).

As several RR-MADD patients present low mitochondrial levels of flavins, it has been suggested that disease states could rather be attributed to disturbances in flavin homeostasis. Recent reports on patients with MADD biochemical profiles show that these can also be due to defects in riboflavin transport and FAD metabolism (Bosch et al., 2011; Missaglia et al., 2018; Olsen et al., 2016). These findings can help to understand the molecular mechanism behind riboflavin responsiveness in MADD cases, as decreased flavin content impairs flavin-dependent FAO enzymes. Moreover, a compilation of a large number of patients with *ETFDH* mutations that respond to vitamin B2 supplementation and their corresponding structural analysis allowed us to note that these mutations do not affect cofactor binding directly, but that they may rather cause destabilization of local interactions leading to long-distance conformational changes that indirectly affect FAD binding (Rodrigues et al., 2012).

12.3.2 Glutaric aciduria type 1

Glutaric aciduria type 1 (GA-1), a rare autosomal recessive inherited neurometabolic disorder, was one of the first cases of β-oxidation disorders to be demonstrated to benefit from riboflavin supplementation. Brandt et al. reported three cases of GA-1 patients that, after riboflavin therapy, showed a reduction in urinary glutaric acid levels, a hallmark metabolite in GA-1 (Brandt et al., 1979). In 1984 another case was reported, in which neurological deterioration was prevented after treatment with riboflavin and a γ-aminobutyric acid (GABA) analog (Dunger and Snodgrass, 1984). Since then other isolated cases have been reported, such as that by Lipkin et al. (1988) of a patient that after vitamin B2 treatment showed reduced levels of GABA in the cerebrospinal fluid. Another case reports an heterozygous

GA-1 patient with the GCDH p.Ser139Leu and p.Pro248Leu variants with only 20% of GCDH activity as measured in fibroblasts (Chalmers et al., 2006). Riboflavin treatment resulted in an increase in enzymatic activity. The authors suggested that this effect could be related to the fact that since Ser-139 is located within the FAD binding pocket, an increase in FAD levels would stabilize the GCDH functional homotetramer through ligand-stabilizing effects (as reviewed in Gomes, 2012). In another case, a child with GA-1 under restricted protein diet and carnitine and prescribed riboflavin supplementation, regained head control and sitting ability with support following vitamin B2 treatment (Pusti et al., 2014). Another recent case is that of a 13-month-old boy with microcephaly, developmental delay, and progressive spasticity, who after a first wrong diagnostic was confirmed to suffer from GA-1 (Sharawat and Dawman, 2018). The child initiated a treatment with trihexyphenidyl, L-carnitine, and high-dose riboflavin (100 mg/day), and the subsequent clinical improvement led the authors to suggest that a prompt initiation of riboflavin therapy can limit the neurologic insult in children with GA-1. We recently undertook an in vitro assessment of the effect of riboflavin and FAD on the stability and activity of β-oxidation dehydrogenases, including GCDH (Lucas et al., 2011). In this report we demonstrated a positive shift in GCDH stability in the presence of increasing FAD levels, as denoted by an increase in the thermal denaturation temperature of the protein. This stabilizing effect was specific for FAD, as no effect was observed upon incubation with riboflavin, which indicates that the stabilizing biomolecule is the flavin and not its precursor. This in vitro study supports the view that upon vitamin B2 supplementation, increased FAD levels in the mitochondria will have pharmacological chaperone effects on β-oxidation flavoproteins. However, in spite of this molecular rational for the beneficial effects of riboflavin supplementation and the increasing number of reported clinical cases, the fact is that there is still no clear recommendation or standard protocol for therapeutic use and dosage to manage GA-1 (Boy et al., 2017).

12.3.3 Fatty acid acyl-CoA dehydrogenase disorders

Riboflavin responsiveness in disorders of single fatty acid acyl-CoA dehydrogenases is still a debatable issue, and although the therapeutic effect of this vitamin has gained interest in recent years, there are still few reported studies for these disorders. To the best of our knowledge, for VLCADD there is only one study reporting improvement of disease symptoms upon riboflavin treatment (Scalais et al., 2015). The authors describe a child patient from a family with a story of repeated neonatal deaths associated with VLCADD, who started riboflavin therapy (50 mg/day) and dietary restrictions very early in life, which improved the management of metabolic crisis (Scalais et al., 2015). In the case of MCAD deficiency, a report of five patients who received riboflavin treatment at 50–150 mg/day showed increased enzymatic activity as determined from catalytic assays in lymphocytes (Duran et al., 1992). SCAD deficiency (SCADD) is a more special case as it is nowadays viewed rather as a biochemical phenotype than as a disease, considering that most infants detected by expanded newborn screening studies are asymptomatic and therefore have no therapeutic recommendation (Wolfe et al., 2011). However, in a recent review Nochi et al. (2017) suggested that SCADD seems to be an oxidative stress disorder rather than an energy deficiency disease, like the other ACADs deficiencies. Nevertheless, a recent study analyzing 10 individuals with SCADD compatible phenotypes, identified through newborn screening by their altered metabolite levels, started immediate riboflavin therapy and remained asymptomatic (Tonin et al., 2016). Notoriously, three of these patients exhibited hypotonia which improved and completely reverted following riboflavin treatment. Similar beneficial effects of riboflavin had also been previously reported by van Maldegem et al., (2010) in a cohort of 16 patients with SCAD deficiency. In this study, FAD blood levels were significantly lower both in homozygous or heterozygous patients with the SCAD p.Gly209Ser variant, when compared with patients with two rare *ACADS* mutations. In these cases a riboflavin supplementation at 150 mg/day, divided into three doses, resulted in clinical notorious improvements (van Maldegem et al., 2010). As already mentioned, in vitro studies helped to clarify the biochemical basis for the therapeutic effects of vitamin B2 in FAO disorders. Studies on MCAD have shown that, under FAD depletion conditions, enzyme tetramerization was hampered and that the resulting misfolded MCAD becomes chaperonin associated (Saijo and Tanaka, 1995). FAD has also been shown to improve thermal stability of MCAD, SCAD-wild type, and SCAD p.Gly209Ser variants (Lucas et al., 2011).

12.4 Respiratory chain deficiencies

Oxidative phosphorylation involves four respiratory complexes (complex I: NADH dehydrogenase-ubiquinone oxidase; complex II: succinate dehydrogenase-ubiquinone oxidoreductase; complex III: ubiquinone cytochrome c oxidoreductase; and complex IV: cytochrome c oxidase) and ATPase (complex V: ATP synthase) that function in synergy to produce ATP. Briefly, complexes I–IV receive electrons from the catabolism of carbohydrates, fats, and proteins and generate a proton gradient across the inner mitochondrial membrane, which is used by complex V for ATP production from ADP and inorganic phosphate. In aerobic organisms this biochemical process is the major source of ATP production. In altered conditions ATP production can be impaired and energy will not be enough for proper cell function, and these situations can lead to mitochondrial disease often involving abnormalities of the central nervous system, muscle, heart, eyes, and renal and hematological systems (Scaglia et al., 2004). RC deficiencies are hallmarks of mitochondrial disease and can be caused by mutation on mitochondrial DNA or in nuclear genes that encode for mitochondrial proteins. The most prevalent RC deficiency is complex I deficiency, which includes NADH:ubiquinone oxidoreductase defects, mutations on complex I assembly genes, and mutations in other nuclear-encoded genes (Skladal et al., 2003). In recent decades, sporadic cases of patients diagnosed with myopathies associated with complex I deficiencies have been reported to benefit from riboflavin supplementation (Bernsen et al., 1993; Garone et al., 2013; Gerards et al., 2011; Scholte et al., 1995). In this genetically heterogeneous disorder, a special attention to the cases associated with *ACAD9* gene mutations should be taken. This gene encodes for acyl-CoA dehydrogenase family member 9 (ACAD9), an enzyme that has been described as an assembly factor for complex I, and which also presents acyl-CoA dehydrogenase activity. ACAD9 is a flavoprotein homologous to VLCAD, and therefore it has been suggested that riboflavin supplementation could have an effect similar to the one observed in VLCADD patients. Recently, a report on a cohort of 70 patients with ACAD9 deficiency showed that riboflavin treatment improves complex I activity in the majority of patient-derived fibroblasts under study (Repp et al., 2018). Most patients showed a clinical beneficial effect and, in particular, patients presenting symptoms during the first year of life had improved survival (Repp et al., 2018). Based on this large cohort it is possible to suggest that riboflavin-responsive complex I deficiency cases are associated with ACAD9 deficiency. Moreover, the molecular mechanism underlying this beneficial effect could be due to an increase in FAD cellular concentration that increases the folding, stability, and activity of ACAD9 (Garone et al., 2013).

Deficiencies in complex II, succinate:ubiquinone oxidoreductase, have also been reported to improve upon vitamin B2 dietary supplementation. One case was reported for a patient with Leigh syndrome and a missense mutation on the *SDHA* gene, for whom riboflavin supplementation resulted in the regression of neurological impairment (Pinard et al., 1999). In a study by Bugiani et al. (2006), patients with complex II deficiency taking riboflavin presented a twofold increase in succinate dehydrogenase activity, as measured in patient-derived fibroblasts, that was in agreement with better symptomatology. Recently two patients presenting mitochondrial myopathy were reported to have riboflavin-responsive complex II deficiency (Nimmo et al., 2018). A detailed genetic study was performed leading to the identification of two missense mutations on a riboflavin transporter as the cause of the disease phenotype. Mutations on riboflavin transporters had already been reported to be associated with complex I and complex IV deficiencies (Foley et al., 2014), as well as complex II deficiency (Schiff et al., 2016) or MADD (Olsen et al., 2016; Wang et al., 2016), for which riboflavin supplementation resulted in clinical improvements. In these cases, the beneficial effect results essentially from an increase in vitamin absorption due to higher intake, and a consequent increase in the availability of flavin in the cell. Overall these reports suggest that patients presenting with mitochondrial encephalomyopathy should have differential diagnosis comprising riboflavin transporter deficiencies, and that riboflavin treatment should be promptly considered.

12.5 Concluding remarks

Vitamin B2, also known as riboflavin, is the precursor of flavin cofactors which are essential for flavoenzymes involved in mitochondrial energy production. Lower levels of riboflavin, due to insufficient intake or deficiencies of riboflavin metabolism, affect flavin concentration in the cell and the quality of flavoenzymes. Mitochondrial energy is deeply affected by the impairment of flavoenzymes, including the several flavoenzymes involved in mitochondrial β-oxidation processes and in membrane-bound RC complexes. Therapeutic intake of vitamin B2 has been reported to improve several mitochondrial pathologies, essentially due to the increase in cellular concentration of the cofactor. At the molecular level FAD will have a pharmacological chaperone effect over the structure and function of such faulty enzymes. Two disorders deserved a special attention, RR-MADD and ACAD9 deficiency, for which the number of well-established riboflavin-responsive cases is substantial. The majority of RR-MADD patients have mutations on the *ETFDH* gene, and these do not necessarily result in amino acid changes that directly affect the protein–flavin association; therefore we hypothesize that the beneficial effects of riboflavin supplementation result from effects on folding efficiency and/or native conformation stability of ETF:QO protein. In the case of ACAD9 deficiency, flavinylation probably has a similar effect to that observed for FAO patients. Finally, advances in the identification and characterization of different human riboflavin transporters have also improved the diagnosis of mitochondrial diseases and helped to elucidate riboflavin therapeutic effects for some mitochondrial disorders.

Acknowledgements

This work was supported by the Fundação para a Ciência e Tecnologia (FCT/MCTES, Portugal) through fellowships to B.J.H. (SFRH/BPD/74475/2010), and grants PTDC/BBB-BQB/5366/2014 and PTDC/BIA-BQM/29963/2017 (to B.J.H.) and PTDC/NEU-NMC/2138/2014 (to C.M.G.). The Gomes laboratory is partly supported by UID/MULTI/04046/2019 Research Unit grant from FCT, Portugal (to BioISI).

References

Alves, E., Henriques, B.J., Rodrigues, J.V., Prudencio, P., Rocha, H., Vilarinho, L., et al., 2012. Mutations at the flavin binding site of ETF:QO yield a MADD-like severe phenotype in drosophila. Biochim. Biophys. Acta 1822, 1284–1292.

Angelini, C., Federico, A., Reichmann, H., Lombes, A., Chinnery, P., Turnbull, D., 2006. Task force guidelines handbook: EFNS guidelines on diagnosis and management of fatty acid mitochondrial disorders. Eur. J. Neurol. 13, 923–929.

Barile, M., Giancaspero, T.A., Brizio, C., Panebianco, C., Indiveri, C., Galluccio, M., et al., 2013. Biosynthesis of flavin cofactors in man: implications in health and disease. Curr. Pharm. Des. 19, 2649–2675.

Bernsen, P.L., Gabreels, F.J., Ruitenbeek, W., Hamburger, H.L., 1993. Treatment of complex I deficiency with riboflavin. J. Neurol. Sci. 118, 181–187.

Bosch, A.M., Abeling, N.G., Ijlst, L., Knoester, H., van der Pol, W.L., Stroomer, A.E., et al., 2011. Brown–Vialetto–Van Laere and Fazio Londe syndrome is associated with a riboflavin transporter defect mimicking mild MADD: a new inborn error of metabolism with potential treatment. J. Inherit. Metab. Dis. 34, 159–164.

Boy, N., Muhlhausen, C., Maier, E.M., Heringer, J., Assmann, B., Burgard, P., et al., 2017. Proposed recommendations for diagnosing and managing individuals with glutaric aciduria type I: second revision. J. Inherit. Metab. Dis. 40, 75–101.

Brandt, N.J., Gregersen, N., Christensen, E., Gron, I.H., Rasmussen, K., 1979. Treatment of glutaryl-CoA dehydrogenase deficiency (glutaric aciduria). Experience with diet, riboflavin, and GABA analogue. J Pediatr. 94, 669–673.

Bratic, I., Trifunovic, A., 2010. Mitochondrial energy metabolism and ageing. Biochim. Biophys. Acta 1797, 961–967.

Bugiani, M., Lamantea, E., Invernizzi, F., Moroni, I., Bizzi, A., Zeviani, M., et al., 2006. Effects of riboflavin in children with complex II deficiency. Brain Dev. 28, 576–581.
Chalmers, R.A., Bain, M.D., Zschocke, J., 2006. Riboflavin-responsive glutaryl CoA dehydrogenase deficiency. Mol. Genet. Metab. 88, 29–37.
Chiong, M.A., Sim, K.G., Carpenter, K., Rhead, W., Ho, G., Olsen, R.K., et al., 2007. Transient multiple acyl-CoA dehydrogenation deficiency in a newborn female caused by maternal riboflavin deficiency. Mol. Genet. Metab. 92, 109–114.
De Colibus, L., Mattevi, A., 2006. New frontiers in structural flavoenzymology. Curr. Opin. Struct. Biol. 16, 722–728.
Depeint, F., Bruce, W.R., Shangari, N., Mehta, R., O'Brien, P.J., 2006. Mitochondrial function and toxicity: role of the B vitamin family on mitochondrial energy metabolism. Chem. Biol. Interact. 163, 94–112.
Dunger, D.B., Snodgrass, G.J., 1984. Glutaric aciduria type I presenting with hypoglycaemia. J. Inherit. Metab. Dis. 7, 122–124.
Duran, M., Cleutjens, C.B., Ketting, D., Dorland, L., de Klerk, J.B., van Sprang, F.J., et al., 1992. Diagnosis of medium-chain acyl-CoA dehydrogenase deficiency in lymphocytes and liver by a gas chromatographic method: the effect of oral riboflavin supplementation. Pediatr. Res. 31, 39–42.
Fan, X., Xie, B., Zou, J., Luo, J., Qin, Z., D'Gama, A.M., et al., 2018. Novel ETFDH mutations in four cases of riboflavin responsive multiple acyl-CoA dehydrogenase deficiency. Mol. Genet. Metab. Rep. 16, 15–19.
Foley, A.R., Menezes, M.P., Pandraud, A., Gonzalez, M.A., Al-Odaib, A., Abrams, A.J., et al., 2014. Treatable childhood neuronopathy caused by mutations in riboflavin transporter RFVT2. Brain 137, 44–56.
Food and Nutrition Board Washington, D.C, 1998. Dietary Reference Intakes for Thiamin, Riboflavin, Niacin, Vitamin B6, Folate, Vitamin B12, Pantothenic Acid, Biotin, and Choline. Institute of Medicine (US), National Academies Press (US).
Garone, C., Donati, M.A., Sacchini, M., Garcia-Diaz, B., Bruno, C., Calvo, S., et al., 2013. Mitochondrial encephalomyopathy due to a novel mutation in ACAD9. JAMA Neurol. 70, 1177–1179.
Gempel, K., Topaloglu, H., Talim, B., Schneiderat, P., Schoser, B.G., Hans, V.H., et al., 2007. The myopathic form of coenzyme Q10 deficiency is caused by mutations in the electron-transferring-flavoprotein dehydrogenase (ETFDH) gene. Brain 130, 2037–2044.
Gerards, M., van den Bosch, B.J., Danhauser, K., Serre, V., van Weeghel, M., Wanders, R.J., et al., 2011. Riboflavin-responsive oxidative phosphorylation complex I deficiency caused by defective ACAD9: new function for an old gene. Brain 134, 210–219.
Gianazza, E., Vergani, L., Wait, R., Brizio, C., Brambilla, D., Begum, S., et al., 2006. Coordinated and reversible reduction of enzymes involved in terminal oxidative metabolism in skeletal muscle mitochondria from a riboflavin-responsive, multiple acyl-CoA dehydrogenase deficiency patient. Electrophoresis 27, 1182–1198.
Goh, L.L., Lee, Y., Tan, E.S., Lim, J.S.C., Lim, C.W., Dalan, R., 2018. Patient with multiple acyl-CoA dehydrogenase deficiency disease and ETFDH mutations benefits from riboflavin therapy: a case report. BMC. Med. Genomics. 11, 37.
Gomes, C.M., 2012. Protein misfolding in disease and small molecule therapies. Curr. Top. Med. Chem. 12, 2460–2469.
Gregersen, N., Wintzensen, H., Christensen, S.K., Christensen, M.F., Brandt, N.J., Rasmussen, K., 1982. C6-C10-dicarboxylic aciduria: investigations of a patient with riboflavin responsive multiple acyl-CoA dehydrogenation defects. Pediatr. Res. 16, 861–868.
Grosch, B.A., 1999. Food Chemistry, second ed. Springer.

Grunert, S.C., 2014. Clinical and genetical heterogeneity of late-onset multiple acyl-coenzyme A dehydrogenase deficiency. Orphanet. J. Rare Dis. 9, 117.

Harpey, J.P., Charpentier, C., Goodman, S.I., Darbois, Y., Lefebvre, G., Sebbah, J., 1983. Multiple acyl-CoA dehydrogenase deficiency occurring in pregnancy and caused by a defect in riboflavin metabolism in the mother. Study of a kindred with seven deaths in infancy: value of riboflavin therapy in preventing this syndrome. J. Pediatr. 103, 394–398.

Henriques, B.J., Rodrigues, J.V., Olsen, R.K., Bross, P., Gomes, C.M., 2009. Role of flavinylation in a mild variant of multiple acyl-CoA dehydrogenation deficiency: a molecular rationale for the effects of riboflavin supplementation. J. Biol. Chem. 284, 4222–4229.

Henriques, B.J., Olsen, R.K., Bross, P., Gomes, C.M., 2010a. Emerging roles for riboflavin in functional rescue of mitochondrial beta-oxidation flavoenzymes. Curr. Med. Chem. 17, 3842–3854.

Henriques, B.J., Bross, P., Gomes, C.M., 2010b. Mutational hotspots in electron transfer flavoprotein underlie defective folding and function in multiple acyl-CoA dehydrogenase deficiency. Biochim. Biophys. Acta 1802, 1070–1077.

Henriques, B.J., Fisher, M.T., Bross, P., Gomes, C.M., 2011. A polymorphic position in electron transfer flavoprotein modulates kinetic stability as evidenced by thermal stress. FEBS Lett. 585, 505–510.

Henriques, B.J., Lucas, T.G., Gomes, C.M., 2016. Therapeutic approaches using riboflavin in mitochondrial energy metabolism disorders. Curr. Drug Targets 17, 1527–1534.

Hoppel, C., DiMarco, J.P., Tandler, B., 1979. Riboflavin and rat hepatic cell structure and function. mitochondrial oxidative metabolism in deficiency states. J. Biol. Chem. 254, 4164–4170.

Hustad, S., McKinley, M.C., McNulty, H., Schneede, J., Strain, J.J., Scott, J.M., et al., 2002. Riboflavin, flavin mononucleotide, and flavin adenine dinucleotide in human plasma and erythrocytes at baseline and after low-dose riboflavin supplementation. Clin. Chem. 48, 1571–1577.

Kucharská, J., 2008. Vitamins in mitochondrial function. In: Gvozdjáková, A. (Ed.), Mitochondrial Medicine: Mitochondrial Metabolism, Diseases, Diagnosis and Therapy. Springer, Dordrecht, pp. 367–384.

Lammer, A.B., Rolinski, B., Ahting, U., Heuss, D., 2011. Multiple acyl-CoA-dehydrogenase deficiency (MADD)—a novel mutation of electron-transferring-flavoprotein dehydrogenase ETFDH. J. Neurol. Sci. 307, 166–167.

Lan, M.Y., Fu, M.H., Liu, Y.F., Huang, C.C., Chang, Y.Y., Liu, J.S., et al., 2010. High frequency of ETFDH c.250G > A mutation in taiwanese patients with late-onset lipid storage myopathy. Clin. Genet. 78, 565–569.

Law, L.K., Tang, N.L., Hui, J., Fung, S.L., Ruiter, J., Wanders, R.J., et al., 2009. Novel mutations in ETFDH gene in Chinese patients with riboflavin-responsive multiple acyl-CoA dehydrogenase deficiency. Clin. Chim. Acta 404, 95–99.

Liang, W.C., Ohkuma, A., Hayashi, Y.K., Lopez, L.C., Hirano, M., Nonaka, I., et al., 2009. ETFDH mutations, CoQ10 levels, and respiratory chain activities in patients with riboflavin-responsive multiple acyl-CoA dehydrogenase deficiency. Neuromuscul. Disord. 19, 212–216.

Lipkin, P.H., Roe, C.R., Goodman, S.I., Batshaw, M.L., 1988. A case of glutaric acidemia type I: effect of riboflavin and carnitine. J. Pediatr. 112, 62–65.

Lucas, T.G., Henriques, B.J., Rodrigues, J.V., Bross, P., Gregersen, N., Gomes, C.M., 2011. Cofactors and metabolites as potential stabilizers of mitochondrial acyl-CoA dehydrogenases. Biochim. Biophys. Acta 1812, 1658–1663.

Merrill Jr., A.H., Lambeth, J.D., Edmondson, D.E., McCormick, D.B., 1981. Formation and mode of action of flavoproteins. Annu. Rev. Nutr. 1, 281–317.

Missaglia, S., Tavian, D., Moro, L., Angelini, C., 2018. Characterization of two ETFDH mutations in a novel case of riboflavin-responsive multiple acyl-CoA dehydrogenase deficiency. Lipids Health Dis. 17, 254.
Nagao, M., Tanaka, K., 1992. FAD-dependent regulation of transcription, translation, post-translational processing, and post-processing stability of various mitochondrial acyl-CoA dehydrogenases and of electron transfer flavoprotein and the site of holoenzyme formation. J. Biol. Chem. 267, 17925–17932.
Nimmo, G.A.M., Ejaz, R., Cordeiro, D., Kannu, P., Mercimek-Andrews, S., 2018. Riboflavin transporter deficiency mimicking mitochondrial myopathy caused by complex II deficiency. Am. J. Med. Genet. A. 176, 399–403.
Nochi, Z., Olsen, R.K.J., Gregersen, N., 2017. Short-chain acyl-CoA dehydrogenase deficiency: from gene to cell pathology and possible disease mechanisms. J. Inherit. Metab. Dis. 40, 641–655.
Olsen, R.K., Olpin, S.E., Andresen, B.S., Miedzybrodzka, Z.H., Pourfarzam, M., Merinero, B., et al., 2007. ETFDH mutations as a major cause of riboflavin-responsive multiple acyl-CoA dehydrogenation deficiency. Brain 130, 2045–2054.
Olsen, R.K.J., Konarikova, E., Giancaspero, T.A., Mosegaard, S., Boczonadi, V., Matakovic, L., et al., 2016. Riboflavin-responsive and -non-responsive mutations in FAD synthase cause multiple acyl-CoA dehydrogenase and combined respiratory-chain deficiency. Am. J. Hum. Genet. 98, 1130–1145.
Pinard, J.M., Marsac, C., Barkaoui, E., Desguerre, I., Birch-Machin, M., Reinert, P., et al., 1999. Leigh syndrome and leukodystrophy due to partial succinate dehydrogenase deficiency: regression with riboflavin. Arch. Pediatr. 6, 421–426.
Powers, H.J., 2003. Riboflavin (vitamin B-2) and health. Am. J. Clin. Nutr. 77, 1352–1360.
Pusti, S., Das, N., Nayek, K., Biswas, S., 2014. A treatable neurometabolic disorder: glutaric aciduria type 1. Case Rep. Pediatr. 2014, 256356.
Repp, B.M., Mastantuono, E., Alston, C.L., Schiff, M., Haack, T.B., Rotig, A., et al., 2018. Clinical, biochemical and genetic spectrum of 70 patients with ACAD9 deficiency: is riboflavin supplementation effective? Orphanet. J. Rare Dis. 13, 120.
Rodrigues, J.V., Henriques, B.J., Lucas, T.G., Gomes, C.M., 2012. Cofactors and metabolites as protein folding helpers in metabolic diseases. Curr. Top. Med. Chem. 12, 2546–2559.
Ross, N.S., Hansen, T.P., 1992. Riboflavin deficiency is associated with selective preservation of critical flavoenzyme-dependent metabolic pathways. Biofactors 3, 185–190.
Saijo, T., Tanaka, K., 1995. Isoalloxazine ring of FAD is required for the formation of the core in the Hsp60-assisted folding of medium chain acyl-CoA dehydrogenase subunit into the assembly competent conformation in mitochondria. J. Biol. Chem. 270, 1899–1907.
Scaglia, F., Towbin, J.A., Craigen, W.J., Belmont, J.W., Smith, E.O., Neish, S.R., et al., 2004. Clinical spectrum, morbidity, and mortality in 113 pediatric patients with mitochondrial disease. Pediatrics 114, 925–931.
Scalais, E., Bottu, J., Wanders, R.J., Ferdinandusse, S., Waterham, H.R., De Meirleir, L., 2015. Familial very long chain acyl-CoA dehydrogenase deficiency as a cause of neonatal sudden infant death: improved survival by prompt diagnosis. Am. J. Med. Genet. A 167A, 211–214.
Schiff, M., Veauville-Merllie, A., Su, C.H., Tzagoloff, A., Rak, M., Ogier de Baulny, H., et al., 2016. SLC25A32 mutations and riboflavin-responsive exercise intolerance. N. Engl. J. Med. 374, 795–797.
Scholte, H.R., Busch, H.F., Bakker, H.D., Bogaard, J.M., Luyt-Houwen, I.E., Kuyt, L.P., 1995. Riboflavin-responsive complex I deficiency. Biochim. Biophys. Acta 1271, 75–83.

Sharawat, I.K., Dawman, L., 2018. Glutaric aciduria type 1 with microcephaly: masquerading as spastic cerebral palsy. J. Pediatr. Neurosci. 13, 349–351.
Skladal, D., Halliday, J., Thorburn, D.R., 2003. Minimum birth prevalence of mitochondrial respiratory chain disorders in children. Brain 126, 1905–1912.
Tonin, R., Caciotti, A., Funghini, S., Pasquini, E., Mooney, S.D., Cai, B., et al., 2016. Clinical relevance of short-chain acyl-CoA dehydrogenase (SCAD) deficiency: exploring the role of new variants including the first SCAD-disease-causing allele carrying a synonymous mutation. BBA Clin. 5, 114–119.
van Maldegem, B.T., Duran, M., Wanders, R.J., Waterham, H.R., Wijburg, F.A., 2010. Flavin adenine dinucleotide status and the effects of high-dose riboflavin treatment in short-chain acyl-CoA dehydrogenase deficiency. Pediatr. Res. 67, 304–308.
Vergani, L., Barile, M., Angelini, C., Burlina, A.B., Nijtmans, L., Freda, M.P., et al., 1999. Riboflavin therapy. biochemical heterogeneity in two adult lipid storage myopathies. Brain 122 (Pt 12), 2401–2411.
Wang, Z.Q., Chen, X.J., Murong, S.X., Wang, N., Wu, Z.Y., 2011. Molecular analysis of 51 unrelated pedigrees with late-onset multiple acyl-CoA dehydrogenation deficiency (MADD) in southern China confirmed the most common ETFDH mutation and high carrier frequency of c.250G > A. J. Mol. Med. (Berl.) 89, 569–576.
Wang, Z., Hong, D., Zhang, W., Li, W., Shi, X., Zhao, D., et al., 2016. Severe sensory neuropathy in patients with adult-onset multiple acyl-CoA dehydrogenase deficiency. Neuromuscul. Disord. 26, 170–175.
Wen, B., Dai, T., Li, W., Zhao, Y., Liu, S., Zhang, C., et al., 2010. Riboflavin-responsive lipid-storage myopathy caused by ETFDH gene mutations. J. Neurol. Neurosurg. Psychiatry 81, 231–236.
Wolfe, L., Jethva, R., Oglesbee, D., et al., 2011. Short-chain acyl-CoA dehydrogenase deficiency. In: Adam, M.P., Ardinger, H.H., Pagon, R.A., et al.,GeneReviews® [Internet]. University of Washington, Seattle, WA.

CHAPTER 13

Linking homocysteine, B vitamins, and choline to ischemic stroke risk

Mahira Moftah[1], Joshua T. Emmerson[1] and Nafisa M. Jadavji[1,2]
[1]Department of Neuroscience, Carleton University, Ottawa, ON, Canada
[2]Department of Biomedical Sciences, Midwestern University, Glendale, AZ, United States

Contents

Key facts

- Stroke is a leading cause of death in the world, however, therapeutic interventions are limited and those people affected typically suffer from a permanent loss of motor function.
- As the world's population is aging, the prevalence of stroke is increasing.
- While there are several risk factors for stroke, nutrition is a modifiable risk factor for stroke.
- Higher levels of homocysteine, a nonprotein amino acid, are linked to increased risk of stroke.
- B vitamins, including folic acid and vitamin B12, reduce the levels of homocysteine in the body.

Molecular Nutrition
DOI: https://doi.org/10.1016/B978-0-12-811907-5.00010-5

- Choline is a nutrient that is involved in reducing the levels of homocysteine. In the brain it is also involved in lipid metabolism and the generation of acetylcholine.
- Results of clinical trials to lower levels of homocysteine through B vitamin supplementation remain unclear with recent advancements in the field.
- Work using model systems reports that reduced levels of B vitamins and increased homocysteine levels impair brain function and make tissue more vulnerable to damage.
- Reducing stroke risk is paramount. Personalized medicine and combination therapies may be more effective.

Abbreviations

MTHFR Methylenetetrahydrofolate reductase
BHMT Betaine-homocysteine *S*-methyltransferase
SAM *S*-adenosylmethionine
tPA Tissue plasminogen activator

13.1 Introduction

Stroke is a leading cause of death globally (Feigin et al., 2015; Mozaffarian et al., 2015). Currently there is a lack of translational research, such that almost none of the reported neuroprotective therapies that were beneficial in animal models have benefited in stroke-affected patients (Dirnagl, 2016). An approved treatment for stroke is the administration of intravenous tissue plasminogen activator (tPA) (Jauch et al., 2013), which breaks down clots (Bonaventura et al., 2016). However, a major limitation for tPA use is that it needs to be administered within 4 hours of stroke onset after which its use may induce hemorrhaging (Jauch et al., 2013). Unfortunately, most stroke patients do not arrive at the hospital until it is too late for treatment (Leibson et al., 1994). Recent research reported that thrombectomy may be a viable therapeutic approach and patients can be treated up to 16 hours after onset of stroke. However, performing a thrombectomy is dependent on the location of the stroke and the size of damage (Albers et al., 2018). The current treatments for stroke, tPA and a thrombectomy, can be used to restore blood flow shortly after a stroke. Preventative approaches to minimize both the risk and severity of a stroke event are attainable from a better understanding of the risk factors and mechanisms involved in the regulation of stroke outcomes.

13.2 Understanding stroke

Stroke represents a major subset of cardiovascular cases. It is a broad term that encompasses several different types of physiological events, each causing neurological dysfunction from ischemic conditions in the brain (Sacco et al., 2013). Generally, stroke occurs when a significant blood clot, termed a thrombus, forms in the circulatory system and this prevents adequate delivery of oxygen and nutrients to the brain, which are essential for proper function (Kolb and Whishaw, 2011). As a result, neurons and glial cells begin to die, ultimately leading to significant brain damage and behavioral impairments. More specifically, stroke is categorized as either ischemic or hemorrhagic (Sacco et al., 2013). An ischemic stroke occurs when a blood clot forms inside of the vasculature within the brain, such as a cerebral artery. This type of stroke event is the most common, occurring in ~87% of all stroke cases (Mozaffarian et al., 2015). Alternatively, hemorrhagic stroke is when a weakened blood vessel ruptures causing bleeding in the brain. The leaked blood accumulates and compresses the surrounding brain tissue (Kumar et al., 2016). A stroke can also be silent which means that there is evidence of damage in the brain, but there are no visible impairments in function (Sacco et al., 2013).

After an ischemic stroke there is a patterned area of damaged cells consisting of two unique features: the ischemic core and the penumbra (Fig. 13.1). The core is the central area of damage that has severely ischemic tissue and this area consists of dying neurons and glia as well as cellular debris. The penumbra is the area that surrounds the core, has mild to moderate ischemic tissue, and is partially salvageable after reperfusion. The duration, severity of blockage, and location of the ischemic stroke all affect the overall severity of damage to the brain. For example, ischemic stroke can either be focal or global. Focal strokes, which are more common, are specific to a small area of the brain, whereas global strokes affect several or all parts of the brain. Nonetheless, after a stroke event where the motor cortex is damaged, motor function of the body becomes compromised contralateral to the damage in the brain. Because there is decussation of sensory neurons at the midbrain, stroke in the right hemisphere affects sensation and movement on the left side of the body.

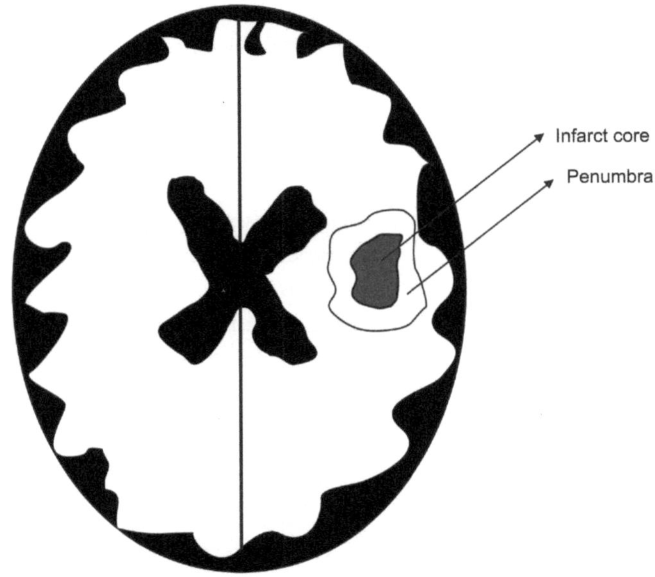

Figure 13.1 ***Dorsal view of brain.*** Right hemisphere showing ischemic stroke damage. The infarct core (*dark gray*) and penumbra (*white*). The core is the central area of damage that has severely ischemic tissue and this area consists of dying neurons and glia. The penumbra is the area that surrounds the core and has mild to moderate ischemic tissue.

Despite understanding the process of a stroke, how it causes neurodegenerative pathology is not completely understood (Busl and Greer, 2010). For example, the amount of functional damage that a stroke can cause varies between people and can range from mild to moderate to severe (Heart and Stroke Foundation, 2016). It is important to consider the possible influence of other factors that contribute to the prevalence of stroke.

13.3 Nutrition

Nutrition is a modifiable risk factor for stroke (Kumar et al., 2016; Mozaffarian et al., 2015). A recent report from the American Health Association described that poor dietary habits (e.g., low consumptions of fruits and vegetables) contribute to the onset of stroke (Benjamin et al., 2018). A component of nutrition is vitamins. For example, folic acid is an important B vitamin in the brain for nucleotide synthesis, methylation, DNA repair, second messenger systems, ion channels, protein and

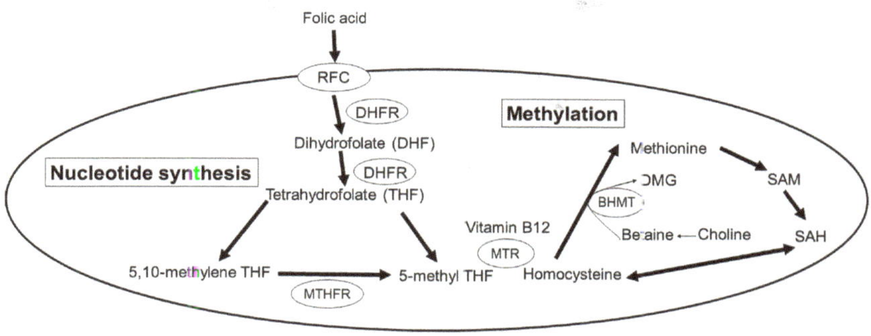

Figure 13.2 ***One-carbon metabolism in the cell.*** *BHMT*, Betaine-homocysteine *S*-methyltransferase; *DHR*, dihydrofolate; *DHFR*, dihydrofolate reductase; *DMG*, dimethylglycine; *MTR*, methionine synthase reductase; *MTHFR*, methylenetetrahydrofolate reductase; *RFC*, reduced folate carrier; *SAH*, *S*-adenosylhomocysteine; *SAM*, *S*-adenosylmethionine; *THF*, tetrahydrofolate reductase.

neurotransmitter synthesis, as well as the metabolism of homocysteine (Murray et al., 2017). One-carbon metabolism, including folic acid metabolism in the cell, is summarized in Fig. 13.2.

13.4 Homocysteine and stroke

High levels of homocysteine have been linked to increased risk of cardiovascular disease (Castro et al., 2006; Santilli et al., 2015; Spence, 2016). In 1969 a report described children with severe homocystinuria as having increased susceptibility to premature death via atherosclerosis and thrombotic occlusions (McCully, 1969). In fact, an elevated level of plasma homocysteine, >12 μmol/L compared to ~5–10 μmol/L in healthy adults (Hainsworth et al., 2015; Obeid et al., 2007), termed hyperhomocysteinemia, is considered an independent risk factor for stroke (Brattstrom et al., 1992).

Homocysteine is a nonprotein amino acid product of methylation reactions in cells that can be measured easily in blood plasma. Homocysteine can be removed from cells in three methods. In all cells, most importantly in the brain, homocysteine is primarily recycled into methionine using folate as a methyl donor. Interestingly, homocysteine metabolism in the brain is different than other organs because the second method, called the transsulfuration pathway, does not occur and remethylation of homocysteine via betaine, the third method, is absent (Lehotsky et al., 2014). Homocysteine is removed by transsulfuration only in liver, pancreatic, and renal tissue (Brosnan et al., 2004). This process requires pyridoxal (vitamin B6) as a coenzyme, serine, and cystathionine β-synthase to convert homocysteine into cystathionine.

The Homocysteine Studies Collaboration published in 2002 compiled and reviewed literature from over 30 prospective or retrospective studies, totaling 1113 stroke patients, associating a 25% reduction in plasma homocysteine levels with a 19% reduction in risk for stroke (The Homocysteine Studies Collaboration, 2002). Recently this association was emphasized in European countries including Italy and Poland, as well as Asian countries such as China, Korea, and Japan (Fu et al., 2015). Of these 13 studies, the initial results from a total of 1206 stroke patients and 1202 controls, having cofactors of stroke risk unaccounted for, reported mixed relationships between plasma homocysteine and stroke. Interestingly, when cofactors such as age, smoking status, and history of cardiovascular disease among others were accounted for, the overall association between plasma homocysteine levels and risk for stroke is positively correlated. Genetic deficiencies in folate metabolism also increase levels of homocysteine, for example, a common polymorphism in methylenetetrahydrofolate reductase (*MTHFR* 677C→T) has been implicated in an increased risk for stroke (Song et al., 2016), possibly through increased levels of homocysteine.

Despite finding a significant association between elevated homocysteine levels and risk of stroke, the mechanism by which this association promotes stroke occurrence remains unclear (Castro et al., 2006; Christopher et al., 2007). This is, in part, because multiple factors and processes are associated with elevated levels of homocysteine and, as a result, homocysteine is prevalent in multiple neurodegenerative pathologies of the central nervous system (Ansari et al., 2014; Obeid et al., 2007). Among these findings, it appears as though hyperhomocysteinemia may promote an increased risk of stroke from downstream effects of decreased global DNA methylation (Baccarelli et al., 2010), increased endothelial dysfunction (Castro et al., 2006; Spence, 2016), and/or increased oxidative damage of cells (Kim and Pae, 1996; Obeid and Herrmann, 2006; Pniewski et al., 2003), making normally functional systems more susceptible to damage. Increased levels of homocysteine result in more reactive oxygen species production via arachidonic acid (Lehotsky et al., 2014).

A stroke sets off a cascade of cellular events in the cells of the brain. An example is epigenetic changes, which include DNA methylation, histone modification, as well as noncoding RNAs (Thompson et al.,

2013). One-carbon metabolism is involved in the generation of methyl groups, through MTHFR and *S*-adenosylmethionine (SAM). Altered levels of SAM, the global methyl donor, have been reported in patients with vascular disease (Castro et al., 2003). In stroke patients, global DNA methylation (LINE1) levels are also reduced (Baccarelli et al., 2010). Interestingly, DNA methyltransferases are abundant in the brain, especially in postmitotic neurons (Goto et al., 1994). Increased activity in these enzymes and more methylation have been reported to result in worse outcomes after ischemic damage in a mouse model (Endres et al., 2000).

Endothelial dysfunction can be described as an imbalance between vasodilator and vasoconstrictor produced by the endothelium. Vascular dilatation depends on nitric oxide (NO), and endothelium-derived relaxing factor. Several reports have outlined that elevated levels of homocysteine impair endothelial-dependent dilatation (Lai and Kan, 2015). Elevated homocysteine levels have been reported to increase oxidative stress uncoupling of NO synthase activity and quenching of NO. Endoplasmic reticulum stress leads to endothelial cell apoptosis and chronic inflammation resulting in prothrombotic conditions (Lai and Kan, 2015). Increasing levels of folic acid in patients with high levels of homocysteine show some positive effects. Folic acid supplementation (5–10 mg per day for 6–8 weeks) in patients with high levels of homocysteine has been reported to result in reduced levels of plasma homocysteine and improved endothelium-dependent dilation and function (Bellamy et al., 1999; Woo et al., 1999).

13.5 Clinical trials to reduce levels of homocysteine

Several clinical trials were conducted to assess whether lowering homocysteine levels by vitamin B supplementation is a viable option to reduce the risk of cardiovascular diseases, such as stroke (Hankey, 2018). The Vitamin Intervention for Stroke Prevention (VISP) trial was a randomized and double-blind study that showed no benefit of vitamin therapy for homocysteine lowering on reoccurring cardiovascular events (Toole et al., 2004). It is important to note that this VISP trial also coincided with the initiation of the mandatory folic acid fortification in North America. The Norwegian Vitamin Study (NORVIT) study investigated the impact of homocysteine lowering in patients with acute myocardial infarction and not ischemic stroke. The NORVIT study also reported that there was no benefit to homocysteine lowering with B vitamins for reducing myocardial infarction risk (Bonaa, 2006).

The Heart Outcomes Prevention Evaluation 2 study reported that the administration of folic acid, vitamin B6, and vitamin B12 did in fact did lower homocysteine levels in patients with vascular disease, but it did not reduce the incidence of cardiovascular disease (Lonn et al., 2006). In 2010 a randomized placebo control, with folic acid, vitamins B6 and B12, and/or omega-3 fatty acids also did not show a reduction in the risk for cardiovascular disease (Galan et al., 2010). The Diabetic Intervention with Vitamins in Nephropathy trial reported that high doses of B vitamins were actually harmful and increased cardiovascular disease in patients with diabetic nephropathy (House et al., 2010). The vitamins to prevent stroke trial showed a reduction in vascular events when lowering homocysteine levels and vitamin B supplementation was combined with antiplatelet therapy. In 2015 a double-blind trial in China reported a 21% reduction in stroke when patients were given enalapril in combination with folic acid (Huo et al., 2015). Further analysis of this study also reported that hypertensive patients with high cholesterol (Qin et al., 2016) and a polymorphism in *MTHFR* at base pair 677 (Zhao et al., 2017) benefited from folic acid supplementation in terms of reducing their risk of cardiovascular disease. It is important to note that China does not have a mandatory government folic acid fortification program in place.

The clinical trials described above indicate that vitamin B supplementation to lower levels of homocysteine is ineffective when the outcome measurement is the onset of cardiovascular disease. Interestingly in 2011 when homocysteine was included in the National Health and Nutrition Examination Survey III study it improved risk prediction for cardiovascular disease (Veeranna et al., 2011). It is important to keep in mind that the question of whether vitamin B supplementation is beneficial for stroke is more complicated than originally thought, especially when different patient populations are considered (Spence and Stampfer, 2011). For example, cyanocobalamin may accelerate a decline in renal function and this could then result in an increased risk for cardiovascular disease, through the build-up of cyanide which could interfere with the decyanation of cyanocobalmin (Spence et al., 2017). When considering vitamin B supplementation, using folic acid and methylcobalamin or hydroxycobalamin to lower homocysteine levels may be more appropriate, rather than cyanocobalamin (Spence, 2017). It could also be plausible that vitamin B12 may play a key role in stroke prevention. Stroke occurs in individuals who are mostly older and intriguingly approximately 20% are vitamin B12 deficient (Andrès et al., 2004,) but only 5%–10% are detectable (Clarke et al., 2004). A serum B12 level within the normal range does not exclude metabolic B12 deficiency (Spence and Stampfer, 2011). In North America and other countries folic acid is in the grain supply because of mandatory folic acid fortification, during times when folic acid is increased vitamin B12 deficiencies are often looked over (Spence, 2013).

The long-term effects of administering B vitamins is a reduction in the levels of homocysteine, but not the markers associated with inflammation or endothelial dysfunction (Christen et al., 2018; Sibani et al., 2000). A recent study in people over the age of 65 reported that supplementation of folic acid and vitamin B12 did indeed reduce levels of homocysteine, but there were no changes in arterial stiffness and atherosclerosis (Van Dijk et al., 2015). Several meta-analyses have reported that lowering homocysteine through vitamin B supplementation does indeed reduce the number of stroke events (Ji et al., 2013; Martí-Carvajal et al., 2017; Tian et al., 2017; Wang et al., 2017). A study in Korea reported that the intake of antioxidants, in combination with B vitamins, is inversely associated with ischemic stroke (Choe et al., 2016). Dietary supplementation of B vitamins to reduce homocysteine levels is a complex question. There are benefits to reduced levels of homocysteine, but a number of factors need to be considered, such as patient population, comorbidities, and government fortification programs (Debreceni and Debreceni, 2014; Hsu et al., 2018; Jenkins et al., 2018; Zeng et al., 2015).

13.6 Mechanisms explaining folate and homocysteine metabolism as a modulator of stroke outcome

Model systems have been developed to study the in vivo mechanisms of hyperhomocysteinemia (Azad et al., 2017). Murine models are recommended for basic research on cardiovascular disease, but large animal models are better for biomedical research since they have many physiological and anatomical similarities to humans (Azad et al., 2017). Using animal model systems these studies have shown that folic acid deficiency increases damage after cerebral ischemia (Hwang et al., 2008). This is through increased neuronal damage, autophagy, and gliosis (Hwang et al., 2008; Jadavji et al., 2018; Škovierová et al., 2016; Zhao et al., 2016).

Ischemic preconditioning, which increases the body's resistance to oxygen loss, may preserve neuronal tissue from the damaging effects of stroke (Kovalska et al., 2015; Pavlikova et al., 2017). Both *in vivo* and *in vitro* data indicate that ischemic preconditioning is beneficial for patients with hyperhomocysteinemia and cerebral ischemia (Kovalska et al., 2015; Pavlikova et al., 2017). Therefore ischemic preconditioning could be used as a preventive measure against stroke and to protect against neurodegeneration associated with stroke. Furthermore, increasing levels of folic acid may be crucial for protecting the brain against damage.

Dietary supplementation could contribute to stroke recovery. A study using in vivo and in vitro model systems found that folic acid enhances the stimulation of Notch signaling and neurogenesis in the brain after ischemic stroke (Zhang et al., 2012). Another study with similar mouse models has also found that B vitamins and choline improve motor functions and enhance neuroplasticity after cerebral ischemia (Jadavji et al., 2017). Such findings point to the dietary supplementation of those nutrients along with other stroke therapies (Jadavji et al., 2017; Zhang et al., 2012).

13.7 Choline

Choline and folic acid are linked through the metabolism of homocysteine (Fig. 13.2). Choline is an essential nutrient, and in the brain it is involved in the synthesis of acetylcholine, as well as being a major component of cell membranes. For example, phosphatidylcholine a metabolite of choline, is a brain phospholipid. Using betaine-homocysteine *S*-methyltransferase(BHMT) choline is converted to betaine which remethylates homocysteine (Fig. 13.2). BHMT is restrictively expressed in the liver and kidney and is also present in the brain tissue of bats (Zhang et al., 2013) and mice (Prieur et al., 2017). In addition, betaine levels are reduced in hyperhomocysteinemic patients and rodent models, highlighting the role of choline metabolism in homocysteine metabolism (Imbard et al., 2015; Jadavji et al., 2012). Increasing the levels of choline through dietary supplementation has been reported to have positive effects on brain function after damage in humans (Zeisel et al., 1991) and in an animal model of stroke (Jadavji et al., 2017).

Citicoline is a choline molecule bonded to a cysteine residue, and, when used in animal models of stoke, it has been reported to reduce neurological impairment after damage (Kakihana et al., 1988), decrease infarct volume and reduce inflammation (Adibhatla et al., 2005; Gutiérrez-Fernández et al., 2012a), as well as increase neuroplasticity (Gutiérrez-Fernández et al., 2012b; Hurtado et al., 2007). In human clinical trials positive effects of citicoline have been reported (Overgaard, 2014), but the results are not clear in all the populations studied (Adibhatla et al., 2005). More investigations are required to understand the impact of citicoline on stroke in humans. It is important to note that combination therapies are beneficial for stroke-affected patients (Wang et al., 2015). It may be that citicoline when combined with a thrombotic agent or lifestyle changes could be more effective in promoting recovery after stroke.

Recent studies have reported that there is an important interaction between the gut microbiome and the brain (Sudo et al., 2004). This is an interesting area of research, especially when applied to neurological diseases, such as stroke. The microbiome has been linked to inflammation, depression, and stress in the brain (Winek et al., 2016). Interactions between dietary intake of choline and related metabolites have been shown to influence risk of cardiovascular diseases, such as stroke (Wang et al., 2011; Zhu et al., 2017). In the context of stroke, the mechanism through which dietary choline changes the bacteria in the gut still needs to be dissected.

13.8 Future directions

This chapter provided an overview of how homocysteine, B vitamins, and choline are implicated in the onset of ischemic stroke. It is still a complex question to answer. However, the movement toward personalized medicine has been facilitated by the advancement of technology. Evidence supporting nutrition as a way to circumvent the risk of stroke is growing. Because the risk and outcomes of stroke are highly variable, future therapeutics will likely involve personalized medicine. In addition, several studies suggest that combining therapeutics, including pharmaceuticals, is more effective for promoting recovery from stroke; a combinational therapy approach may also provide the best therapeutic options for stroke patients.

Considering the data, when dietary supplementation is implemented to reduce the risk of stroke, folic acid combined with methylcobalamin or hydroxycobalamin as well as choline is the most likely candidate therapeutic. Countries that have mandatory folic acid fortification laws should not disregard dietary supplementation, since vitamin B12 deficiency is prevalent in the aging population. Further studies, including multicountry double-blind placebo trials are required to understand the full impact of dietary supplementation with B vitamins and choline for stroke risk.

References

Adibhatla, R.M., Hatcher, J.F., Arenth, P.M., Russell, K.C., Ricker, J.H., Zafonte, R.D., 2005. Cytidine 5′-diphosphocholine (CDP-choline) in stroke and other CNS disorders. Neurochem. Res. 30, 15–23. Available from: https://doi.org/10.1007/s11064-004-9681-8.

Albers, G.W., Marks, M.P., Kemp, S., Christensen, S., Tsai, J.P., Ortega-Gutierrez, S., et al., 2018. Thrombectomy for stroke at 6 to 16 hours with selection by perfusion imaging. N. Engl. J. Med. 378, 708–718. Available from: https://doi.org/10.1056/NEJMoa1713973.

Andrès, E., Loukili, N.H., Noel, E., Kaltenbach, G., Ben Abdelgheni, M., Perrin, A.E., et al., 2004. Vitamin B12 (cobalamin) deficiency in elderly patients. CMAJ. 171, 251–259. Available from: https://doi.org/10.1503/cmaj.1031155.

Ansari, R., Mahta, A., Mallack, E., Luo, J.J., 2014. Hyperhomocysteinemia and neurologic disorders: a review. J. Clin. Neurol. 10, 281–288. Available from: https://doi.org/10.3988/jcn.2014.10.4.281.

Azad, M.A.K., Huang, P., Liu, G., Ren, W., Teklebrh, T., Yan, W., et al., 2017. Hyperhomocysteinemia and cardiovascular disease in animal model. Amino Acids . Available from: https://doi.org/10.1007/s00726-017-2503-5.

Baccarelli, A., Wright, R., Bollati, V., Litonjua, A., Zanobetti, A., Tarantini, L., et al., 2010. Ischemic heart disease and stroke in relation to blood DNA methylation. Epidemiology 21, 819–828. Available from: https://doi.org/10.1097/EDE.0b013e3181f20457.

Bellamy, M.F., McDowell, I.F.W., Ramsey, M.W., Brownlee, M., Newcombe, R.G., Lewis, M.J., 1999. Oral folate enhances endothelial function in hyperhomocysteinaemic subjects. Eur. J. Clin. Invest. 29, 659–662. Available from: https://doi.org/10.1046/j.1365-2362.1999.00527.x.

Benjamin, E.J., Virani, S.S., Callaway, C.W., Chang, A.R., Cheng, S., Chiuve, S.E., et al., 2018. Heart disease and stroke statistics—2018 update: a report from the American Heart Association. Circulation . Available from: https://doi.org/10.1161/CIR.0000000000000558.

Bonaa, K., 2006. Homocysteine lowering and cardiovascular events after acute myocardial infarction. N. Engl. J. Med. 354, 1578–1588.

Bonaventura, A., Montecucco, F., Dallegri, F., 2016. Update on the effects of treatment with recombinant tissue-type plasminogen activator (rt-PA) in acute ischemic stroke. Expert Opin. Biol. Ther. 16 (11), 1323–1340. Available from: https://doi.org/10.1080/14712598.2016.1227779.

Brattstrom, L., Lindgren, A., Israelsson, B., Malinow, M.R., Norrving, B., Upson, B., et al., 1992. Hyperhomocysteinaemia in stroke: prevalence, cause, and relationships to type of stroke and stroke risk factors. Eur. J. Clin. Invest. 22, 214–221.

Brosnan, J.T., Jacobs, R.L., Stead, L.M., Brosnan, M.E., 2004. Methylation demand: a key determinant of homocysteine metabolism. Acta Biochim. Pol. 51, 405–413. Available from: https://doi.org/035001405.

Busl, K.M., Greer, D.M., 2010. Hypoxic-ischemic brain injury: pathophysiology, neuropathology and mechanisms. NeuroRehabilitation. 26, 5–13. Available from: https://doi.org/10.3233/NRE-2010-0531.

Castro, R., Rivera, I., Struys, E.A., Jansen, E.E.W., Ravasco, P., Camilo, M.E., et al., 2003. Increased homocysteine and *S*-adenosylhomocysteine concentrations and DNA hypomethylation in vascular disease. Clin. Chem. 49, 1292–1296. Available from: https://doi.org/10.1373/49.8.1292.

Castro, R., Rivera, I., Blom, H.J., Jakobs, C., Tavares de Almeida, I., 2006. Homocysteine metabolism, hyperhomocysteinaemia and vascular disease: an overview. J. Inherit. Metab. Dis. 29, 3–20. Available from: https://doi.org/10.1007/s10545-006-0106-5.

Choe, H., Hwang, J.-Y., Yun, J.A., Kim, J.-M., Song, T.-J., Chang, N., et al., 2016. Intake of antioxidants and B vitamins is inversely associated with ischemic stroke and cerebral atherosclerosis. Nutr. Res. Pract. 10, 516. Available from: https://doi.org/10.4162/nrp.2016.10.5.516.

Christen, W.G., Cook, N.R., Van Denburgh, M., Zaharris, E., Albert, C.M., Manson, J.E., 2018. Effect of combined treatment with folic acid, vitamin B_6, and vitamin B_{12} on plasma biomarkers of inflammation and endothelial dysfunction in women. J. Am. Heart Assoc. 7, e008517. Available from: https://doi.org/10.1161/JAHA.117.008517.

Christopher, R., Nagaraja, D., Shankar, S.K., 2007. Homocysteine and cerebral stroke in developing countries. Curr. Med. Chem. 14, 2393–2401. Available from: https://doi.org/10.2174/092986707781745613.

Clarke, R., Grimley Evans, J., Schneede, J., Nexo, E., Bates, C., Fletcher, A., et al., 2004. Vitamin B12 and folate deficiency in later life. Age Ageing 33, 34–41. Available from: https://doi.org/10.1093/ageing/afg109.

Debreceni, B., Debreceni, L., 2014. The role of homocysteine-lowering B-vitamins in the primary prevention of cardiovascular disease. Cardiovasc. Ther. 32, 130–138. Available from: https://doi.org/10.1111/1755-5922.12064.

Dirnagl, U., 2016. Thomas Willis lecture: is translational stroke research broken, and if so, how can we fix it? Stroke 47, 2148–2153. Available from: https://doi.org/10.1161/STROKEAHA.116.013244.

Endres, M., Meisel, a, Biniszkiewicz, D., Namura, S., Prass, K., Ruscher, K., et al., 2000. DNA methyltransferase contributes to delayed ischemic brain injury. J. Neurosci. 20, 3175–3181.

Feigin, V.L., Mensah, G.A., Norrving, B., Murray, C.J.L., Roth, G.A., 2015. Atlas of the Global Burden of Stroke (1990–2013): the GBD 2013 study. Neuroepidemiology 45, 230–236. Available from: https://doi.org/10.1159/000441106.

Fu, H.J., Zhao, L.B., Xue, J.J., Wu, Z.X., Huang, Y.P., Liu, W., et al., 2015. Elevated serum homocysteine (Hcy) levels may contribute to the pathogenesis of cerebral infarction. J. Mol. Neurosci. 56, 553–561. Available from: https://doi.org/10.1007/s12031-015-0497-6.

Galan, P., Kesse-Guyot, E., Czernichow, S., Briancon, S., Blacher, J., Hercberg, S., 2010. Effects of B vitamins and omega 3 fatty acids on cardiovascular diseases: a randomised placebo controlled trial. BMJ 341, c6273. Available from: https://doi.org/10.1136/bmj.c6273.

Goto, K., Numata, M., Komura, J.I., Ono, T., Bestor, T.H., Kondo, H., 1994. Expression of DNA methyltransferase gene in mature and immature neurons as well as proliferating cells in mice. Differentiation 56, 39–44. Available from: https://doi.org/10.1046/j.1432-0436.1994.56120039.x.

Gutiérrez-Fernández, M., Leciñana, M.A., de Rodríguez-Frutos, B., Ramos-Cejudo, J., Roda, J.M., Díez-Tejedor, E., 2012a. CDP-choline at high doses is as effective as i.v. thrombolysis in experimental animal stroke. Neurol. Res. 34, 649–656. Available from: https://doi.org/10.1179/1743132812Y.0000000058.

Gutiérrez-Fernández, M., Rodríguez-Frutos, B., Fuentes, B., Vallejo-Cremades, M.T., Álvarez-Grech, J., Expósito-Alcaide, M., et al., 2012b. CDP-choline treatment induces brain plasticity markers expression in experimental animal stroke. Neurochem. Int. 60, 310–317. Available from: https://doi.org/10.1016/j.neuint.2011.12.015.

Hainsworth, A.H., Yeo, N.E., Weekman, E.M., Wilcock, D.M., 2015. Homocysteine, hyperhomocysteinemia and vascular contributions to cognitive impairment and dementia (VCID). Biochim. Biophys. Acta Mol. Basis Dis . Available from: https://doi.org/10.1016/j.bbadis.2015.11.015.

Hankey, G.J., 2018. B vitamins for stroke prevention. Stroke Vasc Neurol 3 (2), 51–58. Available from: https://doi.org/10.1136/svn-2018-000156.
Heart and Stroke Foundation. The burden of heart failure, 2016. Available from: https://www.heartandstroke.ca/-/media/pdf-files/canada/2017-heart-month/heartandstroke-reporton-health-2016.ashx?la=en&hash=91708486C1BC014E24AB4E719B47AEEB8C5EB93E
House, A.A., Eliasziw, M., Cattran, D.C., Churchill, D.N., Oliver, M.J., Fine, A., et al., 2010. Effect of B-vitamin therapy on progression of diabetic nephropathy: a randomized controlled trial. JAMA 303, 1603–1609. Available from: https://doi.org/10.1001/jama.2010.490.
Hsu, C., Chiu, S., Hong, K., Saver, J.L., Wu, Y., Lee, J., 2018. Folic acid in stroke prevention in countries without mandatory folic acid food fortification : a meta-analysis of randomized controlled trials. J. Stroke 20, 99–109.
Huo, Y., Li, J., Qin, X., Huang, Y., Wang, X., Gottesman, R.F., et al., 2015. Efficacy of folic acid therapy in primary prevention of stroke among adults with hypertension in China. JAMA 313, 1325–1335. Available from: https://doi.org/10.1001/jama.2015.2274.
Hurtado, O., Cárdenas, A., Pradillo, J.M., Morales, J.R., Ortego, F., Sobrino, T., et al., 2007. A chronic treatment with CDP-choline improves functional recovery and increases neuronal plasticity after experimental stroke. Neurobiol. Dis. 26, 105–111. Available from: https://doi.org/10.1016/j.nbd.2006.12.005.
Hwang, I.K., Yoo, K.-Y., Suh, H.-W., Kim, Y.S., Kwon, D.Y., Kwon, Y.-G., et al., 2008. Folic acid deficiency increases delayed neuronal death, DNA damage, platelet endothelial cell adhesion molecule-1 immunoreactivity, and gliosis in the hippocampus after transient cerebral ischemia. J. Neurosci. Res. 86, 2003–2015. Available from: https://doi.org/10.1002/jnr.21647.
Imbard, A., Benoist, J.-F., Esse, R., Gupta, S., Lebon, S., De Vriese, A.S., et al., 2015. High homocysteine induces betaine depletion. Biosci. Rep. 35, e00222. Available from: https://doi.org/10.1042/BSR20150094.
Jadavji, N.M., Deng, L., Leclerc, D., Malysheva, O., Bedell, B.J., Caudill, M.A., et al., 2012. Severe methylenetetrahydrofolate reductase deficiency in mice results in behavioral anomalies with morphological and biochemical changes in hippocampus. Mol. Genet. Metab. 106, 149–159. Available from: https://doi.org/10.1016/j.ymgme.2012.03.020.
Jadavji, N.M., Emmerson, J., Willmore, W.G., MacFarlane, A.J., Smith, P., 2017. B-vitamin and choline supplementation increases neuroplasticity and recovery after stroke. Neurobiol. Dis. 103, 89–100.
Jadavji, N.M., Emmerson, J.T., Shanmugalingam, U., Willmore, W.G., Macfarlane, A.J., Smith, P.D., 2018. A genetic deficiency in folic acid metabolism impairs recovery after ischemic stroke. Exp. Neurol. 309, 14–22.
Jauch, E.C., Saver, J.L., Adams, H.P., Bruno, A., Connors, J.J.B., Demaerschalk, B.M., et al., 2013. Guidelines for the early management of patients with acute ischemic stroke: a guideline for healthcare professionals from the American Heart Association/American Stroke Association. Stroke 44, 870–947. Available from: https://doi.org/10.1161/STR.0b013e318284056a.
Jenkins, D.J.A., Spence, J.D., Giovannucci, E.L., Kim, Y., Josse, R., Vieth, R., et al., 2018. Supplemental vitamins and minerals for CVD prevention and treatment. J. Am. Coll. Cardiol. 71, 2570–2584. Available from: https://doi.org/10.1016/j.jacc.2018.04.020.
Ji, Y., Tan, S., Xu, Y., Chandra, A., Shi, C., Song, B., et al., 2013. Vitamin B supplementation, homocysteine levels, and the risk of cerebrovascular disease: a meta-analysis. Neurology 81, 1298–1307. Available from: https://doi.org/10.1212/WNL.0b013e3182a823cc.
Kakihana, M., Fukuda, N., Suno, M., Nagaoka, A., 1988. Effects of CDP-choline on neurologic deficits and cerebral glucose metabolism in a rat model of cerebral ischemia. Stroke 19, 217–222. Available from: https://doi.org/10.1161/01.STR.19.2.217.

Kim, W.K., Pae, Y.S., 1996. Involvement of *N*-methyl-D-aspartate receptor and free radical in homocysteine-mediated toxicity on rat cerebellar granule cells in culture. Neurosci. Lett. 216, 117–120.

Kolb, B., Whishaw, I.Q., 2011. An Introduction to Brain and Behavior, third ed. Worth Publishers, New York. Available from: https://doi.org/10.1017/CBO9780511623806.

Kovalska, M., Kovalska, L., Tothova, B., Mahmood, S., Adamkov, M., Lehotsky, J., et al., 2015. Combination of hyperhomocysteinemia and ischemic tolerance in experimental model of global ischemia in rats. J. Physiol. Pharmacol. 66, 887–897.

Kumar, A., Aakriti, Gupta, V., 2016. A review on animal models of stroke: an update. Brain Res. Bull. Available from: https://doi.org/10.1016/j.brainresbull.2016.02.016.

Lai, W.K.C., Kan, M.Y., 2015. Homocysteine-induced endothelial dysfunction. Ann. Nutr. Metab. 67, 1–12. Available from: https://doi.org/10.1159/000437098.

Lehotsky, J., Petras, M., Kovalska, M., Tothova, B., Drgova, A., Kaplan, P., 2014. Mechanisms involved in the ischemic tolerance in brain: effect of the homocysteine. Cell. Mol. Neurobiol. 35, 7–15. Available from: https://doi.org/10.1007/s10571-014-0112-3.

Leibson, C.L., Naessens, J.M., Brown, R.D., Whisnant, J.P., Olson, D.M., Fonarow, G. C., et al., 1994. Accuracy of hospital discharge abstracts for identifying stroke. Stroke 25, 2348–2355. Available from: https://doi.org/10.1161/01.str.25.12.2348.

Lonn, E., Yusuf, S., Arnold, M.J., Sheridan, P., Pogue, J., Micks, M., et al., 2006. Homocysteine lowering with folic acid and B vitamins in vascular disease. N. Engl. J. Med. 354, 1567–1577. Available from: https://doi.org/10.1056/NEJMoa060900.

Martí-Carvajal, A.J., Solà, I., Lathyris, D., Dayer, M., 2017. Homocysteine-lowering interventions for preventing cardiovascular events. Cochrane Database Syst. Rev. 2017, 10–12. Available from: https://doi.org/10.1002/14651858.CD006612.pub5.

McCully, K.S., 1969. Vascular pathology of homocysteinemia: implications for the pathogenesis of arteriosclerosis. Am. J. Pathol. 56, 111–128.

Mozaffarian, D., Benjamin, E.J., Go, A.S., Arnett, D.K., Blaha, M.J., Cushman, M., et al., 2015. Heart disease and stroke statistics—2016 update: a report from the American Heart Association. Circulation 133, e38–e360. Available from: https://doi.org/10.1161/CIR.0000000000000350.

Murray, L., Emmerson, J., Jadavji, N.M., 2017. Roles of folate in neurological function. Folic Acid: Sources, Health Effects and Role in Disease. Nova Publishers Science Inc.

Obeid, R., Herrmann, W., 2006. Mechanisms of homocysteine neurotoxicity in neurodegenerative diseases with special reference to dementia. FEBS Lett. 580, 2994–3005. Available from: https://doi.org/10.1016/j.febslet.2006.04.088.

Obeid, R., McCaddon, A., Herrmann, W., 2007. The role of hyperhomocysteinemia and B-vitamin deficiency in neurological and psychiatric diseases. Clin. Chem. Lab. Med. 45, 1590–1606. Available from: https://doi.org/10.1515/CCLM.2007.356.

Overgaard, K., 2014. The effects of citicoline on acute ischemic stroke: a review. J. Stroke Cerebrovasc. Dis. 23, 1764–1769. Available from: https://doi.org/10.1016/j.jstrokecerebrovasdis.2014.01.020.

Pavlikova, V., Vidomanova, E., Balharek, T., Marcinek, J., Kudela, E., Hanysova, S., et al., 2017. DNA methylation as mechanism of apoptotic resistance development in endometrial cancer patients. Gen. Physiol. Biophys. 36, 521–529. Available from: https://doi.org/10.4149/gpb.

Pniewski, J., Chodakowska-Zebrowska, M., Wozniak, R., Stepien, K., Stafiej, A., 2003. Plasma homocysteine level and the course of ischemic stroke. Acta Neurobiol. Exp. (Wars) 63, 127–130.

Prieur, E.A.K., Pjetri, E., Zeisel, S.H., Jadavji, N.M., 2017. Reduced brain volume and impaired memory in betaine homocysteine *S*-methyltransferase knockout mice. Appl. Physiol. Nutr. Metab. 42. Available from: https://doi.org/10.1139/apnm-2017-0182.

Qin, X., Li, J., Spence, J.D., Zhang, Y., Li, Y., Wang, X., et al., 2016. Folic acid therapy reduces the first stroke risk associated with hypercholesterolemia among hypertensive patients. Stroke 47, 2805–2812. Available from: https://doi.org/10.1161/STROKEAHA.116.014578.

Sacco, R.L., Kasner, S.E., Broderick, J.P., Caplan, L.R., Connors, J.J., Culebras, A., et al., 2013. An updated definition of stroke for the 21st century: a statement for healthcare professionals from the American Heart Association/American Stroke Association. Stroke 44, 2064–2089. Available from: https://doi.org/10.1161/STR.0b013e318296aeca.

Santilli, F., Davì, G., Patrono, C., 2015. Homocysteine, methylenetetrahydrofolate reductase, folate status and atherothrombosis: a mechanistic and clinical perspective. Vascul. Pharmacol. 78, 1–9. Available from: https://doi.org/10.1016/j.vph.2015.06.009.

Sibani, S., Christensen, B., Ferrall, E.O., Saadi, I., Hiou-tim, F., Rosenblatt, D.S., et al., 2000. Characterization of six novel mutations in the methylenetetrahydrofolate reductase (MTHFR) gene in patients with homocystinuria. Hum. Mutat. 287, 280–287.

Škovierová, H., Vidomanová, E., Mahmood, S., Sopková, J., Drgová, A., Červeňová, T., et al., 2016. The molecular and cellular effect of homocysteine metabolism imbalance on human health. Int. J. Mol. Sci. 17, 1733. Available from: https://doi.org/10.3390/ijms17101733.

Song, Y., Li, B., Wang, C., Wang, P., Gao, X., Liu, G., 2016. Association between 5,10-methylenetetrahydrofolate reductase C677T gene polymorphism and risk of ischemic stroke: a meta-analysis. J. Stroke Cerebrovasc. Dis. 1–9. Available from: https://doi.org/10.1016/j.jstrokecerebrovasdis.2015.11.041.

Spence, J.D., 2013. B vitamin therapy for homocysteine: renal function and vitamin B12 determine cardiovascular outcomes. Clin. Chem. Lab. Med. 51, 633–637. Available from: https://doi.org/10.1515/cclm-2012-0465.

Spence, J.D., 2016. Homocysteine lowering for stroke prevention: unravelling the complexity of the evidence. Int. J. Stroke 11, 744–747. Available from: https://doi.org/10.1177/1747493016662038.

Spence, J.D., 2017. Nutrition in stroke prevention. Semin. Neurol. 37 (3), 259–266. Available from: https://doi.org/10.1055/s-0037-1603470.

Spence, J.D., Stampfer, M.J., 2011. Understanding the complexity of homocysteine lowering with vitamins: the potential role of subgroup analyses. JAMA 306, 2610–2611. Available from: https://doi.org/10.1001/jama.2011.1834.

Spence, J.D., Yi, Q., Hankey, G.J., 2017. B vitamins in stroke prevention: time to reconsider. Lancet. Neurol. 16, 750–760. Available from: https://doi.org/10.1016/S1474-4422(17)30180-1.

Sudo, N., Chida, Y., Aiba, Y., Sonoda, J., Oyama, N., Yu, X.N., et al., 2004. Postnatal microbial colonization programs the hypothalamic–pituitary–adrenal system for stress response in mice. J. Physiol. 558, 263–275. Available from: https://doi.org/10.1113/jphysiol.2004.063388.

The Homocysteine Studies Collaboration, 2002. Homocysteine and risk of ischemic heart disease and stroke. Am. Med. Assoc. 288, 2015–2023.

Thompson, J.W., Dave, K.R., Young, J.I., Perez-Pinzon, M.A., 2013. Ischemic preconditioning alters the epigenetic profile of the brain from ischemic intolerance to ischemic tolerance. Neurotherapeutics 10, 789–797. Available from: https://doi.org/10.1007/s13311-013-0202-9.

Tian, T., Yang, K.Q., Cui, J.G., Zhou, L.L., Zhou, X.L., 2017. Folic acid supplementation for stroke prevention in patients with cardiovascular disease. Am. J. Med. Sci. 354, 379–387. Available from: https://doi.org/10.1016/j.amjms.2017.05.020.

Toole, J.F., Rene, M., Chambless, L.E., Spence, J.D., Pettigrew, L.C., Howard, V.J., et al., 2004. Lowering homocysteine in patients with ischemic stroke to prevent recurrent stroke J. Am. Med. Assoc. 291, 565–575. Available from: https://doi.org/10.1001/jama.291.5.565.

Van Dijk, S.C., Enneman, A.W., Swart, K.M.A., Van Wijngaarden, J.P., Ham, A.C., Brouwer-Brolsma, E.M., et al., 2015. Effects of 2-year vitamin B12 and folic acid supplementation in hyperhomocysteinemic elderly on arterial stiffness and cardiovascular outcomes within the B-PROOF trial. J. Hypertens. 33, 1897–1906. Available from: https://doi.org/10.1097/HJH.0000000000000647.

Veeranna, V., Zalawadiya, S.K., Niraj, A., Pradhan, J., Ference, B., Burack, R.C., et al., 2011. Homocysteine and reclassification of cardiovascular disease risk. J. Am. Coll. Cardiol. 58, 1025–1033. Available from: https://doi.org/10.1016/j.jacc.2011.05.028.

Wang, Z., Klipfell, E., Bennett, B.J., Koeth, R., Levison, B.S., DuGar, B., et al., 2011. Gut flora metabolism of phosphatidylcholine promotes cardiovascular disease. Nature 472, 57–63. Available from: https://doi.org/10.1038/nature09922.

Wang, Y., Li, Q., Wang, J., Zhuang, Q.K., Zhang, Y.Y., 2015. Combination of thrombolytic therapy and neuroprotective therapy in acute ischemic stroke: is it important? Eur. Rev. Med. Pharmacol. Sci. 19, 416–422.

Wang, W.-W., Wang, X.-S., Zhang, Z.-R., He, J.-C., Xie, C.-L., 2017. A meta-analysis of folic acid in combination with anti-hypertension drugs in patients with hypertension and hyperhomocysteinemia. Front. Pharmacol. 8, 585. Available from: https://doi.org/10.3389/fphar.2017.00585.

Winek, K., Dirnagl, U., Meisel, A., 2016. The gut microbiome as therapeutic target in central nervous system diseases: implications for stroke. Neurotherapeutics 13, 762–774. Available from: https://doi.org/10.1007/s13311-016-0475-x.

Woo, K.S., Chook, P., Lolin, Y.I., Sanderson, J.E., Metreweli, C., Celermajer, D.S., 1999. Folic acid improves arterial endothelial function in adults with hyperhomocystinemia. J. Am. Coll. Cardiol. 34, 2002–2006. Available from: https://doi.org/10.1016/S0735-1097(99)00469-6.

Zeisel, S.H., Da Costa, K.A., Franklin, P.D., Alexander, E.A., Lamont, J.T., Sheard, N.F., et al., 1991. Choline, an essential nutrient for humans. FASEB J. 5, 2093–2098. Available from: https://doi.org/10.1096/FASEBJ.5.7.2010061.

Zeng, R., Xu, C.-H., Xu, Y.-N., Wang, Y.-L., Wang, M., 2015. The effect of folate fortification on folic acid-based homocysteine-lowering intervention and stroke risk: a meta-analysis. Public Health Nutr. 18. Available from: https://doi.org/10.1017/S1368980014002134.

Zhang, X., Huang, G., Liu, H., Chang, H., Wilson, J.X., 2012. Folic acid enhances Notch signaling, hippocampal neurogenesis, and cognitive function in a rat model of cerebral ischemia. Nutr. Neurosci. 15, 55–61. Available from: https://doi.org/10.1179/1476830511Y.0000000025.

Zhang, Y., Zhu, T., Wang, L., Pan, Y.-H.H., Zhang, S., 2013. Homocysteine homeostasis and betaine-homocysteine *S*-methyltransferase expression in the brain of hibernating bats. PLoS One 8, e85632. Available from: https://doi.org/10.1371/journal.pone.0085632.

Zhao, Y., Huang, G., Chen, S., Gou, Y., Dong, Z., Zhang, X., 2016. Folic acid deficiency increases brain cell injury via autophagy enhancement after focal cerebral ischemia. J. Nutr. Biochem. Available from: https://doi.org/10.1016/j.jnutbio.2016.08.009.

Zhao, M., Wang, X., He, M., Qin, X., Tang, G., Huo, Y., et al., 2017. Homocysteine and stroke risk. Stroke 48, 1183–1190. Available from: https://doi.org/10.1161/STROKEAHA.116.015324.

Zhu, W., Wang, Z., Tang, W.H.W., Hazen, S.L., 2017. Gut microbe-generated trimethylamine N-oxide from dietary choline is prothrombotic in subjects. Circulation 135, 1671–1673. Available from: https://doi.org/10.1161/CIRCULATIONAHA.116.025338.

CHAPTER 14

Niacin and hyperlipidemia

Maria C. Naranjo[1], Maria C. Millan-Linares[2] and Sergio Montserrat-de la Paz[3]
[1]Department of Food Technology, School of Agricultural and Forest Engineering, University of Lleida, Lleida, Spain
[2]Cell Biology Unit, Instituto de la Grasa, CSIC, Seville, Spain
[3]Department of Medical Biochemistry, Molecular Biology, and Immunology, School of Medicine, University of Seville, Seville, Spain

Contents

Key facts

- This chapter focuses on the effects of niacin (vitamin B3) in disorders related to hyperlipidemia.
- Postprandial hyperlipidemia is a transitory and normal physiological event, which emerges from the response to the ingestion of a fatty meal.
- Zilversmit defined the concept of postprandial hyperlipidemia for the first time as an atherogenic phenomenon in 1979.
- Niacin has been defined as a broad spectrum lipid-modulating drug that raises fasting levels of plasma high-density lipoprotein cholesterol and reduces fasting levels of plasma triglycerides, low-density lipoprotein cholesterol, and lipoprotein [a].
- Growing evidence supports niacin leading to positive changes in fasting levels of plasma lipids and lipoproteins

Molecular Nutrition
DOI: https://doi.org/10.1016/B978-0-12-811907-5.00008-7

Abbreviations

CVDs	Cardiovascular diseases
FAs	Fatty acids
HCA_2	Hydroxycarboxylic acid receptor 2
HDL-C	High-density lipoprotein cholesterol
LDL-C	Low-density lipoprotein cholesterol
Lp[a]	Lipoprotein [a]
PGD_2	Prostaglandin D2
TG	Triglycerides
TRLs	Triglyceride-rich lipoproteins
VLDL	Very-low-density lipoproteins

14.1 Introduction

Cardiovascular diseases (CVDs) contribute to about 50% of deaths in Europe in spite of the considerable improvement in medical care (Chapman et al., 2011). Treatment of hyperlipoproteinemias, mainly caused by elevated fasting levels of plasma low-density lipoprotein cholesterol (LDL-C), and treatment of arterial hypertension are among the principal therapeutic goals in CVDs (Zeman et al., 2015). Although the objective for LDL-C is accomplished, the risk of suffering cardiovascular events (residual cardiovascular risk) remains raised ranging from 65% to 70% (Kearny et al., 2008). The residual cardiovascular risk has special significance in patients with high fasting levels of plasma triglyceride (TG) [very-low-density lipoprotein (VLDL)], apoB(100), small-dense low-density lipoprotein (LDL) particles, and lipoprotein (a) (Lp[a]), and low fasting levels of plasma high-density lipoprotein cholesterol (HDL-C) (Chapman et al., 2011).

Niacin has been applied for many years to prevent and treat CVDs (Song and FitzGerald, 2013). The well-known antiatherogenic activity of this drug is thought to result from its antidyslipidemic effects, which occur with unwanted adverse effects, for instance, flush (which is characterized by warmth, redness, itching, or tingling of the skin, especially on the face and neck). The detection of a niacin receptor expressed in immune cells, adipocytes, epidermal Langerhans cell, and retinal pigmented epithelium (Martin et al., 2009) has helped to clarify the mechanisms underlying the advantages while minimizing the side effects of niacin. Hence this chapter provides updated data on the pharmacological effects of niacin and discusses the function of niacin in disorders related to postprandial (nonfasting) hyperlipidemia.

14.2 Postprandial hyperlipidemia

Postprandial hyperlipidemia is a transitory and normal physiological event, which emerges from the response to the ingestion of a fatty meal. Dietary fat is absorbed by the enterocytes via specific transporters, such as cluster of differentiation 36 (CD36) for fatty acids (FAs), or passive diffusion. TG and other lipids have the assistance of apoB48 together with apolipoprotein IV and apolipoprotein AI to form postprandial TG-rich lipoproteins (TRLs) inside the enterocytes, in a process involving the microsomal TG transfer protein and FAs transport proteins. The intestinal secreted TRLs have the function of balancing the absorbed dietary lipids for transport in the aqueous plasma and to supply cells with exogenous FAs by receptors, such as the apoB48 receptor, LDL receptor, and LDL receptor-related protein, or nonreceptor-dependent mechanisms for energy and several metabolic pathways (Varela et al., 2013; Bermudez et al., 2011). The levels of plasma TG commonly peak 3 or 4 hours after a fat meal and are prone to return to baseline within 6–8 hours. Nonetheless, postprandial hyperlipidemia can become pathological when the dimension and length of the TRLs' response is exacerbated, with the accumulation of postprandial TRLs and their remnants in the circulation (Chan et al., 2013). In this sense, the postprandial hyperlipidemic peak may be two- or threefold greater and be extended, even up to 10–12 hours after the dietary fat ingestion (Cohn, 2006).

Zilversmit defined the concept of postprandial hyperlipidemia for the first time as an atherogenic phenomenon in 1979 (Zilversmit, 1979). This idea received greater awareness after the discovery of postprandial TRLs as cholesterol-independent atherogenic particles (Sniderman, 2000) and postprandial abnormalities in the TG metabolism as a hallmark of patients with established coronary heart disease (Patsch et al., 1992). The detection of postprandial TRLs, via apoB48, in human atheroma has supplied further evidence for their direct role in atherogenesis (Proctor et al., 2002). The greater the dimension and length of the postprandial TRLs' response, the greater the exposure of the arterial wall to postprandial TRLs and their remnants. Therefore the probability of TG replacing cholesteryl esters in LDL-C and HDL-C particles will be increased. Postprandial TRLs can penetrate the arterial wall and arrive at the subendothelial area, causing endothelial lipid (remarkably TG) deposits, the attraction of monocytes, the production of inflammatory markers, and oxidative stress (Pirillo et al., 2014). The role of TG in atherosclerosis-mediated inflammation depends on their direct vascular effects, but it is also associated with changes in the functionality of HDL-C. These modifications include protection against vessel inflammation or disorders of immune response (Patel et al., 2009). Prospective epidemiology on nonfasting levels of plasma TG in response to normal food intake includes three large-scale studies: the Copenhagen City Heart study (Lindman et al., 2010), Women's Health study (Boren et al., 2014), and the Norwegian counties study (Miller et al., 2008); all of them have revealed the following information: (1) nonfasting levels of plasma TG are raised among populations with established CVDs or with multiple risk factors predisposing to CVDs and (2) long-term follow-up of subjects in prospective, population-based studies related nonfasting and (less robustly) fasting TG to the incidence of CVDs events or deaths (Nordestgaard et al., 2007). Numerous patients with CVDs remain at high risk for CVDs events even if the LDL-C objective has been reached with lipid-lowering therapy (Bansal et al., 2007). This evidence suggests that nonfasting levels of plasma TG may be predictive and independent of traditional LDL-C related risk of CVDs.

The better understanding of the physiology and genetic regulation of postprandial TG metabolism could lead to new targets for therapy (Varbo et al., 2013). Nevertheless, the facts from randomized clinical trials on the benefits of lowering TG are far less robust than for the benefits of lowering LDL-C with statins (Miller et al., 2011; Catapano et al., 2011). This condition may be due to the lack of high-quality evidence for the advantages of TG-lowering drugs due to the absence of specific target objectives for both nonfasting and fasting levels of plasma TG. Suitable dietary changes, such as limited fat content, caloric restriction, restriction of alcohol intake, and increased exercise, could be essential for the management of high nonfasting (Lopez et al., 2008, 2011; Pacheco et al., 2006) and fasting (Chan et al., 2013; Berglund et al., 2012; Watts et al., 2013) levels of plasma TG. Current guidelines do not specify the atherogenic lipid profile in the postprandial period as a target for therapy, nor do they mention any target values for the parameters of postprandial hyperlipidemia. The first recommended pharmacological step to decrease prominent levels of plasma TG in individuals with high or very high CVDs risk based on global risk assessment is statin therapy, especially in subjects with metabolic syndrome and type 2 diabetes (Ryden et al., 2013). Statins also reduce nonfasting levels of plasma TG according to available data (Kolovou et al., 2011). It has been reported that ezetimibe decreases apoB48 secretion in the human intestine, suggesting a straight effect of this drug on the assembly of postprandial TRLs in enterocytes (Tremblay et al., 2009). Studies on fibrates have reported significant lowering of nonfasting levels of plasma TG in response to a standardized fat challenge (Chan et al., 2013; Kolovou et al., 2011). Additionally, fenofibrate also decreases the levels of plasma apoB48 and biomarkers for postprandial TRLs remnants (Chan et al., 2012).

Dual peroxisome proliferator-activated receptor (PPAR)α/PPARδ agonists, dietary oils rich in diacylglycerols, inhibitors of diacylglycerol-O-acyltransferase-1, and microsomal TG transfer protein, antisense oligonucleotides for apoB100, apoB48, and apolipoprotein CIII (apoCIII), and incretin-based treatments are new pharmacological and nonpharmacological approaches which could be applied alone or in combination with traditional therapies to maximize treatment for management of dyslipidemia due to high fasting and nonfasting levels of plasma TG (Chan et al., 2013). Nevertheless, these emerging agents require further testing in clinical trials in order to study in detail their clinical efficacy, mechanisms of action, safety, and tolerability.

14.3 Effects of niacin and mechanisms of action

Niacin, generally known as nicotinic acid or vitamin B3, is a water-soluble vitamin that belongs to the vitamin B complex. This vitamin is converted in vivo to a coenzyme involved in lipid catabolism, nicotinamide adenine dinucleotide (NAD +) (Liu et al., 2015). The US recommended Daily Allowance for adults ranges between 16 and 18 mg/day in accordance with the National Institutes of Health, which is far away from the pharmacologically active hypolipidemic dosage, 1–3 g/day (Zeman et al., 2015). Altschul et al. (1955) was the first to report the cholesterol-lowering effects of niacin. Since then, niacin has been defined as a broad spectrum lipid-modulating drug that raises fasting levels of plasma HDL-C and reduces fasting levels of plasma TG, LDL-C, and Lp[a] (Vosper, 2009). Indeed niacin was the first cholesterol-lowering drug shown to reduce cardiovascular events, cardiovascular mortality, and all-cause mortality (Canner et al., 1986). Nonetheless, these lipid-modifying effects have been accompanied by side effects such as cephalea, gastrointestinal discomfort, pruritus, and flush possibly mediated by prostaglandin D2 (PGD_2) and prostaglandin E2 and are among the mainly inconvenient of the niacin administration declining compliance with the treatment

(Rhodes et al., 2013). Flushing depends on the tolerance and compromises the activation of various members of the transient receptor potential vanilloid (TRPV) subfamily of TRP ion channels, called TRPV1 and TRPV3, which appear analogous to the consumption of spicy food (for instance, in response to the capsaicin of chili peppers) (Clifton et al., 2015; Ma et al., 2014, 2015). These new findings reexamine the earlier issues of how to mitigate flushing in the maintenance of niacin therapy (Cooper et al., 2015a,b). Table 14.1 displays a detailed description of the main effects of niacin on fasting levels of plasma lipids and cardiovascular events from randomized controlled trials (Canner et al., 1986; Anonymous, 1975: 36, 37, Creider et al., 2012; Carlson et al., 1977; Blankenhorm et al., 1987; Brown et al., 2001; Taylor et al., 2004, 2009; Whitney et al., 2005; Boden et al., 2011; Landray et al., 2014). The smaller scale studies led to the testing of the multiple beneficial effects of niacin monotherapy on circulating lipoproteins, principally on increasing fasting levels of plasma HDL-C (Blankenhorm et al., 1987; Brown et al., 2001; Taylor et al., 2004, 2009; Whitney et al., 2005), and two large randomized trials studied the clinical efficacy and safety of a high dose (up to 2 g) of niacin alone (AIM-HIGH Study) (Boden et al., 2011) or in combination with the PGD_2 receptor-1 antagonist laropiprant (HPS2-THRIVE Study) (Landray et al., 2014) in the setting of intensive statin therapy to keep low levels of plasma LDL-C. The addition of niacin or niacin/laropiprant to the statin treatment had no additional clinical benefits in spite of the improvement in the plasma lipid profile, including the increase in the fasting levels of plasma HDL-C. However, a large number of adverse effects were reported (Anderson et al., 2014). This discordance between niacin and statins seems to be an unresolved concern. The findings of the niacin receptor GPR109A, recently recalled hydroxycarboxylic acid receptor 2 (HCA_2) (Offermanns et al., 2011) has opened up new research lines into the mechanisms through which niacin may exert its pharmacological effects (Yasuda et al., 2015). The role of statins on HCA_2-mediated signaling networks at both fasting and nonfasting conditions would be an interesting issue to study the negative interaction mentioned above in future research. In the HPS2-THRIVE trial, laropiprant was employed to delay flushing, which is at least mediated by HCA_2 and the capsaicin receptor TRPV1 ion channel. The stimulation of HCA_2 by niacin triggers a cascade of distal connected enzymes which include the cytosolic phospholipase A_2 for the liberation of endogenous arachidonic acid from the cell membrane, the constitutive cyclooxygenase isoform 1

Table 14.1 Basic characteristics of controlled clinical studies with niacin.

Study[a]	Study population	Duration	Treatment	Changes in lipids	Cardiovascular effects
CDP [a]	8341 M after MI	6 years	Niacin or clofibrate versus placebo	TC ↓ by 9.9% TAG ↓ by 26.1%	↓ Nonfatal MI by 27% ↓ Cerebrovascular events by 24%
Stockholm trial [b]	558 patients after MI, aged <70	4 years	Clofibrate 2 × 1 g + niacin 3 × 1 g versus placebo	TC ↓ by 26% TAG ↓ by 30%	↓ Nonfatal MI by 50%
CDP follow-up [c]		15 years			↓ Mortality by 11%
CLAS [d]	162 M after CABG	2 years 4 years	Niacin 3–12 g/day + colestipol 30 g/day versus placebo	TC ↓ 15%–20 % LDL-C ↓ by 43% HDL-C ↑ by 31%	In 16.2% of patients net atherosclerotic regression at 2 years and 17.9% at 4 years, compared with 2.4% and 6.4%, respectively in the placebo group ($P = .002$ and $P = .04$)
HATS [e]	160 patients with CAD and low HDL-C[b]	3 years	Group A: simvastatin 10–20 mg/day plus niacin 2–4 g/day Group B: antioxidant Group C: simvastatin + niacin + antioxidant Group D: placebo	↓LDL-C by 42% ↑ HDL-C by 42% (group A)	Group A: regression of the most severe stenosis in proximal coronary segments by 0.4% versus placebo ($P < .0001$); ↓ the composite clinical end point[a] by 88% ($P = .03$)
ARBITER-2 [f]	167 patients with CAD and HDL-C <1.17 mmol/L	1 years	ER-niacin 1 g/day versus placebo + stable statin therapy	↑ HDL-C by 21%	↓ Progression of cIMT in niacin group without insulin resistance ($P = .026$)

(*Continued*)

Table 14.1 (Continued)

Study[a]	Study population	Duration	Treatment	Changes in lipids	Cardiovascular effects
ARBITER-6 [g]	208 patients (30 years) with CAD or equivalent of CAD risk	1.2 years	ER-niacin versus ezetimibe + preexisting statin therapy	↓ LDL-C more pronounced in EZE (20% vs 12%, $P = .01$) ↑ HDL-C more pronounced in ERN (+18% vs −7% in EZE, $P = .001$)	↓ Incidence of cardiovascular events by 5% in ERN versus 1% in EZE ($P = .04$)
AFREGS [h]	143 patients (<76 years) with low HDL-C and coronary disease	30 months	Niacin 0.25−3 g gemfibrozil 1.2 g cholestyramine 2 g versus placebo	26% decrease in LDL-C and 36% increase in HDL-C	13.7% decrease of combined cardiovascular events (MI, hospitalization for angina, TIA, stroke, death, and cardiovascular procedures ($P = .04$)
AIM-HIGH [i]	3414 patients (45 years) with CVD	3 years	ER-niacin (1.5−2.0 g/day) versus placebo (+ preexisting statin therapy with/without ezetimibe)	Higher decrease in LDL-C and TAG (14% vs 8% and 31% vs 10%) and higher increase in HDL-C (25% vs 12%) in ERN	No significant difference in the incidence of cardiovascular events

HPS2-THRIVE [j]	25,673 patients (aged 50–80) with history of MI/stroke/PAD, or DM with CAD	3.9 years	Baseline therapy: simvastatin 40 mg with/without ezetimibe ER-niacin/laropiprant (2 g/40 mg) or placebo	ERN/LPT: decrease in LDL-C by 10%, TAG by 33%, increase in HDL-C by 6%	No evidence for benefit in addition of ERN/LPT to effective LDL lowering statin therapy on primary cardiovascular end points[c,d]

[a]Citation follows the study acronym: *apoB*, Apolipoprotein B; *CABG*, coronary artery bypass grafting; *CAD*, coronary artery disease; *CVD*, cardiovascular diseases; *DM*, diabetes mellitus; *ER*, extended release; *MI*, myocardial infarction; *PAD*, peripheral arterial disease.

[b]For men < 0.9 mmol/L, for women < 1.04 mmol/L.

[c]Coronary death, MI or stroke, or revascularization.

[d]Nonfatal MI or coronary death, stroke, or revascularization. *apoB*, Apolipoprotein B; *cIMT*, carotid intima-media thickness; *ERN*, ER-niacin; *EZE*. ezetimibe; *LPT*, laropiprant; *MI*, myocardial infarction; ↓ – decrease; ↑ – increase.

[a]Anonymous, 1975
[b]Carlson et al., 1977
[c]Canner et al., 1986
[d]Blankenhorm et al., 1987
[e]Brown et al., 2001
[f]Taylor et al., 2004
[g]Taylor et al., 2009
[h]Whitney et al., 2005
[i]Boden et al., 2011
[j]Landray et al., 2014

Source: Adapted from Montserrat-de la Paz, S., Bermudez, B., Naranjo, M.C., Lopez, S., Abia, R., Muriana, F.J.G., 2016. Pharmacological effects of niacin on acute hyperlipidemia. Curr. Med. Chem. 23, 2826–2835.

and the inducible cyclooxygenase isoform 2 as the rate-limiting stage for the conversion of arachidonic acid into the unsteady cyclic endoperoxide prostaglandin H_2 (PGH_2), and the prostaglandin synthase for the isomerization of PGH_2 to be transformed into PGD_2 (Fig. 14.1; Montserrat-de la Paz et al., 2016).

Niacin decreases the levels of plasma TG and apoB100-containing lipoproteins (VLDL and LDL-C), chiefly by the partial inhibition of lipolysis from the adipose tissue, leading to a lower flux of free FAs to the liver (Fig. 14.2; Montserrat-de la Paz et al., 2016). The exact mechanism by which this is accomplished remains unidentified, but upon binding to niacin, HCA_2 is activated via the G_i family members of heterotrimeric G proteins. This step triggers an inhibitory effect on adenylyl cyclases and a reduction of intracellular cyclic adenosine monophosphate (cAMP) levels. The activity of the cAMP-dependent protein kinase A is decreased, and the phosphorylation of its target hormone-sensitive lipase, which is the primary lipase responsible for the hydrolysis of TG, is damaged (Linke et al., 2009). A decrease in free FAs to the liver inhibits the hepatic expression of PPARγ coactivator-1b (PGC-1b) and apoCIII. Reduced PGC-1b expression decreases the formation and secretion of VLDL (Barroso et al., 2011). The decreased expression of apoCIII may reduce the levels of plasma VLDL and LDL-C by a quick turnover. Moreover, niacin decreases the liver fat contents and VLDL synthesis via the inhibition of microsomal diacylglycerol O-acyltransferase 2, a key enzyme which catalyzes the last reaction in TG synthesis (Kamanna et al., 2013; Le Bloc'h et al., 2010). Niacin has been reported to transiently upregulate CD36, FATP2, and FATP4 gene expression in human enterocyte-like Caco-2 cells at intestinal levels, supporting the idea that niacin may promote the FAs uptake (Riedel et al., 2014).

HDL-C has an essential role in reverse cholesterol transport but its antiinflammatory, antioxidative, antithrombotic, and antiapoptotic functions must also be highlighted (Navab et al., 2007). Niacin is one of the most effective molecules for increasing low levels of plasma HDL-C (Vosper, 2009; Vega and Grundy, 1994). Apart from its effects on the levels of plasma VLDL, niacin drives a change toward larger HDL subpopulations particles, indicating a modulation of the HDL-TG metabolism (Lamon-Fava et al., 2008). This effect is partially due to an increase of HDL apoAI production; the mechanism of action is still under debate, but the liver and adipose tissue seem to be key players. Hepatic apoAI secretion by niacin has been proposed to take place via the activation of

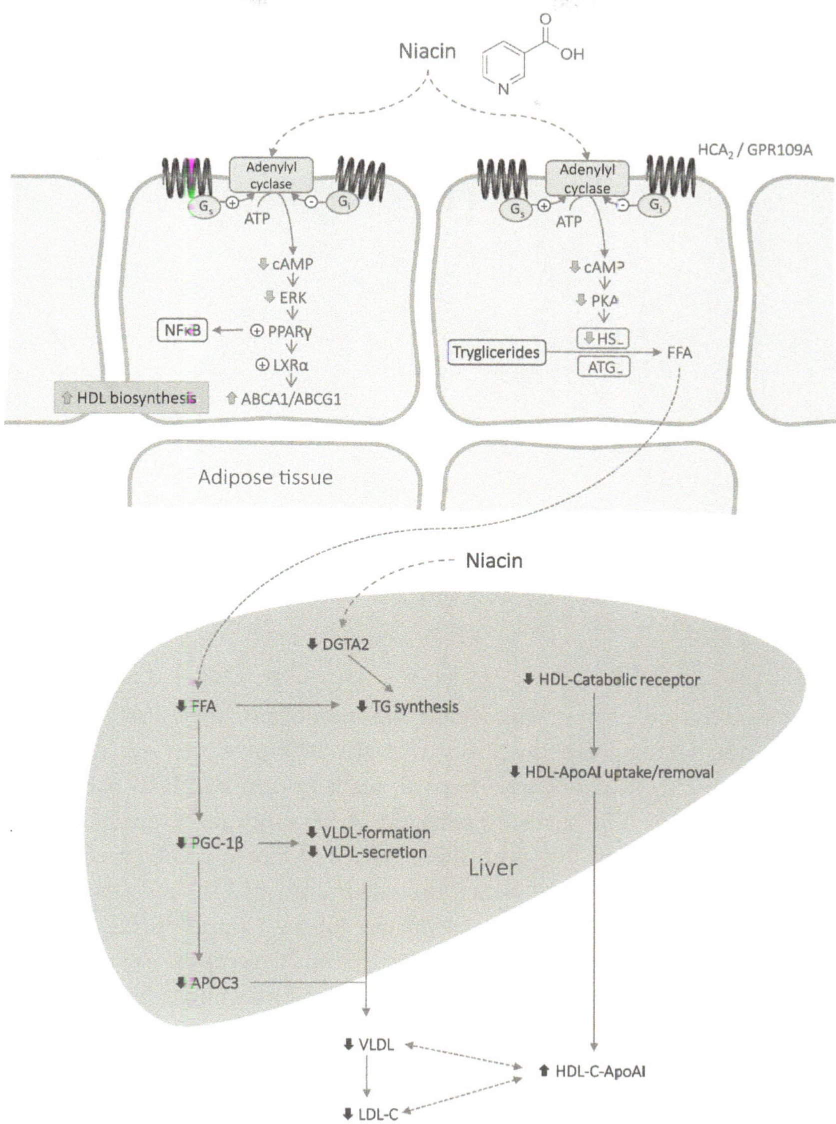

Figure 14.1 Mechanism of niacin-induced flushing by activation of HCA_2 on epidermal Langerhans cells and keratinocytes. *Adapted from Montserrat-de la Paz, S., Bermudez, B., Naranjo, M.C., Lopez, S., Abia, R., Muriana, F.J.G., 2016. Pharmacological effects of niacin on acute hyperlipidemia. Curr. Med. Chem. 23, 2826–2835.*

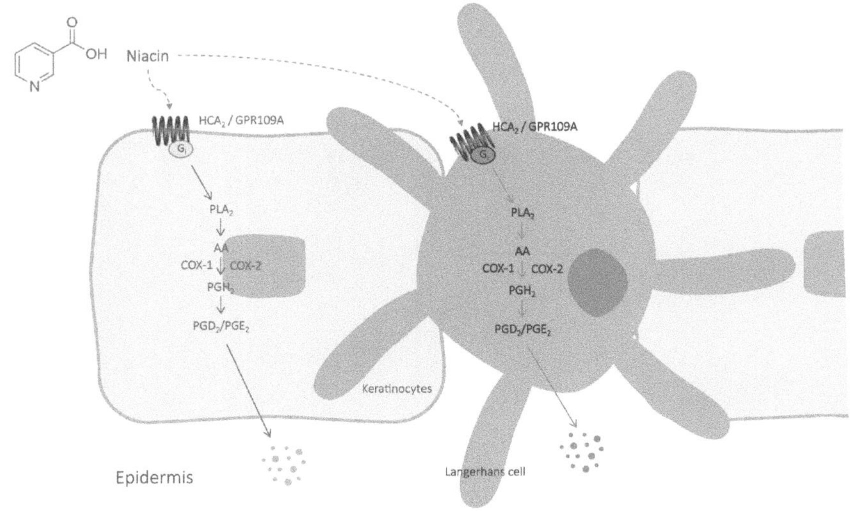

Figure 14.2 Potential mechanisms underlying the antidyslipidemic effects of niacin. *Adapted from Montserrat-de la Paz, S., Bermudez, B., Naranjo, M.C., Lopez, S., Abia, R., Muriana, F.J.G., 2016. Pharmacological effects of niacin on acute hyperlipidemia. Curr. Med. Chem. 23, 2826–2835.*

mitogen-activated protein kinase and the member of the PPAR family of transcription factors (van der Hoorn et al., 2008). Moreover, niacin has been demonstrated to decrease hepatic reabsorption of HDL particles by the inhibition of the surface-expressed ATP-synthase β-chains (Zhang et al., 2008). This is in line with the capacity of niacin to block the apoAI fractional catabolic rate and hence the catabolism of HDL-C (Pang et al., 2014). It is worth pointing out that niacin (up to 1 mmol/L for 24 hours) can provoke the expression of PPARγ, liver X receptor α, and ATP-binding cassette transport A1 in adipocytes, and the cholesterol efflux to apoAI from the cells (Wu and Zhao, 2009).

In previous studies, the applications of immediate- (King et al., 1994) or extended- (O'Keefe et al., 1995) release forms of niacin were demonstrated to concern the postprandial metabolism of dietary fats in subjects with normal or high fasting levels of plasma TG. Niacin (3 g/day) was supplied for 12 weeks and later a postprandial study was performed. Both treatments led to a significant diminution in the nonfasting levels of plasma TG. It is worth pointing out that postprandial hyperlipidemia was instantly enhanced after the start of the treatment, whereas the effects on fasting levels of plasma total cholesterol were evident after various days of treatment (Carlson et al., 1968). Additionally, it has been recently found out that 2 g of a single dose of extended-release niacin 1 hour prior to a high-fat meal, also decreases nonfasting levels of plasma TG in healthy subjects (Usman et al., 2012).

An inherent characteristic of diabetic dyslipidemia is a high nonfasting level of plasma TG, via exaggerated peak level or delayed clearance, and this condition regularly appears even in diabetic patients with normal fasting levels of plasma TG (Tentolouris et al., 2007). A recent study evaluated the effect of niacin on postprandial hyperlipidemia in men with type 2 diabetes and high fasting levels of plasma TG to estimate the residual risk in the dyslipidemic diabetic population (Ooi et al., 2015). The subjects had lower levels of plasma TG during the postprandial state after 12 weeks of treatment with the extended-release form of niacin (1–2 g/day). The reduction of TG postprandial reflected the growth in the levels of plasma HDL-C. The effects of both niacin and aerobic exercise on postprandial TG and insulin have been investigated in men with metabolic syndrome (Plaisance et al., 2008), which is the collection of three or more cardiovascular risk factors, including obesity, insulin resistance, hypertension, and dyslipidemia (Lusis et al., 2008). It is usual that individuals with metabolic syndrome have elevated fasting levels of plasma TG. Surprisingly, 6 weeks of extended-release niacin decreased the peak of TG by 18% and the total area-under-the-curve for TG by 23%, but mitigated the postprandial TG-lowering effect of moderate-intensity aerobic exercise execution 1 hour prior to the ingestion of a high-fat meal. The buffering effect of niacin on aerobic exercise-induced reduction of nonfasting levels of plasma TG emphasizes the limitations of pharmacological and nonpharmacological approaches for the control of hyperlipidemia when homeostatic mechanisms are overwhelmed in lipid metabolism.

The kinetics of apoB100 and apoB48 have been studied in different lipoprotein fractions of individuals with combined hyperlipidemia in order to clarify the mechanistic effects of niacin on nonfasting levels of plasma TG (Lamon-Fava et al., 2008). Treatment with extended-release niacin (2 g/day) for 12 weeks resulted in a decrease of plasma TG but also in an increase of apoB100 and apoB48 fractional catabolic values in TRLs, both in fasting and nonfasting states. ApoB100 or apoB48 production rate were not affected by niacin, indicating that the hepatic catabolism of postprandial TRLs is a substantial mechanism in the regulation of acute hyperlipidemia by niacin. Supporting the intensified catabolism of TRLs, earlier in vitro studies in HepG2 cells have exhibited that niacin (up to

3 mmol/L for 2 hours) may support the posttranslational degradation of apoB in hepatocytes (Jin et al., 1999). Nevertheless, further studies are required to understand the accurate dynamic mechanism whereby niacin modulates the postprandial metabolism of dietary fats.

14.4 Conclusion

The control of hyperlipidemia is an urgent necessity due to the progressive relationship between the overstated nonfasting levels of plasma TG, which are a feature of impaired metabolism of dietary fats, and CVDs. There is not a clear limit for harmful effects connected to hyperlipidemia during the postprandial period. Hence early treatment of an excessive increase of TG and/or delayed TG clearance is of the utmost importance, specifically in diseases linked with abnormalities of lipid metabolism. According to this data, growing evidence supports niacin leading to positive changes in fasting levels of plasma lipids and lipoproteins. Additionally, niacin has been shown to improve the levels of plasma TG during the postprandial state. Further research at the molecular level is needed to delimit the relationship between the clinical evidence of niacin benefits on postprandial lipid profile and the mechanisms implicated to maintain correctly the health.

Acknowledgments

S.M. acknowledges financial support from "V Own Research Plan" (University of Seville).

References

Altschul, R., Hoffer, A., Stephen, J.D., 1955. Influence of nicotinic acid on serum cholesterol in man. Arch. Biochem. Biophys. 54, 558–559.

Anderson, T.J., Boden, W.E., Desvigne-Nickens, P., Fleg, J.L., Kashyap, M.L., McBride, R., et al., 2014. Safety profile of extended-release niacin in the AIM-HIGH trial. N. Engl. J. Med. 371, 288–290.

Anonymous, 1975. Clofibrate and niacin in coronary heart disease. JAMA 231, 360–381.

Bansal, S., Buring, J.E., Rifai, N., Mora, S., Sacks, F.M., Ridker, P.M., 2007. Fasting compared with nonfasting triglycerides and risk of cardiovascular events in women. JAMA 298, 309–316.

Barroso, E., Rodríguez-Calvo, R., Serrano-Marco, L., Astudillo, A.M., Balsinde, J., Palomer, X., et al., 2011. The PPARβ/δ activator GW501516 prevents the downregulation of AMPK caused by a high-fat diet in liver and amplifies the PGC-1α-lipin 1-PPARα pathway leading to increased fatty acid oxidation. Endocrinology 152, 1848–1859.

Berglund, L., Brunzell, J.D., Goldberg, A.C., Goldberg, I.J., Sacks, F., Murad, M.H., et al., 2012. Endocrine Society. Evaluation and treatment of hypertriglyceridemia: an Endocrine Society clinical practice guideline. J. Clin. Endocrinol. Metab. 97, 2969–2989.
Bermudez, B., Lopez, S., Ortega, A., Varela, L.M., Pacheco, Y.M., Abia, R., et al., 2011. Oleic acid in olive oil: from a metabolic framework toward a clinical perspective. Curr. Pharm. Des. 17, 831–843.
Blankenhorn, D.H., Nessim, S.A., Johnson, R.L., Sanmarco, M.E., Azen, S.P., Cashin-Hemphill, L., 1987. Beneficial effects of combined colestipol-niacin therapy on coronary atherosclerosis and coronary venous bypass grafts. JAMA 257, 3233–3240.
Boden, W.E., Probstfield, I.L., Anderson, T., Chaitman, B.R., Desvignes-Nickens, P., Koprowicz, K., et al., 2011. Niacin in patients with low HDL cholesterol levels receiving intensive statin therapy. N. Engl. J. Med. 365, 2255–2267.
Boren, J., Matikainen, N., Adiels, M., Taskinen, M.R., 2014. Postprandial hypertriglyceridemia as a coronary risk factor. Clin. Chim. Acta 431, 131–142.
Brown, B.G., Zhao, X.Q., Chait, A., Fisher, L.D., Cheung, M.C., Morse, J.S., et al., 2001. Simvastatin and niacin, antioxidant vitamins, or the combination for the prevention of coronary disease. N. Engl. J. Med. 345, 1583–1589.
Canner, P.L., Berger, K.G., Wenger, N.K., Stamler, J., Friedman, L., Prineas, R.J., et al., 1986. Fifteen year mortality in Coronary Drug Project patients: long-term benefit with niacin. J. Am. Coll. Cardiol. 8, 1245–1255.
Carlson, L.A., Oro, L., Ostman, J., 1968. Effect of nicotinic acid on plasma lipids in patients with hyperlipoproteinemia during the first week of treatment. J. Atheroscler. Res. 8, 667–677.
Carlson, L.A., Danielson, M., Ekberg, I., Klintermar, B., Rosenhamer, G., 1977. Reduction of myocardial reinfarction by the combined treatment with clofibrate and nicotinic acid. Atherosclerosis. 28, 81–86.
Catapano, A.L., Reiner, Z., De Backer, G., Graham, I., Taskinen, M.R., Wiklund, O., et al., 2011. European Society of Cardiology (ESC); and the European Atherosclerosis Society (EAS). ESC/EAS guidelines for the management of dyslipidaemias: the Task Force for the management of dyslipidaemias of the European Society of Cardiology (ESC) and the European Atherosclerosis Society (EAS). Atherosclerosis 217, 3–46.
Chan, D.C., Wong, A.T., Yamashita, S., Watts, G.F., 2012. Apolipoprotein B-48 as a determinant of endothelial function in obese subjects with type 2 diabetes mellitus: effect of fenofibrate treatment. Atherosclerosis. 221, 484–489.
Chan, D.C., Pang, J., Romic, G., Watts, G.F., 2013. Postprandial hypertriglyceridemia and cardiovascular disease: current and future therapies. Curr. Atheroscler. Rep. 15, 309–317.
Chapman, M.J., Ginsberg, H.N., Amarenco, P., Andreotti, F., Boren, J., Catapano, A.L., et al., 2011. Triglyceride-rich lipoproteins and high-density lipoprotein cholesterol in patients at high risk of cardiovascular disease: evidence and guidance for management. Eur. Heart J. 32, 1345–1361.
Clifton, H.L., Inceoglu, B., Ma, L., Zheng, J., Schaefer, S., 2015. TRPV1 channels are involved in niacin-induced cutaneous vasodilation in mice. J. Cardiovasc. Pharmacol. 65, 184–191.
Cohn, J.S., 2006. Postprandial lipemia and remnant lipoproteins. Clin. Lab. Med. 26, 773–786.
Cooper, D.L., Murrell, D.E., Roane, D.S., Harirforoosh, S., 2015a. Effects of formulation design on niacin therapeutics: mechanism of action, metabolism, and drug delivery. Int. J. Pharm. 490, 55–64.
Cooper, D.L., Carmical, J.A., Panus, P.C., Harirforoosh, S., 2015b. Formulation and in vitro evaluation of niacin-loaded nanoparticles to reduce prostaglandin mediated vasodilatory flushing. Eur. Rev. Med. Pharmacol. Sci. 19, 3977–3988.

Creider, J.C., Hegele, R.A., Joy, T.R., 2012. Niacin: another look at underutilized lipid-lowering medication. Nat. Rev. Endocrinol. 8, 517–528.

Jin, F.Y., Kamanna, V.S., Kashyap, M.L., 1999. Niacin accelerates intracellular apoB degradation by inhibiting triacylglycerol synthesis in human hepatoblastoma (HepG2) cells. Arterioscler. Thromb. Vasc. Biol. 19, 1051–1059.

Kamanna, V.S., Ganji, S.H., Kashyap, M.L., 2013. Recent advances in niacin and lipid metabolism. Curr. Opin. Lipidol. 24, 239–245.

Kearny, P.M., Blackwell, L., Collins, R., Keech, A., Simes, J., Peto, R., et al., 2008. Efficacy of cholesterol-lowering therapy in 18686 people with diabetes in 14 randomised trials of statins: a meta-analysis. Lancet 371, 117–125.

King, J., Crouse, J., Terry, J., Morgan, T., Spray, B., Miller, N., 1994. Evaluation of effects of unmodified niacin on fasting and postprandial plasma lipids in normolipidemic men with hypoalphalipoproteinemia. Am. J. Med. 97, 323–331.

Kolovou, G.D., Mikhailidis, D.P., Kovar, J., Lairon, D., Nordestgaard, B.G., Ooi, T.C., et al., 2011. Assessment and clinical relevance of non-fasting and postprandial triglycerides: an expert panel statement. Curr. Vasc. Pharmacol. 9, 258–270.

Lamon-Fava, S., Diffenderfer, M.R., Barrett, P.H.R., Buchsbaum, A., Nyaku, M., Horvath, K.V., et al., 2008. Extended-release niacin alters the metabolism of plasma apolipoprotein (apo) A-I and apoB-containing lipoproteins. Arterioscler. Thromb. Vasc. Biol. 28, 1672–1678.

Landray, M.J., Haynes, R., Hopewell, J.C., Parish, S., Aung, T., Tomson, J., et al., 2014. Effects of extended-release niacin with laropiprant in high-risk patients. N. Engl. J. Med. 371, 203–212.

Le Bloc'h, J., Leray, V., Chetiveaux, M., Freuchet, B., Magot, T., Krempf, M., et al., 2010. Nicotinic acid decreases apolipoprotein B100-containing lipoprotein levels by reducing hepatic very low density lipoprotein secretion through a possible diacylglycerol acyltransferase 2 inhibition in obese dogs. J. Pharmacol. Exp. Ther. 334, 583–589.

Lindman, A.S., Veierod, M.B., Tverdal, A., Pedersen, J.L., Selmer, R., 2010. Nonfasting triglycerides and risk of cardiovascular death in men and women from the Norwegian counties study. Eur. J. Epidemiol. 25, 789–798.

Linke, A., Sonnabend, M., Fasshauer, M., Hollriegel, R., Schuler, G., Niebauer, J., et al., 2009. Effects of extended-release niacin on lipid profile and adipocyte biology in patients with impaired glucose tolerance. Atherosclerosis 205, 207–213.

Liu, D., Wang, X., Kong, L., Chen, Z., 2015. Nicotinic acid regulates glucose and lipi metabolism through lipid independent pathways. Curr. Pharm. Biotechnol. 16, 3–10.

Lopez, S., Bermudez, B., Pacheco, Y.M., Villar, J., Abia, R., Muriana, F.J., 2008. Distinctive postprandial modulation of beta cell function and insulin sensitivity by dietary fats: monounsaturated compared with saturated fatty acids. Am. J. Clin. Nutr. 88, 638–644.

Lopez, S., Bermudez, B., Ortega, A., Varela, L.M., Pacheco, Y.M., Villar, J., et al., 2011. Effects of meals rich in either monounsaturated or saturated fat on lipid concentrations and on insulin secretion and action in subjects with high fasting triglyceride concentrations. Am. J. Clin. Nutr. 93, 494–499.

Lusis, A.J., Attie, A.D., Reue, K., 2008. Metabolic syndrome: from epidemiology to systems biology. Nat. Rev. Genet. 9, 819–830.

Ma, L., Lee, B.H., Mao, R., Cai, A., Jia, Y., Clifton, H., et al., 2014. Nicotinic acid activates the capsaicin receptor TRPV1. Potential mechanism for cutaneous flushing. Arterioscler. Thromb. Vasc. Biol. 34, 1272–1280.

Ma, L., Lee, B.H., Clifton, H., Schaefer, S., Zheng, J., 2015. Nicotinic acid is a common regulator of heat-sensing TRPV1-4 ion channels. Sci. Rep. 5, 8906.

Martin, P.M., Ananth, S., Cresci, G., Roon, P., Smith, S., Ganapathy, V., 2009. Expression and localization of GPR109A (PUMA-G/HM74A) mRNA and protein in mammalian retinal pigment epithelium. Mol. Vis. 15, 362–372.

Miller, M., Cannon, C.P., Murphy, S.A., Qin, J., Ray, K.K., Braunwald, E., 2008. Impact of triglyceride levels beyond low-density lipoprotein cholesterol after acute coronary syndrome in the PROVE IT-TIMI 22 trial. J. Am. Coll. Cardiol. 51, 724–730.

Miller, M., Stone, N.J., Ballantyne, C., Bittner, V., Criqui, M.H., Ginsberg, H.N., et al., 2011. Triglycerides and cardiovascular disease. Circulation 123, 2292–2333.

Montserrat-de la Paz, S., Bermudez, B., Naranjo, M.C., Lopez, S., Abia, R., Muriana, F.J. G., 2016. Pharmacological effects of niacin on acute hyperlipidemia. Curr. Med. Chem. 23, 2826–2835.

Navab, M., Yu, R., Gharavi, N., Huang, W., Ezra, N., Lotfizadeh, A., et al., 2007. High-density lipoprotein: antioxidant and anti-inflammatory properties. Curr. Atheroscler. Rep. 9, 244–248.

Nordestgaard, B.G., Benn, M., Schnohr, P., Tybjaerg-Hansen, A., 2007. Nonfasting triglycerides and risk of myocardial infarction, ischemic heart disease, and death in men and women. JAMA 298, 299–308.

Offermanns, S., Colletti, S.L., Lovenberg, T.W., Semple, G., Wise, A., IJzerman, A.P., 2011. International Union of Basic and Clinical Pharmacology. LXXXII: nomenclature and classification of hydroxy-carboxylic acid receptors (GPR81, GPR109A, and GPR109B). Pharmacol. Rev. 63, 269–290.

O'Keefe, J., Harris, W., Nelson, J., Windsor, S., 1995. Effects of pravastatin with niacin or magnesium on lipid levels and postprandial lipemia. Am. J. Cardiol. 76, 480–484.

Ooi, E.M., Watts, G.F., Chan, D.C., Pang, J., Tenneti, V.S., Hamilton, S.J., et al., 2015. Effects of extended-release niacin on postprandial metabolism of Lp(a) and ApoB-100-containing lipoproteins in statin-treated men with type 2 diabetes mellitus. Arterioscler. Thromb. Vasc. Biol. 35, 2686–2693.

Pacheco, Y.M., Bermudez, B., Lopez, S., Abia, R., Villar, J., Muriana, F.J., 2006. Ratio of oleic to palmitic acid is a dietary determinant of thrombogenic and fibrinolytic factors during the postprandial state in men. Am. J. Clin. Nutr. 84, 342–349.

Pang, J., Chan, D.C., Hamilton, S.J., Tenneti, V.S., Watts, G.F., Barrett, P.H., 2014. Effect of niacin on high-density lipoprotein apolipoprotein A-I kinetics in statin-treated patients with type 2 diabetes mellitus. Arterioscler. Thromb. Vasc. Biol. 34, 427–432.

Patel, S., Puranik, R., Nakhla, S., Lundman, P., Stocker, R., Wang, X.S., et al., 2009. Acute hypertriglyceridaemia in humans increases the triglyceride content and decreases the anti-inflammatory capacity of high density lipoproteins. Atherosclerosis 204, 424–428.

Patsch, J.R., Miesenbock, G., Hopferwieser, T., Muhlberger, V., Knapp, E., Dunn, J.K., et al., 1992. Relation of triglyceride metabolism and coronary artery disease. Studies in the postprandial state. Arterioscler. Thromb. 12, 1336–1345.

Pirillo, A., Norata, G.D., Catapano, A.L., 2014. Postprandial lipemia as a cardiometabolic risk factor. Curr. Med. Res. Opin. 30, 1489–1503.

Plaisance, E.P., Mestek, M.L., Mahurin, A.J., Taylor, J.K., Moncada-Jimenez, J., Grandjean, P.W., 2008. Postprandial triglyceride responses to aerobic exercise and extended-release niacin. Am. J. Clin. Nutr. 88, 30–37.

Proctor, S.D., Vine, D.F., Mamo, J.C., 2002. Arterial retention of apolipoprotein B(48)- and B(100)-containing lipoproteins in atherogenesis. Curr. Opin. Lipidol. 13, 461–470.

Rhodes, T., Norquist, J.M., Sisk, C.M., McQuarrie, K., Trovato, A., Liao, J., et al., 2013. The association of flushing bother, impact, treatment satisfaction and discontinuation of niacin therapy. Int. J. Clin. Pract. 67, 1238–1246.

Riedel, A., Lang, R., Rohm, B., Rubach, M., Hofmann, T., Somoza, V., 2014. Structure-dependent effects of pyridine derivatives on mechanisms of intestinal fatty acid uptake: regulation of nicotinic acid receptor and fatty acid transporter expression. J. Nutr. Biochem. 25, 750–757.

Ryden, L., Grant, P.J., Anker, S.D., Berne, C., Cosentino, F., Danchin, N., et al., 2013. ESC Guidelines on diabetes, pre-diabetes, and cardiovascular diseases developed in collaboration with the EASD: the Task Force on diabetes, pre-diabetes, and cardiovascular diseases of the European Society of Cardiology (ESC) and developed in collaboration with the European Association for the Study of Diabetes (EASD). Eur. Heart J. 34, 3035–3087.

Sniderman, A.D., 2000. Postprandial hypertriglyceridemia(s): time to enlarge our pathophysiologic perspective. Eur. J. Clin. Invest. 30, 935–937.

Song, W.L., FitzGerald, G.A., 2013. Niacin, an old drug with a new twist. J. Lipid Res. 54, 2586–2594.

Taylor, A.J., Sullenberger, L.E., Lee, H.J., Grace, K.A., 2004. Arterial biology for the investigation of the treatment effects of reducing cholesterol (ARBITER) 2: a double-blind, placebo-controlled study of extended release niacin on atherosclerosis progression in secondary prevention patients treated with statins. Circulation 110, 3512–3517.

Taylor, A.J., Villines, T.C., Stanek, E.J., Devine, P.J., Griffen, L., Miller, M., et al., 2009. Extended-release niacin or ezetimibe and carotid intima-media thickness. N. Engl. J. Med. 361, 2113–2122.

Tentolouris, N., Stylianou, A., Lourida, E., Perrea, D., Kyriaki, D., Papavasiliou, E.C., et al., 2007. High postprandial triglyceridemia in patients with type 2 diabetes and microalbuminuria. J. Lipid Res. 48, 218–225.

Tremblay, A.J., Lamarche, B., Hogue, J.C., Couture, P., 2009. Effects of ezetimibe and simvastatin on apolipoprotein B metabolism in males with mixed hyperlipidemia. J. Lipid Res. 50, 1463–1471.

Usman, M.H.U., Qamar, A., Gadi, R., Lilly, S., Goel, H., Hampson, J., et al., 2012. Extended-release niacin acutely suppresses postprandial triglyceridemia. Am. J. Med. 125, 1026–1035.

van der Hoorn, J.W., de Haan, W., Berbee, J.F., Havekes, L.M., Jukema, J.W., Rensen, P.C., et al., 2008. Niacin increases HDL by reducing hepatic expression and plasma levels of cholesteryl ester transfer protein in APOE*3Leiden.CETP mice. Arterioscler. Thromb. Vasc. Biol. 28, 2016–2022.

Varbo, A., Benn, M., Tybjaerg-Hansen, A., Jorgensen, A.B., Frikke-Schmidt, R., Nordestgaard, B.G., 2013. Remnant cholesterol as a causal risk factor for ischemic heart disease. J. Am. Coll. Cardiol. 61, 427–436.

Varela, L.M., Ortega-Gomez, A., Lopez, S., Abia, R., Muriana, F.J., Bermudez, B., 2013. The effects of dietary fatty acids on the postprandial triglyceride-rich lipoprotein/apoB48 receptor axis in human monocyte/macrophage cells. J. Nutr. Biochem. 24, 2031–2039.

Vega, G.L., Grundy, S.M., 1994. Lipoprotein responses to treatment with lovastatin, gemfibrozil, and nicotinic acid in normolipidemic patients with hypoalphalipoproteinemia. Arch. Intern. Med. 154, 73–82.

Vosper, H., 2009. Niacin: a re-emerging pharmaceutical for the treatment of dyslipidaemia. Br. J. Pharmacol. 158, 429–441.

Watts, G.F., Ooi, E.M., Chan, D.C., 2013. Demystifying the management of hypertriglyceridaemia. Nat. Rev. Cardiol. 10, 648–661.

Whitney, E.J., Krasuski, R.A., Personius, B.E., Michalek, J.E., Maranian, A.M., Kolasa, M.W., et al., 2005. Randomized trial of a strategy for increasing high-density lipoprotein cholesterol levels: effect on progression of coronary heart disease and clinical events. Ann. Intern. Med. 142, 95–104.

Wu, Z.H., Zhao, S.P., 2009. Niacin promotes cholesterol efflux through stimulation of the PPARgamma-LXRalpha-ABCA1 pathway in 3T3-L1 adipocytes. Pharmacology 84, 282–287.

Yasuda, D., Imura, Y., Ishii, S., Shimizu, T., Nakamura, M., 2015. The atypical N-glycosylation motif, Asn-Cys-Cys, in human GPR109A is required for normal cell surface expression and intracellular signaling. FASEB J. 29, 2412–2422.

Zeman, M., Vecka, M., Perlik, F., Hromadka, R., Stankova, B., Tvrzicka, E., et al., 2015. Niacin in the treatment of hyperlipidemias in light of new clinical trials: has niacin lost its place? Med. Sci. Monit. 21, 2156–2162.

Zhang, L.H., Kamanna, V.S., Zhang, M.C., Kashyap, M.L., 2008. Niacin inhibits surface expression of ATP synthase beta chain in HepG2 cells: implications for raising HDL. J. Lipid Res. 49, 1195–1201.

Zilversmit, D.B., 1979. Atherogenesis: a postprandial phenomenon. Circulation 60, 473–485.

Further reading

Lukasova, M., Hanson, J., Tunaru, S., Offermanns, S., 2011. Nicotinic acid (niacin): new lipid-independent mechanisms of action and therapeutic potentials. Trends Pharmacol. Sci. 32, 700–707.

CHAPTER 15

Novel preventive mechanisms of vitamin B6 against inflammation, inflammasome, and chronic diseases

Peipei Zhang[1], Takashi Suda[2], Sofya Suidasari[3], Thanutchaporn Kumrungsee[3], Noriyuki Yanaka[3] and Norihisa Kato[3]
[1]State Key Laboratory of Cellular Stress Biology, School of Medicine & School of Life Science, Xiamen University, Xiamen, Fujian, China
[2]Department of Immunology and Molecular Biology, Cancer Research Institute, Kanazawa University, Kanazawa, Japan
[3]Graduate School of Integrated Sciences for Life, Hiroshima University, Higashi-Hiroshima, Japan

Contents

Key facts of inflammasome

1. The inflammasome was discovered by Dr. Jürg Tschopp at University of Lausanne in 2002.
2. The inflammasomes are multiprotein complexes responsible for the activation of caspase-1.

DOI: https://doi.org/10.1016/B978-0-12-811907-5.00032-4

3. Inflammasomes fight against infection.
4. Inflammasomes play a central role in sepsis and in a subset of autoinflammatory syndromes, such as cryopyrin-associated periodic syndromes, familial Mediterranean fever, and gout. Inflammasomes have also been implicated in other diseases including diabetes, inflammatory bowel disease, arteriosclerosis, and Alzheimer disease.
5. Vitamin B6, vitamin C, and unsaturated fatty acids can suppress NLRP3 inflammasome activation, while cholesterol can activate the NLRP3 inflammasome.

Key facts of carnosine

1. Carnosine, imidazole dipeptide (β-alanyl-L-histidine), was discovered by Dr. Vladimir Gulevic at University of Charkow in 1900.
2. Carnosine is highly concentrated in cardiac and skeletal muscles and brain.
3. Carnosine exerts antioxidant, antiinflammation antiglycation, and antiaging effects.
4. Carnosine has pH-buffering and metal ion-chelation activities.
5. Carnosine is a regulator of intracellular calcium and contractility in cardiac muscles.
6. Consumption of carnosine enhances the recovery of fatigue and prevents chronic diseases such as diabetes, atherosclerosis, and cognitive impairment.
7. Inadequate vitamin B6 intake lowers cardiac and skeletal muscle carnosine levels.

Summary points

- Vitamin B6 plays a role in amino acid metabolism as a coenzyme, pyridoxal 5′-phosphate.
- Lower vitamin B6 status is associated with higher risk of chronic diseases such as cardiovascular disease and cancers.
- Vitamin B6 may prevent such diseases by lowering inflammation.
- As possible mechanisms for the antiinflammation effect, vitamin B6 may modulate the kynurenine pathway and sphingosine-1-phosphate, and inhibit NF-κB activation.

- Recent studies have further suggested vitamin B6 may suppress inflammation by inhibition of the NLRP3 inflammasome and by elevation of the levels of carnosine and anserine, antiinflammation dipeptides.
- In this chapter, we review the currently available knowledge about the role of vitamin B6 in the modulations of inflammation, inflammasomes, and the imidazole dipeptides in relation to chronic diseases.

Definitions of words and terms

Vitamin B6 Vitamin B6 is a water-soluble vitamin. Vitamin B6 has an important role in the metabolism of amino acids as a coenzyme, pyridoxal 5'-phosphate. Vitamin B6 exerts a preventive effect against cardiovascular disease and cancers.

Cardiovascular disease Cardiovascular disease is a disease of the heart and blood vessels that includes numerous problems, many of which are related to a process called atherosclerosis.

Cancer Cancer is a disease in which abnormal cells grow without control and, in some cases, invade nearby tissues, often causing death.

Inflammation Inflammation is the body's immune system's natural response to harmful stimuli. It works to heal wounds or against infection, but it can also play an important role in some chronic diseases.

Inflammasomes The inflammasomes are cytoplasmic multiprotein complexes that serve as platforms for the activation of caspase-1, which converts proinflammatory cytokines (interleukin-1β and interleukin-18) from their inactive forms to active forms. Caspase-1 also induces pyroptosis, an inflammatory mode of programmed cell death.

Carnosine Carnosine is an imidazole dipeptide (β-alanyl-L-histidine) and is found at high concentrations in skeletal and cardiac muscles, and in brain. Carnosine exerts antioxidant, antiinflammation, antiglycation, antiaging, and ergogenic functions.

Abbreviations

AIM2	absent in melanoma 2
AOM	azoxymethane
ASC	apoptosis-associated speck-like protein containing a caspase recruitment domain
B6	vitamin B6
CRP	C-reactive protein
CVD	cardiovascular disease
DMH	1,2-dimethylhydrazine
DSS	dextran sulfate sodium
HSP70	heart shock protein 70
IκB	I kappa B
LPS	lipopolysaccharide
NF-κB	nuclear factor-kappa B
NLRC4	NLR family card domain-containing 4
NLRP1b	NLR family pyrin domain-containing 1b
NLRP3	NLR family pyrin domain-containing 3

NO	nitric oxide
8-OHdG	8-hydroxy-2′-deoxyguanosine
PL	pyridoxal
PLP	pyridoxal 5′-phospate
PM	pyridoxamine
PMP	pyridoxamine 5′-phosphate
PN	pyridoxine
PNP	pyridoxine 5′-phosphate
S1P	sphingosine-1-phosphate
STAT3	signal transducer and activator of transcription-3
TLRs	toll-like receptors

15.1 Introduction

15.1.1 Metabolism and functions of vitamin B6

Vitamin B6 (B6) is a water-soluble vitamin, which can be found in various foods such as fish, poultry, whole grains, legumes, banana, nuts, and sesame. There are six isoforms of B6 vitamers, which are pyridoxine (PN), pyridoxal (PL), and pyridoxamine (PM), and their phosphorylated forms of pyridoxine 5′-phosphate (PNP), pyridoxal 5′-phosphate (PLP), and pyridoxamine 5′-phosphate (PMP). Among the six isoforms, PLP is the most active form that acts as a coenzyme in more than 150 enzymatic reactions, including amino acid and carbohydrate metabolisms. Beyond the role of B6 as the coenzyme of several PLP enzymes, from 1990s, there is growing evidence indicating the role of B6 as a preventive factor against chronic diseases such as cardiovascular disease (CVD) and cancers.

15.1.2 Vitamin B6 and chronic diseases

In developed countries, severe dietary B6-deficiency is rare. Meanwhile, low B6 status, or marginal B6-deficiency has been reported in a limited number of people, including users of oral contraceptives and some drugs (Spinneker et al., 2017), and smokers (Ulvik et al., 2010).

There is growing evidence that low plasma PLP is associated with high risk of CVD (Page et al., 2009; Sakakeeny et al., 2012; Shen et al., 2009), stroke (Dierkes et al., 2007), and thrombosis (Hron et al., 2007). Low plasma PLP is linked to elevation of the inflammation marker C-reactive protein (CRP) (Fig. 15.1) (Friso et al., 2001). Also PLP may exert an antiischemic effect in the heart by blocking purinergic receptors (Dhalla et al., 2013). In the transsulfuration pathway, PLP plays a crucial role as a coenzyme of cystathionine β-synthetase for the conversion of homocysteine to cystathionine and as a coenzyme of cystathionase for the

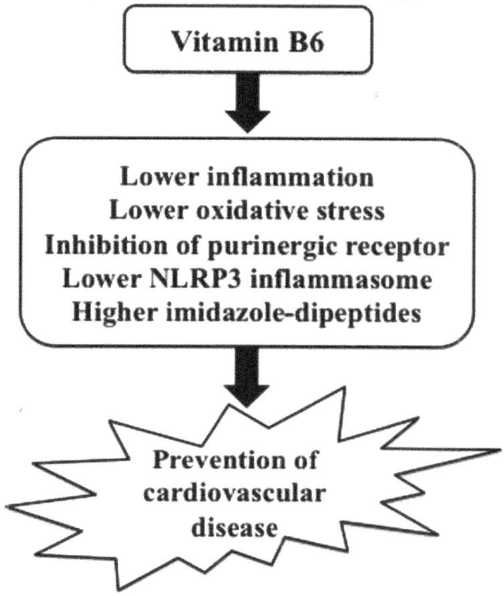

Figure 15.1 Possible mechanisms of the preventive effects of vitamin B6 against coronary heart disease.

synthesis of cysteine from cystathionine. Homocysteine has been involved in the pathophysiology of atherosclerosis (Ganguly and Alam, 2015). However, studies on the preventive role of B6 against atherosclerosis—with the hypothesis that supplemental B6 prevents atherosclerosis by suppressing homocysteine accumulation—have yielded controversial results (Bostom and Lathrop, 1997; Friso et al., 2001; Shen et al., 2009). Shen et al. reported a plasma PLP association with circulating CRP and 8-hydroxy-2′-deoxyguanosine (8-OHdG, oxidative stress marker) independent of the homocysteine-mediated pathway in older Puerto Ricans living in Massachusetts (Shen et al., 2009). In addition, B6 vitamers are capable of reducing the superoxide radical and lipid peroxide levels induced by H_2O_2 in vascular endothelial cells (Mahfouz et al., 2009). Inadequate B6 status decreases the production of glutathione and thus impairs the antioxidant defense system (Dalto and Matte, 2017). Thus oxidative stress may represent another mechanistic pathway through which low B6 may lead to CVD (Fig. 15.1).

A recent meta-analysis by Mocellin et al. (2017) showed low B6 intake or low plasma PLP have been associated with several cancers, including colorectal, gastrointestinal, stomach, lung, liver, pancreas, breast, and kidney cancers. Especially, there is increasing evidence for the association of risk of colorectal and gastrointestinal cancers with plasma PLP or B6 intake (Mocellin et al., 2017). Studies with rodents and cell cultures have suggested that supplemental B6 may exhibit antitumor effects by reducing cell proliferation, inflammation, oxidative stress, and angiogenesis (Fig. 15.2) (Matsubara et al., 2003). Actually, PLP is a selective inhibitor of DNA polymerase alpha and epsilon responsible for cell proliferation (Mizushina et al., 2003). Another antitumor mechanism may result from the reduction of sphingosine-1-phosphate (S1P) levels by PLP. S1P, a sphingolipid metabolite, activates nuclear factor-kappa B (NF-κB) and signal transducer and activator of transcription-3 (STAT3), two transcriptional regulators that serve as master switches in inflammation and carcinogenesis (Aoki et al., 2016; Liang et al., 2013). The irreversible degradation of S1P is catalyzed by the PLP-dependent S1P lyase, an enzyme that regulates the steady state S1P concentration in tissues and circulation. Zhang et al. reported that supplemental B6 plays a role in increasing gene expression of p21 (suppressor of cell cycle progression) via p53 activation in several cancer cells and the mouse colon (Zhang et al., 2014). B6 may exert an anticolon tumor effect by the protection of the colon epithelium

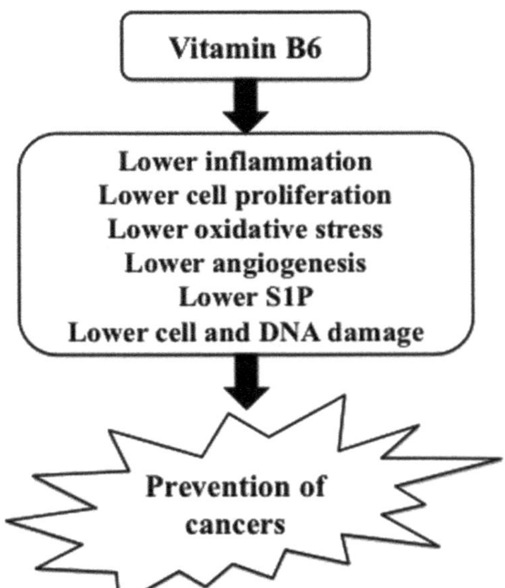

Figure 15.2 Possible mechanisms of the preventive effects of vitamin B6 against carcinogenesis.

from damage in rats treated with 1,2-dimethylhidrazine (DMH) (Kayashima et al., 2011) and to decreased lithocholic acid, a colon carcinogen (Okazaki et al., 2012). Additionally, PLP has been also reported to prevent DNA lesions (Fig. 15.2) (Kanellis et al., 2007).

15.1.3 Vitamin B6 and inflammation

B6 has been considered to play a preventive role in CVD through lowering inflammation, a crucial mechanism underlying atherosclerosis and heart disease progression (Lotto et al., 2011). Epidemiological studies have demonstrated a relationship between B6 status and inflammation, in which plasma PLP concentrations are inversely correlated with inflammation markers such as CRP (Sakakeeny et al., 2012).

B6-dependent antiinflammatory pathways are not completely clear. One of the main pathways is the kynurenine pathway involved in tryptophan metabolism (Fig. 15.3) (Wang et al., 2015). In this pathway, PLP acts as a cofactor of enzymes that convert kynurenine into a variety of compounds, including kynurenic acid, anthranilic acid, xanthurenic acid, and 3-hydroxyanthranilic acid. These kynurenine-related metabolites have been suggested to have antiinflammatory beneficial effects (Wang et al., 2015; Ueland et al., 2016). It has been also considered that the reduction of S1P by PLP may lead to lower inflammation (Fig. 15.3). Dietary

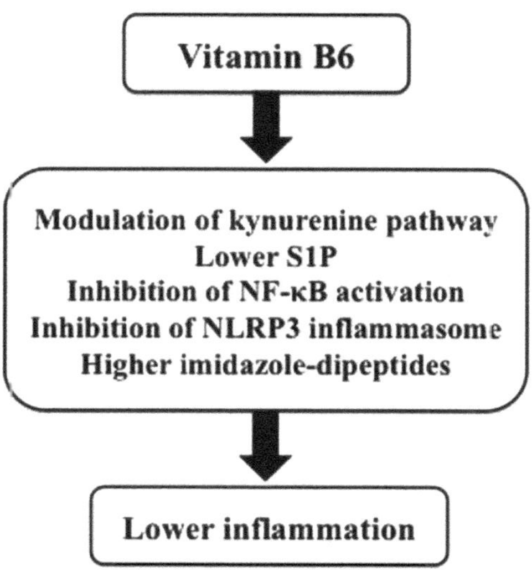

Figure 15.3 Possible mechanisms of the inhibitory effects of vitamin B6 against inflammation.

supplemental B6 increases heart levels of carnosine and anserine, antioxidant and antiinflammatory imidazole dipeptides (Fig. 15.3) (Suidasari et al., 2015). This topic will be discussed later.

With a different mechanism, Yanaka et al. (2005) have indicated an inhibitory effect of the B6 vitamer PL on the NF-κB activation in lipopolysaccharide (LPS)-treated macrophages. This inhibitory effect was associated with suppression of the expression of proinflammatory mediators such as cyclooxygenase-2 and inducible nitric oxide synthase. Intriguingly the inhibition of NF-κB activation is mediated by suppression of I kappa B (IκB) degradation through the inhibition of its ubiquitination (Yanaka et al., 2011). Consistent with these studies, dietary supplemental B6 suppresses gene expressions of several inflammatory mediators in the colon of rodents treated with colon carcinogen (Toya et al., 2012; Yanaka et al., 2011). Moreover, recently, it was found that B6 inhibits the NLR family pyrin domain-containing 3 (NLRP3) inflammasome that activates inflammation (Zhang et al., 2016). This finding will be described next.

15.1.4 Vitamin B6 and inflammasomes

The recent study by Zhang et al. (2016) indicates that B6 reduces the production of interleukin-1β (IL-1β), a pleiotropic inflammatory cytokine, by suppressing the NLRP3 inflammasome. IL-1β is synthesized as its biologically inactive precursor (pro-IL-1β), which is then proteolytically converted by caspase-1 to its mature form. Production of pro-IL-1β is predominantly regulated by NF-κB, which can be activated by multiple stimuli, including Toll-like receptors (TLRs) (signal 1 in Fig. 15.4). On the other hand, caspase-1 is activated by inflammasomes (signal 2 in Fig. 15.4) (Schroder and Tschopp, 2010). Many members of the nucleotide-binding domain and leucine-rich repeat (NLR) family of proteins, including NLR family pyrin domain-containing 1 (NLRP1), NLRP3, NLR family CARD domain-containing 4 (NLRC4), and other pyrin domain-containing proteins, such as pyrin and absent in melanoma 2 (AIM2), have been shown to form an inflammasome, together with the adaptor protein apoptosis-associated speck-like protein containing a caspase recruitment domain (ASC) and caspase-1. Among these, the NLRP3 inflammasome is the most intensively studied, because it responds to a large variety of stimuli, such as viral and bacterial RNA, bacterial ionophores, pore-forming toxins, adenosine triphosphate (ATP), urate crystals, cholesterol crystals, β-amyloids, high glucose concentrations, asbestos, and

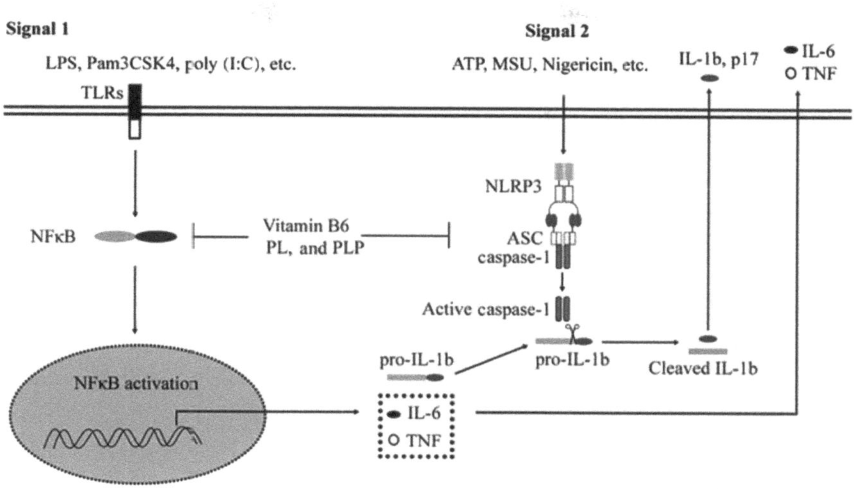

Figure 15.4 Possible mechanisms underlying the inhibitory effects of vitamin B6 on interleukin-1β (IL-1β) production. Production of IL-1β is a two-step process. "Signal 1" occurs after stimulation of toll-like receptors (TLRs) by microbial or endogenous ligands leading to nuclear factor-kappa B (NF-κB)-dependent upregulation of pro-IL-1β. "Signal 2" is provided by the inflammasome(s). The NLRP3 inflammasome is activated by a wide array of substances such as adenosine triphosphate (ATP), monosodium urate, and nigericin. Activated NLRP3 recruits procaspase-1 through the adaptor protein ASC to form the NLRP3 inflammasome complex, leading to activation of caspase-1, which then cleaves pro-IL-1β to generate mature IL-1β. Yanaka et al. showed that vitamin B6 inhibits NF-κB activation. Zhang et al. reported that PL and PLP inhibit both "signal 1" and the NLRP3-mediated "signal 2," thereby leading to a reduction in the release of mature IL-1β from macrophages and resistance to a lethal dose of LPS in mice.

silica (Duewell et al., 2010; Martinon et al., 2006; Schroder and Tschopp, 2010). Thus NLRP3 has been implicated in a variety of inflammatory diseases, including IBD, gout, arteriosclerosis, Alzheimer disease, and diabetes (Bauer et al., 2010; Duewell et al., 2010; Heneka et al., 2013; Martinon et al., 2006; Masters et al., 2010; Stienstra et al., 2010; Villani et al., 2009). Additionally, gain-of-function mutations in NLRP3 have been shown to cause hereditary autoinflammatory diseases called cryopyrin-associated periodic syndromes (Hoffman et al., 2001).

To investigate the possible influence of B6 on inflammasomes, we have previously evaluated the effects of B6 vitamers (PL, PLP, PM, and PN) on IL-1β production by mouse peritoneal macrophages in response to sequential stimulation with LPS (providing signal 1 through TLR4) and ATP (providing signal 2 through NLRP3) (Fig. 15.4) (Zhang et al.,

2016). When macrophages were treated with B6 vitamers before LPS stimulation, IL-1β production and IL-6 and TNF-α production were inhibited at the mRNA level by PL and PLP but not by PM and PN; these effects of PL and PLP can be explained by their inhibition of NF-κB activation. Further, under these conditions, PL and PLP sharply inhibited the phosphorylation-dependent activation of TAK and IKKs kinases, which play important roles in the NF-κB pathway. Interestingly, when macrophages were treated with B6 vitamers after LPS stimulation but before ATP stimulation, IL-1β production was again inhibited by PL and PLP, but not by PM and PN. Further, under these conditions, the expression of pro-IL-1β was not affected by PL and PLP, but proteolytic maturation of both caspase-1 and IL-1β was inhibited. In addition, PL and PLP inhibited the production of IL-18, another caspase-1-dependent cytokine, but not IL-6. Additionally, IL-1β production, induced by other NLRP3 activators including crystals and nigericin (bacterial ionophore), was also suppressed by PL and PLP. Moreover, both PL and PLP inhibited IL-1β production induced by infection with *Staphylococcus aureus*, which activates the NLRP3 inflammasome. In contrast, neither PL nor PLP significantly affected IL-1β production induced by infection with either *Salmonella typhimurium*, which activates the NLRC4 inflammasome, or with *Listeria monocytogenes*, which activates the AIM2 inflammasome. We also found that PL and PLP inhibited nigericin-induced IL-1β production by LPS-primed cells of the THP-1 human monocytic cell line. These results indicate that both PL and PLP inhibit the NLRP3 inflammasome pathway in humans and mice.

There is growing evidence that supplemental B6 attenuates the progression of chronic diseases like rheumatoid arthritis, Alzheimer disease, atherosclerosis, and colon cancer (Heneka, 2017; Huang et al., 2010; Komatsu et al., 2001; Till et al., 2005; Zhang et al., 2006; Zschabitz et al., 2013). Importantly, activation of the NLRP3 inflammasome is known to contribute to the development of rheumatoid arthritis, Alzheimer disease, and atherosclerosis, as deletion of NLRP3 dramatically reduces inflammation and protects against the incidence of these diseases (Duewell et al., 2010; Heneka et al., 2013; Vande et al., 2014). In our experience, PL or PLP, when injected intraperitonially into mice, can counter the increase in serum and peritoneal fluid IL-1β levels that are induced by a low dose of LPS and ATP or a high dose of LPS alone (Zhang et al., 2016). Further, intraperitoneal injection of PL and PLP improved survival in mice administered a lethal dose of LPS. Collectively, these findings suggest that the beneficial effects of B6 vitamers in inflammatory diseases can be explained at least in part by their inhibitory effects against the NLRP3 inflammasome.

15.1.5 Vitamin B6 and imidazole dipeptides

Suidasari et al. provided the first evidence that dietary supplemental B6 to a marginal B6-deficient diet markedly elevates heart concentrations of L-carnosine (β-alanyl-L-histidine) and L-anserine (β-alanyl-N-methyl-L-histidine) in rats (Figs. 15.5 and 15.6) (Suidasari et al., 2015). A subsequent study has indicated that supplemental B6 significantly increases carnosine and anserine in skeletal muscles of rats (Suidasari et al., 2016). The levels of their precursor, β-alanine, were also increased by supplemental B6 in parallel with the levels of carnosine and anserine (Suidasari et al., 2015, 2016). Meanwhile, dietary supplemental B6 markedly decreased ornithine concentrations in the muscles. Ornithine decarboxylase, PLP enzyme, metabolizes ornithine to polyamines, which are further metabolized to β-alanine. Thus the increased imidazole dipeptides may be at least in part, ascribed to increased production of β-alanine from ornithine by increased activity of PLP enzyme.

Carnosine is found at highest concentrations in skeletal and cardiac muscles and in the brain. The levels of carnosine in the brain, liver, and colon were unaffected by supplemental B6 (Suidasari et al., unpublished results). Studies have shown the role of carnosine as an intracellular pH buffer important for athletic performance and capacity (Artioli et al.,

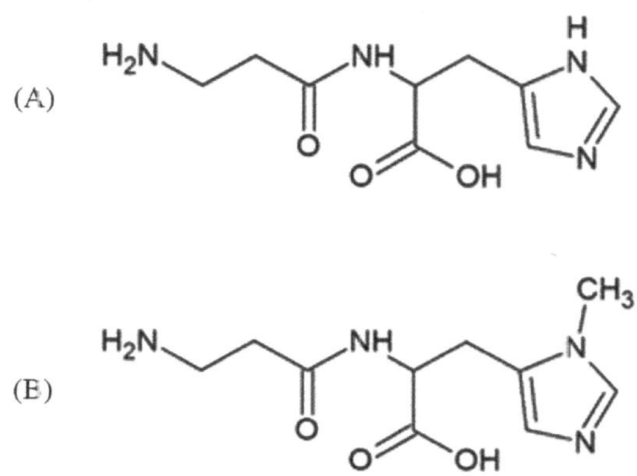

Figure 15.5 Chemical structures of L-carnosine (β-alanyl-L-histidine) (A) and L-anserine (β-alanyl-*N*-methyl-L-histidine) (B).

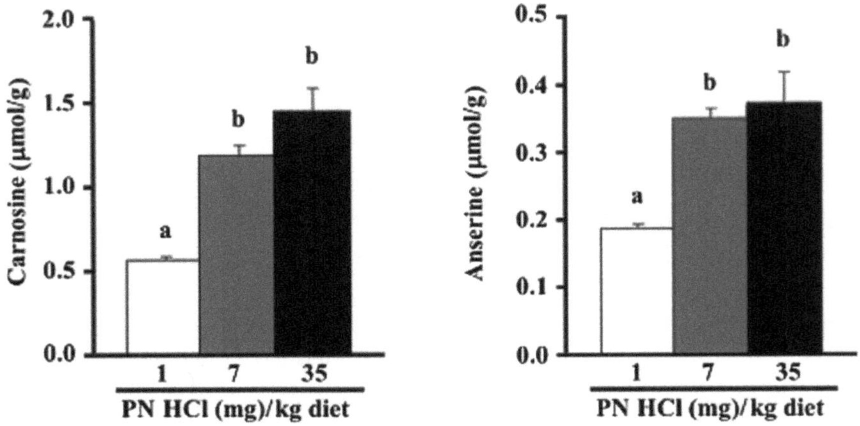

Figure 15.6 Effect of dietary levels of vitamin B6 on concentrations of carnosine and anserine in rat hearts. Mean ± SE ($n = 4$ for carnosine and anserine). The 7 mg PN HCl/kg diet is the recommended level of dietary B6. The 1 mg PN HCl/kg diet is a marginal B6-deficient level. *Values with different superscript* are significantly different by Tukey's multiple-range test ($P < .05$). *Data from Suidasari, S., Hasegawa, T., Yanaka, N., Kato, N., 2015. Dietary supplemental vitamin B6 increases carnosine and anserine concentrations in the heart of rats. Springerplus 4, 280.*

2018; Caruso et al., 2012). Power athletes have higher carnosine levels than untrained individuals (Artioli et al., 2018; Parkhouse et al., 1985). Carnosine activates muscle phosphorylase, a PLP enzyme, responsible for the degradation of glycogen (Johnson et al., 1982). Carnosine elevates the expression of heat shock protein 70 (HSP70), a protector of cell function by the prevention of irreversible protein damage (Hipkiss et al., 2013).

Carnosine and anserine are thought to exert antioxidant, antiinflammatory, antiglycation, and antiischemic effects on the heart (Baye et al., 2016; Boldyrev et al., 2013). They have biochemical capacities, such as metal ion chelation, as well as pH buffering (Boldyrev et al., 2013). In cardiac myocytes, carnosine is suggested to be a modulator of intracellular calcium and contractility (Roberts and Zaloga, 2000; Zaloga et al., 1997). A study by de Courten et al. has shown skeletal muscle carnosine is associated with insulin resistance, energy expenditure, dynamic physical activity, and atherogenic index (de Courten et al., 2015). Thus dietary supplemental B6, in correcting low B6 status, might have a positive effect on cardiovascular disease by elevating the imidazole dipeptides.

Excess nitric oxide (NO) production occurs in several pathological states, including ischemia and inflammation, and is generally accompanied by increased oxidative/nitrosative stress. Caruso et al. indicated that carnosine caused a suppression of total NO production by LPS-stimulated macrophages accompanied by a simultaneous drastic increase in their intracellular low toxicity end product, nitrite, with no inhibition of iNOS (Caruso et al., 2017). Analysis in a cell-free system showed the formation of multiple adducts of carnosine–NO and carnosine–nitrite, thus providing a possible mechanism for the changes in free NO and nitrite in the presence of carnosine. In the stimulated macrophages, the addition of carnosine was also characterized by a suppressed release of proinflammatory mediators (Caruso et al., 2017). These results provide evidence for the property of carnosine that modulates the production of NO by stimulated macrophages.

Suidasari et al. (2015) indicated B6 supplementation increases serum concentrations of carnosine. It has been suggested that higher concentrations of carnosine due to exercise decrease blood pressure in rats and humans (Nagai et al., 2012). It has been suggested that plasma carnosine is involved in preventing early-stage lipid oxidation in the circulation (Stegen et al., 2015). Carnosine also has been suggested as an antiaging factor (Hipkiss et al., 2016). Thus elevated serum carnosine following B6 supplementation may be favorable for the circulation as well as the cardiac and skeletal muscles.

15.2 Conclusions

There is growing evidence that low B6 status is associated with the risk of chronic diseases such as CVD and cancers. The link between B6 and inflammation may be at least in part due to the mechanism by which B6 suppresses the risk of such diseases. Studies have revealed the antiinflammatory effects of B6 by modulation of the kynurenine pathway, the S1P levels, and NF-κB activation. Recent studies have further delineated modulation of the NLRP3 inflammasome and imidazole dipeptides by B6, leading to decreased inflammation. However, the information is still limited on the antiinflammatory mechanisms of B6 and their possible links to chronic diseases. Further study with metabolomics analyses of B6-responsive metabolites related to chronic diseases may be necessary because of the enormous number of PLP-dependent enzymatic reactions.

References

Aoki, M., Aoki, H., Rmanathan, R., Hait, N.C., Takabe, K., 2016. Sphingsine-1-phosphate signaling in immune cells and inflammation: Roles and Therapeutic Potential. Mediat. Inflamm. 2016, 11.

Artioli, G.G., Sale, C., Jones, R.L., 2018. Carnosine in health and disease. Eur. J. Sport Sci. 4, 1–10.

Bauer, C., Duewell, P., Mayer, C., Lehr, H.A., Fitzgerald, K.A., Dauer, M., et al., 2010. Colitis induced in mice with dextran sulfate sodium (DSS) is mediated by the NLRP3 inflammasome. Gut 59, 1192–1199.

Baye, E., Ukropcova, B., Ukropec, J., Hipkiss, A., Aldini, G., de Courten, B., 2016. Physiological and therapeutic effects of carnosine on cardiometabolic risk and disease. Amino Acids 48, 1131–1149.

Boldyrev, A.A., Aldini, G., Derave, W., 2013. Physiology and pathophysiology of carnosine. Physiol. Rev. 93, 1803–1845.

Bostom, A.G., Lathrop, L., 1997. Hyperhomocysteinemia in end-stage renal disease (ESRD): prevalence, etiology, and potential relationship to arteriosclerotic outcomes. Kidney Int. 52, 10–20.

Caruso, J., Charles, J., Unruh, K., Giebel, R., Learmonth, L., Potter, W., 2012. Ergogenic effects of β-alanine and carnosine: proposed future research to quantify their efficacy. Nutrients 4, 585–601.

Caruso, G., Fresta, C.G., Martinez-Becerra, F., Antonio, L., Johnson, R.T., de Campos, R.P.S., et al., 2017. Carnosine modulates nitric oxide in stimulated murine RAW 264.7 macrophages. Mol. Cell. Biochem. 431, 197–210.

Dalto, D.B., Matte, J.J., 2017. Pyridoxine (vitamin B) and the glutathione peroxidase system; a link between one-carbon metabolism and antioxidation. Nutrients 9, 189.

de Courten, B., Kurdiova, T., de Courten, M.P., Belan, V., Everaert, I., Vician, M., et al., 2015. Muscle carnosine is associated with cardiometabolic risk factors in humans. PLoS One 10, e0138707.

Dhalla, N.S., Takeda, S., Elimban, V., 2013. Mechanisms of the beneficial effects of vitamin B6 and pyridoxal 5-phosphate on cardiac performance in ischemic heart disease. Clin. Chem. Lab. Med. 51, 535–543.

Dierkes, J., Weikert, C., Klipstein-Grobusch, K., Westphal, S., Luley, C., Möhlig, M., et al., 2007. Plasma pyridoxal-5-phosphate and future risk of myocardial infarction in the European Prospective Investigation into Cancer and Nutrition Potsdam cohort. Am. J. Clin. Nutr. 86, 214–220.

Duewell, P., Kono, H., Rayner, K.J., Sirois, C.M., Vladimer, G., Bauernfeind, F.G., et al., 2010. NLRP3 inflammasomes are required for atherogenesis and activated by cholesterol crystals. Nature 464, 1357–1361.

Friso, S., Jacques, P.F., Wilson, P.W., Rosenberg, I.H., Selhub, J., 2001. Low circulating vitamin B(6) is associated with elevation of the inflammation marker C-reactive protein independently of plasma homocysteine levels. Circulation 103, 2788–2791.

Ganguly, P., Alam, S.F., 2015. Role of homocysteine in the development of cardiovascular disease. Nutr. J. 14, 6.

Hoffman, H.M., Mueller, J.L., Broide, D.H., Wanderer, A.A., Kolodner, R.D., 2001. Mutation of a new gene encoding a putative pyrin-like protein causes familial cold autoinflammatory syndrome and Muckle-Wells syndrome. Nat. Genet. 29, 301–305.

Heneka, M.T., 2017. Inflammasome activation and innate immunity in Alzheimer's disease. Brain Pathol. 27, 220–222.

Heneka, M.T., Kummer, M.P., Stutz, A., Delekate, A., Schwartz, S., Vieira-Saecker, A., et al., 2013. NLRP3 is activated in Alzheimer's disease and contributes to pathology in APP/PS1 mice. Nature 493, 674–678.

Hipkiss, A.R., Cartwright, S.P., Bromley, C., Gross, S.R., Bill, R.M., 2013. Carnosine: can understanding its actions on energy metabolism and protein homeostasis inform its therapeutic potential? Chem. Cent. J. 7, 38.
Hipkiss, A.R., Baye, E., de Courten, B., 2016. Carnosine and the processes of ageing. Maturitas 93, 28–33.
Hron, G., Lombardi, R., Eichinger, S., Lecchi, A., Kyrle, P.A., Cattaneo, M., 2007. Low vitamin B6 levels and the risk of recurrent venous thromboembolism. Haematologica 92, 1250–1253.
Huang, S.C., Wei, J.C., Wu, D.J., Huang, Y.C., 2010. Vitamin B(6) supplementation improves pro-inflammatory responses in patients with rheumatoid arthritis. Eur. J. Clin. Nutr. 64, 1007–1013.
Johnson, P., Fedyna, J.S., Schindzielorz, A., Smith, C.M., Kasvinsky, P.J., 1982. Regulation of muscle phosphorylase activity by carnosine and anserine. Biochem. Biophys. Res. Commun. 109, 769–775.
Kanellis, P., Gagliardi, M., Banath, J.P., Szilard, R.K., Nakada, S., Galicia, S., et al., 2007. A screen for suppressors of gross chromosomal rearrangements identifies a conserved role for PLP in preventing DNA lesions. PLoS Genet. 3, e134.
Kayashima, T., Tanaka, K., Okazaki, Y., Matsubara, K., Yanaka, N., Kato, N., 2011. Consumption of vitamin B6 reduces colonic damage and protein expression of HSP70 and HO-1, the anti-tumor targets, in rats exposed to 1,2-dimethylhydrazine. Oncol. Lett. 2, 1243–1246.
Komatsu, S., Watanabe, H., Oka, T., Tsuge, H., Nii, H., Kato, N., 2001. Vitamin B-6-supplemented diets compared with a low vitamin B-6 diet suppress azoxymethane-induced colon tumorigenesis in mice by reducing cell proliferation. J. Nutr. 131, 2204–2207.
Liang, J., Nagahashi, M., Kim, E.Y., Harikumar, K.B., Yamada, A., Huang, W.C., et al., 2013. Sphingosine-1-phosphate links persistent STAT3 activation, chronic intestinal inflammation, and development of colitis-associated cancer. Cancer Cell 23, 107–120.
Lotto, V., Choi, S.-W., Friso, S., 2011. Vitamin B6: a challenging link between nutrition and inflammation in CVD. Br. J. Nutr. 106, 183–195.
Mahfouz, M.M., Zhou, S.Q., Kummerow, F.A., 2009. Vitamin B_6 compounds are capable of reducing the superoxide radical and lipid peroxide levels induced by H_2O_2 in vascular endothelial cells in culture. Int. J. Vit. Nutr. Res. 79, 218–229.
Martinon, F., Petrilli, V., Mayor, A., Tardivel, A., Tschopp, J., 2006. Gout-associated uric acid crystals activate the NALP3 inflammasome. Nature 440, 237–241.
Masters, S.L., Dunne, A., Subramanian, S.L., Hull, R.L., Tannahill, G.M., Sharp, F.A., et al., 2010. Activation of the NLRP3 inflammasome by islet amyloid polypeptide provides a mechanism for enhanced IL-1beta in type 2 diabetes. Nat. Immunol. 11, 897–904.
Matsubara, K., Komatsu, S., Oka, T., Kato, N., 2003. Vitamin B6-mediated suppression of colon tumorigenesis, cell proliferation, and angiogenesis (review). J. Nutr. Biochem. 14, 246–250.
Mizushina, Y., Xu, X., Matsubara, K., Murakami, C., Kuriyama, I., Oshige, M., et al., 2003. Pyridoxal 5'-phosphate is a selective inhibitor in vivo of DNA polymerase alpha and epsilon. Biochem. Biophys. Res. Commun. 312, 1025–1032.
Mocellin, S., Briarava, M., Pilati, P., 2017. Vitamin B6 and cancer risk: a field synopsis and meta-analysis. J. Natl. Cancer. Inst. 109, 1–9.
Nagai, K., Tanida, M., Niijima, A., Tsuruoka, N., Kiso, Y., Horii, Y., et al., 2012. Role of l-carnosine in the control of blood glucose, blood pressure, thermogenesis, and lipolysis by autonomic nerves in rats: involvement of the circadian clock and histamine. Amino Acids 43, 97–109.

Okazaki, Y., Utama, Z., Suidasari, S., Zhang, P., Yanaka, N., Tomotake, H., et al., 2012. Consumption of vitamin B(6) reduces fecal ratio of lithocholic acid to deoxycholic acid, a risk factor for colon cancer, in rats fed a high-fat diet. J. Nutr. Sci. Vitaminol. 58, 366–370.

Page, J.H., Ma, J., Chiuve, S.E., Stampfer, M.J., Selhub, J., Manson, J.E., et al., 2009. Plasma vitamin B(6) and risk of myocardial infarction in women. Circulation 120, 649–655.

Parkhouse, W.S., McKenzie, D.C., Hochachka, P.W., Ovalle, W.K., 1985. Buffering capacity of deproteinized human vastus lateralis muscle. J. Appl. Physiol. 58, 14–17.

Roberts, P.R., Zaloga, G.P., 2000. Cardiovascular effects of carnosine. Biochemistry (Mosc.) 65, 856–861.

Sakakeeny, L., Roubenoff, R., Obin, M., Fontes, J.D., Benjamin, E.J., Bujanover, Y., et al., 2012. Plasma pyridoxal-5-phosphate is inversely associated with systemic markers of inflammation in a population of U.S. adults. J. Nutr. 142, 1280–1285.

Schroder, K., Tschopp, J., 2010. The inflammasomes. Cell 140, 821–832.

Shen, J., Lai, C., Mattei, J., Ordovas, J.M., Tucker, K.L., 2009. Association of vitamin B-6 status with inflammation, oxidative stress, and chronic inflammatory conditions: the Boston Puerto Rican Health Study. Am. J. Clin. Nutr. 91, 337–342.

Spinneker, A., Sola, R., Lemmen, V., Castillo, M.J., Pietrzik, K., González-Gross, M., 2017. Vitamin B_6 status, deficiency and its consequences-an overview. Nutr. Hosp. 22, 7–24.

Stegen, S., Stegen, B., Aldini, G., Altomare, A., Cannizzaro, L., Orioli, M., et al., 2015. Plasma carnosine, but not muscle carnosine, attenuates high-fat diet-induced metabolic stress. Appl. Physiol. Nutr. Metab. 40, 868–876.

Stienstra, R., Joosten, L.A., Koenen, T., van Tits, B., van Diepen, J.A., van den Berg, S. A., et al., 2010. The inflammasome-mediated caspase-1 activation controls adipocyte differentiation and insulin sensitivity. Cell. Metab. 12, 593–605.

Suidasari, S., Hasegawa, T., Yanaka, N., Kato, N., 2015. Dietary supplemental vitamin B6 increases carnosine and anserine concentrations in the heart of rats. Springerplus 4, 280.

Suidasari, S., Stautemas, J., Uragami, S., Yanaka, N., Derave, W., Kato, N., 2016. Carnosine content in skeletal muscle is dependent on vitamin B6 status in rats. Front. Nutr. 2, 39.

Till, U., Rohl, P., Jentsch, A., Till, H., Muller, A., Bellstedt, K., et al., 2005. Decrease of carotid intima-media thickness in patients at risk to cerebral ischemia after supplementation with folic acid, vitamins B6 and B12. Atherosclerosis 181, 131–135.

Toya, K., Hirata, A., Ohata, T., Sanada, Y., Kato, N., Yanaka, N., 2012. Regulation of colon gene expression by vitamin B6 supplementation. Mol. Nutr. Food Res. 56, 641–652.

Ueland, P.M., McCann, A., Midttun, O., Ulvik, A., 2016. Inflammation, vitamin B6 and related pathways. Mol. Asp. Med. 53, 10–27.

Ulvik, A., Ebbing, M., Steinar Hustad, S., Midttun, Ø., Nygård, O., Vollset, S.E., et al., 2010. Long- and short-term effects of tobacco smoking on circulating concentrations of B vitamins. Clin. Chem. 56, 5.

Vande, W.L., Van, O.N., Jacques, P., Fossoul, A., Verheugen, E., Vogel, P., et al., 2014. Negative regulation of the NLRP3 inflammasome by A20 protects against arthritis. Nature 512, 69–73.

Villani, A.C., Lemire, M., Fortin, G., Louis, E., Silverberg, M.S., Collette, C., et al., 2009. Common variants in the NLRP3 region contribute to Crohn's disease susceptibility. Nat. Genet. 41, 71–76.

Wang, Q., Liu, D., Song, P., Zou, M.H., 2015. Tryptophan-kynurenine pathway is dysregulated in inflammation, and immune activation. Front. Biosci. 20, 1116–1143.

Yanaka, N., Koyama, T.A., Komatsu, S., Nakamura, E., Kanda, M., Kato, N., 2005. Vitamin B6 suppresses NF-kappaB activation in LPS-stimulated mouse macrophages. Int. J. Mol. Med. 16, 1071–1075.

Yanaka, N., Ohata, T., Toya, K., Kanda, M., Hirata, A., Kato, N., 2011. Vitamin B6 suppresses serine protease inhibitor 3 expression in the colon of rats and in TNF-α-stimulated HT-29 cells. Mol. Nutr. Food Res. 55, 635–643.

Zaloga, G.P., Roberts, P.R., Black, K.W., Lin, M., Zapata-Sudo, G., Sudo, R.T., et al., 1997. Carnosine is a novel peptide modulator of intracellular calcium and contractility in cardiac cells. Am. J. Physiol. 272, H462–H468.

Zhang, S.M., Moore, S.C., Lin, J., Cook, N.R., Manson, J.E., Lee, I.M., et al., 2006. Folate, vitamin B6, multivitamin supplements, and colorectal cancer risk in women. Am. J. Epidemiol. 163, 108–115.

Zhang, P., Suidasari, S., Hasegawa, T., Yanaka, N., Kato, N., 2014. Vitamin B activates p53 and elevates p21 gene expression in cancer cells and the mouse colon. Oncol. Rep. 31, 2371–2376.

Zhang, P., Tsuchiya, K., Kinoshita, T., Kushiyama, H., Suidasari, S., Hatakeyama, M., et al., 2016. Vitamin B6 prevents IL-1 beta protein production by inhibiting NLRP3 inflammasome activation. J. Biol. Chem. 291, 24517–24527.

Zschabitz, S., Cheng, T.Y., Neuhouser, M.L., Zheng, Y., Ray, R.M., Miller, J.W., et al., 2013. B vitamin intakes and incidence of colorectal cancer: results from the Women's Health Initiative Observational Study cohort. Am. J. Clin. Nutr. 97, 332–343.

Further reading

Komatsu, S., Watanabe, H., Oka, T., Tsuge, H., Kato, N., 2002. Dietary vitamin B6 suppresses colon tumorigenesis, 8-hydroxyguanosine, 4-hydroxynonenal, and inducible nitric oxide synthase protein in azoxymethane-treated mice. J. Nutr. Sci. Vitaminol. 48, 65–68.

Kumrungsee, T., Nirmagustina, D.E., Arima, T., Onishi, K., Sato, K., Kato, N., et al., 2019. Novel metabolic disturbances in marginal vitamin B_6-deficient rat heart. J. Nutr. Biochem. 65, 26–34.

CHAPTER 16

New properties of vitamin B6 or pyridoxine in experimental oxidative stress in the brain

K.E. Danielyan and S.G. Chailyan
H Buniatian Institute of Biochemistry, National Academy of Science of Armenia, Yerevan, Armenia

Contents

Key facts

- Thiamine, pyridoxine, riboflavin, and nicotinamide are responsible for cell development.
- Pyridoxine and thiamine are important during the early stages of cell development.
- Riboflavin and nicotinamide are important during the late stages of cell development.
- Inhibition of xanthine oxidoreductase (XO) is a key process in the proliferation of the cells.
- XO activity in the presence of pyridoxine is specifically inhibited.
- XO activity in the presence of pyridoxine is specifically inhibited by allopurinol.

Molecular Nutrition
DOI: https://doi.org/10.1016/B978-0-12-811907-5.00017-8

- We have delineated the existence of nonprimer xanthine oxidoreductase (XOR) substrates in rat liver, making it regulative and a key enzyme for purine catabolism.
- Inhibition of XOR suppresses the entire purine catabolism in rat liver.
- Purified XOR doesn't have any activity in the presence of nonprimer substrate.
- Timely inhibition with allopurinol of XO might stimulate the growth of cells and their proliferation, as well as their death, presumably because of the inhibition of purine catabolism by a feedback mechanism as well as the prevention of reactive oxygen species formation.
- A low concentration of allopurinol effectively decreases the number of dead cells and promotes proliferation
- Inhibition of XOR with pyridoxine might interfere with the cell proliferation processes in dose-dependent and time-dependent manners.
- Pyridoxine, acting as a coenzyme in the processes of epinephrine synthesis, might activate XO via epinephrine.
- XO might be used for regenerative treatment after stroke, for neurogenesis, or heart infarction.
- B6 might promote cell survival in vitro in neuronal cells culture during oxidative stress.
- B6 prevents BBB disruption in vivo in the conditions of hydrogen peroxide-determined oxidative stress.

Abbreviations

ADMA	asymmetric dimethylarginine
ARE	antioxidant response elements
AT-II	angiotensin II
eNOS	nitric oxide synthase
ER	endoplasmic reticulum
ERO1	ER oxidoreductin 1
ETC	electron transport chain
FAD	flavin adenine dinucleotide
GTP	Guanosine-5'-triphosphate
HGPRT	hypoxanthine-guanine phosphoribosyltransferase
KATP	ATP-sensitive potassium channel L-DOPA L-3,4-dihydroxyphenylalanine
mitoTEMPO	mitochondria-targeted antioxidants
Mo-pt	molybdopterin center
mPTP	permeability transition pore
mtJ	mitochondrial membrane potential
NOXs	NADPH oxidases

Nrf2	nuclear factor erythroid 2-related factor 2
O^{2-}	superoxide anion
PD	Parkinson disease
PDI	protein disulfide isomerase
Prdx6	peroxiredoxin 6
Prxs	peroxiredoxin
ROS	reactive oxygen species
XO	xanthine oxidase
XOR	xanthine oxidoreductase
UTP	Uridine-5'-triphosphate
ZnCys3	zinc—sulfur clusters

16.1 Introduction

It is very well documented that after forebrain ischemia/reperfusion, the generation of thane excessive amount of superoxide anion radicals occurs. Evidence exists that allopurinol, a xanthine oxidase inhibitor, reduces delayed cell death in animal models (Mink et al., 1991) of perinatal asphyxia and in human patients with other forms of organ reperfusion injury. Thus, allopurinol pretreatment suppresses the generation of superoxide anion radicals, making xanthine oxidoreductase enzyme (XOR; EC 1.17.3.2), the main one responsible for the oxidative damage caused after oxidative stress, early inflammation, and endothelial injury (Ono et al., 2009).

XOR, which is the last and regulatory enzyme in purine catabolism, might induce the generation of a purines pool in the cells and trigger the generation of the new cells, that is, regenerative processes.

We found out that pyridoxine or vitamin B is the inhibitor of XOR. We proposed and experimentally proved that the regenerative abilities of vitamin B are mediated via the inhibition of XOR.

16.2 Description of the free radical-producing systems in the organism

Reactive oxygen species (ROS) generation is a vitally important process. However, oxidative stress is determined by the misbalance between the formation and utilization of ROS. The generation of ROS in the normally functioning cells occurs in the organelles and transfers into the cytoplasm. An overwhelming amount of ROS might trigger nonreversible cell death.

It is supposed that mitochondria are the major reservoirs for ROS generation in most mammalian cells. During respiration an estimated 1%—2%

of O_2 gains an electron and it is reduced to superoxide anion (O^{2-}) (Cadenas et al., 1977), which is the source for the generation of hydrogen peroxide (H_2O_2) (Boveris et al., 1972). This percentage may be even lower (0.15%) according to a recent study (St-Pierre et al., 2002). The oxygen is also the source for the formation of the highly reactive molecules of hydroxyl anions. In comparison with the O^{2-} and hydroxyl anions, the hydrogen peroxide formed, particularly in mitochondria, is much more stable and can serve as a signaling molecule triggering the intracellular cascades (Bienert et al., 2006; Lee and Thevenod, 2006).

The respiratory chain is mainly localized in the inner membrane of the mitochondria and it is proved that the complexes I and III are the main components of the chain responsible for the production of the free radicals

Protein folding is another process which might be accompanied with the formation of the free radicals. It was proven, 25% of generated ROS might occur in endoplasmic reticulum (ER) due to the formation of disulfide bonds (Malhotra and Kaufman, 2007; Tu and Weissman, 2004).

NADPH oxidases (NOXs) are enzymes, which may function as the key regulators in pathological processes, such as ischemia–reperfusion, diabetes, neurodegenerative diseases, and atherosclerosis, as well as other vessel-related diseases (Ray and Shah, 2005; Cave et al., 2006; Bedard and Krause, 2007; Pendyala et al., 2009b), due to the formation of O_2, which forms the superoxide anion (O^{2-}) (Leto et al., 2009; Pendyala et al., 2009a).

Hemoglobin and myoglobins might serve as a source for the formation of free radicals. The reduction of nitrite to •NO under hypoxic conditions serves as a putative autoregulatory mechanism for capillaries and muscle (Kumar et al., 2012). Nitric oxide synthases also might serve as a source of the •NO (Kumar et al., 2012).

The other enzyme, which will be highlighted in this chapter is XOR. Under normal circumstances most of this enzyme exists in the form of NAD-dependent cytosolic dehydrogenase (XDH).

16.3 General description of the xanthine oxidase enzyme

Xanthine oxidase (XO) as well as the XDH are two enzymes responsible for the last steps of purine metabolism, and the hydroxylation of a wide variety pyrimidine, pterin, and aldehyde substrates. XOR enzymes have been isolated from a wide range of organisms, from bacteria to man. All of these proteins have similar molecular weights and composition of redox centers (Hille and Nishino, 1995; Moriwaki et al., 1999). The mammalian enzymes, which catalyze the hydroxylation of hypoxanthine and xanthine, the last two steps in the formation of urate, are synthesized as the dehydrogenase form. XDH exists mostly as such in the cell but can be readily converted to the oxidase form XO by oxidation of sulfhydryl residues or by proteolysis. XDH shows a preference for NADH reduction at the flavin adenine dinucleotide (FAD) reaction site, whereas XO fails to react with NADH and exclusively uses dioxygen as its substrate, leading to the formation of superoxide anions and hydrogen peroxide (Hille and Nishino, 1995). The active form of the enzyme is that of a homodimer of molecular mass 290 kDa, with each of the monomers acting independently in catalysis. Each subunit contains one molybdopterin cofactor, two spectroscopically distinct (2Fe−2S) centers, and one FAD cofactor. The oxidation of xanthine takes place at the molybdopterin center (Mo-pt) and the electrons thus introduced are rapidly distributed to the other centers by intramolecular electron transfer (Olson et al., 1974). The full amino acid sequences of XOR enzymes from various sources have been deduced by sequencing of the respective cDNAs or genes. They all consist of approximately 1330 amino acids and are highly homologous with, for example, the bovine milk enzyme (1332 residues), and show 90% sequence identity to the human liver enzyme (1333 residues) (Ichida et al., 1993).

16.4 Xanthine oxidase regulates purine catabolism by feedback mechanism

There are numerous publications providing evidence on the primer, the regulating role of the presence of hypoxanthine/xanthine, and its catabolism in the purine metabolic pathway.

For instance, Edwards et al. performed the small clinical trial with the infusion of the radiolabeled (8-^{14}C) adenine to four patients with gout as well as to the patients suffering from Lesch−Nyhan syndrome. Five days after infusion it became clear that the mean cumulative excretion of radioactivity after adenine administration to patients not receiving and receiving (off and on) allopurinol therapy was 6.1%-3.6% of infused radioactivity for gouty subjects and 15.9%-20.8% for the Lesch−Nyhan patients.

This is the important works, which proved the existence of the feedback mechanism, where the inhibition of the regulative enzyme XOR might prevent release of the radioactivity from the organism due to the degradation of radiolabeled adenine (Edwards et al., 1981).

Edwards et al. (1979) suggested that purine salvage is a major contributor to increased purine excretion and that the purine catabolic pathway responds differently to an increased substrate load in hypoxanthine-guanine phosphoribosyltransferase deficiency.

Another group has shown that allopurinol treatment might promote the excretion of xanthine/hypoxanthine, as well as the 8-hydroxy-7-methyl guanine, but not any other minor purines into the bloodstream (Simmonds and Bowyer, 1974).

Bleisch et al. (1994) have shown that allopurinol, besides inhibiting uric acid synthesis, reduced the rate of degradation of adenosine monophosphate.

Another group has demonstrated that orotic acid excretion was increased with a dose of allopurinol and reduced by the addition of purines (Löffler and Gröbner, 1988).

This finding proves our suggestion that there is a tight interaction between the catabolism of purines and pyrimidines and inhibition of one of them might stimulate the activation of the other one.

It was suggested that not only ammonium but also hypoxanthine accumulation might control the regulation not only of the adenylate but also the guanylate pool sizes (Leung and Schramm, 1978; Sabina et al., 1979).

In contrast to the inhibition of purine catabolism it was demonstrated that adenine, orotic acid, and azaserine inhibited purine synthesis, but hypoxanthine and allopurinol did not in the platelets (Jerushalmy et al., 1980). However, experiments performed with the different organs of the rat have demonstrated that allopurinol enhances the synthesis of adenine nucleotides from the administered inosine in the brain and liver of rats in contrast to the heart and kidneys (Pechán and Zimmer, 1989).

Extremely valuable work has shown that a decrease of PP-ribose-P availability in the presence of allopurinol is due to competition between adenine and hypoxanthine salvage pathways into nucleotides, and not to the synthesis of inosine (Lalanne and Lafleur, 1980).

In astroglia derived from the Lesch–Nyhan syndrome-carrying mice with the deficiency of the purine salvage enzyme hypoxanthine-guanine phosphoribosyltransferase (HGPRT) it was demonstrated existence of low cellular levels of adenine dinucleotide phosphate, adenine triphosphate (ATP), and guanosine-5'-triphosphate (GTP), indicating that the accelerated de novo purine synthesis does not compensate adequately for the deficiency of salvage nucleotide synthesis, and higher level of uridine-5'-triphosphate (UTP), probably due to enhanced de novo synthesis of pyrimidine nucleotides (Pelled et al., 1999).

Interesting work was related to the influence of the purines and pyrimidines metabolism on cells' differentiation processes.

Authors thought that since purine and pyrimidine nucleotides play an important role in the synthesis of important macromolecules, it can be suggested that the depletion of guanine ribonucleotide as a result of the inhibition of early de novo purine biosynthesis, or due to specific inhibition of de novo guanine nucleotide biosynthesis, may be an obligatory step in the initiation of the differentiation in mycophenolic acid and acivicin-treated HL60 cells (Gladden et al., 2011).

Based on our studies we were able, by the use of allopurinol and a different nonprimer for XOR substrates, entering into the purine catabolism chain at the upstream points, to prove the existence of a feedback mechanism of purine catabolism regulation via XOR (Gyongyan et al., 2013).

The specific activity of XO in the rat liver in the presence of different substrates was the following (1) in comparison with the control: blank control 0.96 ± 0.05; xanthine 2.12 ± 0.08; allopurinol in low concentration 1.70 ± 0.12; allopurinol in high concentration 1.52 ± 0.06, $P < .05$; (2) for histidine-3.30 ± 0.19, in the presence of allopurinol in low and high concentrations 2.28 ± 0.13, 1.78 ± 0.08; (3) for riboflavin 1.26 ± 0.06; with allopurinol in low concentration 0.72 ± 0.13; in high concentration 0.99 ± 0.19; (4) for adenosine-2.94 ± 0.07; with allopurinol in low and high concentrations 1.90 ± 0.23 and 2.12 ± 0.10; and (5) for desoxyadenosine 2.41 ± 0.37; with allopurinol 2.03 ± 0.10, 2.03 ± 0.06. In comparison with the control all the substrates elevated the XOR activity in a statistically significant way, whereas the specific inhibitor—allopurinol—diminished that activity.

Taking into the consideration that the use of allopurinol allows activity of XOR to be significantly reduced, we have proved that XOR is the key regulative enzyme in the purine catabolism pathway. In our previous studies we have demonstrated that the inhibition of XOR activity with allopurinol might stimulate the in vitro process of cells proliferation, whereas the inhibition of dihydropyrimidine dehydrogenase might prevent brain-derived cells from death. After all we have proved and presented the fundamental mechanism of such phenomenon, which might be utilized for regenerative processes and the prevention of cell proliferation in the setting of cancer development (Danielyan, 2013a).

Also to prove whether the pure enzyme is able to react with the non-primer substrates we have checked the activity of the purified enzyme from the rat liver XOR in the presence of histidine, one of the substrates, which stimulated the activity of the enzyme very strongly.

We have noticed a 10-fold elevation of XOR activity in a statistically significant way (control 1.63 ± 0.20; xanthine 2.16 ± 0.11; allopurinol 1.81 ± 0.05, $P < .05$). However, when instead of the primer substrate (xanthine), histidine was added, the activity of XOR disappeared (histidine 1.77 ± 0.30; allopurinol 1.15 ± 0.20).

16.5 Antioxidant systems

In the conditions of oxidative stress organisms over the course of evolution developed protective mechanisms which include the regulation of gene expression and biochemical levels as the first step to trigger defense. As soon as ROS production is enhanced three main components are activated, which are Kelch-like ECH-associated protein 1, nuclear factor erythroid 2-related factor 2 (Nrf2), and antioxidant response elements (ARE). The binding of Nrf2 to the DNA sequences present in ARE induces transcription of cytoprotective, antioxidant genes including superoxide dismutase (SOD), glutathione peroxidase (GPx), catalase (CAT), gamma-GCS, and glutathione *S*-transferase (GST). In addition, several other cytoprotective genes (heme oxygenase) are induced (Kalyanaraman, 2013).

These antioxidant enzymes are subject to posttranslational modifications that temporally control their H_2O_2-degrading activity to represent a mechanism to govern transient changes in local H_2O_2 levels, which is important for redox signaling in response to specific stimuli or conditions.

A redox-signaling role for antioxidant enzymes is exemplified by peroxiredoxin (Prxs). Prxs show high reactivity for H_2O_2 when compared with other thiol oxidants and exhibits a rate constant (1.3×10^7 M/s) sufficiently high to outcompete CAT and GPx for H_2O_2.

Fisher in his work talks about peroxiredoxin 6s (Prdx6) antioxidative abilities. In accordance with his work data, Prdx6 is the prototype and the only mammalian 1-Cys member of the Prdx family (Chatterjee et al., 2011).

The reversion of redox signaling requires reductive repair of reactive cysteines in proteins. An antioxidant enzyme responsible for the repair of oxidized protein cysteines is the 12-kDa oxidoreductase Trx (Holmgren et al., 2005).

A deficit in the formation of ROS highlights the chronic granulomatous disease (Dinauer, 2007), which is caused by an underactive NOX system, in which the capacity of phagocytic leukocytes to generate a microbicide burst of ROS is impaired, leaving the individual susceptible to severe, life-threatening infections by opportunistic microbes. By contrast, it has only recently emerged that excessive ROS production by an overactive NOX system, both in phagocytic and nonphagocytic cell types of the artery wall, may set in motion a vicious cycle of radical and nonradical oxidant generation in various cellular compartments, which disrupts redox circuits that are normally controlled by thiol-dependent antioxidant defenses (Jones, 2008; Santos et al., 2009).

Most of the vasculature diseases related to ROS generation are treated with antioxidants, which are not too effective (vitamins C and E, and β-carotene). However, it is necessary to mention that these compounds are able to chemically remove excessive amount of ROS from the model systems of vascular diseases (Morris and Carson, 2003).

Explanations of why vitamin E is ineffective during the clinical trials have been perfectly suggested and described by Drummond et al. (2011).

Along with the existing known antioxidants in our publications we are proposing and proving data about the XOR-mediated antioxidant abilities of pyridoxine, one of the subcomponents of the vitamin B complex. We were also able to prove that pyridoxine. by suppressing the XO activity. might influence the proliferative activity of the human brain-derived primer cell culture as well as in in vivo experimental pathological settings (Danielyan, 2013b; Aganyants et al., 2014).

16.6 Comparison of the influence of pyridoxine ability to trigger cells generation with the nicotinamide, riboflavin, and thiamine

In one of our investigations (Danielyan, 2013b) we have determined the growth and development of the human embryo brain-derived cell culture, as well as death of the cells in the presence of single components of vitamin B complex: nicotinamide, riboflavin, pyridoxine, and thiamine.

During the early period of the growth, important components responsible for the development of the cells were thiamine, pyridoxine, riboflavin, and nicotinamide. However, the most vivid difference we were able to detect was between the groups treated with the pyridoxine and thiamine.

The size of the embryonic bodies, as well as smaller cells, were sensitive to all the components of vitamin B subcomponents. At day 12 the size of the small cells' fraction treated with the subcomponents of vitamin B complex was smaller in comparison with the control groups. However, the average size of the embryonic bodies in comparison with day 4 increased by 20% in the groups treated with the subcomponents, indicating that small cells were gathering together and forming larger embryonic bodies.

.Our previous results (Danielyan and Kevorkian, 2011) indicated that the early stage inhibition of the XO in the human brain-derived cell culture by allopurinol initiated the increase of cells number in comparison with the later stage of inhibition.

In comparison with the all other subcomponents of vitamin B complex, only in pyridoxine-containing samples was XO activity specifically inhibited by allopurinol. Moreover, pyridoxine by itself inhibited the formation of uric acid. In all the other samples XO activity wasn't inhibited with any concentrations of allopurinol, probably due to the initiation of the alternative pathways of uric acid formation.

Similarly to allopurinol, the pyridoxine treatment during the early stages of the treatment initiated the increase in the number of the cells, whereas in the late stages that process was suppressed. During the late stages the most effective components were riboflavin and nicotinamide.

16.7 Pyridoxine

The biologically active form of the B6 vitamers is pyridoxal-5′'-phosphate (PLP), which plays a coenzymatic role in several distinct enzymatic activities ranging from the synthesis, interconversion, and degradation of amino acids to the replenishment of one-carbon units, synthesis and degradation of biogenic amines, synthesis of tetrapyrrolic compounds, and metabolism of amino-sugars. Pyridoxal-5'-phosphate is the metabolically active form and is involved in 100 enzymatic reactions including carbohydrate, amino acid, and fatty acid metabolism. In the catalytic process of PLP-dependent enzymes, the substrate amino acid forms a Schiff base with PLP and the electrophilicity of the PLP pyridine ring plays important roles in the subsequent catalytic steps. While the essential role of PLP in the acquisition of biological activity of many proteins has been long recognized, the finding that some PLP enzymes require the coenzyme for refolding in vitro points to an additional role of PLP as a chaperone in the folding process (Cellini et al., 2014).

Vitamin B6 or pyridoxine has an important role in the function of the human nervous system. Experimental data are not generally available on the role in human development, but significant conclusions may be made from studies of the effect of disorders of B6 vitamin metabolism. The common active form in human tissue is PLP, most of which is found in muscle, bound to phosphorylase. There is evidence that in some situations B6 vitamers can function as antioxidants. The fetus is dependent on the placenta for the supply of vitamin B6 and the demand correlates with amino acid metabolism. Few reports are available on the role of B6 in embryogenesis. Studies of human disorders, where B6 metabolism is blocked, show a major role in neurotransmitter function with secondary cerebral and cerebellar hypoplasia. Pyridoxine potentiates vitamin A teratogenicity and an excess leads to peripheral nerve cell degeneration (Slaughter et al., 2014).

Thus the literature data show evidence on the vitally important role of this compound in the functioning and development of the human brain. In our work we have clarified some possible biochemical mechanisms mediated by B6 in the abovementioned physiological processes as well as delineated the role of XOR in B-dependent cells regenerative processes.

In addition, we have highlighted the regulating abilities of XO for the entire purine catabolism and the dependence of this ability on another compound, in this case the activator, epinephrine.

It was shown that allopurinol is able to decrease the metabolic rate of dopamine in the striatum of MPTP-treated rats (Miele et al., 1995). Allen et al. (1994) have reported that catecholamines might interact with the released iron and xanthine oxidase to produce highly reactive hydroxyl radicals. Another group had published results where they demonstrated that glutathione transferase in microsomes might be activated by the epinephrine and norepinephrine and that due to interactions ROS might be formed, which activate XO via the proteolysis of the latter. Activated XO might further interact with glutathione transferase (Lundqvist and Morgenstern, 1992). There is a work with evidence that xanthine-dependent oxidation of NADH might be inhibited by the epinephrine

(Khandke et al., 1986). Yonetani and Iwaki (1981) have shown that in eviscerated rats with functional hepatectomy the infusion of epinephrine induces hyperuricemia and this effect was abolished by pretreatment with allopurinol. On the other hand, it was also demonstrated that XO is able to oxidize epinephrine (Valerino and McCormack, 1971; McCord and Fridovich, 1970).

Thus there is a tight interaction between the activity of the XO and epinephrine and this interaction might have a reversible nature. We have obtained similar results in our laboratory, which are presented below.

It is necessary to add the notion about B6 and its role in the processes of XO and epinephrine interaction. Pyridoxine phosphate is the cofactor of DOPA-carboxylase, which is one of the enzymes responsible for the formation of dopamine from L-DOPA (L-3,4-dihydroxyphenylalanine) in the chain of adrenaline synthesis from phenylalanine (Bukreev, 1978). To delineate the link between pyridine and XO we have treated animals with theophylline, which induces B6 deficiency in rats (Bukreev, 1978; Ubbink et al., 1989; Weir et al., 1990; Shimizu et al., 1994; Barnes and Pauwels, 1994; Aganyants et al., 2014).

Clarification of XO–pyridoxine–epinephrine interdependence might highlight the mechanisms of the induction or suppression of cell proliferation during neurogenesis or cancer. The addressed points can be beneficial also for the studies related to the treatment of Parkinson disease (PD).

In our work we were able to prove the influence of these two compounds—epinephrine and pyridoxine—as activator and inhibitor of XO, on the biochemistry of XO, the proliferative abilities of the human brain-derived cells (E 90) in vitro, and also the interdependence of XO from pyridoxine in vivo (Aganyants et al., 2014).

The experiments clearly show that the addition of pyridoxine into the mixture did provoke the inhibition of the XO. In comparison with the blank control (5.0299e − 3 ± 1.4215e − 3) the addition of the riboflavin along with the pyridoxine inhibited the enzyme activity (2.2715e − 3 ± 1.1444e − 3). Similarly the inhibition of the enzyme was noticed in the presence of the adenosine (2.6610e − 3 ± 6.1656e − 4), desoxyadenosine (7.6259e − 4 ± 4.4994e − 4), as well as aspartate (8.1127e − -4 ± 3.5362e − 4).

The activity of purified enzyme from the liver XOR was also evaluated in the presence of four different concentrations of pyridoxine: 5.9, 14.75, 59, and 147.17 μM. The K_m for the enzyme and xanthine as a substrate was equal to 0.051 nM, $V_{max} = 0.0279$, whereas the K_i for pyridoxine was equal to 0.0076 mM (Aganyants et al., 2014).

Theophylline is the compound depleting the amount of B6 in the organism

In our experiments we treated the animals via water with theophylline (water was prewarmed to increase the solubility of theophylline) over 10 days. XO activity was compared with the scheme animals' brains. The activity of XO in the subcortical parts of the brain were higher in a statistically significant way in comparison with the cortex in both groups of the animals. We were expecting that theophylline pretreatment would activate XO, whereas the obtained results were evidence of the opposite. We suggest that the dose of the theophylline wasn't sufficient for the total inhibition of XO and just provoked its activity as the enzyme responsible for elimination of toxic compounds.

The evaluation of XO-specific activity in the presence of epinephrine or initial compounds responsible for epinephrine synthesis was assessed in our experiments too.

In comparison with the control ($9.0519e-3 \pm 9.1319e-4$) the addition of the epinephrine in a statistically significant way stimulated the activity of XO (0.1281 ± 0.0121). Allopurinol in the presence of epinephrine was able to diminish that activity ($0.0694 \pm 7.7637e-3$). We also tried to determine the influence of continuously synthesizing epinephrine from tyrosine in the presence of cofactors pyridoxine and phenylalanine on the activity of XO or on the final formation of uric acid (0.0221 ± 0.0115; $0.0101 \pm 9.7123e-4$, respectively). Both these effects were inhibited in the presence of allopurinol ($7.2137e-3 \pm 1.0007e-3$; $7.2415e-3 \pm 2.7852e-4$, respectively).

We also evaluated the influence of the epinephrine on the process of the purine catabolism.

In comparison with the blank control (0.031 ± 0.016), in the presence of the nonprimer substrates, riboflavin $0.049 \pm 1.947e-3$, adenosine 0.05 ± 0.013, and desoxyadenosine $0.063 \pm 4.366e-3$ ($P < .05$), epinephrine was able to activate XO activity (2016).

We evaluated also the impact of pyridoxine and epinephrine treatment of the human brain-derived cell culture over different time periods.

In our previous experiments we were using low concentrations of pyridoxine for cell culture treatment and were able to detect a high proliferative rate of the cells (Danielyan, 2013b). We used a high concentration and found out a slight increase in cell death and no proproliferative effect. Epinephrine was able to elevate the number of the cells in the Petri dishes during all treatment periods. However, it is necessary to mention that along with this positive effect, an elevation of the cell death was also noticed in comparison with control groups.

Activation of XO by epinephrine triggers cells proliferation as evidenced by study results. In some studies α-2-agonists are able to stimulate the proliferation of breast tumor cells (Szpunar et al., 2013). We think that in a pathological state and even during different aggravating conditions XO might be activated differently. Also it is necessary to take into consideration that XOR acts as a dual enzyme: it is performing its action as a dehydrogenase and as an oxidase, mostly in pathological conditions (Stark et al., 1989). The coefficient of inhibition for this enzyme by different inhibitors vary widely, as do the V_{max} of the reactions (http://www.brenda-enzymes.org/enzyme.php?ecno = 1.17.3.2), assuming different mechanisms of their regulation. However, during biochemical experiments we have proved once again that XO is the rate-limiting enzyme and activation of it might have an impact on the entire purine catabolism.

Pyridoxine had no statistically significant effect on cell growth in experiments. Previously we have noticed proproliferative effects of pyridoxine, however, the implied concentrations (100 × higher) didn't have any impact on the significance of the obtained current results. In our previous studies we have also demonstrated that inhibition of XOR activity with allopurinol might stimulate in vitro cell proliferation processes (Danielyan and Kevorkian, 2011), whereas the inhibition of dihydropyrimidine dehydrogenase might prevent brain-derived cells from death (Danielyan, 2013a,b; Danielyan and Chailyan, 2013).

In the comparable concentration to epinephrine, pyridoxine had no any effect. We need to mention that pyridoxine behaves as a dual effect compound for XO: at a low concentration it inhibits the enzyme, whereas at a high concentration it doesn't possess such an effect or even activate it. We have tried to delineate the pyridoxine–XO link with the use of theophylline, assuming that it will deplete the pyridoxine and we will observe activation of XO. However, in vivo results reflected the exact opposite picture, which means that we must consider even more complicated interactions between these compounds. In addition to the above presented note, we can just speculate that theophylline by triggering ATP synthesis might also initiate activation of purine catabolism and pyridoxine quantity depletion is the secondary for this vitally important process.

We have proved and presented that the fundamental mechanism of purine catabolism regulation via XO in the presence of epinephrine and

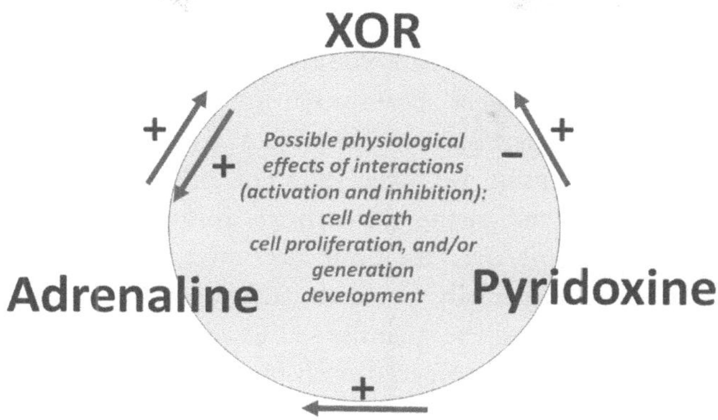

Figure 16.1 Purine catabolism regulation via xanthine oxidoreductase (XOR)/xanthine oxidase (XO) in the presence of epinephrine and pyridoxine.

pyridoxine is inhibited. This phenomenon might be utilized for regenerative processes, the prevention of cell proliferation in cancer development, and PD treatment (interdependent interactions of these compounds are presented in (Fig. 16.1).

16.8 The role of pyridoxine in pathological conditions in vitro and in vivo

Cystein is a compound contributing to the synthesis of reduced glutathione (GSH). The GSH-dependent antioxidant system, including GPx, glutathione reductase (GR), and GST, plays a fundamental role in cellular defense against reactive free radicals and other oxidant species (Wu et al., 2004; Keles et al., 2010). Some studies indicate that in liver tissue of vitamin B6-deficient rats the malondialdehyde level and GR activity is increased, whereas GSH synthesis, GPx, and GSH activities are decreased (Taysi, 2005). In some other studies it is shown that GSH concentrations and GR activities are unchanged in the liver, kidney, brain, lung, spleen, and plasma, and that GPx activities is increased in the liver of vitamin B6-deficient rats when compared to control rats (Takeuchi et al., 1991). Thus deficiency of vitamin B6 might directly as well as indirectly exacerbate the antioxidative defense mechanism and promote oxidative stress

To delineate the impact of B6 in experimental oxidative stress conditions we used peroxide as the compound which might have deleterious effects and induce cell death via apoptosis and necrosis. We treated neuronal cells containing cell culture with 3% hydrogen peroxide for 24 hours and detected results by counting the cell number in the field as well as staining the dead cells with Trypan blue dye.

Similar experiments were performed in vivo. The animals were injected with the hydrogen peroxide intracranially either alone or in combination with the vitamin B6 over different time periods (days 1–6, 6–12, 1–12). At the end of the experiments animals were intravenously injected with Evans blue dye. An hour later after circulation of the dye the animals were intracranially perfused and the brains were dissected. The dye was extracted and the quantity of it was determined spectrophotometrically. Results were compared with the XO classical inhibitor allopurinol (Danielyan and Simonyan, 2017).

The human brain-derived neuronal cells-containing culture was maintained for 7 days. On day 7 the culture was treated with the 3% hydrogen peroxide for 24 hours.

In comparison with the control (2680.00 ± 45.34) in the peroxide-treated group (1631.89 ± 111.77) the number of the cells was dramatically decreased (Fig. 16.2). Allopurinol treatment 15 minutes before (1852.38 ± 94.79) and 15 minutes after (1950.38 ± 33.67) increased the cells number but in a not statistically significant way. The addition of pyridoxine into the cells media increased the number of the cells in a statistically significant way, moreover, treatment with pyridoxine before peroxide addition was less efficient (2106.88 ± 79.64) than after (2392.38 ± 104.01), ($P < .05$).

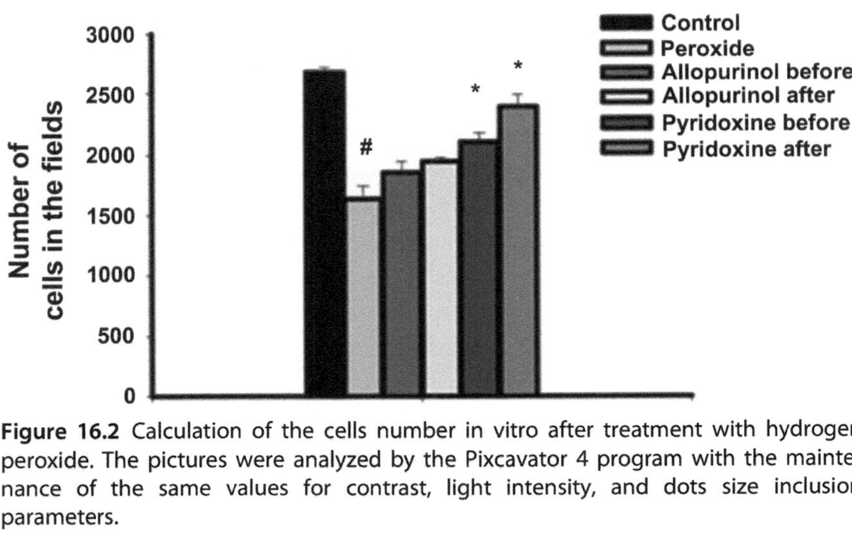

Figure 16.2 Calculation of the cells number in vitro after treatment with hydrogen peroxide. The pictures were analyzed by the Pixcavator 4 program with the maintenance of the same values for contrast, light intensity, and dots size inclusion parameters.

One-hour treatment of the cells culture with hydrogen peroxide (740.33 ± 86.16) in comparison with the control group (245.90 ± 31.72) strongly increased the number of dead cells in the culture in a statistically significant way ($P < .05$), (Fig. 16.3). Treatment with the allopurinol before (556.78 ± 16.17), as well as after (536.70 ± 49.79) addition of hydrogen peroxide, and treatment with pyridoxine after modeling of oxidative stress (630.22 ± 71.84) were less effective in comparison with the treatment with the B6 before oxidative stress initiation (231.50 ± 53.77), ($P < .05$, ONE WAY ANOVA for the comparison of the peroxide control group with the treatment all four groups) ($P < .05$, *t*-test for the comparison of control vs. peroxide negative control group).

In vivo studies were performed by injection of the hydrogen peroxide into the cortical layers of the brain. To address the question related to the involvement of XOR and B6 in the processes of BBB disruption, animals were intravenously injected with Evans blue (Danielyan and Simonyan, 2017).

After Evans blue extraction the values of the ipsilateral hemisphere were extracted from the numbers of the contralateral hemisphere to exclude the brain perfusion experimental errors (Fig. 16.4). Animals were treated over three different time periods: days 1–12, 1–6, and 6–12. In comparison with the control, all treatment periods were effective for allopurinol as well as pyridoxine (control 0.029756 ± 0.010616; 1–12

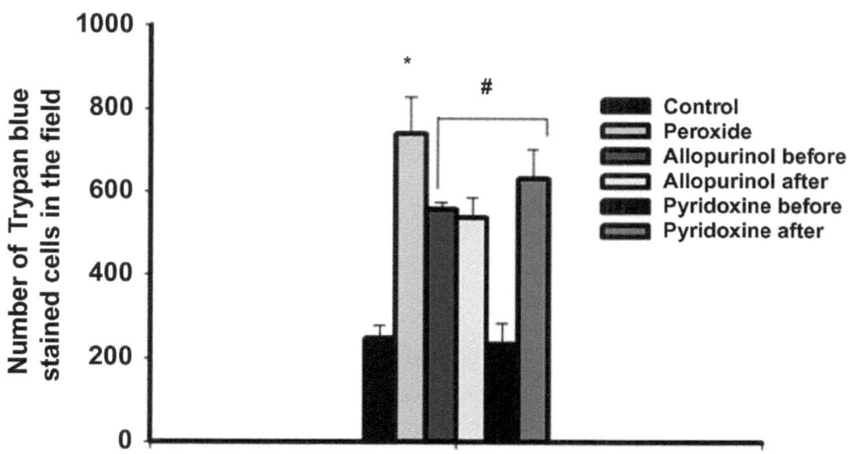

Figure 16.3 Calculation of the death cells number in the culture. The cells were stained with Trypan blue (0.04%) solution and their numbers were calculated.

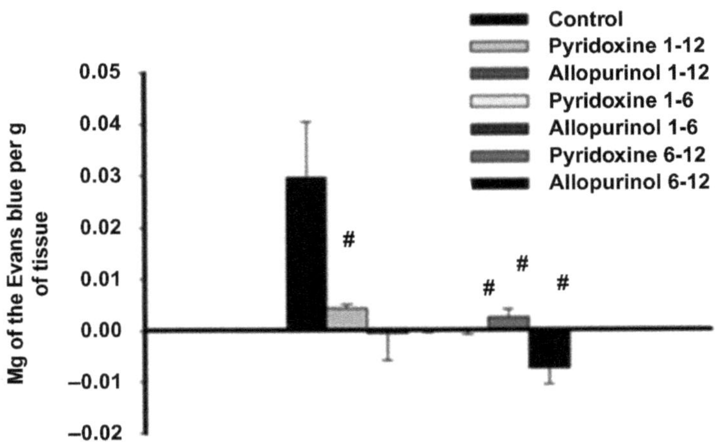

Figure 16.4 Evans blue extraction values from the animal's brains represented as μg/g of the tissue.

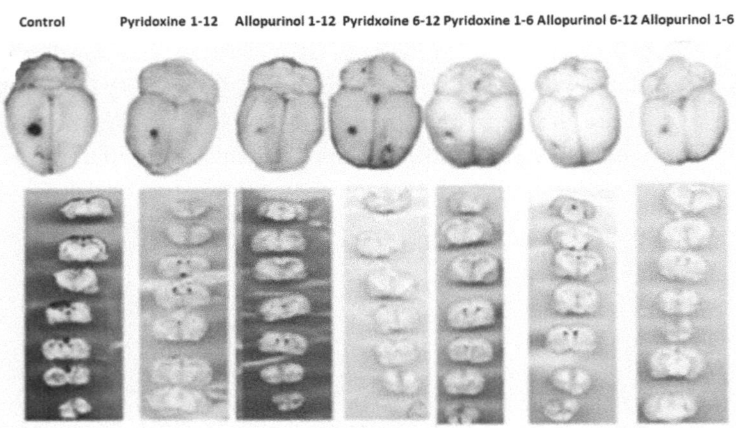

Figure 16.5 In vivo evaluation of new and classical inhibitors of xanthine oxidase (XO). Representative pictures of the whole brains of the animals.

pyridoxine 0.004131 ± 0.000803; 1−12 allopurinol 0.00062 ± 0.042976; 1−6 pyridoxine 8.5E − 05 ± 0.000353; 1−6 allopurinol −8.9e − 05 ± 0.000816; 6−12 pyridoxine 0.002451 ± 0.001573; 6−12 allopurinol −0.00742 ± 0.003123), ($P < .05$) (Figs. 16.4 and 16.5).

The use of allopurinol as well as pyridoxine over different time periods after brain damage has significant effects on the protection of BBB from peroxide-determined damage.

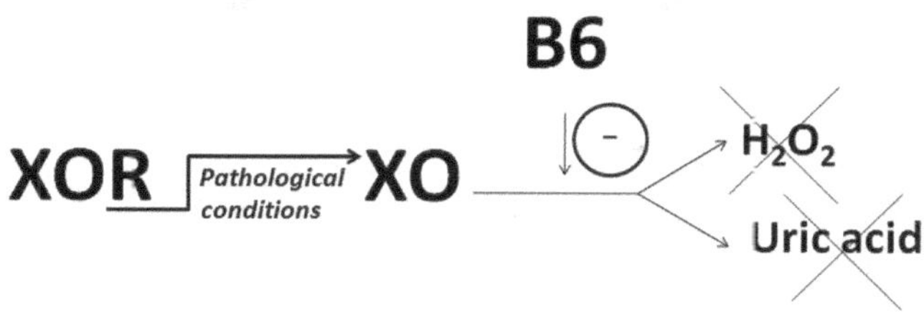

Figure 16.6 Schematic representation of the B6 impact on xanthine oxidoreductase (XOR).

The antioxidative abilities of pyridoxine that are proposed by our work might be applicable for the treatment of stroke in the future (Danielyan and Simonyan, 2017) (Fig. 16.6).

References

International Ethical Guidelines for Health-related Research Involving Humans. Prepared by the Council for International Organizations of Medical Sciences (CIOMS) in Collaboration with the World Health Organization (WHO). Geneva, 2016, 122 pp.

Aganyants, H.A., Abrahamyan, R.A., Chailyan, S.G., Danielyan, K.E., 2014. New highlights in the regulation of cells proliferation. Neurosci. Biomed. Eng. 2, 81–86.

Allen, D.R., Wallis, G.L., McCay, P.B., 1994. Catechol adrenergic agents enhance hydroxyl radical generation in xanthine oxidase systems containing ferritin: implications for ischemia/reperfusion. Arch. Biochem. Biophys. 315 (2), 235–243.

Barnes, P.J., Pauwels, R.A., 1994. Theophylline in the management of asthma: time for reappraisal? Eur. Respir. J. 7 (3), 579–591.

Bedard, K., Krause, K.H., 2007. The NOX family of ROS-generating NADPH oxidases: physiology and pathophysiology. Physiol. Rev. 87, 245–313.

Bienert, G.P., Schjoerring, J.K., Jahn, T.P., 2006. Membrane transport of hydrogen peroxide. Biochim. Biophys. Acta 1758, 994–1003.

Bleisch, S., Sillero, M.A., Torrecilla, A., Sillero, A., 1994. Uric acid synthesis by rat liver supernatants from purine bases, nucleosides and nucleotides. Effect of allopurinol. Cell Biochem. Funct. 12 (4), 237–245.

Boveris, A., Oshino, N., Chance, B., 1972. The cellular production of hydrogen peroxide. Biochem. J. 128, 617–630.

Bukreev, V.I., 1978. Effect of pyridoxine on the psychopathology and pathochemistry of involutional depressions. Zh. Nevropatol. Psikhiatr. Im. S. S. Korsakova 78 (3), 402–408.

Cadenas, E., Boveris, A., Ragan, C.I., Stoppani, A.O., 1977. Production of superoxide radicals and hydrogen peroxide by NADH-ubiquinone reductase and ubiquinol-cytochrome c reductase from beef-heart mitochondria. Arch. Biochem. Biophys. 180, 248–257.

Cave, A.C., Brewer, A.C., Narayanapanicker, A., Ray, R., Grieve, D.J., Walker, S., et al., 2006. NADPH oxidases in cardiovascular health and disease. Antioxid. Redox Signal. 8, 691–728.

Cellini, B., Montioli, R., Oppici, E., Astegno, A., Voltattorni, C.B., 2014. The chaperone role of the pyridoxal 5′-phosphate and its implications for rare diseases involving B6-dependent enzymes. Clin. Biochem. 47 (3), 158–165.

Chatterjee, S., Feinstein, S.I., Dodia, C., Sorokina, E., Lien, Y.C., Nguyen, S., et al., 2011. Peroxiredoxin 6 phosphorylation and subsequent phospholipase A2 activity are required for agonist-mediated activation of NADPH oxidase in mouse pulmonary microvascular endothelium and alveolar macrophages. J. Biol. Chem. 286 (13), 11696–11706.

Danielyan, K.E., 2013a. Dependence of cells survival from xanthine oxidase and dihydopyrimidine dehydrogenase correlative activities in human brain derived cell culture. Cent. Nerv. Syst. Agents Med. Chem. 13 (2), 108–113.

Danielyan, K.E., 2013b. Subcomponents of vitamine B complex regulate the growth and development of human brain derived cells. Am. J. Biomed. Res. 1 (2), 28–34.

Danielyan, K.E., Kevorkian, G.A., 2011. Xanthine oxidase activity regulates human embryonic brain cells growth. Biopolym. Cell 27 (5), 350–353.

Danielyan, K.E., Chailyan, S.G., 2013. Xanthine dehydrogenase inhibition stimulates growth and development of human brain derived cells. Am. J. Med. Biol. Res. 1 (4), 95–98.

Danielyan, K.E., Simonyan, A.A., 2017. Protective abilities of pyridoxine in experimental oxidative stress settings in vivo and in vitro. Biomed. Pharmacother. 86, 537–540.

Dinauer, M.C., 2007. Disorders of neutrophil function: an overview. Methods Mol. Biol. 412, 489–504.

Drummond, G.R., Selemidis, S., Griendling, K.K., Sobey, C.G., 2011. Combating oxidative stress in vascular disease: NADPH oxidases as therapeutic targets. Nat. Rev. Drug Discov. 10 (6), 453–471.

Edwards, N.L., Recker, D., Fox, I.H., 1979. Overproduction of uric acid in hypoxanthine-guanine phosphoribosyltransferase deficiency. Contribution by impaired purine salvage. J. Clin. Invest. 63 (5), 922–930.

Edwards, N.L., Recker, D., Airozo, D., Fox, I.H., 1981. Enhanced purine salvage during allopurinol therapy: an important pharmacologic property in humans. J. Lab. Clin. Med. 98 (5), 673–683.

Gladden, J.D., Zelickson, B.R., Wei, C.C., Ulasova, E., Zheng, J., Ahmed, M.I., et al., 2011. Novel insights into interactions between mitochondria and xanthine oxidase in acute cardiac volume overload. Free Radic. Biol. Med. 51, 1975–1984.

Gyongyan, S.A., Manucharyan, T.G., Danielyan, K.E., Kevorkyan, G.A., Chailyan, S.G., 2013. Xanthine oxidoreductase is a key enzyme of purine catabolism regulation. Electron. J. Nat. Sci. 5, 17.

Hille, R., Nishino, T., 1995. Flavoprotein structure and mechanism. 4. Xanthine oxidase and xanthine dehydrogenase. FASEB J. 9 (11), 995–1003.

Holmgren, A., Johansson, C., Berndt, C., Lonn, M.E., Hudemann, C., Lillig, C.H., 2005. Thiol redox control via thioredoxin and glutaredoxin systems. Biochem. Soc. Trans. 33, 1375–1377.

Ichida, K., Amaya, Y., Noda, K., Minoshima, S., Hosoya, T., Sakai, O., et al., 1993. Cloning of the cDNA encoding human xanthine dehydrogenase (oxidase): structural analysis of the protein and chromosomal location of the gene. Gene 133 (2), 279–284.

Jerushalmy, Z., Patya, M., Boer, P., Sperling, O., 1980. De novo synthesis of purine nucleotides in human blood platelets. Haemostasis 9 (1), 20–27.

Jones, D.P., 2008. Radical-free biology of oxidative stress. Am. J. Physiol. Cell Physiol. 295, C849–C868.

Kalyanaraman, B., 2013. Teaching the basics of redox biology to medical and graduate students: oxidants, antioxidants and disease mechanisms. Redox Biol. 1 (1), 244–257.

Keles, M., Al, B., Gumustekin, K., Demircan, B., Ozbey, I., Akyuz, M., et al., 2010. Antioxidant status and lipid peroxidation in kidney tissue of rats fed with vitamin B6-deficient diet. Ren. Fail. 32, 618–622.

Khandke, L., Gullapalli, S., Patole, M.S., Ramasarma, T., 1986. Vanadate-stimulated NADH oxidation by xanthine oxidase: an intrinsic property. Arch. Biochem. Biophys. 244 (2), 742–749.

Kumar, V., Calamaras, T.D., Haeussler, D., Colucci, W.S., Cohen, R.A., McComb, M. E., et al., 2012. Cardiovascular redox and ox stress proteomics. Antioxid Redox Signal 17 (11), 1528–1559.

Lalanne, M., Lafleur, F., 1980. Inosine synthesis and phosphoribosylpyrophosphate availability in rat liver cells in the presence of allopurinol. Can. J. Biochem. 58 (8), 607–613.

Lee, W.K., Thevenod, F., 2006. A role for mitochondrial aquaporins in cellular life-and-death decisions? Am. J. Physiol. Cell. Physiol. 291, C195–C202.

Leto, T.L., Morand, S., Hurt, D., Ueyama, T.T., 2009. Targeting and regulation of reactive oxygen species generation by Nox family NADPH oxidases. Antioxid Redox Signal 11, 2607–2619.

Leung, H.B., Schramm, V.L., 1978. The role of adenosine monophosphate nucleosidase in the regulation of adenine nucleotide levels in *Azotobacter vinelandii* during aerobic–anaerobic transitions. Arch. Biochem. Biophys. 190 (1), 46–56.

Löffler, W., Gröbner, W., 1988. A study of dose-response relationships of allopurinol in the presence of low or high purine turnover. Klin. Wochenschr. 66 (4), 153–159.

Lundqvist, G., Morgenstern, R., 1992. Mechanism of activation of rat liver microsomal glutathione transferase by noradrenaline and xanthine oxidase. Biochem. Pharmacol. 43 (8), 1725–1728.

Malhotra, J.D., Kaufman, R.J., 2007. Endoplasmic reticulum stress and oxidative stress: a vicious cycle or a doubleedged sword? Antioxid. Redox Signal. 9, 2277–2293.

McCord, J.M., Fridovich, I., 1970. The utility of superoxide dismutase in studying free radical reactions. II. The mechanism of the mediation of cytochrome c reduction by a variety of electron carriers. J. Biol. Chem. 245 (6), 1374–1377.

Miele, M., Esposito, G., Migheli, R., Sircana, S., Zangani, D., Fresu, G.L., et al., 1995. Effects of allopurinol on 1-methyl-4-phenyl-1,2,3,6-tetrahydropyridine (MPTP)-induced neurochemical changes in the striatum and in the brainstem of the rat. Neurosci. Lett. 183 (3), 155–159.

Mink, R.B., Dutka, A.J., Hallenbeck, J.M., 1991. Allopurinol pretreatment improves evoked response recovery following global cerebral ischemia in dogs. Stroke 22, 660–665.

Moriwaki, Y., Yamamoto, T., Higashino, K., 1999. Enzymes involved in purine metabolism—a review of histochemical localization and functional implications. Histol. Histopathol. 14, 1321–1340.

Morris, C.D., Carson, S., 2003. Routine vitaminsupplementation to prevent cardiovascular disease: a summary of the evidence for the U.S. Preventive Services Task Force. Ann. Intern. Med. 139, 56–70.

Olson, J.S., Ballou, D.P., Palmer, G., Massey, V., 1974. The mechanism of action of xanthine oxidase. J. Biol. Chem. 249 (14), 4363–4382.

Ono, T., Tsuruta, R., Fujita, M., Aki, H.S., Kutsuna, S., Kawamura, Y., et al., 2009. Xanthine oxidase is one of the major sources of superoxide anion radicals in blood after reperfusion in rats with forebrain ischemia/reperfusion. Brain Res. 1305, 158–167.

Pechán, I., Zimmer, H.G., 1989. The effect of allopurinol on the synthesis of adenine nucleotides and ribonucleic acid from inosine via a salvage pathway in the brain of rats. Cesk. Neurol. Neurochir. 52 (6), 378–383.

Pelled, D., Sperling, O., Zoref-Shani, E., 1999. Abnormal purine and pyrimidine nucleotide content in primary astroglia cultures from hypoxanthine-guanine phosphoribosyltransferase-deficient transgenic mice. J. Neurochem. 72 (3), 1139–1145.

Pendyala, S., Usatyuk, P.V., Gorshkova, I.A., Garcia, J.G., Natarajan, V., 2009a. Regulation of NADPH oxidase in vascular endothelium: the role of phospholipases, protein kinases, and cytoskeletal proteins. Antioxid. Redox Signal. 11, 841–860.
Pendyala, S., Usatyuk, P.V., Gorshkova, I.A., Garcia, J.G., Natarajan, V., 2009b. Regulation of NADPH oxidase in vascular endothelium: the role of phospholipases, protein kinases, and cytoskeletal proteins. Antioxid. Redox Signal. 11, 841–860.
Ray, R., Shah, A.M., 2005. NADPH oxidase and endothelial cell function. Clin. Sci. (Lond.) 109, 217–226.
Sabina, R.L., Hanks, A.R., Magill, J.M., Magill, C.W., 1979. Role of purine base excretion in regulation of purine pools. Mol. Gen. Genet. 173 (1), 31–38.
Santos, C.X., Tanaka, L.Y., Wosniak, J., Laurindo, F.R., 2009. Mechanisms and implications of reactive oxygen species generation during the unfolded protein response: roles of endoplasmic reticulum oxidoreductases, mitochondrial electron transport, and NADPH oxidase. Antioxid. Redox Signal. 11, 2409–2427.
Shimizu, T., Maeda, S., Mochizuki, H., Tokuyama, K., Morikawa, A., 1994. Theophylline attenuates circulating vitamin B6 levels in children with asthma. Pharmacology 49 (6), 392–397.
Simmonds, H.A., Bowyer, A., 1974. Purine and pyrimidine excretion in psoriasis: a comparison with healthy controls during allopurinol therapy. Br. J. Clin. Pharmacol. 1 (2), 107–111.
Slaughter, S.R., Hearns-Stokes, R., van der Vlugt, T., Joffe, H.V., 2014. FDA approval of doxylamine-pyridoxine therapy for use in pregnancy. N. Engl. J. Med. 370 (12), 1081–1083.
St-Pierre, J., Buckingham, J.A., Roebuck, S.J., Brand, M.D., 2002. Topology of superoxide production from different sites in the mitochondrial electron transport chain. J. Biol. Chem. 277, 44784–44790.
Stark, K., Seubert, P., Lynch, G., Baudry, M., 1989. Proteolytic conversion of xanthine dehydrogenase to xanthine oxidase: evidence against a role for calcium-activated protease (calpain). Biochem. Biophys. Res. Commun. 165 (2), 858–864.
Szpunar, M.J., Burke, K.A., Dawes, R.P., Brown, E.B., Madden, K.S., 2013. The antidepressant desipramine and α2-adrenergic receptor activation promote breast tumor progression in association with altered collagen structure. Cancer Prev. Res. (Phila.) 6 (12), 1262–1272.
Takeuchi, F., Izuta, S., Tsubouchi, R., Shibata, Y., 1991. Glutathione levels and related enzyme activities in vitamin B-6 deficient rats fed a high methionine and low cysteine diet. J. Nutr. 121, 1366–1373.
Taysi, S., 2005. Oxidant/antioxidant status in liver tissue of vitamin B6 deficient rats. Clin. Nutr. 24, 35–39.
Tu, B.P., Weissman, J.S., 2004. Oxidative protein folding in eukaryotes: mechanisms and consequences. J. Cell Biol. 164, 341–346.
Ubbink, J.B., Delport, R., Becker, P.J., Bissbort, S., 1989. Evidence of a theophylline-induced vitamin B6 deficiency caused by noncompetitive inhibition of pyridoxal kinase. J. Lab. Clin. Med. 113 (1), 15–22.
Valerino, D.M., McCormack, J.J., 1971. Xanthine oxidase-mediated oxidation of epinephrine. Biochem. Pharmacol. 20 (1), 47–55.
Weir, M.R., Keniston, R.C., Enriquez, J.I., McNamee, G.A., 1990. Depression of vitamin B6 levels due to theophylline. Ann. Allergy 65 (1), 59–62.
Wu, G., Fang, Y.Z., Yang, S., Lupton, J.R., Turner, N.D., 2004. Glutathione metabolism and its implications for health. J. Nutr. 134, 489–492.
Yonetani, Y., Iwaki, K., 1981. Catecholamine-induced hyperuricemia in eviscerated rats with functional hepatectomy. Jpn. J. Pharmacol. 31 (3), 323–332.

CHAPTER 17

Nonalcoholic fatty liver disease and use of folate

O Karmin[1,2,3], Connie W.H. Woo[4], Victoria Sid[2,3] and Yaw L. Siow[2,5,6]

[1]Department of Animal Science, University of Manitoba, Winnipeg, MB, Canada
[2]Department of Physiology and Pathophysiology, University of Manitoba, Winnipeg, MB, Canada
[3]Laboratory of Integrative Biology, St. Boniface Hospital Research Centre, Winnipeg, MB, Canada
[4]Department of Pharmacology and Pharmacy, Li Ka Shing Faculty of Medicine, University of Hong Kong, Hong Kong, SAR, China
[5]Agriculture and Agri-Food Canada, Canadian Centre for Agri-Food Research in Health and Medicine, Winnipeg, MB, Canada
[6]Innovative Therapy Research Laboratory, St. Boniface Hospital Research Centre, Winnipeg, MB, Canada

Contents

Molecular Nutrition
DOI: https://doi.org/10.1016/B978-0-12-811907-5.00028-2

Key facts of Fig. 17.1

- Absorption of dietary folate and folic acid in the small intestine is mediated through folate transporters: reduced folate carrier and proton-coupled folate transporter (PCFT).
- Dietary folate is mainly in the form of polyglutamate that is hydrolyzed to monoglutamate [10-formyl-tetrahydrofolate (10-formyl-THF) and 5-methyl tetrahydrofolate (5-MTHF)] prior to absorption.
- Folic acid is a monoglutamate that is readily transported into intestinal epithelial cells, where it is slowly converted to 5-MTHF.
- PCFT is the primary transporter for dietary folate/folic acid absorption in the small intestine with a more favorable acidic microenvironment.
- Upon intestinal absorption, monoglutamate forms of folic acid are delivered via the hepatic portal system to the liver where they undergo intracellular polyglutamylation.
- Liver is the primary organ for folate storage, metabolism, and redistribution to the circulation and bile.

Key facts of Fig. 17.2

- Folate-dependent one-carbon transfer reactions can occur in the cytoplasm, nucleus, and mitochondria.
- 10-Formyl-tetrahydrofolate (10-formyl-THF) and 5-methyl tetrahydrofolate (5-MTHF) are the major coenzymes in these pathways: purine nucleotide synthesis, interconversion of glycine and serine, and homocysteine remethylation to methionine.

Key facts of Fig. 17.3

- Folate regulates sulfur-containing amino acid metabolism through the interaction between the methionine cycle, transsulfuration, and desulfuration reactions.
- Homocysteine is an intermediate amino acid formed during the metabolism of methionine to cysteine. It can be metabolized via the remethylation pathway and the transsulfuration pathway.
- Remethylation of homocysteine to methionine requires 5-methyl tetrahydrofolate (5-MTHF) and vitamin B12.
- Metabolism of homocysteine to cysteine through the transsulfuration pathway is catalyzed by cystathionine-β-synthase (CBS) and

cystathionine-γ-lyase (CSE); both of which require vitamin B6 as a coenzyme in their activities.
- Cysteine serves as a precursor for the biosynthesis of glutathione, a major endogenous antioxidant.
- CBS and CSE are also responsible for the biosynthesis of hydrogen sulfide through desulfuration reactions.

Summary points

- This chapter focuses on the role of folate in nonalcoholic fatty liver disease.
- Folate is vitamin B9 and is naturally occurring, while folic acid is the synthetic form.
- Folate plays a key role in one-carbon transfer reactions that are essential for nucleic acid biosynthesis, methylation reaction, and sulfur-containing amino acid metabolism.
- Nonalcoholic fatty liver disease (NAFLD) is the most common chronic liver disease that is associated with obesity and type 2 diabetes.
- Folate deficiency is uncommon in the general population in countries with mandatory folate fortification policies. However, low serum folate levels are detected in NAFLD patients with adequate dietary intake of folate.
- Chronic high-fat diet feeding induces fatty liver and impairs hepatic metabolism in rodents. Serum and liver folate levels are decreased in high-fat diet-induced obese mice.
- In a rodent model of NAFLD, folic acid supplementation (1) protects against oxidative stress and increased inflammatory cytokine production in the liver, and (2) improves hepatic lipid and glucose metabolism through restoration of AMP-activated protein kinase.
- Clinical studies of folate supplementation in NAFLD patients are warranted.

17.1 Introduction

Folate (vitamin B9) is an important micronutrient that plays a key role in one-carbon transfer reactions that are essential for nucleic acid biosynthesis, methylation reactions, and sulfur-containing amino acid metabolism (Tibbetts and Appling, 2010; Stover and Field, 2011). Dysregulation of folate-dependent one-carbon metabolism has been implicated in metabolic diseases such as obesity, type 2 diabetes mellitus, hyperhomocysteinemia, and nonalcoholic fatty liver disease (NAFLD) (Da Silva et al., 2014; Nilsson et al., 2015; Sid et al., 2017). NAFLD represents a broad spectrum of liver disorders ranging from steatosis (hepatic lipid accumulation) to its advanced forms such as nonalcoholic steatohepatitis (NASH) and cirrhosis, the latter can further progress to hepatocellular carcinoma (HCC) (Cohen et al., 2011). NAFLD is often found in patients with obesity, hyperlipidemia, hyperglycemia, insulin resistance, or hypertension (Farrell and Larter, 2006). The prevalence of NAFLD is in parallel with a global increase in obesity and type 2 diabetes (Loomba and Sanyal, 2013). Currently, there are no pharmacological agents approved for NAFLD, and only supportive therapies are available to prevent the progression to the advanced conditions (Chalasani et al., 2012). Nutritional approaches are emerging as a promising management strategy for obesity and NAFLD (Veena et al., 2014). Vitamins are essential micronutrients that play important roles in growth and metabolism. Low serum folate levels are associated with obesity, NAFLD, or type 2 diabetes (Mahabir et al., 2008; Nilsson et al., 2015; Xia et al., 2018). The role of folate in NAFLD is currently being evaluated in animal studies and clinical trials. This chapter will focus on the current knowledge regarding the role of folate in NAFLD.

17.2 Folate and folic acid

17.2.1 Folate and folic acid in diet—food and supplements

Folic acid is a synthetic form of natural folate and is used in supplements, fortified foods, and feeds. The basic structure of folate comprises three components: (1) a pteridine ring that is attached via a methylene group to (2) *p*-amino benzoic acid to form pteroic acid, and (3) L-glutamic acid. Folate exists in many forms that differ in the oxidation state of the pteridine ring at the N5 and N10 position and/or in the number of glutamic acid residues conjugated by γ-glutamyl bonds at the end of the molecule (Stover, 2004; Zhao et al., 2009). Mammals lack the enzymatic capacity to synthesize folate; therefore, the intake of dietary folate is necessary to meet their physiological requirements (Zhao et al., 2009). The recommended daily allowance (RDA) for folic acid in healthy individuals is 400 μg of dietary folate equivalents (DFEs) per day. In pregnant women, the RDA increases to 600 μg of DFEs per day to ensure both maternal well-being and healthy fetal development (Institute of Medicine

Standing Committee on the Scientific Evaluation of Dietary Reference Intakes and Its Panel on Folate, Others B Vitamins and Choline, 1998). Folate is widely distributed in foods. Dark green leafy vegetables, animal liver, and citrus fruits are the most abundant source of naturally occurring folate. Dietary folate often exists in reduced and polyglutamated form. Folic acid is the synthetic (stable) form of folate that is used for dietary supplementation and fortification (Iyer and Tomar, 2009). It is an oxidized monoglutamate with higher bioavailability than its natural counterpart. In North America, cereals and grain products are also important sources of folate due to the mandatory fortification in these foods. In addition to dietary folate and folic acid, folate-producing bacteria in the intestine may serve as an endogenous source of folate (Rong et al., 1991). However, the contribution of intestinal bacteria to whole body folate homeostasis in mammals is significantly less than the dietary source of folate (Visentin et al., 2014).

17.2.2 Folate absorption and metabolism

Dietary folate absorption is mediated through folate transporters in the small intestine (Visentin et al., 2014; Sid et al., 2017) (Fig. 17.1). The reduced folate carrier (RFC/SLC19A1) and proton-coupled folate transporter (PCFT/SLC46A1) are abundantly expressed along the apical membrane of enterocytes (Visentin et al., 2014; Zhao et al., 2011). PCFT has been identified as the primary transporter for folate/folic acid absorption in the proximal intestine, which has a more favorable acidic microenvironment (Visentin et al., 2014). Dietary folate is mainly in the reduced form as formyl- or methyl-polyglutamate (Wright et al., 2007), and requires hydrolysis to monoglutamate by either glutamate carboxypeptidase II (in human intestine) or γ-glutamyl hydrolases (in rodent intestine) prior to the absorption at the intestinal brush border membrane. Conversely, synthetic folic acid is a monoglutamate and therefore does not require hydrolysis for intestinal absorption (Hu et al., 2016). Folic acid approaches 100% bioavailability when it is consumed in an empty stomach. However, only 85% of folic acid is absorbed when taken with food, possibly due to its adsorption or chelation with food matrix (Caudill, 2010). Dietary folate is heat labile and susceptible to destruction in the gastrointestinal tract. In addition, incomplete hydrolysis of the polyglutamate chain of folate may hinder the absorption of food folate. Therefore only 50% of naturally occurring food folate is bioavailable

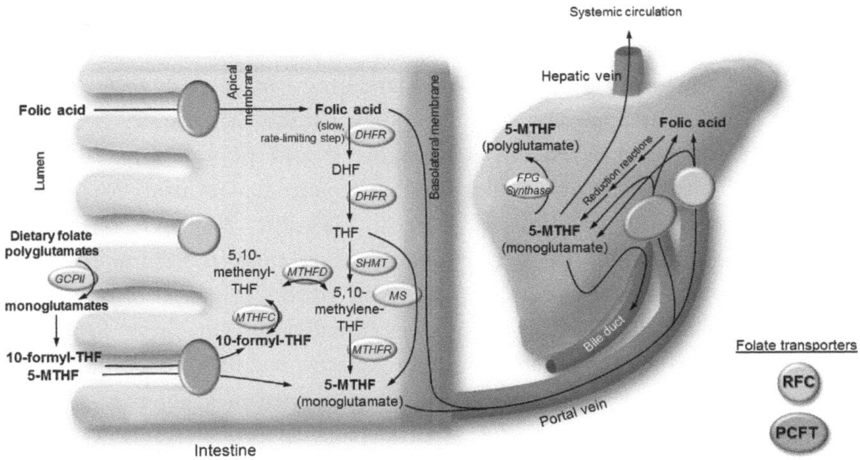

Figure 17.1 Folate absorption and metabolism in the intestine and liver. The major routes of folate absorption and metabolism in the intestine and liver are illustrated. The key forms of folate that enter these organs are shown in *bold*. *PCFT*, Proton-coupled folate transporter; *RFC*, reduced folate transporter. Horizontal ovals denote enzymes and overlap the pathways they catalyze. *DHF*, dihydrofolate; *THF*, Tetrahydrofolate; *5-MTHF*, 5-methyltetrahydrofolate; *DHFR*, dihydrofolate reductase; *SHMT*, serine hydroxymethyltransferase; *MTHFR*, methylenetetrahydrofolate reductase; *MTHFD*, methylenetetrahydrofolate dehydrogenase; *MTHFC*, methylenetetrahydrofolate cyclohydrolase; *MS*, methionine synthase; *GCPII*, glutamate carboxypeptidase II; *FPG* synthase, folylpolyglutamate synthase. *Modified image based on Sid, V., Siow, Y.L., O, K., 2017. Role of folate in nonalcoholic fatty liver disease. Can. J. Physiol. Pharmacol. 95, 1141–1148.*

(Institute of Medicine Standing Committee on the Scientific Evaluation of Dietary Reference Intakes and Its Panel on Folate, Others B Vitamins and Choline, 1998; Caudill, 2010).

Upon absorption by enterocytes, folic acid is reduced to dihydrofolate (DHF) that is subsequently reduced to tetrahydrofolate (THF), the biologically active form of folate (Wright et al., 2007). Because both reactions are catalyzed by DHF reductase (DHFR), the first enzymatic reduction of folic acid to DHF becomes the rate-limiting step. The addition of a one-carbon moiety to THF by serine hydroxymethyltransferase (SHMT) generates 5,10-methylene-tetrahydrofolate (5,10-methylene-THF). Pyridoxal-5′-phosphate (PLP; active form of vitamin B6) is an essential cofactor for SHMT activity. The 5,10-methylene-THF is further reduced to 5-methyl THF (5-MTHF) by 5,10-methylene-THF reductase (Tibbetts and Appling, 2010). The 5-MTHF is the main form of folate that is transported across the basolateral membrane of enterocytes and enters the portal circulation (Wright et al., 2007). However, a high intake of folic acid may exceed the metabolic capacity of enterocytes, leading to its accumulation in the portal circulation (Pietrzik et al., 2010; Hu et al., 2016).

The folic acid and 5-MTHF derived from intestine are subsequently delivered to liver via the portal vein (Wright et al., 2007; Hu et al., 2016; Sid et al., 2017) (Fig. 17.1). Liver is the major organ for folate storage and metabolism (Wright et al., 2007). It plays an important role in maintaining the folate homeostasis (Steinberg et al., 1979). Both RFC and PCFT are expressed on the basolateral membrane of hepatocytes (Zhao et al., 2011). Once inside hepatocytes, folic acid is metabolized to 5-MTHF that undergoes polyglutamation by folylpolyglutamate synthase. The polyglutamate form is the preferential form for storage in hepatocytes and is the reactive form for folate-dependent enzymatic reactions relative to the monoglutamate form (Zhao et al., 2009). While up to 20% of 5-MTHF is retained in the liver, the rest is delivered to the extrahepatic tissues through the systemic circulation or secreted into the bile via the bile duct. Bile folate can be reabsorbed into the liver for storage and redistribution to other tissues (Steinberg et al., 1979).

17.2.3 Folate-mediated one-carbon transfer reactions

Folate serves as a cofactor to facilitate the transfer of one-carbon units. Sarcosine, *N,N*-dimethylglycine (derived from choline), glycine, histidine, and serine (mainly through its conversion to formate in the mitochondria) are the common sources of one-carbon units. The folate-mediated one-carbon transfer reactions take place in various cellular compartments including the cytoplasm, nucleus, and mitochondria (Tibbetts and Appling, 2010; Sid et al., 2017). Intracellular one-carbon transfers are mediated by coenzymatic forms of THF, which carries a one-carbon unit for amino acid metabolism, nucleotide biosynthesis, and methylation reactions (Stover and Field, 2011; Sid et al., 2017) (Fig. 17.2). In the cytoplasm and the nucleus, 5,10-methylene-THF serves as a substrate for the biosynthesis of deoxythymidylate (dTMP) from deoxyuridylate (dUMP) and for the interconversion of glycine and serine (Tibbetts and Appling, 2010). These reactions may also occur in the mitochondria. The de novo purine nucleotide biosynthesis and the remethylation of homocysteine to methionine are folate-dependent reactions that take place in the cytoplasm

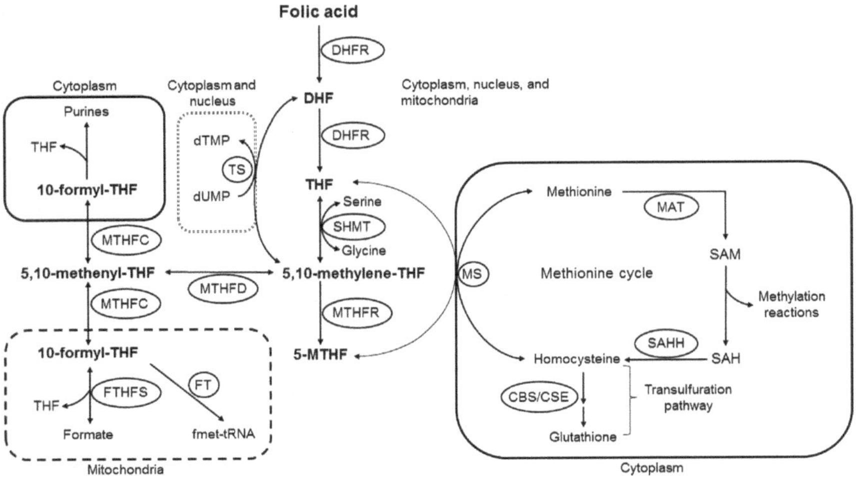

Figure 17.2 Compartmentalization of folate-dependent one-carbon metabolism. One-carbon metabolism for nucleotide biosynthesis, amino acid metabolism, and methylation reactions are distributed within intracellular compartments such as the cytoplasm, nucleus, and mitochondria. The box with solid lines denotes reactions that only occur in the cytoplasm, the box with dotted lines denotes reactions that mainly occur in the mitochondria, and the box with double dotted lines denotes reactions that occur in both the cytoplasm and nucleus. The other one-carbon metabolism reactions may occur in all three cellular compartments. *DHF*, Dihydrofolate; *THF*, tetrahydrofolate; *5-MTHF*, 5-methyltetrahydrofolate; *DHFR*, dihydrofolate reductase; *SHMT*, serine hydroxymethyltransferase; *MTHFR*, methylenetetrahydrofolate reductase; *MTHFD*, methylenetetrahydrofolate dehydrogenase; *MTHFC*, methylenetetrahydrofolate cyclohydrolase; *FTHFS*, formyltetrahydrofolate synthetase; *TS*, thymidylate synthase; *dTMP*, deoxythymidylate; *dUMP*, deoxyuridylate; *MS*, methionine synthase; *MAT*, methionine adenosyltransferase; *CBS*, cystathionine-β-synthase; *CSE*, cystathionine-Y-lyase; *SAM*, *S*-adenosylmethionine; *SAH*, *S*-adenosylhomocysteine; *SAHH*, adenosylhomocysteine hydrolase; fmet-*tRNA*, formylmethionine-tRNA; *FT*, formyltransferase. *Reproduced with permission from Sid, V., Siow, Y.L., O, K., 2017. Role of folate in nonalcoholic fatty liver disease. Can. J. Physiol. Pharmacol. 95, 1141–1148.*

(Stover and Field, 2011). The 5,10-methylene-THF is reversibly converted to 5,10-methenyl-THF, a precursor for 10-formyl-tetrahydrofolate (10-formyl-THF) by methylenetetrahydrofolate dehydrogenase (Herbig et al., 2002). The 10-formyl-THF provides one-carbon moieties for the biosynthesis of purine nucleotides while 5-MTHF donates carbon units for the biosynthesis of methionine (Tibbetts and Appling, 2010). Methionine is an essential precursor for the biosynthesis of *S*-adenosylmethionine (SAM), a principal methyl donor that regulates a number of fundamental cellular processes involved in cell signaling, protein localization, degradation of molecules, and gene expression. Folate deficiency impairs dTMP synthesis and homocysteine remethylation. Accumulation of homocysteine is associated with increased *S*-adenosylhomocysteine (SAH), a potent inhibitor of SAM-dependent methylation reactions (Stover, 2004).

17.2.4 Metabolic interconnection of B vitamins

Folate and several other B vitamins (i.e., vitamin B6 and B12) are essential cofactors in one-carbon transfer reactions and sulfur-containing amino acid metabolism. Deficiency in folate and vitamin B12 leads to impaired DNA/protein methylation by SAM, which has an important implication in the development of cognitive and metabolic disorders. One of the key products generated during one-carbon metabolism is homocysteine (Selhub, 2002; Stover, 2004). Homocysteine is an intermediate amino acid formed during the metabolism of methionine to cysteine. It can be metabolized via the remethylation pathway and the transsulfuration pathway (Sarna et al., 2015) (Fig. 17.3). Under physiological conditions, remethylation of homocysteine to methionine is catalyzed by methionine synthase that utilizes 5-MTHF as a substrate and vitamin B12 as a cofactor. Vitamin B12 deficiency can result in an accumulation of 5-MTHF, which is often known as a "methyl folate trap." Too much 5-MTHF depletes the other forms of folate, leading to the inhibition of purine, thymidylate, and methionine synthesis. Another major source of methyl groups is choline, which is primarily obtained from the diet. Choline is oxidized to betaine that serves as a methyl donor for remethylation of homocysteine to methionine via betaine hydroxymethyltransferase (BHMT) (Tibbetts and Appling, 2010) (Fig. 17.3). This reaction occurs when the activity of methionine synthase is compromised.

In the transsulfuration pathway, homocysteine is metabolized to cysteine through enzymatic reactions catalyzed by cystathionine-β-synthase (CBS) and cystathionine-γ-lyase (CSE) (Sarna et al., 2015) (Fig. 17.3). Metabolism of homocysteine through the transsulfuration pathway is increased under oxidative stress. Cysteine is the precursor for the synthesis of glutathione, a potent antioxidant tripeptide (Mosharov et al., 2000; Sarna et al., 2015). Approximately 50% of the glutathione pool in hepatocytes is derived from cysteine that is synthesized through the transsulfuration pathway (Mosharov et al., 2000). Homocysteine and cysteine also serve as substrates for CBS and CSE-mediated desulfuration reactions to

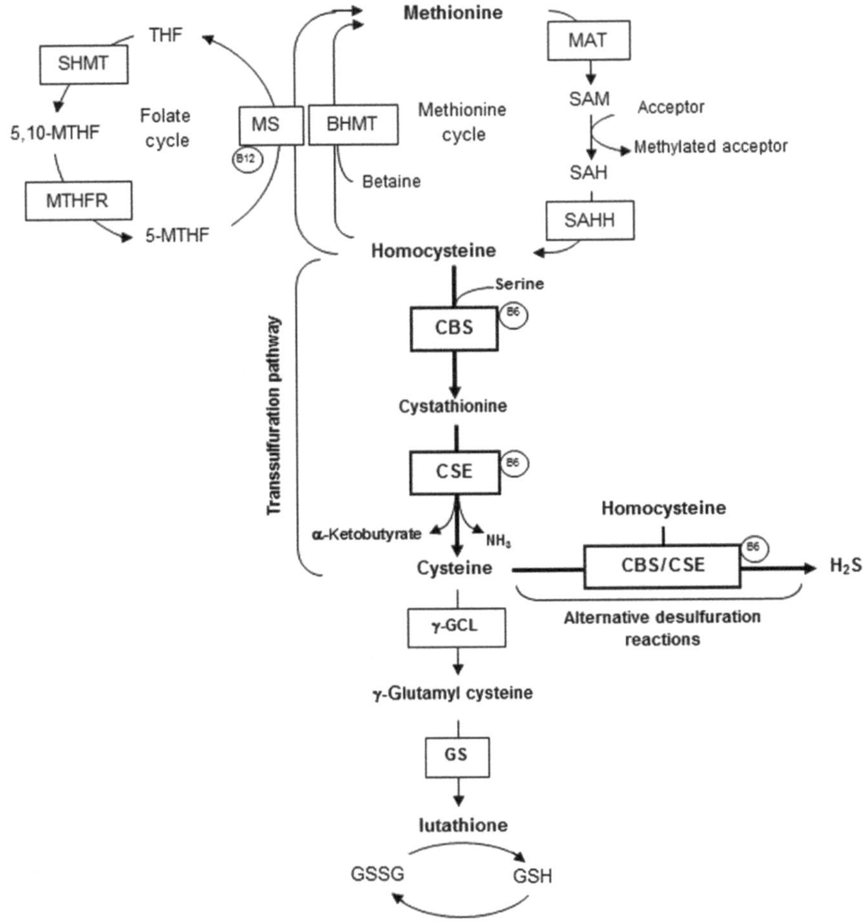

Figure 17.3 The hepatic cystathionine-β-synthase/cystathionine-γ-lyase (CBS/CSE) system. Through regulation of the transsulfuration pathway and performance of alternative desulfuration reactions, the hepatic *CBS/CSE* system converges homocysteine and cysteine metabolism with H_2S biosynthesis. The transsulfuration pathway is linked to the methionine cycle via the intermediate sulfur-containing amino acid, homocysteine. Homocysteine may be remethylated to regenerate methionine, primarily via a folate-dependent reaction, or homocysteine may be irreversibly metabolized by the transsulfuration pathway. *CBS* and *CSE* regulate the transsulfuration pathway, consecutively catabolizing homocysteine to produce the sulfur-containing amino acid cysteine. Cysteine, in turn, may be used for protein synthesis or may be stored as glutathione following integration into the glutathione biosynthetic pathway. Alternatively, both cysteine and homocysteine may serve as substrate for *CBS*- and *CSE*-mediated desulfuration reactions which lead to the endogenous synthesis of H_2S. (*Boxes* denote enzymes). *MAT,* Methionine adenosyltransferase; *SAM, S*-adenosylmethionine; *SAH, S*-adenosylhomocysteine; *SAHH,* adenosylhomocysteine hydrolase; *BHMT,* betaine homocysteine methyltransferase; *MS,* methionine synthase; *THF,* tetrahydrofolate; *SHMT,* serine hydroxymethylase; *5,10-MTHF* 5,10-methylene-tetrahydrofolate; *MTHFR,* methylenetetrahydrofolate reductase; *5-MTHF,* 5-methyltetrahydrofolate; *CBS,* cystathionine-β-synthase; *CSE,* cystathionine-γ-lyase; H_2S, hydrogen sulfide; *γ-GCL,* γ-glutamate-cysteine ligase; *GS,* glutathione synthetase. *Reproduced with permission from Sarna, L.K., Siow, Y.L., O, K., 2015. The CBS/CSE system: a potential therapeutic target in NAFLD? Can. J. Physiol. Pharmacol. 93, 1–11.*

produce hydrogen sulfide (H_2S) (Sarna et al., 2015) (Fig. 17.3). Both the CBS and CSE reactions require PLP (active form of vitamin B6) as an essential cofactor. In addition, vitamin B6 also contributes to the synthesis of 5-MTHF mediated by SHMT. Deficiency of vitamin B6 is correlated with low levels of vitamin B12 and folate (Parra et al., 2018). Therefore depletion of vitamin B6, B12, and/or folate can impair one-carbon transfer reactions and sulfur-containing amino acid metabolism.

17.2.5 Folate deficiency

In North America mandatory folic acid fortification of cereal grain products was established in 1998 to reduce the incidence of neural tube defects in newborns (CDC, 2010). General populations in Canada and the United States have achieved adequate intakes of folate since the implementation of the folic acid fortification policy (Bailey et al., 2010). However, folate deficiency may still present in some European, African, and Asian countries that do not impose mandatory folic acid fortification policies (Dhonukshe-Rutten et al., 2009). Folate deficiency can also be caused by gene mutations and environmental factors that impair folate absorption or metabolism. DHFR deficiency can compromise folate status in red blood cells and cause megaloblastic anemia, a condition of large abnormal red blood cells (Cario et al., 2011). Chronic alcohol consumption can lead to folate deficiency due to intestinal malabsorption, reduced hepatic storage, and increased urinary excretion of folate (Medici and Halsted, 2013). Folate deficiency has been linked to dysregulation of intracellular metabolic processes (Da Silva et al., 2014). Emerging evidence indicates that low circulating folate levels are associated with metabolic disorders including hyperhomocysteinemia, obesity, and NAFLD. An elevation of homocysteine in the circulation is a common biomarker of folate deficiency.

17.2.6 Folate and metabolic disease

A study based on the US National Health and Nutrition Examination Survey (NHANES, 2003–2006) reported that serum folate levels were significantly reduced in obese patients (12.4 g/L) compared with normal-weight individuals (13.1 g/L) (Bird et al., 2015). Regression analysis revealed that the serum folate level is negatively correlated with body mass index (BMI) regardless of adjustment for vitamin intakes and demographic variables such as gender, age, ethnicity, smoking status, and alcohol use. However, the BMI values were positively associated with folate levels in red blood cells (Bird et al., 2015). The mechanism and clinical significance of such a discrepancy in the correlations between BMI and folate levels in serum and RBC remain to be investigated. In another study, gastric bypass surgery significantly improved folate status in morbidly obese patients (Updegraff and Neufeld, 1981). It is plausible that obesity may be one of the underlying causes for the imbalance of endogenous folate levels. Low circulating folate levels were detected in patients with type 2 diabetes (Nilsson et al., 2015). The low blood folate levels were correlated to high levels of fasting blood glucose and increased expression of hepatic genes involved in the development of diabetes. Folate depletion also caused epigenetic and transcriptional alterations in the liver, which might contribute to the pathogenesis of type 2 diabetes (Nilsson et al., 2015). The reduction of serum folate levels found in patients with metabolic disease suggests a potential relationship between the abnormal metabolic processes and perturbed folate status.

17.2.7 Folate status and NAFLD

Several reports have indicated the association between the circulating folate level and NAFLD. Obese female patients with severe NAFLD showed significantly reduced serum folate levels compared with individuals with normal liver morphology or minimal liver damage (21 vs 27 nmol/L) (Hirsch et al., 2005). Another cohort study showed a correlation of low serum folic acid levels with the presence and severity of steatosis (Xia et al., 2018). Such a correlation was independent of gender, BMI, insulin resistance, and parameters of metabolic syndrome. Low serum folate and vitamin B12 levels were also correlated with increased NASH severity (Mahamid et al., 2018). While clinical evidence suggests that patients with NAFLD may be at a higher risk for folate deficiency, a causal relationship has yet to be confirmed. Further clinical investigation is necessary to establish proper folate intake guidelines for patients with NAFLD.

Animal models that mimic the histology and pathology of NAFLD have been established. High-fat diets can induce histopathological changes that resemble the NAFLD features including hepatic lipid accumulation, oxidative stress, and inflammation in rodents (Sarna et al., 2012; Nakamura and Terauchi, 2013; Sid et al., 2018a,b). In a recent study, a high-fat diet feeding caused a significant decrease in serum and liver folate levels in mice (Sid et al., 2018b). This was attributed to impaired expression of hepatic folate transporters (PCFT and RFC). It appears that prolonged consumption of diets that are rich in fat may exert a negative impact on folate homeostasis (Sid et al., 2018b). Another study reported that a depletion of dietary folate in rodents was associated with an increased expression of lipid biosynthetic genes, which contributed to abnormal lipid metabolism in the liver (Champier et al., 2012). Hepatic lipid transport via very low density lipoprotein (VLDL) was impaired in folate-deficient mice leading to hepatic lipid accumulation (Christensen et al., 2010). These results suggest that alterations in folate metabolism may have an important implication in NAFLD.

17.3 Nonalcoholic fatty liver disease

17.3.1 Prevalence and pathogenesis of NAFLD

The global prevalence of NAFLD is approximately 20%–30% and increases to 70%–90% in patients with obesity and type 2 diabetes (Younossi et al., 2016, 2018a). NAFLD is considered as the hepatic manifestation of metabolic syndrome. Patients with NAFLD tend to be obese (BMI > 30 kg/m^2) and often exhibit comorbidities associated with insulin resistance, dyslipidemia, hypertriglyceridemia, and hypertension (Farrell and Larter, 2006). Although insulin resistance is an independent risk factor for NAFLD, some patients may have normal insulin function (Cohen et al., 2011). Aside from metabolic risk factors, other nonmodifiable risk factors such as age, gender, ethnicity, and certain gene variants may also influence the susceptibility to NAFLD. Men are more likely to accumulate abdominal fat, which increases their risk towards NAFLD development. Moreover, Hispanics and Asians are more likely to develop fatty liver compared to individuals of African descent (Browning et al., 2004). Hispanic individuals often carry a gene variant of patatin-like phospholipase domain-containing protein 3, which results in a twofold increase in hepatic triglyceride content and confers susceptibility towards NAFLD. In addition, mutations in other genes involved in lipid metabolism can also increase the risk of NAFLD (Birkenfeld and Shulman, 2014).

Steatosis is the main histological feature of NAFLD which is defined as lipid accumulation in more than 5% of hepatocytes (Tiniakos et al., 2010). Steatosis is often a self-limiting condition; however, it can advance to NASH that is characterized by steatosis, inflammation, and hepatocyte injury (Cohen et al., 2011). Hepatocyte ballooning is a form of hepatocellular injury that is characterized by cell swelling, which is an essential feature that distinguishes NASH from steatosis. Liver fibrosis is frequently detected in NASH patients (Yeh and Brunt, 2014). The presence of advanced hepatic fibrosis increases the risk for cirrhosis and HCC. Although the progression of steatosis to NASH is reversible, NASH may irreversibly advance to cirrhosis that is increasingly susceptible to the development of portal hypertension and HCC (Kessoku et al., 2014). The pathogenesis of NAFLD is complex and incompletely understood. The two-hit hypothesis was initially proposed to describe NAFLD pathogenesis. This hypothesis suggests that perturbations in lipid metabolism lead to steatosis (first hit), which sensitizes the liver to the secondary hit, such as inflammation, oxidative stress, and cell injury (Day, 2005). However, steatosis may not always precede inflammation. It is plausible that inflammation could precede lipid accumulation in NASH patients (Tiniakos et al., 2010). Furthermore, the two-hit theory does not account for many other metabolic changes that occur in NAFLD. This has led to the development of the multiple-parallel-hit hypothesis, which suggests that multiple factors such as insulin resistance, lipotoxicity, oxidative stress, inflammation, gut-derived endotoxins, adipokines, or genetic factors may simultaneously induce NAFLD (Tilg and Moschen, 2010). As NAFLD is a multifaceted disease associated with several metabolic abnormalities, there are currently no therapeutic drugs approved for its treatment. Novel therapeutic strategies are urgently required for the management of NAFLD (Younossi et al., 2018b).

17.3.2 Current treatment for nonalcoholic fatty liver disease

Lifestyle modifications such as increasing physical activity and healthy diet are considered to be the most safe and effective strategies for NAFLD management. Such modifications can promote weight loss, alleviate steatosis, and improve liver function (Chalasani et al., 2012). Minimal weight loss (3%–5%) is sufficient to reduce hepatic lipid accumulation in NAFLD patients. However, greater than 7% weight reduction is required to improve histological features associated with NASH (Glass et al., 2015). Patients who receive bariatric surgery have profound weight loss, which is associated with improved liver histology and insulin sensitivity (Mechanick et al., 2009). However, bariatric surgery is not recommended for cirrhotic patients due to concerns of liver failure after a rapid weight loss. Although gradual weight loss appears to be beneficial for NAFLD patients, lifestyle changes and adherence to healthy diets can be a challenge. Several pharmacological agents that target certain metabolic risk factors have been proposed for the treatment of NAFLD (Chalasani et al., 2012). Metformin, a first line antidiabetic agent, reduces insulin resistance and alanine transaminase levels but has limited effects on inflammation and steatosis in NAFLD patients (Bugianesi et al., 2005). Thiazolidinediones are insulin sensitizers and have been shown to improve liver function and histology in patients with NASH (Neuschwander-Tetri et al., 2003). However, their long-term safety and efficacy for NAFLD treatment have not been established (Chalasani et al., 2012). Oxidative stress is a key mediator in liver injury in NAFLD. While treatment with antioxidants such as vitamin E has been shown to ameliorate steatosis, inflammation, and hepatocyte ballooning, further investigation is required to determine the effectiveness of antioxidants in NAFLD treatment (Sanyal et al., 2004). NAFLD patients have a high cardiovascular risk and therefore statins have been used to treat dyslipidemia and improve cardiovascular outcomes in these patients. The use of statins appears to be safe and effective for correcting lipid abnormalities in NAFLD patients (Chalasani et al., 2012). There is currently no single agent that can target all metabolic risk factors associated with NAFLD. Researchers are still searching for therapeutic agents that can target multiple pathways associated with NAFLD pathogenesis (Younossi et al., 2018b).

17.3.3 Role of folic acid supplementation in nonalcoholic fatty liver disease

It was reported that folic acid supplementation during high-fat diet feeding in mice could effectively improve lipid and glucose metabolism in the liver (Sid et al., 2015). Such effects were mediated through the regulation of AMP-activated protein kinase, a key regulator of whole body energy balance and metabolic homeostasis (Sid et al., 2015). Folate and folic acid exhibit antioxidant functions due to their ability to directly scavenge reactive oxygen species (ROS) (Gliszczynska-Swiglo and Muzolf, 2007) and regulate ROS-generating or metabolizing enzymes (Woo et al., 2006; Hwang et al., 2011; Sarna et al., 2012). It was shown in rodents that folic acid supplementation could confer protective effects against oxidative stress in the liver (Woo et al., 2006; Sarna et al., 2012) and kidney (Hwang et al., 2011). Hepatic oxidative stress is associated with increased expression of reduced nicotinamide adenine dinucleotide phosphate (NADPH) oxidase in animal models of obesity, metabolic syndrome, and NAFLD. Folic acid supplementation effectively inhibited NADPH oxidase-mediated superoxide production, restoring the antioxidant response in hyperhomocysteinemic rats and in high-fat diet-induced obese mice (Woo et al., 2006; Hwang et al., 2011; Sarna et al., 2012). Patients with NAFLD also have elevated levels of proinflammatory cytokines in the circulation, immune cells, liver, and adipose tissue (Day, 2006; Braunersreuther et al., 2012). Macrophages grown in a folate-depleted medium had high expression of proinflammatory cytokines including interleukin-1β, monocyte chemoattractant protein-1, interleukin-6 (IL-6), and tumor necrosis factor-α (TNF-α) (Kolb and Petrie, 2013). Incubation of macrophages with folic acid attenuated homocysteine-induced proinflammatory cytokine expression (Au-Yeung et al., 2006). Folic acid supplementation in high-fat diet-fed mice significantly decreased the expression of hepatic proinflammatory cytokines (IL-6, TNF-α) through inhibition of nuclear factor kappa B, a key transcriptional factor of proinflammatory cytokine genes (Sid et al., 2018a). Folic acid supplementation in overweight individuals or hyperhomocysteinemic patients was associated with a reduction of proinflammatory cytokine levels (Wang et al., 2005; Solini et al., 2006). Those results indicate that folic acid possesses lipid and glucose lowering effects, as well as antioxidant and antiinflammatory functions, which makes it a promising candidate for managing NAFLD. Although folic acid supplementation appears to be beneficial for alleviating metabolic abnormalities, clinical studies are required to further validate the effect of folic acid supplementation in patients with NAFLD.

17.4 Conclusions

Vitamins are micronutrients that support physiological functions in the body. Folate (vitamin B9) plays a fundamental role in one-carbon metabolism that is essential for gene expression and sulfur-containing amino acid homeostasis. Although low folate status is observed in patients with malabsorption, kidney dysfunction, or liver disease, dietary folate deficiency is uncommon in generally healthy populations in countries that have implemented mandatory folate fortification policies. However, obese individuals with NAFLD are reported to have low folate levels in the serum despite the adequate intake of folate from diets and/or supplements (Hirsch et al., 2005; Xia et al., 2018; Mahamid et al., 2018). A recent study has revealed that fatty liver is associated with impaired folate transporter expression and low folate levels in diet-induced obese mice (Sid et al., 2018b). In animal studies, folic acid supplementation can restore hepatic redox balance, improve lipid and glucose metabolism, and attenuate inflammatory cytokine production in rodents with diet-induced metabolic abnormalities (i.e., overweight, fatty liver, hyperglycemia) (Woo et al., 2006; Sarna et al., 2012; Sid et al., 2015, 2018a). Nutritional therapy including folic acid supplementation appears to be an alternative approach for the management of metabolic diseases, such as NAFLD and diabetes. Future research is warranted to address whether the regulation of folate homeostasis can improve the clinical outcomes in patients with NAFLD or other metabolic diseases. If proven effective, folic acid supplementation may be an economical and effective approach to control this emerging public health threat (NAFLD) globally.

Acknowledgements

This work was supported, in part, by grants from the Natural Sciences and Engineering Research Council of Canada and St. Boniface Hospital Foundation.

References

Au-Yeung, K.K., Yip, J.C., Siow, Y.L., O, K., 2006. Folic acid inhibits homocysteine-induced superoxide anion production and nuclear factor kappa B activation in macrophages. Can. J. Physiol. Pharmacol. 84, 141–147.

Bailey, R.L., Dodd, K.W., Gahche, J.J., Dwyer, J.T., McDowell, M.A., Yetley, E.A., et al., 2010. Total folate and folic acid intake from foods and dietary supplements in the United States: 2003–2006. Am. J. Clin. Nutr. 91, 231–237.

Bird, J.K., Ronnenberg, A.G., Choi, S.W., Du, F., Mason, J.B., Liu, Z., 2015. Obesity is associated with increased red blood cell folate despite lower dietary intakes and serum concentrations. J. Nutr. 145, 79–86.

Birkenfeld, A.L., Shulman, G.I., 2014. Nonalcoholic fatty liver disease, hepatic insulin resistance, and type 2 diabetes. Hepatology 59, 713–723.

Braunersreuther, V., Viviani, G.L., Mach, F., Montecucco, F., 2012. Role of cytokines and chemokines in non-alcoholic fatty liver disease. World J. Gastroenterol. 18, 727–735.

Browning, J.D., Szczepaniak, L.S., Dobbins, R., Nuremberg, P., Horton, J.D., Cohen, J. C., et al., 2004. Prevalence of hepatic steatosis in an urban population in the United States: impact of ethnicity. Hepatology 40, 1387–1395.

Bugianesi, E., Gentilcore, E., Manini, R., Natale, S., Vanni, E., Villanova, N., et al., 2005. A randomized controlled trial of metformin versus vitamin E or prescriptive diet in nonalcoholic fatty liver disease. Am. J. Gastroenterol. 100, 1082–1090.

Cario, H., Smith, D.E., Blom, H., Blau, N., Bode, H., Holzmann, K., et al., 2011. Dihydrofolate reductase deficiency due to a homozygous DHFR mutation causes megaloblastic anemia and cerebral folate deficiency leading to severe neurologic disease. Am. J. Hum. Genet. 88, 226–231.

Caudill, M.A., 2010. Folate bioavailability: implications for establishing dietary recommendations and optimizing status. Am. J. Clin. Nutr. 91, 1455s–1460s.

CDC, 2010. CDC Grand Rounds: additional opportunities to prevent neural tube defects with folic acid fortification. Morb. Mortal. Wkly. Rep. (MMWR) 59, 980–984.

Chalasani, N., Younossi, Z., Lavine, J.E., Diehl, A.M., Brunt, E.M., Cusi, K., et al., 2012. The diagnosis and management of non-alcoholic fatty liver disease: practice guideline by the American Gastroenterological Association, American Association for the Study of Liver Diseases, and American College of Gastroenterology. Gastroenterology 142, 1592–1609.

Champier, J., Claustrat, F., Nazaret, N., Fevre Montange, M., Claustrat, B., 2012. Folate depletion changes gene expression of fatty acid metabolism, DNA synthesis, and circadian cycle in male mice. Nutr. Res. 32, 124–132.

Christensen, K.E., Wu, Q., Wang, X., Deng, L., Caudill, M.A., Rozen, R., 2010. Steatosis in mice is associated with gender, folate intake, and expression of genes of one-carbon metabolism. J. Nutr. 140, 1736–1741.

Cohen, J.C., Horton, J.D., Hobbs, H.H., 2011. Human fatty liver disease: old questions and new insights. Science 332, 1519–1523.

Da Silva, R.P., Kelly, K.B., Al Rajabi, A., Jacobs, R.L., 2014. Novel insights on interactions between folate and lipid metabolism. Biofactors 40, 277–283.

Day, C.P., 2005. Natural history of NAFLD: remarkably benign in the absence of cirrhosis. Gastroenterology 129, 375–378.

Day, C.P., 2006. From fat to inflammation. Gastroenterology 130, 207–210.

Dhonukshe-Rutten, R.A., De Vries, J.H., De Bree, A., Van Der Put, N., Van Staveren, W.A., De Groot, L.C., 2009. Dietary intake and status of folate and vitamin B12 and their association with homocysteine and cardiovascular disease in European populations. Eur. J. Clin. Nutr. 63, 18–30.

Farrell, G.C., Larter, C.Z., 2006. Nonalcoholic fatty liver disease: from steatosis to cirrhosis. Hepatology 43, S99–S112.

Glass, L.M., Dickson, R.C., Anderson, J.C., Suriawinata, A.A., Putra, J., Berk, B.S., et al., 2015. Total body weight loss of ≥ 10% is associated with improved hepatic fibrosis in patients with nonalcoholic steatohepatitis. Dig. Dis. Sci. 60, 1024–1030.

Gliszczynska-Swiglo, A., Muzolf, M., 2007. pH-Dependent radical scavenging activity of folates. J. Agric. Food Chem. 55, 8237–8242.

Herbig, K., Chiang, E.P., Lee, L.R., Hills, J., Shane, B., Stover, P.J., 2002. Cytoplasmic serine hydroxymethyltransferase mediates competition between folate-dependent deoxyribonucleotide and *S*-adenosylmethionine biosyntheses. J. Biol. Chem. 277, 38381–38389.

Hirsch, S., Poniachick, J., Avendano, M., Csendes, A., Burdiles, P., Smok, G., et al., 2005. Serum folate and homocysteine levels in obese females with non-alcoholic fatty liver. Nutrition 21, 137–141.

Hu, J., Wang, B., Sahyoun, N.R., 2016. Application of the key events dose-response framework to folate metabolism. Crit. Rev. Food Sci. Nutr. 56, 1325–1333.

Hwang, S.Y., Siow, Y.L., Au-Yeung, K.K., House, J., O, K., 2011. Folic acid supplementation inhibits NADPH oxidase-mediated superoxide anion production in the kidney. Am. J. Physiol. Renal. Physiol. 300, F189–F198.

Institute of Medicine Standing Committee on the Scientific Evaluation of Dietary Reference Intakes andIts Panel on Folate, Others B Vitamins and Choline, 1998. The National Academies Collection: Reports funded by National Institutes of Health. Dietary Reference Intakes for Thiamin, Riboflavin, Niacin, Vitamin B6, Folate, Vitamin B12, Pantothenic Acid, Biotin, and Choline. National Academies Press (US) National Academy of Sciences, Washington, DC.

Iyer, R., Tomar, S.K., 2009. Folate: a functional food constituent. J. Food Sci. 74, R114–R122.
Kessoku, T., Ogawa, Y., Yoneda, M., Imajo, K., Sumida, Y., Eguchi, Y., et al., 2014. Simple scoring system for predicting cirrhosis in nonalcoholic fatty liver disease. World J. Gastroenterol. 20, 10108–10114.
Kolb, A.F., Petrie, L., 2013. Folate deficiency enhances the inflammatory response of macrophages. Mol. Immunol. 54, 164–172.
Loomba, R., Sanyal, A.J., 2013. The global NAFLD epidemic. Nat. Rev. Gastroenterol. Hepatol. 10, 686–690.
Mahabir, S., Ettinger, S., Johnson, L., Baer, D.J., Clevidence, B.A., Hartman, T.J., et al., 2008. Measures of adiposity and body fat distribution in relation to serum folate levels in postmenopausal women in a feeding study. Eur. J. Clin. Nutr. 62, 644–650.
Mahamid, M., Mahroum, N., Bragazzi, N.L., Shalaata, K., Yavne, Y., Adawi, M., et al., 2018. Folate and B12 levels correlate with histological severity in NASH patients. Nutrients 10, E440.
Mechanick, J.I., Kushner, R.F., Sugerman, H.J., Gonzalez-Campoy, J.M., Collazo-Clavell, M.L., Spitz, A.F., et al., 2009. American Association of Clinical Endocrinologists, The Obesity Society, and American Society for Metabolic & Bariatric Surgery medical guidelines for clinical practice for the perioperative nutritional, metabolic, and nonsurgical support of the bariatric surgery patient. Obesity (Silver Spring) 17 (Suppl. 1), S1–S70.
Medici, V., Halsted, C.H., 2013. Folate, alcohol, and liver disease. Mol. Nutr. Food Res. 57, 596–606.
Mosharov, E., Cranford, M.R., Banerjee, R., 2000. The quantitatively important relationship between homocysteine metabolism and glutathione synthesis by the transsulfuration pathway and its regulation by redox changes. Biochemistry 39, 13005–13011.
Nakamura, A., Terauchi, Y., 2013. Lessons from mouse models of high-fat diet-induced NAFLD. Int. J. Mol. Sci. 14, 21240–21257.
Neuschwander-Tetri, B.A., Brunt, E.M., Wehmeier, K.R., Oliver, D., Bacon, B.R., 2003. Improved nonalcoholic steatohepatitis after 48 weeks of treatment with the PPAR-gamma ligand rosiglitazone. Hepatology 38, 1008–1017.
Nilsson, E., Matte, A., Perfilyev, A., De Mello, V.D., Kakela, P., Pihlajamaki, J., et al., 2015. Epigenetic alterations in human liver from subjects with type 2 diabetes in parallel with reduced folate levels. J. Clin. Endocrinol. Metab. 100, E1491–E1501.
Parra, M., Stahl, S., Hellmann, H., 2018. Vitamin B(6) and its role in cell metabolism and physiology. Cells 7 (7), 84.
Pietrzik, K., Bailey, L., Shane, B., 2010. Folic acid and L-5-methyltetrahydrofolate: comparison of clinical pharmacokinetics and pharmacodynamics. Clin. Pharmacokinet. 49, 535–548.
Rong, N., Selhub, J., Goldin, B.R., Rosenberg, I.H., 1991. Bacterially synthesized folate in rat large intestine is incorporated into host tissue folyl polyglutamates. J. Nutr. 121, 1955–1959.
Sanyal, A.J., Mofrad, P.S., Contos, M.J., Sargeant, C., Luketic, V.A., Sterling, R.K., et al., 2004. A pilot study of vitamin E versus vitamin E and pioglitazone for the treatment of nonalcoholic steatohepatitis. Clin. Gastroenterol. Hepatol. 2, 1107–1115.
Sarna, L.K., Wu, N., Wang, P., Hwang, S.Y., Siow, Y.L., O, K., 2012. Folic acid supplementation attenuates high fat diet induced hepatic oxidative stress via regulation of NADPH oxidase. Can. J. Physiol. Pharmacol. 90, 155–165.
Sarna, L.K., Siow, Y.L., O, K., 2015. The CBS/CSE system: a potential therapeutic target in NAFLD? Can. J. Physiol. Pharmacol. 93, 1–11.
Selhub, J., 2002. Folate, vitamin B12 and vitamin B6 and one carbon metabolism. J. Nutr. Health Aging 6, 39–42.

Sid, V., Wu, N., Sarna, L.K., Siow, Y.L., House, J.D., O, K., 2015. Folic acid supplementation during high-fat diet feeding restores AMPK activation via an AMP-LKB1-dependent mechanism. Am. J. Physiol. Regul. Integr. Comp. Physiol. 309, R1215–R1225.

Sid, V., Siow, Y.L., O, K., 2017. Role of folate in nonalcoholic fatty liver disease. Can. J. Physiol. Pharmacol. 95, 1141–1148.

Sid, V., Shang, Y., Siow, Y.L., Hewage, S.M., House, J.D., O, K., 2018a. Folic acid supplementation attenuates chronic hepatic inflammation in high-fat diet fed mice. Lipids 53, 709–716.

Sid, V., Siow, Y.L., Shang, Y., Woo, C.W., O, K., 2018b. High-fat diet consumption reduces hepatic folate transporter expression via nuclear respiratory factor-1. J. Mol. Med. (Berl.) 96 (11), 1203–1213.

Solini, A., Santini, E., Ferrannini, E., 2006. Effect of short-term folic acid supplementation on insulin sensitivity and inflammatory markers in overweight subjects. Int. J. Obes. (Lond.) 30, 1197–1202.

Steinberg, S.E., Campbell, C.L., Hillman, R.S., 1979. Kinetics of the normal folate enterohepatic cycle. J. Clin. Invest. 64, 83–88.

Stover, P.J., 2004. Physiology of folate and vitamin B12 in health and disease. Nutr. Rev. 62, S3–12 (Discussion S13).

Stover, P.J., Field, M.S., 2011. Trafficking of intracellular folates. Adv. Nutr. 2, 325–331.

Tibbetts, A.S., Appling, D.R., 2010. Compartmentalization of mammalian folate-mediated one-carbon metabolism. Annu. Rev. Nutr. 30, 57–81.

Tilg, H., Moschen, A.R., 2010. Evolution of inflammation in nonalcoholic fatty liver disease: the multiple parallel hits hypothesis. Hepatology 52, 1836–1846.

Tiniakos, D.G., Vos, M.B., Brunt, E.M., 2010. Nonalcoholic fatty liver disease: pathology and pathogenesis. Annu. Rev. Pathol. 5, 145–171.

Updegraff, T.A., Neufeld, N.J., 1981. Protein, iron, and folate status of patients prior to and following surgery for morbid obesity. J. Am. Diet. Assoc. 78, 135–140.

Veena, J., Muragundla, A., Sidgiddi, S., Subramaniam, S., 2014. Non-alcoholic fatty liver disease: need for a balanced nutritional source. Br. J. Nutr. 112, 1858–1872.

Visentin, M., Diop-Bove, N., Zhao, R., Goldman, I.D., 2014. The intestinal absorption of folates. Annu. Rev. Physiol. 76, 251–274.

Wang, G., Dai, J., Mao, J., Zeng, X., Yang, X., Wang, X., 2005. Folic acid reverses hyper-responsiveness of LPS-induced chemokine secretion from monocytes in patients with hyperhomocysteinemia. Atherosclerosis 179, 395–402.

Woo, C.W., Prathapasinghe, G.A., Siow, Y.L., O, K., 2006. Hyperhomocysteinemia induces liver injury in rat: protective effect of folic acid supplementation. Biochim. Biophys. Acta 1762, 656–665.

Wright, A.J., Dainty, J.R., Finglas, P.M., 2007. Folic acid metabolism in human subjects revisited: potential implications for proposed mandatory folic acid fortification in the UK. Br. J. Nutr. 98, 667–675.

Xia, M.F., Bian, H., Zhu, X.P., Yan, H.M., Chang, X.X., Zhang, L.S., et al., 2018. Serum folic acid levels are associated with the presence and severity of liver steatosis in Chinese adults. Clin. Nutr. 37, 1752–1758.

Yeh, M.M., Brunt, E.M., 2014. Pathological features of fatty liver disease. Gastroenterology 147, 754–764.

Younossi, Z.M., Koenig, A.B., Abdelatif, D., Fazel, Y., Henry, L., Wymer, M., 2016. Global epidemiology of nonalcoholic fatty liver disease-meta-analytic assessment of prevalence, incidence, and outcomes. Hepatology 64, 73–84.

Younossi, Z., Anstee, Q.M., Marietti, M., Hardy, T., Henry, L., Eslam, M., et al., 2018a. Global burden of NAFLD and NASH: trends, predictions, risk factors and prevention. Nat. Rev. Gastroenterol. Hepatol. 15, 11–20.

Younossi, Z.M., Loomba, R., Rinella, M.E., Bugianesi, E., Marchesini, G., Neuschwander-Tetri, B.A., et al., 2018b. Current and future therapeutic regimens for nonalcoholic fatty liver disease and nonalcoholic steatohepatitis. Hepatology 68, 361–371.

Zhao, R., Matherly, L.H., Goldman, I.D., 2009. Membrane transporters and folate homeostasis: intestinal absorption and transport into systemic compartments and tissues. Expert. Rev. Mol. Med. 11, e4.

Zhao, R., Diop-Bove, N., Visentin, M., Goldman, I.D., 2011. Mechanisms of membrane transport of folates into cells and across epithelia. Annu. Rev. Nutr. 31, 177–201.

CHAPTER 18

Folates transport in placentas

Erika Castaño-Moreno[1], Raúl Piñuñuri[2], Reyna Peñailillo[1], Paola Casanello[3], Miguel Llanos[1] and Ana María Ronco[1]
[1]Laboratory of Nutrition and Metabolic Regulation, Human Nutrition Unit, Institute of Nutrition and Food Technology (INTA), University of Chile, Santiago, Chile
[2]School of Nutrition and Dietetics, Faculty of Health, University of Bernardo O'Higgins, Santiago, Chile
[3]Department of Obstetrics, Department of Neonatology, School of Medicine, Pontificia Universidad Católica de Chile, Santiago, Chile

Contents

Key facts of folates and pregnancy

- Folate (vitamin B9) is an essential vitamin in all periods of life, but it is crucial during the preconceptional and early period of pregnancy to guarantee adequate placental and fetal growth.
- Insufficient or deficient folate supply before pregnancy and during the first trimester of pregnancy leads to an increased risk of neural tube defects.
- The essential necessity of folate requirements for a normal fetal development has led to several countries adopting a public policy of food fortification with folic acid (FA), the synthetic form of folates.

Molecular Nutrition
DOI: https://doi.org/10.1016/B978-0-12-811907-5.00009-9

- From the Americas (33 countries, plus the United States and Canada), through Africa, India, and Australia, countries that have mandated the fortification of wheat flour with FA have reduced the incidence of neural tube disease. In Europe, only in England is it a legal requirement, in the other 27 European countries, the fortification is voluntary.
- In relation to the amount of fortification, the Centers for Disease Control recommended a fortification of 1.4 mg of FA/kg product, although in some countries the level of fortification can be higher (2.5 mg FA/kg product).
- The WHO recommends to all women who want to get pregnant a consumption of 400 μg/day of FA, in addition to folate of natural foods, 3 months before conception and during the first trimester of pregnancy.
- It is recommended that the additional consumption of FA by the pregnant women be balanced with the intake of other vitamins (mainly B12) to avoid imbalances in placental concentrations of vitamins that could alter the placental function and long-term offspring outcomes.

Summary points

- This chapter focuses on folate transport in the placenta, an important process for fetal growth and development.
- Folate is an essential nutrient belonging to the family of hydrosoluble B vitamins (B9) and is contained in some foods like vegetables and fruits, and in fortified foods and supplements (as FA, the synthetic form of folates).
- Fetal folate concentrations are absolutely dependent on the transfer through the placenta and these in turn depend on the intake of folates in the mother's diet and the consumption of fortified foods and supplements.
- Folates are transferred from the mother to the fetus through three specific placental transporters: reduced folate carrier, proton-coupled folate transporter, and folate receptor 1, located in different regions of the placenta.
- Folate transporters' expression in the placenta is related to birth weight and gestational age.
- Folates' concentration in the umbilical cord blood is higher and vitamin B12 is lower in preterm compared to term newborns, leading to a higher folates/B12 ratio.

- Folates in the placenta are sensed by a mechanism mediated by mechanistic target of rapamycin (mTOR), the catalytic subunit of two structurally distinct complexes, mTORC1 and mTORC2, that are considered as positive regulators of folate transporters.
- Folate transport through the placenta may be impaired by several factors like pathophysiological conditions (preeclampsia) and maternal lifestyle (chronic alcohol consumption).
- Folates metabolism is related to the one-carbon cycle which is involved in the DNA methylation reactions, one of the known epigenetic mechanisms.
- Because folates are involved in epigenetic mechanisms, folate concentrations reaching the placenta and fetus should be appropriate (neither excessive nor deficient) and balanced with other micronutrients (such as vitamins B12, B6, choline) to reduce modifications in the methylation reactions that could alter placental function and fetal growth and development, leading to fetal programming.
- Recent reports have found that an excessive consumption of FA ($>$1000 mg/day), when concomitant with low or deficient vitamin B12 intake, may result in a high folates/vitamin B12 ratio that could be deleterious to fetal and long-term development.
- We advocate to introduce cutoff points for folate blood levels and their biomarkers during pregnancy that could be produced due to a possible excessive FA intake.

18.1 Introduction

Folates, also called vitamin B9, belong to the family of hydrosoluble B vitamins and are constituted by chemical structures derived from polyglutamates. Folates are essential micronutrients for cellular functions, growth, and development. During pregnancy, demands for folates increase 5- to 10-fold, due to their importance in processes like vasculogenesis and angiogenesis, both key processes in placental function, fetal growth, and development (Scott, 1999; Tamura and Picciano, 2006). The essential necessity for folates during pregnancy is demonstrated by the fact that maternal deficiency is associated with several adverse outcomes, such as low birth weight, risk of spontaneous abortion, and neural tube defect (NTD). Accumulated evidence indicates that these effects are reverted by adequate supplementation of folate during the preconceptional period and the first trimester of pregnancy (Hoffbrand, 2014; Wilson et al., 2007).

The main investigations in this area have been related to nutritional aspects, since folate deficiency has been associated with numerous diseases, including hematological disorders, oncological disease, and developmental alterations like NTD, including spina bifida, meningocele, and anencephaly in the newborn (Gong et al., 2016). Nowadays, folates have become relevant because of their key involvement in the one-carbon cycle, the main metabolic pathway related to the biological methylations including DNA methylation, one of the most studied epigenetic mechanisms in vertebrates (Scott, 1999). Its relevance during pregnancy has led numerous countries to develop public policies of food fortification to ensure its supply to the fetus, thus avoiding NTD. Until a few years ago, folates transport was mainly studied in the gastrointestinal epithelia, although known folate transporters have been also described in the placenta (Solanky et al., 2010; Yasuda et al., 2008). In this chapter, we will review aspects of placental structure, placental folate transporters, folate requirements, and alterations of folate transport during pregnancy.

18.2 Chemical forms of folates

Folates are water-soluble vitamins of complex B (B9). The term "folates" (polyglutamates) includes all chemical forms of folates. Folates are constituted by the pteridine ring, a methylene group, a *p*-aminobenzoic, an L-glutamic acid residue, and a *p*-aminobenzoic acid with different one-carbon substituents linked at the N_5- and/or N_{10}-position, which give the names to the different chemical forms (Naderi and House, 2018) (Fig. 18.1). Folate is the natural form present in foods, which is the reduced form of folates, and is conjugated to a polyglutamate chain. Folic acid (FA) or pteroylglutamate is the synthetic and the oxidized form of folates with one unit of glutamate; it is the most stable form of folates, and therefore the folate form used in nutritional supplementation and food fortification (Outline et al., 2012; Scaglione and Panzavolta, 2014). After FA absorption, it is metabolized to dihydrofolate (DHF) and then to its active form, tetrahydrofolate. The principal circulating form of folates is 5-methyl tetrahydrofolate (5-MTHF). Both FA and natural folate from foods are converted to 5-MTHF to participate in the folate cycle (Naderi and House, 2018) (Fig. 18.2).

The folate present naturally in foods has a bioavailability near to 50%, lower than the bioavailability of FA which is approximately 85% (Bailey et al., 2015; Institute of Medicine, 1998) going up to almost 100% when

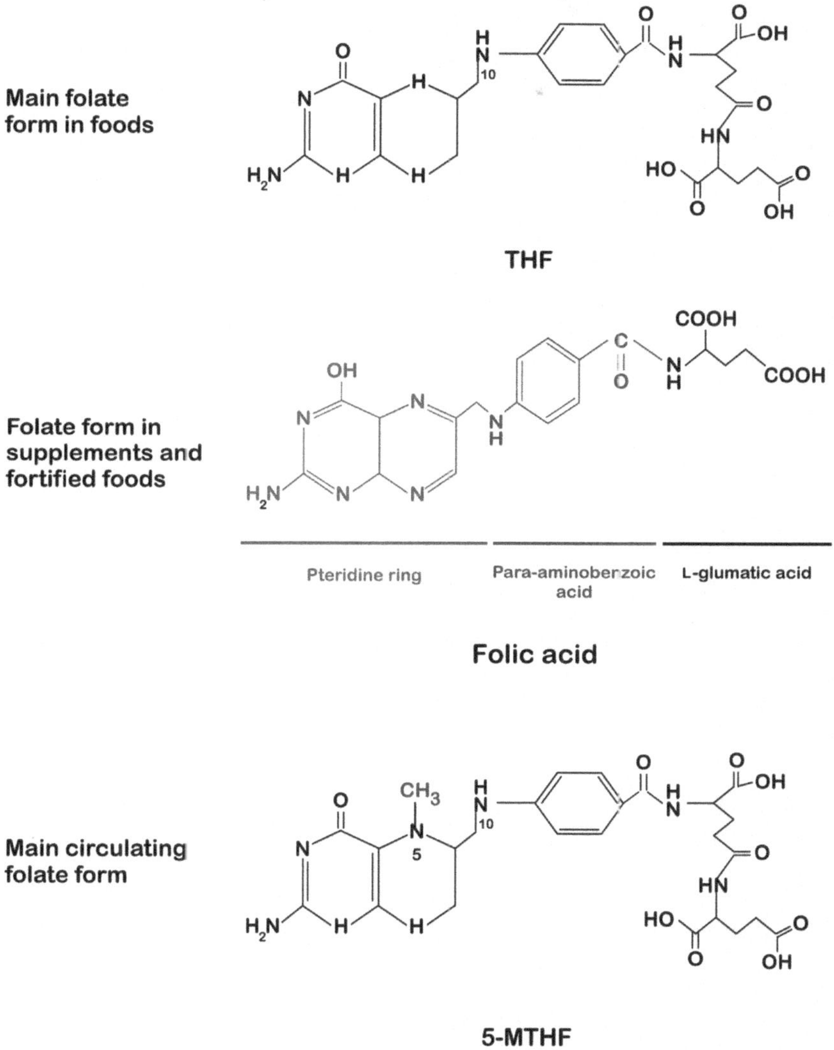

Figure 18.1 Chemical structure of the main forms of folates. THF: tetrahydrofolate; 5-MTHF: 5-methyl tetrahydrofolate.

it is administered as supplements taken on an empty stomach (Allen, 2008). Hence to know the bioavailability of all consumed folates, the term "dietary folate equivalent" (DFE) was coined, because of the different absorption levels between natural and synthetic folates. FA is 1.7 times more bioavailable than folate from foods (85/50 = 1.7); this conversion

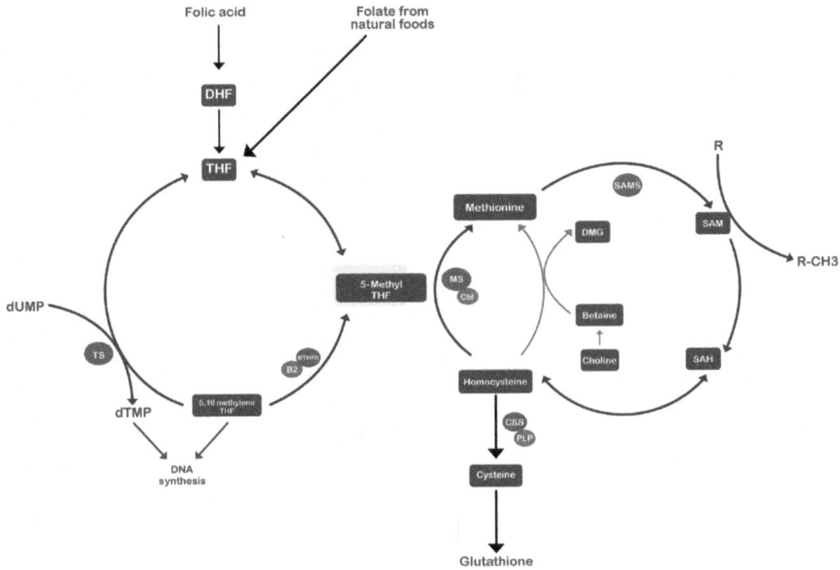

Figure 18.2 Folate cycle. DHF: dihydrofolate; THF: tetrahydrofolate; TS: thymidilate synthetase ; dTMP: deoxythymidine monophosphate; dUMP: deoxyuridine monophosphate; MTHFR: methylenetetrahydrofolate reductase; MS: methionine synthase; Cbl: cobalamine; CβS: cystathionine-β-synthase; PLP:pyridoxal-5′ -phosphate; DMG: dimethylglycine; SAM: S-adenosylmethionine; SAMS: S-adenosyl methionine synthetase; SAH: S-adenosyl homocysteine.

factor is supported by a long-term controlled study with folates intake in women (Yang et al., 2005).

18.3 Requirements of folates during pregnancy

Folates requirements during pregnancy increase 5- to 10-fold, not only due to higher demands for fetal growth and development, but also because of the increased folate catabolism during pregnancy (McPartlin et al., 1993). Inadequate intake of folates leads to decreased levels, first in plasma and subsequently in erythrocytes, increased levels of homocysteine (Hcy), and other clinical complications like megaloblastic anemia (Institute of Medicine, 1998). Folates are taken up by erythrocytes in the bone marrow, and for this reason, folates levels in erythrocytes are considered a good biomarker for long-term status of folates, but not for recent intake (Institute of Medicine, 1998). Hcy is also a biomarker of folate status; under folates deficiency, circulating Hcy levels are increased (de Benoist, 2008). Cutoff points of adequate folates status in adults have been reported, with Hcy levels around 12 and 16 μmol/L according to different reports in the literature (Bailey et al., 2015; Institute of Medicine, 1998; Rasmussen et al., 1996). However, these cutoff points are not applicable to pregnant women for whom there are no reference values for folate status determined through Hcy concentrations.

The estimation of folates requirements is based on the premise of maintaining adequate folate levels in the erythrocytes, which reflect tissue stores in the body. According to different studies, maternal folate levels are reduced by 50% during pregnancy, as a physiological response related to different processes like hemodilution, increased renal excretion, and hormonal changes. In addition, during pregnancy folates are more required by the one-carbon transfer reactions and for nucleotide synthesis in cell division (Institute of Medicine, 1998; Molloy et al., 2008). Several organizations (IOM, FAO, WHO) have established the dietary reference intakes for these vitamins during pregnancy. For this purpose two parameters were coined: the estimated average requirement (EAR), defined as *the recommendations for the 50% of healthy individuals in a group*; and the recommended dietary allowance (RDA), defined as *the average daily dietary intake level that is sufficient to all (97%–98%) healthy individuals*. For pregnant women, the EAR is 520 μg/day of DFE and the RDA is 600 μg/day of DFE (Food and Agriculture Organization of the United States—FAO. World Health Organization—WHO, 2001; Institute of Medicine, 1998) (Table 18.1).

The WHO have established hematological folates levels cutoff points in blood for the nonpregnant population: in serum: high >45.3 nmol/L, normal 13.5–45.3 nmol/L, deficit <6.8 nmol/L; in erythrocytes: depletion <362 nmol/L, anemia 226 nmol/L (WHO, 2012). Adult requirements of folates are 400 μg/day. There is no consensus on cutoff points for folates and their relationship with metabolic alterations during pregnancy (Table 18.2).

Since the status of this vitamin has been strongly associated with NTD (Czeizel and Dudás, 1992), the WHO and the Centers for Disease Control and Prevention recommend food fortification with 1.4 mg of FA/kg of product (Bailey et al., 2015). In addition to fortified foods and dietary folate, the WHO recommends a FA supplementation of 400 μg/day 3 months before pregnancy and during the first trimester to prevent NTD and 5 mg/day if there is a previous history of NTD (Institute of Medicine, 1998; WHO, 2012, 2015). The WHO established that folate

Table 18.1 Folate requirements expressed as dietary folate equivalent (DFE).

Population	EAR (μg/day)	RDA (μg/day)
Infant and children		
0–12 months	65a	80
1–3 years	120	150
4–6 years	160	200
7–13 years (boys and girls)	250	300
14–18 years (boys and girls)	330	400
Adults		
>19 years (men and women)	320	400
Pregnancy	520	600
Lactation	450	500

These values are based on the Institute of Medicine (IOM) and on the Food and Agriculture Organization of the United Nations (FAO). Estimated average requirement (EAR), *the recommendations for the 50% the healthy individuals in a group*. Recommended dietary allowance (RDA) *is the average daily dietary intake level that is sufficient to all (97%–98%) healthy individuals (EAR + 2 standard deviation)*. Folate requirements expressed as DFE.

[a]The adequate intake (IA) a recommended daily intake value based on observed or experimentally determined approximations of nutrient intake by a group (or groups) of healthy people that are assumed to be adequate—used when an RDA cannot be determined (Food and Agriculture Organization of the United States, FAO. World Health Organization, WHO, 2001; Institute of Medicine, 1998).

erythrocyte levels >906 nmol/L represent the optimal level to prevent these malformations, and that these levels are achieved with an intake of 350 μg/day of FA (400 μg/day is the current recommendation), from fortified foods and supplements, in addition to natural folate intake from a varied diet (Crider et al., 2014; Tinker et al., 2015; WHO, 2015). Some countries like the United States, Canada, and Latin American countries, including Chile, have implemented food fortification policies to add FA to wheat flour (1.4–2.5 mg/kg) (Honein et al, 2001; Informe Programa Fortificación de Harinas, 2011; Bailey et al., 2015) (Table 18.2).

18.4 Folate transport in placenta and metabolism

The amount of folate transported to the fetus is determined by the maternal circulating folate concentrations. This is shown by a positive correlation between folate concentrations in the maternal plasma and umbilical cord blood, and by placental concentrations of folates.

Table 18.2 Levels for folate, vitamin B12, homocysteine, and methylmalonic acid references levels.

Biomarker	Tissue	Deficiency	Depletion	Adequate	High	Observation
Total folates	Plasma/serum	<7 nmol/L		13.5–45.3 nmol/L		Indicator to prevent anemia in adults (WHO, 2012)
		<10 nmol/L				Indicator of hyperhomocysteinemia in adults (Alasfoor, 2013)
Total folates	RBC	<226.5 nmol/L				Indicator to prevent anemia in adults (WHO, 2012)
				>906 nmol/L		Indicator to prevent neural tube defects, before pregnancy (WHO, 2015)
		<340 mmol/L				Indicator of hyperhomocysteinemia (Alasfoor, 2013)
Total vitamin B12	Plasma/serum	<148 pmol/L	<221 pmol/L	200–600 pmol/L		Indicator to prevent anemia and neurological complications in adults. (Green et al., 2017)
Total vitamin B12	Plasma/serum	<150 pmol/L				Indicator of hyperhomocysteinemia (Alasfoor, 2013)
Holotranscobalamin	Plasma/serum	<35 pmol/L	<40 pmol/L	40–100 pmol/L		Indicator to prevent anemia in adults (Green et al., 2017)
Homocysteine	Plasma/serum			8–15 μmol/L	>15 μmol/L	Indicator of hyperhomocysteinemia in adults (Green et al., 2017)
Methylmalonic acid	Plasma/serum			0.04–0.037 μmol/L	>0.37 μmol/L	Indicator of vitamin B12 deficiency in adults (Green et al., 2017)

RBC, Red blood cells.

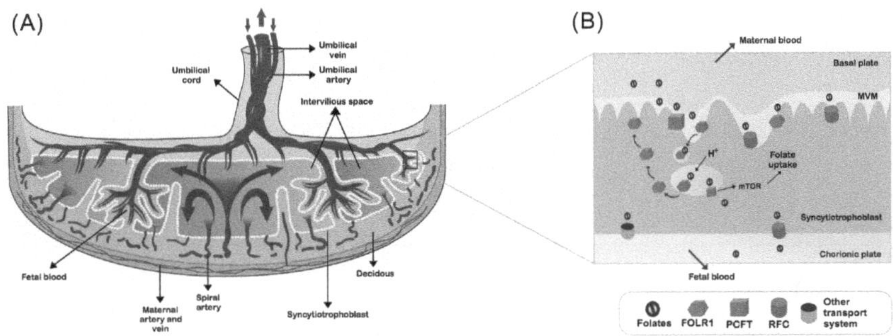

Figure 18.3 Structure of the human placenta (Fig 18.3A). Proposed mechanism for folate transport across human placental syncytiotrophoblast (Fig 18.3B).

The transport of folates from the mother to the fetus has a first concentration component, that is protective to the fetus, since folate-deficient mothers deliver newborns with normal folate stores (Henderson et al., 1995).

The key factors for fetal growth and development, including the supply of nutrients from the mother to the fetus, are carried out by optimal placental functioning. Implantation leads to the proliferation of trophoblast cells, which contribute to the formation of the syncytiotrophoblast (SCT), which represents the interface between the maternal and fetal circulations and plays a critical role in nutrient transport to the fetus to guarantee an adequate fetal growth (Guttmacher et al., 2014; Lager and Powell, 2012; Zhang et al., 2015) (Fig. 18.3A).

The metabolism of folates occurs in most organs, including the placenta (Shin et al., 2014). In the placenta, folates uptake occurs in the SCT (the specialized and multinucleated cell of the placenta) in the form of 5-MTHF (Scott, 1999) or FA, which is first converted into DHF and then into 5-MTHF. Folate and vitamin B12 metabolism includes the remethylation of Hcy to methionine (transmethylation pathways) through methionine synthetase with vitamin B12 (in the form MetCbl or MetB12) as a cofactor and 5-MTHF as a methyl group donor (Hoffbrand, 2014; Scaglione and Panzavolta, 2014). *S*-adenosylmethionine (SAM) is produced in the transmethylation pathways from methionine and ATP (Hoffbrand, 2014); SAM is the main methyl group donor in the methylation reactions in the body, and consequently, participates in epigenetic mechanisms that include DNA and histone methylation (Anderson et al., 2012; Molloy, 2012). Moreover, SAM is an allosteric activator of cystathionine β-synthase (Ereño-Orbea et al., 2014) which requires vitamin B6 as a cofactor in the transsulfuration pathway of Hcy, where cysteine, an important precursor of glutathione (γ-glutamyl-cysteinyl-glycine) is produced (Hoffman, 2011). The transsulfuration constitutes an important pathway for Hcy degradation (Scaglione and Panzavolta, 2014) (Fig. 18.2).

Since vitamin B12 or cobalamin (Cbl) is necessary in folate metabolism, it is important to mention that this vitamin, in the adenosylcobalamin (AdoCbl or AdoB12) form, is a cofactor of the methylmalonyl-CoA mutase (MMCoAM) in the mitochondria (Combs, 2012; Obeid et al., 2015). The enzyme MMCoAM is responsible for the conversion of methylmalonyl-CoA (MMCoA) to succinyl-CoA to enter the Krebs Cycle (Combs, 2012). Those metabolites, MMCoA, propionyl-CoA, and succinyl-CoA, are intermediates of the energetic metabolism in the cell, and they sense and regulate energy balance. On the other hand, MMCoA and MMCoAM are regulators of the enzyme carnitine palmitoyltransferase-1 (López-Viñas et al., 2007; Takahashi-Iñiguez et al., 2012), which is responsible for the transport of fatty acids into the mitochondria to be subsequently β-oxidized (Nsiah-Sefaa and McKenzie, 2016).

At a cellular level, folates are transported from the mother to the fetus through the placenta by three specific transporters: reduced folate carrier (RFC), proton-coupled folate transporter (PCFT)/hem carrier protein 1, and folate receptor α (FOLR1 or FRα) (Solanky et al., 2010). In addition, other nonspecific transporters belonging to the ATP-binding cassette (ABC) superfamily participate in placental folates transport (Keating et al., 2011; Fig. 18.3B).

18.4.1 Reduced folate carrier

RFC is the main folate transporter in different tissues; it is expressed both in the apical and basolateral membranes, has greater affinity for reduced folates, and acts in a neutral pH environment (Zhao et al., 2011). RFC also has affinity for antifolate substances used in different types of cancers, which alter the transport and availability of folate in cells (Visentin et al., 2014; Zhao et al., 2011; Zhao and Goldman, 2013). RFC has a structure of approximately 591 amino acids and 12 transmembrane domains, with N and C terminals located in the cytoplasm (Visentin et al., 2014). In the placenta it is expressed in the apical and basolateral membrane of the SCT, among other cells. RFC transports the reduced folate from the maternal blood, in an anion exchange mechanism with organic phosphate, which is synthesized and retained inside the cell, and then folate is released by RFC from the placental basolateral membrane to the fetal circulation (Visentin et al., 2014; Zhao and Goldman, 2013).

18.4.2 Proton-coupled folate transporter

PCFT is the most recently described solute carrier (SLC) group of membrane transport proteins (*SLC46A1*) (Visentin et al., 2014). PCFT has high affinity for FA and reduced folates. The transport of folate via PCFT is optimal at a pH of 5.0–5.5, and if it increases the uptake of folate by this conveyor is diminished (Visentin et al., 2014; Zhao et al., 2011; Zhao and Goldman, 2013). It is expressed in different tissues, but mainly in the apical membrane of the duodenum and proximal jejunum, in the sinusoidal membrane of the liver, the apical membrane of the kidney, and in the placenta (Zhao and Goldman, 2013). In placental cells, PCFT is expressed not only in the apical membrane, but also in the endosomal vesicles that are formed by the intake of folate by the FRα, which in this case, could be called an exporter of endosomal folate (Zhao et al., 2009). Like RFC, PCFT also presents 12 transmembrane domains.

18.4.3 Folate receptor

FR or FOLR1, like the previous transporters, is expressed in different tissues including the placenta, where it is located in the apical membrane of the SCT. There are four human FR cDNA isoforms (α, β, γ, and δ); FRα is crucial and is highly expressed in the placenta, where it exerts essential functions. Placental FRα, obtained from human placental villi, was cloned in 1989, and was identified as complexly anchored to the membrane (Verma and Antony, 1991). Later, FRα was characterized as a 35 kDa membrane glycoprotein, hydrophobic glycosyl phosphatidylinositol anchored with high binding affinity in the physiologic folates concentrations (in nM range) (Verma et al., 1992). It has greater affinity for 5-MTHF than for other reduced folate forms and its activity is optimal at neutral to moderately acid pH (Carter et al., 2011; Guéant et al., 2013; Zhao et al., 2011; Zhao and Goldman, 2013). Folate binds to the FRα in the cell membrane which leads to an invagination into the cytoplasm, forming a vesicle that circulates in the endosomal compartment, where it is acidified, releasing the receiver from the folate and recycling it back to the apical membrane. The PCFT transporter is also found in the vesicles, where it has a key role in capturing folate to release it into the cytoplasm, while RFC releases folate to the fetal blood (Zhao et al., 2011; Zhao and Goldman, 2013).

It has been shown that the expression of FRα is essential for the development of the embryo (Piedrahita et al., 1999). Despite its necessity for proper fetal development, it is not essential for folate transport; it has been demonstrated that $FR\alpha^{-/-}$ mice are fertile and their progeny viable under adequate folate supplementation. Partial folate supplementation before and during the first trimester of gestation leads to several developmental effects in the fetus (Spiegelstein et al., 2004).

By ex vivo placental perfusion experiments it was demonstrated that FOLR mediate maternal-to-fetal folate transport in a two-stage process. First, maternal circulating folate in the form of 5-MTHF is captured by FRα on the maternally facing chorionic surface, a process favored by a high affinity of FRα for the 5-MTHF (Henderson et al., 1995). The folate bound to receptors is destined for fetal transport; thus a dynamic equilibrium state is created, which may be displaced by incoming circulating folates (from dietary sources) to generate an intervillous blood level approximately three times higher than that of the maternal blood. In the second step, folates are passively transferred to the fetal circulation along a downhill concentration gradient constituting a unique mechanism for transplacental folate transport (Henderson et al., 1995). This mechanism can explain the deleterious effect of maternal folate deficiency on fetal growth and development.

18.4.4 Other folate transporters in placenta

In term placenta, ABC transporters such as P-glycoprotein and multidrug resistance protein (MRP) are expressed to function as efflux transport systems for xenobiotics (Zhao et al., 2011). These ABC superfamily exporters are low-affinity, high-capacity folate transporters and include MRP1, MRP2, MRP3, and ABC G2 transporter; they are all expressed in the apical membrane (maternal side) of the placenta opposing the transport of folate to the fetal circulation (St-Pierre et al., 2000). There is evidence that MRP1 and MRP3 are also expressed in the basolateral membrane of the fetal blood vessel endothelia with some evidence for expression in the apical SCT. MRP2 is localized to the apical SCT membrane (St-Pierre et al., 2000) where it participates in folate homeostasis.

In general, the availability of folate in the fetus depends on the joint and coordinated actions of the receiver and the transporters; changes in their expression or activities may affect such availability. Folate transporters in placenta are highly expressed in the first stages of pregnancy and their expression has been described as decreasing as pregnancy progresses (Solanky et al., 2010).

18.5 Regulation of folate transport in the placenta

18.5.1 Folate sensors

Recently, Silva et al., using cultured primary human trophoblast cells, reported a new folate sensing mechanism mediated by mechanistic target of rapamycin (mTOR) by which folate modulates cell functions such as protein synthesis, nutrient transport, and mitochondrial respiration (Silva et al., 2017). It was found that folate deficiency in pregnant mice inhibited mTORC1 and mTORC2 (part of the mTOR complex) signaling resulting in decreased amino acid transport, protein synthesis, and mitochondrial function, thus explaining the link between folate deficiency and fetal growth restriction. When intracellular folate concentrations are low, mTORC1 is predominantly localized in the cytosol as an inactive form. Increased intracellular folate concentrations sensed by PCFT localized in the lysosomal membrane promote the trafficking of mTORC1 toward the lysosomal membrane initiating mTORC1 signaling and activating several cellular processes including folate uptake (Rosario et al., 2017). Therefore PCFT is necessary for folate sensing by mTOR as demonstrated in cultured primary trophoblast cells (Silva et al., 2017). Furthermore, mTORC1 and mTORC2 regulate trophoblast folate uptake by modulating cell surface expression of FRα and RFC (Rosario et al., 2016) Thus mTORC1 and mTORC2 may be considered positive regulators of folate transporters (Silva et al., 2017).

18.5.2 Pathophysiological conditions and environmental factors

It has been reported that Hcy is a key modulator of the translational upregulation of FOLR and therefore a link between perturbed folate metabolism and coordinated upregulation of FOLR (Antony et al., 2004).

It was observed that some pathophysiological conditions and environmental factors can alter placental folate transport. In preeclampsia, a pathophysiological condition during pregnancy (Goffin et al., 2018), the mRNA of PCFT, FRα, and FRβ decrease at the placental level (Tang et al., 2013; Williams et al., 2012). In human cytotrophoblasts isolated from pregnancies with gestational diabetes mellitus (GDM), ^{3}H-FA uptake was more sensitive to acidic pH, indicating that GDM modulates folate uptake by the SCT (Araújo et al., 2013). In obese women, the protein concentration of FRα in the microvilli membranes increased and RFC was decreased, without modifications of their activities (Carter et al., 2011). On the other hand, in our lab we observed a lower expression of FRα and PCFT in newborns both small and large for gestational age (SGA and LGA), in comparison to newborns adequate for gestational age (Caviedes et al., 2016). In addition, FRα and PCFT placental expression (mRNA) was reduced in preterm newborns (32–36 weeks of gestation) while FRα protein levels were increased (Castaño et al., 2017), suggesting an involvement of epigenetic mechanisms determined by folate levels and vitamin B12 in the umbilical cord.

It was reported that abnormal transport of folate to the developing embryo leads to alterations including craniofacial malformations, cardiac damage, and NTD. In addition, the inhibition of FA binding to FRα may be a risk factor for NTD (Boyles et al., 2011; Piedrahita et al., 1999; Spiegelstein et al., 2004; Tang and Finnell, 2003; Zhu et al., 2007). The aberrant DNA methylation of folate transporter genes in placentas from offspring with NTD has not been demonstrated (Farkas et al., 2013).

In some hereditary diseases, such as the syndrome of systemic and cerebral folate deficiency of infancy, an autosomal recessive disorder, there is a hereditary folate malabsorption characterized by the loss of function of PCFT, which leads to a severe systemic and cerebral folate deficiency. When the FRα loss of function is detected in an autosomal recessive disorder it results solely in a cerebral folate deficiency (Zhao et al., 2017). In in vitro studies in BeWo cells and primary cultured human trophoblasts, progesterone, a steroid hormone produced by the placenta, specifically inhibited the ^{3}H-FA uptake (Keating et al., 2007).

Chronic and heavy alcohol consumption during pregnancy impairs folate transport to the fetus as assessed by the fetal:maternal serum folate ratio in the alcohol-exposed pair which was $\leq$ 1 compared with the control ($\geq$ 1). In cord blood of newborns delivered by alcohol consumers folate levels were lower compared to controls, probably as a consequence of altered folate concentration in placentas (Hutson et al., 2012). Additionally, a decrease in cord folate levels in infants born to smoking mothers compared to nonsmoking mothers has been shown (Stark et al., 2007).

In pregnant rats exposed to cadmium (5 mg/kg of $CdCl_2$), embryonic folate content was decreased and the levels of placental *pcft* mRNA and protein abundance were markedly decreased. However, FRα and RFC expression were not affected. It has been reported that some nutrients are able to regulate folate transport at a placental level like maternal lipopolysaccharide, vitamin D3, and iron (Best et al., 2016; Chen et al., 2015; Zhao et al., 2014).

Altogether the literature to date shows the relevance of pregestational maternal folate status for an adequate fetal development and growth throughout pregnancy. The role of placental folates transporters and binding proteins is essential for this process, mainly regulating fetal levels of these vitamins. Folates availability is key for all the cellular processes in the placenta itself as well as in the maternal and fetal physiology, for example, lipid metabolism and DNA and histone methylation.

References

Alasfoor, D., 2013. WHO technical consultation on folate and vitamin B12 deficiencies. List of participants. Food. Nutr. Bull. 29, 245–246.

Allen, L.H., 2008. Causes of vitamin B12 and folate deficiency. Food. Nutr. Bull. 29, S20–S34. discussion S35–S37.

Anderson, O.S., Sant, K.E., Dolinoy, D.C., 2012. Nutrition and epigenetics: an interplay of dietary methyl donors, one-carbon metabolism and DNA methylation. J. Nutr. Biochem. 23, 853–859. Available from: https://doi.org/10.1016/j.jnutbio.2012.03.003.

Antony, A., Tang, Y.-S., Khan, R.A., Biju, M.P., Xiao, X., Li, Q.-J., et al., 2004. Translational upregulation of folate receptors is mediated by homocysteine via RNA-heterogeneous nuclear ribonucleoprotein E1 interactions. J. Clin. Invest. 113, 285–301. Available from: https://doi.org/10.1172/JCI11548.

Araújo, J.R., Correia-Branco, A., Moreira, L., Ramalho, C., Martel, F., Keating, E., 2013. Folic acid uptake by the human syncytiotrophoblast is affected by gestational diabetes, hyperleptinemia, and TNF-α. Pediatr. Res. 73, 388–394. Available from: https://doi.org/10.1038/pr.2013.14.

Bailey, L.B., Stover, P.J., McNulty, H., Fenech, M.F., Gregory, J.F., Mills, J.L., et al., 2015. Biomarkers of nutrition for development-folate review. J. Nutr. 145, 1636S–1680S. Available from: https://doi.org/10.3945/jn.114.206599.

Best, C.M., Pressman, E.K., Cao, C., Cooper, E., Guillet, R., Yost, O.L., et al., 2016. Maternal iron status during pregnancy compared with neonatal iron status better predicts placental iron transporter expression in humans. FASEB J. 30, 3541–3550. Available from: https://doi.org/10.1096/fj.201600069R.

Boyles, A.L., Ballard, J.L., Gorman, E.B., McConnaughey, D.R., Cabrera, R.M., Wilcox, A.J., et al., 2011. Association between inhibited binding of folic acid to folate receptor alpha in maternal serum and folate-related birth defects in Norway. Hum. Reprod. 26, 2232–2238. Available from: https://doi.org/10.1093/humrep/der144.

Carter, M.F., Powell, T.L., Li, C., Myatt, L., Dudley, D., Nathanielsz, P., et al., 2011. Fetal serum folate concentrations and placental folate transport in obese women.

Am. J. Obstet. Gynecol. 205, . Available from: https://doi.org/10.1016/j.ajog.2011.02.05383.e17-83.e25.

Castaño, E., Caviedes, L., Hirsch, S., Llanos, M., Iñiguez, G., Ronco, A.M., 2017. Folate transporters in placentas from preterm newborns and their relation to cord blood folate and vitamin B12 levels. PLoS One 12, e0170389. Available from: https://doi.org/10.1371/journal.pone.0170389.

Caviedes, L., Iñiguez, G., Hidalgo, P., Castro, J.J., Castaño, E., Llanos, M., et al., 2016. Relationship between folate transporters expression in human placentas at term and birth weights. Placenta 38, 24–28. Available from: https://doi.org/10.1016/j.placenta.2015.12.007.

Chen, Y.-H., Yu, Z., Fu, L., Xia, M.-Z., Zhao, M., Wang, H., et al., 2015. Supplementation with vitamin D3 during pregnancy protects against lipopolysaccharide-induced neural tube defects through improving placental folate transportation. Toxicol. Sci. 145, 90–97. Available from: https://doi.org/10.1093/toxsci/kfv036.

Combs, G.F., 2012. Vitamin B12. The Vitamins. Elsevier, pp. 377–394. Available from: https://doi.org/10.1016/B978-0-12-381980-2.00017-7.

Crider, K.S., Devine, O., Hao, L., Dowling, N.F., Li, S., Molloy, A.M., et al., 2014. Population red blood cell folate concentrations for prevention of neural tube defects: Bayesian model. BMJ 349, g4554. Available from: https://doi.org/10.1136/bmj.g4554.

Czeizel, A.E., Dudás, I., 1992. Prevention of the first occurrence of neural-tube defects by periconceptional vitamin supplementation. N. Engl. J. Med. 327, 1832–1835. Available from: https://doi.org/10.1056/NEJM199212243272602.

de Benoist, B., 2008. Conclusions of a WHO Technical Consultation on folate and vitamin B12 deficiencies. Food. Nutr. Bull. 29, 238–244.

Ereño-Orbea, J., Majtan, T., Oyenarte, I., Kraus, J.P., Martínez-Cruz, L.A., 2014. Structural insight into the molecular mechanism of allosteric activation of human cystathionine β-synthase by *S*-adenosylmethionine. Proc. Natl. Acad. Sci. U.S.A. 111, E3845–E3852. Available from: https://doi.org/10.1073/pnas.1414545111.

Farkas, S.A., Böttiger, A.K., Isaksson, H.S., Finnell, R.H., Ren, A., Nilsson, T.K., 2013. Epigenetic alterations in folate transport genes in placental tissue from fetuses with neural tube defects and in leukocytes from subjects with hyperhomocysteinemia. Epigenetics 8, 303–316. Available from: https://doi.org/10.4161/epi.23988.

Food and Agriculture Organization of the United States—FAO. World Health Organization—WHO, 2001. Human Vitamin and Mineral Requeriments. Food and Nutrition Division—FAO, Rome.

Goffin, S.M., Derraik, J.G.B., Groom, K.M., Cutfield, W.S., 2018. Maternal pre-eclampsia and long-term offspring health: is there a shadow cast? Pregnancy Hypertens. 12, 11–15. Available from: https://doi.org/10.1016/j.preghy.2018.02.003.

Gong, R., Wang, Z.-P., Wang, M., Gao, L.-J., Zhao, Z.-T., 2016. Effects of folic acid supplementation during different pregnancy periods and relationship with the other primary prevention measures to neural tube defects. J. Matern. Fetal Neonatal. Med. 29, 3894–3901. Available from: https://doi.org/10.3109/14767058.2016.1152241.

Green, R., Allen, L.H., Bjørke-Monsen, A.-L., Brito, A., Guéant, J.-L., Miller, J.W., et al., 2017. Vitamin B12 deficiency. Nat. Rev. Dis. Prim. 3, 17040. Available from: https://doi.org/10.1038/nrdp.2017.40.

Guéant, J.-L., Namour, F., Guéant-Rodriguez, R.-M., Daval, J.-L., Gue, R., 2013. Folate and fetal programming: a play in epigenomics? Trends Endocrinol. Metab. 24, 279–289. Available from: https://doi.org/10.1016/j.tem.2013.01.010.

Guttmacher, A.E., Maddox, Y.T., Spong, C.Y., 2014. The Human Placenta Project: placental structure, development, and function in real time. Placenta 35, 303–304. Available from: https://doi.org/10.1016/j.placenta.2014.02.012.

Henderson, G.I., Perez, T., Schenker, S., Mackins, J., Antony, A.C., 1995. Maternal-to-fetal transfer of 5-methyltetrahydrofolate by the perfused human placental cotyledon: evidence for a concentrative role by placental folate receptors in fetal folate delivery. J. Lab. Clin. Med. 126, 184–203.

Honein, M.A., Paulozzi, L.J., Mathews, T.J., et al., 2001. Impact of Folic Acid Fortification of the US Food Supply on the Occurrence of Neural Tube Defects. JAMA. 285 (23), 2981–2986. Available from: https://doi.org/10.1001/jama.285.23.2981.

Hoffbrand, A.V., 2014. Professor John Scott, folate and neural tube defects. Br. J. Haematol. 164, 496–502. Available from: https://doi.org/10.1111/bjh.12654.

Hoffman, M., 2011. Hypothesis: hyperhomocysteinemia is an indicator of oxidant stress. Med. Hypotheses 77, 1088–1093. Available from: https://doi.org/10.1016/j.mehy.2011.09.009.

Hutson, J.R., Stade, B., Lehotay, D.C., Collier, C.P., Kapur, B.M., 2012. Folic acid transport to the human fetus is decreased in pregnancies with chronic alcohol exposure. PLoS One 7, e38057. Available from: https://doi.org/10.1371/journal.pone.0038057.

Informe Programa Fortificación de Harinas. Subsecretaría de Salud Pública, Ministerio de Salud. Instituto de Salud Pública de Chile, 2011, 13 pag.

Institute of Medicine, 1998. Dietary Reference Intakes for Thiamin, Riboflavin, Niacin, Vitamin B6, Folate, Vitamin B12, Pantothenic Acid, Biotin, and Choline. Institute of Medicine, National Academies Press (US), Washington, DC.

Keating, E., Gonçalves, P., Lemos, C., Costa, F., Campos, I., Smith, S.B., et al., 2007. Progesterone inhibits folic acid transport in human trophoblasts. J. Membr. Biol. 216, 143–152. Available from: https://doi.org/10.1007/s00232-007-9057-5.

Keating, E., Araújo, J.R., Martel, F., 2011. The placental transport of folates. Interference by xenobiotics and pathological conditions. Canal BQ 8, 44–48.

Lager, S., Powell, T.L., 2012. Regulation of nutrient transport across the placenta. J. Pregnancy 2012, 1–14. Available from: https://doi.org/10.1155/2012/179827.

López-Viñas, E., Bentebibel, A., Gurunathan, C., Morillas, M., de Arriaga, D., Serra, D., et al., 2007. Definition by functional and structural analysis of two malonyl-CoA sites in carnitine palmitoyltransferase 1A. J. Biol. Chem. 282, 18212–18224. Available from: https://doi.org/10.1074/jbc.M700885200.

McPartlin, J., Halligan, A., Scott, J.M., Darling, M., Weir, D.G., 1993. Accelerated folate breakdown in pregnancy. Lancet 341, 148–149.

Molloy, A.M., 2012. Genetic aspects of folate metabolism. In: Stanger, O. (Ed.), Sub-Cellular Biochemistry. Springer, Berlin, pp. 105–130. Available from: https://doi.org/10.1007/978-94-007-2199-9_7.

Molloy, A.M., Kirke, P.N., Brody, L.C., Scott, J.M., Mills, J.L., 2008. Effects of folate and vitamin B12 deficiencies during pregnancy on fetal, infant, and child development. Food. Nutr. Bull. 29, S101–S111.

Naderi, N., House, J.D., 2018. Recent developments in folate nutrition. Advances in Food and Nutrition Research. Academic Press, pp. 195–213. Available from: https://doi.org/10.1016/BS.AFNR.2017.12.006.

Nsiah-Sefaa, A., McKenzie, M., 2016. Combined defects in oxidative phosphorylation and fatty acid β-oxidation in mitochondrial disease. Biosci. Rep. 36, e00313. Available from: https://doi.org/10.1042/BSR20150295.

Obeid, R., Fedosov, S.N., Nexo, E., 2015. Cobalamin coenzyme forms are not likely to be superior to cyano- and hydroxyl-cobalamin in prevention or treatment of cobalamin deficiency. Mol. Nutr. Food Res. 59, 1364–1372 Available from: https://doi.org/10.1002/mnfr.201500019.

Outline, C., Concepts, A., Mitchell, H.K., Snell, E.S., Williams, R.J., 2012. Folate. The Vitamins 349–375. Available from: https://doi.org/10.1016/B978-0-12-381980-2.00016-5.

Piedrahita, J.A., Oetama, B., Bennett, G.D., van Waes, J., Kamen, B.A., Richardson, J., et al., 1999. Mice lacking the folic acid-binding protein Folbp1 are defective in early embryonic development. Nat. Genet. 23, 228–232. Available from: https://doi.org/10.1038/13861.

Rasmussen, K., Møller, J., Lyngbak, M., Pedersen, A.M., Dybkjaer, L., 1996. Age- and gender-specific reference intervals for total homocysteine and methylmalonic acid in plasma before and after vitamin supplementation. Clin. Chem. 42, 630–636.

Rosario, F.J., Powell, T.L., Jansson, T., 2016. Mechanistic target of rapamycin (mTOR) regulates trophoblast folate uptake by modulating the cell surface expression of FR-α and the RFC. Sci. Rep. 6, 31705. Available from: https://doi.org/10.1038/srep31705.

Rosario, F.J., Nathanielsz, P.W., Powell, T.L., Jansson, T., 2017. Maternal folate deficiency causes inhibition of mTOR signaling, down-regulation of placental amino acid transporters and fetal growth restriction in mice. Sci. Rep. 7, 3982. Available from: https://doi.org/10.1038/s41598-017-03888-2.

Scaglione, F., Panzavolta, G., 2014. Folate, folic acid and 5-methyltetrahydrofolate are not the same thing. Xenobiotica 44, 480–488. Available from: https://doi.org/10.3109/00498254.2013.845705.

Scott, J.M., 1999. Folate and vitamin B12. Proc. Nutr. Soc. 58, 441–448.

Shin, J., Kim, Y., Park, H., Kim, H., Lee, H., 2014. Localization of folate metabolic enzymes, methionine synthase and 5,10-methylenetetrahydrofolate reductase in human placenta. Gynecol. Obstet. Invest. 78, 259–265. Available from: https://doi.org/10.1159/000364866.

Silva, E., Rosario, F.J., Powell, T.L., Jansson, T., 2017. Mechanistic target of rapamycin is a novel molecular mechanism linking folate availability and cell function. J. Nutr. 147, 1237–1242. Available from: https://doi.org/10.3945/jn.117.248823.

Solanky, N., Requena Jimenez, A., D'Souza, S.W., Sibley, C.P., Glazier, J.D., 2010. Expression of folate transporters in human placenta and implications for homocysteine metabolism. Placenta 31, 134–143. Available from: https://doi.org/10.1016/j.placenta.2009.11.017.

Spiegelstein, O., Mitchell, L.E., Merriweather, M.Y., Wicker, N.J., Zhang, Q., Lammer, E.J., et al., 2004. Embryonic development of folate binding protein-1 (Folbp1) knockout mice: effects of the chemical form, dose, and timing of maternal folate supplementation. Dev. Dyn. 231, 221–231. Available from: https://doi.org/10.1002/dvdy.20107.

Stark, K.D., Pawlosky, R.J., Sokol, R.J., Hannigan, J.H., Salem, N., 2007. Maternal smoking is associated with decreased 5-methyltetrahydrofolate in cord plasma. Am. J. Clin. Nutr. 85, 796–802. Available from: https://doi.org/10.1093/ajcn/85.3.796.

St-Pierre, M.V., Serrano, M.A., Macias, R.I., Dubs, U., Hoechli, M., Lauper, U., et al., 2000. Expression of members of the multidrug resistance protein family in human term placenta. Am. J. Physiol. Regul. Integr. Comp. Physiol. 279, R1495–R1503. Available from: https://doi.org/10.1152/ajpregu.2000.279.4.R1495.

Takahashi-Iñiguez, T., García-Hernandez, E., Arreguín-Espinosa, R., Flores, M.E., 2012. Role of vitamin B12 on methylmalonyl-CoA mutase activity. J. Zhejiang Univ. Sci. B 13, 423–437. Available from: https://doi.org/10.1631/jzus.B1100329.

Tamura, T., Picciano, M.F., 2006. Folate and human reproduction. Am. J. Clin. Nutr. 83, 993–1016. Available from: https://doi.org/10.1016/S0370-1573(06)00240-7.

Tang, L.S., Finnell, R.H., 2003. Neural and orofacial defects in Folp1 knockout mice [corrected]. Birth Defects Res. A Clin. Mol. Teratol. 67, 209–218. Available from: https://doi.org/10.1002/bdra.10045.

Tang, Z., Buhimschi, I.A., Buhimschi, C.S., Tadesse, S., Norwitz, E., Niven-Fairchild, T., et al., 2013. Decreased levels of folate receptor-β and reduced numbers of fetal macrophages (Hofbauer cells) in placentas from pregnancies with severe pre-eclampsia. Am. J. Reprod. Immunol. 70, 104–115. Available from: https://doi.org/10.1111/aji.12112.

Tinker, S.C., Hamner, H.C., Qi, Y.P., Crider, K.S., 2015. U.S. women of childbearing age who are at possible increased risk of a neural tube defect-affected pregnancy due to suboptimal red blood cell folate concentrations, National Health and Nutrition Examination Survey 2007 to 2012. Birth Defects Res. A Clin. Mol. Teratol. 103, 517–526. Available from: https://doi.org/10.1002/bdra.23378.

Verma, R.S., Antony, A.C., 1991. Kinetic analysis, isolation, and characterization of hydrophilic folate-binding proteins released from chorionic villi cultured under serum-free conditions. J. Biol. Chem. 266, 12522–12535.

Verma, R.S., Gullapalli, S., Antony, A.C., 1992. Evidence that the hydrophobicity of isolated, in situ, and de novo-synthesized native human placental folate receptors is a function of glycosyl-phosphatidylinositol anchoring to membranes. J. Biol. Chem. 267, 4119–4127.

Visentin, M., Diop-Bove, N., Zhao, R., Goldman, I.D., 2014. The intestinal absorption of folates. Annu. Rev. Physiol. 76, 251–274. Available from: https://doi.org/10.1146/annurev-physiol-020911-153251.

WHO, 2012. Serum and Red Blood Cell Folate Concentrations for Assessing Folate Status in Populations. Vitamin and Mineral Nutrition Information System, Geneva.

WHO, 2015. Guideline: Optimal Serum and Red Blood Cell Folate Concentrations in Women of Reproductive Age for Prevention of Neural Tube Defects. World Health Organization, Geneva.

Williams, P.J., Mistry, H.D., Morgan, L., 2012. Folate transporter expression decreases in the human placenta throughout pregnancy and in pre-eclampsia. Pregnancy Hypertens. 2, 123–131. Available from: https://doi.org/10.1016/j.preghy.2011.12.001.

Wilson, R.D., Wilson, R.D., Désilets, V., Wyatt, P., Langlois, S., Gagnon, A., et al., 2007. Pre-conceptional vitamin/folic acid supplementation 2007: the use of folic acid in combination with a multivitamin supplement for the prevention of neural tube defects and other congenital anomalies. J. Obstet. Gynaecol. Can. 29, 1003–1013. Available from: https://doi.org/10.1016/S1701-2163(16)32685-8.

Yang, T.L., Hung, J., Caudill, M.A., Urrutia, T.F., Alamilla, A., Perry, C.A., et al., 2005. A long-term controlled folate feeding study in young women supports the validity of the 1.7 multiplier in the dietary folate equivalency equation. J. Nutr. 135, 1139–1145. Available from: https://doi.org/10.1093/jn/135.5.1139.

Yasuda, S., Hasui, S., Yamamoto, C., Yoshioka, C., Kobatashi, M., Itagaki, S., et al., 2008. Placental folate transport during pregnancy. Biosci. Biotechnol. Biochem. 72, 2277–2284. Available from: https://doi.org/10.1271/bbb.80112.

Zhang, S., Regnault, T.R.H., Barker, P.L., Botting, K.J., McMillen, I.C., McMillan, C. M., et al., 2015. Placental adaptations in growth restriction. Nutrients 7, 360–389. Available from: https://doi.org/10.3390/nu7010360.

Zhao, R., Goldman, I.D., 2013. Folate and thiamine transporters mediated by facilitative carriers (SLC19A1-3 and SLC46A1) and folate receptors. Mol. Aspects Med. 34, 373–385. Available from: https://doi.org/10.1016/j.mam.2012.07.006.

Zhao, R., Min, S.H., Wang, Y., Campanella, E., Low, P.S., Goldman, I.D., 2009. A role for the proton-coupled folate transporter (PCFT-SLC46A1) in folate receptor-mediated endocytosis. J. Biol. Chem. 284, 4267–4274. Available from: https://doi.org/10.1074/jbc.M807665200.

Zhao, R., Diop-Bove, N., Visentin, M., Goldman, I.D., 2011. Mechanisms of membrane transport of folates into cells and across epithelia. Annu. Rev. Nutr. 31, 177–201. Available from: https://doi.org/10.1146/annurev-nutr-072610-145133.

Zhao, M., Chen, Y.-H., Chen, X., Dong, X.-T., Zhou, J., Wang, H., et al., 2014. Folic acid supplementation during pregnancy protects against lipopolysaccharide-induced neural tube defects in mice. Toxicol. Lett. 224, 201–208. Available from: https://doi.org/10.1016/j.toxlet.2013.10.021.

Zhao, R., Aluri, S., Goldman, I.D., 2017. The proton-coupled folate transporter (PCFT-SLC46A1) and the syndrome of systemic and cerebral folate deficiency of infancy: hereditary folate malabsorption. Mol. Aspects Med. 53, 57–72. Available from: https://doi.org/10.1016/j.mam.2016.09.002.

Zhu, H., Wlodarczyk, B.J., Scott, M., Yu, W., Merriweather, M., Gelineau-van Waes, J., et al., 2007. Cardiovascular abnormalities in Folr1 knockout mice and folate rescue. Birth Defects Res. A Clin. Mol. Teratol. 79, 257–268. Available from: https://doi.org/10.1002/bdra.20347.

Further reading

OMS, 2014. Directriz: Administración diaria de suplementos de hierro y ácido fólico en el embarazo. OMS, Ginebra.

CHAPTER 19

Cobalamin (vitamin B12) malabsorption

Emmanuel Andres[1,2] and Nassim Dali-Youcef[3,4]
[1]Department of Internal Medicine, Diabetes and Metabolic Diseases, Hôpitaux Universitaires de Strasbourg, Strasbourg, France
[2]EA 3072 "Mitochondrie, Stress oxydant et Protection musculaire", Université de Strasbourg, Strasbourg, France
[3]Laboratory of General and Specialized Biochemistry, Hôpitaux Universitaires de Strasbourg, Strasbourg, France
[4]Department of Molecular Science, University Hospital of Strasbourg, University of Strasbourg, Strasbourg, France

Contents

19.1 Introduction

Cobalamin (vitamin B12) is the largest and most complex of all the vitamins (Fig. 19.1A) (Quadros, 2010). The name vitamin B12 is generic for a specific group of cobalt-containing corrinoids with biological activity in humans. Interestingly, it is the only known metabolite to contain cobalt, which gives this water-soluble vitamin its red color. The main cobalamins in humans and animals are hydroxo-, adenosyl-, and methylcobalamin, the latter two being the active coenzyme forms (O'Leary and Samman, 2010). Cobalamin deficiency is relatively frequent, whatever the age of the patients and the phenotype of the studied population (O'Leary and Samman, 2010). Its clinical manifestations are relatively well-known, and

Molecular Nutrition
DOI: https://doi.org/10.1016/B978-0-12-811907-5.00014-2

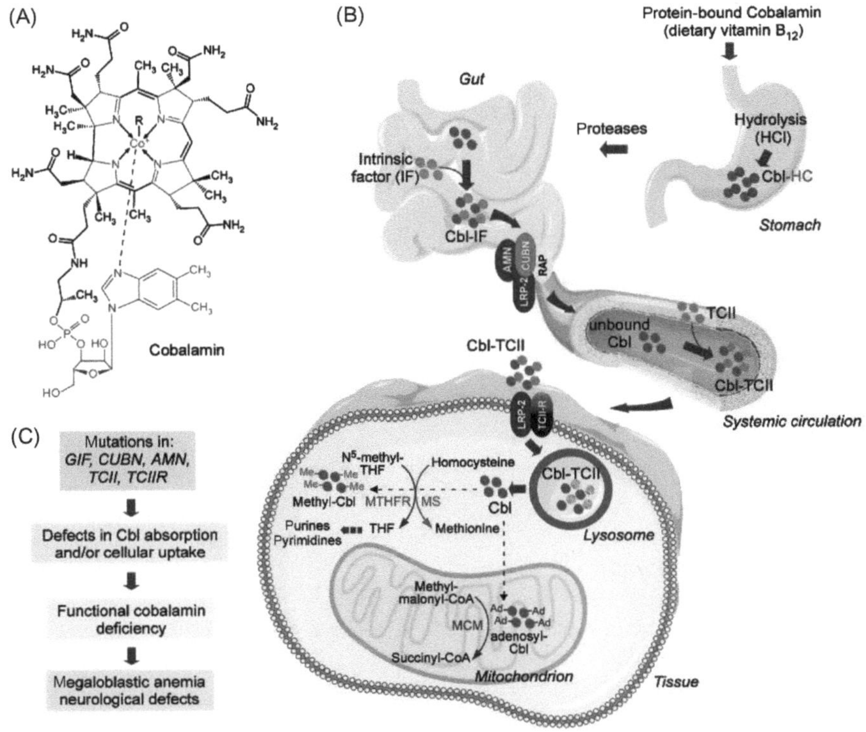

Figure 19.1 Cobalamin (cbl, vitamin B12) absorption and metabolic pathway. (A) Structure of cobalamin (vitamin B_{12}) with a corrin ring bound to a central cobalt atom. (B) The metabolic journey of cbl from nutrient intake to its intestinal absorption. Endocytic receptors and proteins responsible for vitamin B_{12} intestinal absorption include cubilin (CUBN), amnionless (AMN), receptor-associated protein (RAP), and megalin (LRP-2). The membrane megalin/transcobalamin II (TCII) receptor complex allows the cellular uptake of cbl. Lysosomal-mediated degradation of TCII and subsequent release of free cbl is essential for vitamin B_{12} metabolic functions. *MS*, Methionine synthase; *THF*, tetrahydrofolate; *MTHFR*, methyltetrahydrofolate reductase; *MCM*, methylmalonyl coA mutase. (C) Mutations in genes encoding the IF (GIF), CUBN, AMN, TCII, or their receptors provoke defects in cbl absorption and/or cellular uptake which translate into functional cbl deficiency and its clinical manifestations.

are mainly neurological and hematological (hence the old terminology of pernicious anemia) (O'Leary and Samman, 2010; Dali-Youcef and Andrès, 2009). Although cobalamin was isolated almost 60 years ago, its metabolism remains incompletely well-defined (Dali-Youcef and Andrès, 2009). In practice cobalamin metabolism is complex and requires many processes and steps, any one of which, if not present, may lead to cobalamin deficiency. The molecular biology of cobalamin deficiency has been the subject of several studies investigating the genetics of cobalamin metabolism, but to date very few reviews are available (Dali-Youcef and Andrès, 2009; Surendran et al., 2018; Green et al., 2017).

This review summarizes the current knowledge on cobalamin metabolism and metabolic pathway with a clinical perspective, with a focus on cobalamin malabsorption.

19.2 Cobalamin metabolism and function

The average cobalamin content is approximately 1.0 mg in healthy adults, with 20–30 μg found in the kidneys, heart, spleen, and brain (O'Leary and Samman, 2010). Estimates of total cobalamin body content for adults ranges from 0.6 to 3.9 mg with mean values of 2–3 mg. The normal range of cobalamin plasma concentration is 150–750 pg/mL, with peak levels achieved 8–12 hours after ingestion.

The different stages of cobalamin metabolism are shown in Fig. 19.1B (Dali-Youcef and Andrès, 2009; Nicolas and Gueant, 1994). Absorption depends mainly on intrinsic factor, which is secreted by the gastric mucosa. Intrinsic factor binds cobalamin to form a complex that is absorbed by the terminal ileum (Matthews, 1995). This mechanism is responsible for the absorption of at least 60% of oral cobalamin. Cobalamin metabolism is complex and requires many processes, any one of which, if not present, may lead to cobalamin deficiency (Dali-Youcef and Andrès, 2009). Once metabolized, cobalamin is a cofactor and coenzyme in many biochemical reactions, including DNA synthesis, methionine synthesis from homocysteine, and conversion of propionyl into succinyl coenzyme A from methylmalonate.

Table 19.1 describes the different actors of the cobalamin metabolism and the causes of cobalamin deficiency (Andrès et al., 2004). It has been estimated that there is a delay of 5–10 years between the onset of cobalamin deficiency and the appearance of clinical manifestations, due to important hepatic stores (>1.5 mg) and the enterohepatic cycle (Dali-Youcef and Andrès, 2009). In a recent study, we reported the principal causes of cobalamin deficiency in 172 patients (median age 70 years) hospitalized in the University Hospital of Strasbourg, France (Andrès et al., 2000). These causes are represented by food–cobalamin malabsorption (53%), Biermer's disease (pernicious anemia) (33%), insufficient nutritional cobalamin intake (2%), and postsurgical malabsorption (1%). In this study

Table 19.1 Stages of cobalamin metabolism and corresponding causes of cobalamin deficiency (Dali-Youcef and Andrès, 2009; Green et al., 2017; Nicolas and Gueant, 1994).

Stages and actors in cobalamin metabolism	Causes of cobalamin deficiency
Intake solely through food	Strict vegetarianism (patients who are sick in institutions or in psychiatric hospitals)
Digestion brings into play	Gastrectomies
Haptocorrin	Pernicious anemia
Gastric secretions (hydrochloric acid and pepsin)	Food–cobalamin malabsorption
Intrinsic factor	
Pancreatic and biliary secretions	
Enterohepatic cycle	
Absorption brings into play	Ileal resections and malabsorption
Intrinsic factor	Pernicious anemia
Cubilin, amnionless	Food–cobalamin malabsorption
Calcium and energy	
Transport by transcobalamins	Congenital deficiency in transcobalamin II
Intracellular metabolism based on various intracellular enzymes	Congenital deficiency in various intracellular enzymes

over 10% of the patients suffered from cobalamin deficiency of undetermined etiology.

19.3 Vitamin B12 ingestion and its related disorders

Cobalamin is produced exclusively by microbial synthesis in the digestive tract of animals (Watanabe et al., 2014). Therefore animal protein products are the source of vitamin B12 in the human diet, in particular offal (i.e., liver, kidney). Other good sources are fish, eggs, and dairy products. Hydroxo-, methyl-, and 5′-deoxyadenosylcobalamin are the main cobalamins present in foods. A typical Western diet contributes 3–30 mg of cobalamin per day based on the recommended dietary allowance set by the Food and Nutrition Board of the Institute of Medicine (United States) of 2.4 mg/day for adults and from 2.6 to 2.8 mg/day during pregnancy (Institute of Medicine, 1998).

Cobalamin deficiency caused by dietary deficiency (which requires any animal product intake) is rare, even exceptional, in the general population. Dietary causes of deficiency are limited to elderly people who are already malnourished, such as elderly patients, living in institutions (they may consume inadequate amounts of cobalamin-containing foods) or in psychiatric hospitals (Andrès et al., 2004; van Asselt et al., 2000). This is also the case for certain groups of patients who observe strict vegetarian or vegan diets (Rizzo et al., 2016). This is also the case for patients suffering from global and severe malnutrition of the kwashiorkor type (e.g., in underdeveloped countries). Studies focusing on elderly people, particularly those who are in institutions or who are sick and malnourished, have suggested a cobalamin deficiency prevalence of 30%–40%. The Framingham study demonstrated a prevalence of 12% among elderly people living in the community (Lindenbaum et al., 1994). Using a stringent definition, we found that vitamin B12 deficiency had a prevalence of 5% in a group of patients followed or hospitalized in a tertiary reference hospital (Andrès et al., 2005a).

19.4 Food–cobalamin digestion and its related disorders

Dietary cobalamin, which is bound to proteins in food, is released in the acidic environment of the stomach where it is rapidly complexed to the binding protein and transporter haptocorrin (HC), also referred to as the R-binder or transcobalamin I (Fig. 19.1B) (Dali-Youcef and Andrès, 2009). About 80% of circulating cobalamin is bound to HC and serum cobalamin levels have been correlated with serum HC concentrations. Although some unexplained low serum cobalamin concentrations were reported to be caused by mild to severe HC deficiencies, these abnormalities were not accompanied by clinical manifestations of cobalamin deficiency (Carmel, 2003). Cobalamin continues its route in the gastrointestinal track and dissociates from HC under the action of pancreatic proteases, followed by its association in the intestine with the intrinsic factor (also known as the S-binder) which is essential for ileal absorption of cobalamin (Fig. 19.1B) (Dali-Youcef and Andrès, 2009; Green et al., 2017). These different processes are involved as we describe below in the syndrome of food–cobalamin malabsorption.

The syndrome of food–cobalamin malabsorption is a syndrome characterized by the inability of the body to release cobalamin from food or intestinal transport proteins, particularly in the presence of hypochlorhydria (Carmel, 1995). This syndrome is not a "true" malabsorption of the cobalamin but a poor digestion of dietary cobalamins (Andrès et al.,

2003). Authors supporting the existence of this syndrome have employed a modified Schilling test, which uses animal protein-bound radioactive cobalamin (e.g., salmon, trout) and revealed malabsorption when the results of a standard Schilling test were normal (Carmel, 1995; Andrès et al., 2003; Aimone-Gastin et al., 1997). Some authors have speculated about the reality and significance of cobalamin deficiency related to food–cobalamin malabsorption, because many patients displayed mild clinical or hematological features (Carmel, 1995). However, we recently described several patients with serious features classically associated with Biermer's disease, including polyneuropathy, confusion, dementia, medullar-combined sclerosis, anemia, and pancytopenia (Andrès et al., 2005a). Nevertheless, the partial nature of this form of malabsorption may produce a more slowly progressive depletion of cobalamin than does the more complete malabsorption engendered by disruption of the intrinsic factor-mediated absorption. The slower progression of cobalamin depletion probably explains why mild, preclinical deficiency is more frequently associated with food–cobalamin malabsorption than with Biermer's disease (see Table 19.2 for all the clinical manifestations) (Green et al., 2017; Andrès et al., 2005a). In our experience, it currently accounts for

Table 19.2 Food–cobalamin malabsorption syndrome (Carmel, 1995; Andrès et al., 2003; Aimone-Gastin et al., 1997).

Criteria for food–cobalamin malabsorption	Associated conditions or agents
Low serum cobalamin (vitamin B12) levels Normal results of Schilling test using free cyanocobalamin labeled with cobalt-58 or abnormal results of derived Schilling test[a] No antiintrinsic factor antibodies No dietary cobalamin deficiency	Gastric disease: atrophic gastritis, type A atrophic gastritis, gastric disease associated with *Helicobacter pylori* infection, partial gastrectomy, gastric bypass, vagotomy Pancreatic insufficiency: alcohol abuse Gastric or intestinal bacterial overgrowth: achlorhydria, tropical sprue, Ogilvie's syndrome, HIV Drugs: antacids (H2--receptor antagonists and proton pump inhibitors) or biguanides (metformin) Alcohol abuse Sjögren's syndrome, systemic sclerosis Aging or idiopathic

[a]Derived Schilling tests use food-bound cobalamin (e.g., egg yolk, chicken, and fish proteins).

approximately 60%–70% of cases of mild to severe cobalamin deficiency in middle-aged adult and in elderly patients (Andrès et al., 2000). The principal characteristics of this syndrome are listed in Table 19.3 (Andrès et al., 2003, 2005a). In practice food–cobalamin malabsorption is mainly caused by atrophic gastritis (Carmel, 2000). Over 40% of patients older than 80 years have gastric atrophy that might or might not be related to *Helicobacter pylori* infection (Cavalcoli et al., 2017). Other factors that contribute to food–cobalamin malabsorption are chronic carriage of *H. pylori* (Kaptan et al., 2000); intestinal microbial proliferation, situations in which cobalamin deficiency can be corrected by antibiotic treatment (Carmel, 1995); long-term ingestion of antiacids such as Histamine 2-receptor antagonists and proton pump inhibitors, especially among patients with Zollinger–Ellison syndrome (Jung et al., 2015; Maes et al., 2017; Termanini et al., 1998; Miller, 2018); and long-term intake of biguanides (metformin) (Miller, 2018; Andrès et al., 2002; Bauman et al., 2000; Out et al., 2018; Wong et al., 2018). In addition, other food–cobalamin malabsorption inducers include chronic alcoholism, especially in malnourished patients (Carmel, 1995); surgery or gastric reconstruction (e.g., bypass surgery for obesity) (Carmel, 1995); partial exocrine pancreatic failure (Carmel, 1995; Guéant et al., 1990); and rarely Sjögren's syndrome or systemic sclerosis (Andrès et al., 2001a). In this setting, it is to note that patients can absorb "unbound" cobalamin (free or *crystalline* cobalamin) through the intrinsic factor pathway or passive diffusion mechanisms (Andrès et al., 2005a; Carmel, 1995). The recognition of the syndrome has contributed to new developments in the field of oral cobalamin therapy (Kuzminski et al., 1998; Andrès et al., 2001b, 2018).

19.5 Cobalamin absorption and its related disorders

Cobalamin absorption depends mainly on intrinsic factor, which is secreted by the gastric mucosa. Intrinsic factor binds cobalamin forming a complex that is absorbed by the terminal ileum (Fig. 19.1B) (Dali-Youcef and Andrès, 2009).

The absence of intrinsic factor leads to severe cobalamin deficiency (Dali-Youcef and Andrès, 2009; Tanner et al., 2005). This mechanism is responsible for at least 60% of the absorption of oral cobalamin. In practice, this mechanism has been previously explored by the Schilling's test (currently not available in numerous countries). This complex is located at the apical side of brush border membranes (BBMs) of polarized epithelia,

Table 19.3 Main clinical features of cobalamin deficiency (Andrès et al., 2000, 2008; Healton et al., 1991; Miles et al., 2016; Stabler et al., 1990).

Hematological manifestations	Neuropsychiatric manifestations	Digestive manifestations	Other manifestations
Frequent: macrocytosis, neutrophil hypersegmentation, aregenerative macrocytary anemia, and medullar megaloblastosis ("blue spinal cord")	Frequent: polyneuritis (especially sensitive), ataxia, and Babinski's phenomenon	Classic: Hunter's glossitis, jaundice, LDH and bilirubin elevation ("intramedullary destruction")	Frequent: Tiredness, loss of appetite
Rare: isolated thrombocytopenia and neutropenia, pancytopenia	Classic: combined sclerosis of the spinal cord	Debatable: abdominal pain, dyspepsia, nausea, vomiting, diarrhea, and disturbances in intestinal functioning	Under study: atrophy of the vaginal mucosa and chronic vaginal and urinary infections (especially mycosis), hypofertility and repeated miscarriages, venous thromboembolic disease, and angina (hyperhomocysteinemia)
Very rare: hemolytic anemia, thrombotic microangiopathy (presence of schistocytes)	Rare: isolated thrombocytopenia and neutropenia, pancytopenia Under study: changes in the higher functions, dementia, stroke and atherosclerosis (hyperhomocysteinemia), Parkinsonian syndromes, depression, and multiple sclerosis	Rare: resistant and recurring mucocutaneous ulcers	

such as the intestinal apical BBM (Green et al., 2017). It consists of the intrinsic factor–cobalamin receptor named cubilin (CUBN), a 460 kDa peripheral membrane glycoprotein, encoded by the CUBN gene, which was mapped to chromosomal region 10p12.33–p13 (Kozyraki et al., 1998), and the 48 kDa amnionless protein encoded by the amnionless (AMN) gene, a gene essential for mouse gastrulation (Kalantry et al., 2001), and localized on human chromosome 14 (Fyfe et al., 2004). The human megalin/gp330/LRP-2 receptor, encoded by the LRP-2 gene located on chromosome 2q24–q31 (Korenberg et al., 1994), is a giant endocytic receptor (600 kDa) of the low-density lipoprotein receptor (LDLR) family (Saito et al., 1994) that was strongly suggested to play an important role in the stability of the CUBN/AMN complex (Ahuja et al., 2008). It is noteworthy that ligands for megalin include apoE, lipoprotein lipase, lactoferrin, receptor-associated protein (RAP) among other proteins and that this interaction is Ca^{2+} dependent (Orlando et al., 1997; Moestrup et al., 1996; Christensen et al., 1992). Importantly, the endoplasmic reticulum localized 39 kDa protein RAP, which binds to all members of the LDLR family but also in a region contiguous to the cobalamin–intrinsic factor binding region on the CUBN protein (Birn et al., 1997; Kristiansen et al., 1999), allows the processing of megalin where it binds to the newly synthesized megalin receptor in the endoplasmic reticulum and prevents the early binding of ligands and the aggregation of megalin receptors (Christensen and Birn, 2002). Intestinal-specific inactivation of megalin in in vivo animal models would be of particular interest to establish a precise role of megalin in cobalamin–intrinsic factor absorption at the intestinal BBM–blood barrier and its potential relationship with hereditary megaloblastic anemia 1 (MGA1), a rare autosomal recessive disorder affecting human subjects with neurological symptoms and juvenile megaloblastic anemia (Imerslund, 1960; Gräsbeck, 2006).

The endocytic receptor CUBN comprises a short N-terminal region followed by eight epidermal growth factor repeats and a large cluster of 27 CUB domains. Deletion mutant and immunoprecipitation experiments identified the CUB1-8 region as the binding domain for the cobalamin–intrinsic factor complex and the overlapping CUB13 and 14 domains as the binding region for the RAP protein (Kristiansen et al., 1999). Mutations in CUBN were reported to cause hereditary MGA1 (Aminoff et al., 1999). Two principal mutations were identified in Finnish patients (FM), a 3916C→T missense mutation named FM1 changing a highly conserved proline to leucine (P1297L) in CUB domain 8, suggesting that this proline is functionally crucial in CUBN, and one point mutation (FM2) in the intron interrupting CUB domain 6 responsible for in-frame insertions producing truncated CUBN. Interestingly normal size CUBN protein was identified in urine samples from homozygous FM1 patients, whereas a complete absence of the protein was reported in a patient homozygous for the FM2 mutation (Aminoff et al., 1999). Other mutations were also uncovered but were subsequently identified as polymorphisms after their detection in normal individuals in the general population. The CUBN P1297L mutation associated with hereditary MGA1 was reported to cause impaired recognition of the cobalamin–intrinsic factor complex by CUBN (Kristiansen et al., 2000). Moreover, mutation in AMN was reported in recessive hereditary MGA1 (Tanner et al., 2003) and hence was demonstrated to be crucial for a functional cobalamin–IF receptor (Kalantry et al., 2001). This study demonstrated that homozygous mutations affecting exons 1–4 of the human AMN gene translated into selective malabsorption of cobalamin, a phenotype associated with hereditary MGA1. Another study reported AMN deletion mutants in dogs with selective intestinal malabsorption of cobalamin associated with urinary loss of low molecular weight protein reminiscent of the human Imerslund–Gräsbeck syndrome (IGS, also known as MGA1). The authors showed that these mutations in the AMN gene abrogated AMN expression and blocked CUBN processing and targeting to the apical membrane. The essential AMN–CUBN interaction was recapitulated and validated in a heterologous cell-transfection model, hence explaining the molecular basis of intestinal cobalamin malabsorption syndrome (He et al., 2005). In this setting, homozygous nonsense and missense mutations in the gene encoding the gastric intrinsic factor GIF were also reported to cause hereditary juvenile cobalamin deficiency (Dali-Youcef and Andrès, 2009; Tanner et al., 2005).

In middle-aged adults or in elderly patients cobalamin deficiency is classically caused by Biermer's disease, also called Addison's disease or historically pernicious anemia (Andrès et al., 2004). Biermer's disease is an autoimmune disease characterized by the destruction of the gastric mucosa, especially fundal, associated with a primarily cell-mediated autoimmune process (Toh et al., 1997). The latter is responsible for the destruction of gastric parietal cells and the consequent impairment of intrinsic factor's secretion to bind the ingested cobalamin. Asymptomatic autoimmune gastritis, a chronic inflammatory disease of the gastric mucosa, precedes the onset of corpus atrophy by 10–20 years. The gastritis arises from activation of pathologic Th1 CD4+ T cells to gastric H^+/K^+-ATPase that is normally resident on gastric mucosal secretory membranes. The onset of autoimmune gastritis is marked by circulating parietal cell antibody to gastric H^+/K^+-ATPase. Gastric parietal cells produce two essential biologics: intrinsic factor and HCl acid. Biermer's disease is a consequence of intrinsic factor loss and a neutralizing intrinsic factor antibody that impairs cobalamin absorption. Biermer's disease is characterized by the presence of various antibodies, for example, antiintrinsic factor (diagnosis specificity of >90%) and gastric parietal anticell antibodies that target the H^+/K^+-ATPase α and ß subunits (Pruthi and Tefferi, 1994; Li et al., 2018). This disease is also characterized by an abnormal result of the Schilling's test, an abnormal result indicating malabsorption, and corrected at a later stage by the administration of intrinsic factor (currently, this test is not available) (Pruthi and Tefferi, 1994). In our experience, this disease accounted for approximately 40%–50% of cases of cobalamin deficiency according to the population studied (Andrès et al., 2004). In this setting other autoimmune disorders are commonly associated, such as thyroid disease (mainly Hashimoto's disease), Sjögren's syndrome, type 1 diabetes mellitus, vitiligo, and rarely celiac disease (Pruthi and Tefferi, 1994; Li et al., 2018). Epidemiological data showed that patients with Biermer's etiologically linked to autoimmune gastritis are at increased risk of gastric cancer (relative risk of 6.8) (Pruthi and Tefferi, 1994; Li et al., 2018).

In addition to Biermer's disease, there are other causes of "true" malabsorption of cobalamins (malabsorption in relation with digestive tract damages or resections) (Green et al., 2017; Andrès et al., 2004; Markle, 1996). Since the 1980s, these causes have become rarer, owing mainly to the decreasing frequency of gastric and terminal small intestine surgical resection (e.g., total gastrectomy for stomach ulcers, which is currently prevented or treated with antacids) (Andrès et al., 2004; Markle, 1996). To date several disorders might however be associated with cobalamin malabsorption. These disorders include exocrine pancreas' function deficiency following chronic pancreatitis (mainly in relation to alcoholism); lymphomas or tuberculosis of the intestine (with a specific damage of the terminal ileum); celiac disease; Crohn's disease (much rarer with anti-TNFα treatments); and unfrequently Whipple's disease (Green et al., 2017; Andrès et al., 2004; Markle, 1996). At this level, it is also common to mention bothriocephalosis infections (due to *Diphyllobothriose latum*), a disease mainly reported in the Nordic countries (Markle, 1996).

IGS is a rare autosomal recessive disorder characterized by a selective cobalamin malabsorption with proteinuria and megaloblastic anemia, which is responsive to parenteral cobalamin therapy (Gräsbeck, 2006). The cobalamin deficiency appears in childhood and includes other manifestations such as failure to thrive and grow, infections, and neurological damage. Mild proteinuria (with no signs of kidney disease) is present in about half of the patients. The syndrome was first described in Finland and Norway where the prevalence is about 1/200,000. In most cases, the molecular basis of the selective malabsorption and proteinuria involves a mutation in one of two genes, CUBN on chromosome 10 or AMN on chromosome 14 (as seen before) (Gräsbeck, 2006). Both proteins are components of the intestinal receptor for the cobalamin–intrinsic factor complex and the receptor mediating the tubular reabsorption of protein from the primary urine.

19.6 Cobalamin distribution in the tissues and its related disorders

After cobalamin is absorbed at the BBM–blood barrier, it dissociates from the intrinsic factor and reaches the systemic circulation where it associates with transcobalamin II (TC II) (Fig. 19.1B). The kidney represents an essential organ where body cobalamin stores are maintained and studies have demonstrated that the kidney regulates plasma cobalamin levels by maintaining a pool of unbound cobalamin that can be released in case of cobalamin deficiency (Okuda, 1962a,b; Scott et al., 1984; Birn, 2006). The tissular cobalamin–TC II complex uptake is achieved through megalin (LRP-2)- and TC II receptor-mediated endocytosis which plays a crucial role in cobalamin homeostasis (Moestrup et al., 1996; Yammani et al., 2003). It is worth mentioning that TC II is responsible for the cellular uptake of cobalamin in most tissues and that TC II deficiency is associated with severe megaloblastic anemia (Fig. 19.1C) (Li et al., 1994; Teplitsky et al., 2003). Impaired megalin function has not been associated with cobalamin deficiency so far; however inappropriate megalin signaling has been shown to cause deleterious effects as a consequence of cobalamin uptake inhibition in tissues.

Part of the unbound cobalamin serves as a cofactor for methionine synthase-mediated homocysteine catabolism into methionine and methyltetrahydrofolate reductase (MTHFR)-mediated formation of the vitamin

B9 biologically active form, tetrahydrofolate, which is then involved in the synthesis of purines and pyrimidines (Fig. 19.1B) (Green et al., 2017). The other part of free cobalamin is transferred to the mitochondria where it is transformed into adenosylcobalamin, an important cofactor in methylmalonyl-coenzyme A mutase-mediated formation of succinyl-CoA from methylmalonyl-CoA, the product of odd-chain fatty acid and some amino acid catabolism (Dali-Youcef and Andrès, 2009; Green et al., 2017). Hence cobalamin deficiency will cause homocysteine accumulation, increased methylmalonyl−CoA levels and decreased MTHFR activity. These changes translate into several abnormalities including folate deficiency and the subsequent inhibition of the formation of purines and pyrimidines essential for RNA and DNA synthesis (Green et al., 2017).

19.7 Particular points of interest for the clinician

These reactions seen above explain the main clinical manifestations of cobalamin deficiency: megaloblastic anemia and neurocognitive abnormalities seen in adults and elderly patients with cobalamin deficiency, related or not to cobalamin malabsorption (Andrès et al., 2000, 2008; Healton et al., 1991; Miles et al., 2016; Stabler et al., 1990). Other clinical manifestations are highly polymorphic and of varying severity, ranging from milder conditions such as fatigue, common sensory neuropathy, atrophic glossitis (Hunter's glossitis), and isolated macrocytosis or neutrophil hypersegmentation, to severe disorders, including combined sclerosis of the spinal cord, hemolytic anemia, pseudothrombotic microangiopathy, and even pancytopenia (Andrès et al., 2000, 2008; Healton et al., 1991). Table 19.2 includes all the clinical manifestations related to cobalamin deficiency.

The chemical reactions described above also explain the elements of the definition of cobalamin deficiency (Box 19.1) (Andrès et al., 2000; Herrmann and Obeid, 2013; Herrmann et al., 2005; Wickramasinghe, 2006; Nexo and Hoffmann-Lücke, 2011). In practice, the latter is characterized by serum cobalamin levels <150 pmol/L (200 pg/mL) ± serum total homocysteine levels >13 μmol/L or urinary methylmalonic acid >0.4 μmol/L. In addition to this definition, holotranscobalamin (referred to as active vitamin B12) also seems to be a promising marker for cobalamin deficiency (Nexo and Hoffmann-Lücke, 2011).

BOX 19.1 Definitions of cobalamin (vitamin B12) deficiency (Andrès et al., 2000; Herrmann and Obeid, 2013; Herrmann et al., 2005; Wickramasinghe, 2006; Nexo and Hoffmann-Lücke, 2011)

- Serum cobalamin levels <150 pmol/L and clinical features and/or hematological anomalies related to cobalamin deficiency.
- Serum cobalamin levels <150 pmol/L (<200 pg/mL) on two separate occasions.
- Serum cobalamin levels <150 pmol/L and total serum homocysteine levels >13 mmol/L or methylmalonic acid levels >0.4 mmol/L (in the absence of kidney failure or atheroma and of methylene tetra hydro folate reductase (MTHFR) deficiency and in the absence of folate and vitamin B6 deficiencies).
- Low serum holotranscobalamin levels <35 pmol/L.

As seen above, the disappearance of the Schilling's test and the recognition of food–cobalamin malabsorption have changed the approach to the etiological diagnosis of cobalamin deficiency (Andrès et al., 2004). Thus the etiological diagnosis of cobalamin malabsorption has become above all a diagnosis of exclusion: exclusion of malnutrition (with all the difficulties of dietary surveys) and exclusion of Biermer's disease (with gastroscopy results and antibody research). In this context, it is mainly the patient's history and anamnesis that make it possible to evoke this diagnosis of cobalamin malabsorption. Box 19.2 includes all the conditions responsible for the malabsorption of dietary cobalamins (Green et al., 2017; Andrès et al., 2004; Herrmann and Obeid, 2012; Holt, 2007).

The recognition of the food–cobalamin malabsorption and the observation that about 1%–5% of free cobalamin (crystalline) is absorbed along the entire intestine by passive diffusion has led to the development of new routes of cobalamin delivery, such as oral and nasal (Kuzminski et al., 1998; Andrès et al., 2001b; van Asselt et al., 1998). Several recent studies and reviews have documented the efficacy of oral cobalamin (cyanocobalamin) therapy (Andrès et al., 2001b; Wang et al., 2018). In this setting, we have documented the usefulness of oral cobalamin in food–cobalamin malabsorption and even in Biermer's disease (Andrès et al., 2001b, 2005b).

BOX 19.2 Conditions responsible for malabsorption of dietary cobalamins (vitamin B12) (Green et al., 2017; Andrès et al., 2004; Herrmann and Obeid, 2012; Holt, 2007)

- Biermer's disease (pernicious anemia).
- Food–cobalamin malabsorption: atrophic gastritis, gastric disease associated with *Helicobacter pylori* infection, partial gastrectomy, gastric bypass, vagotomy; exocrine pancreas' function deficiency following chronic pancreatitis (mainly in relation with alcoholism); gastric or intestinal bacterial overgrowth (achlorhydria, tropical sprue, Ogilvie's syndrome, HIV); antacids (Histamine 2 receptor antagonists and proton pump inhibitors); biguanides (metformin); alcohol abuse; and systemic autoimmune diseases (Sjögren's syndrome, systemic sclerosis).
- Cobalamin malabsorption related to digestive tract damages: gastrectomy or intestinal resection; lymphomas or tuberculosis of the intestine (with a specific damage of the terminal ileum); celiac disease; Crohn's disease; Whipple's disease and *Diphyllobothriose latum* infection.
- Defects in the cobalamin metabolic pathway, in the step of cobalamin absorption: alterations of the genes and/or proteins (quantitative or qualitative) of the GIF and gastric intrinsic factor, CUBN/AMN and cubilin and amnionless (hereditary megaloblastic anemia 1, juvenile megaloblastic anemia, Imerslund–Gräsbeck syndrome).

19.8 Conclusion

In this chapter we have reviewed different aspects of the cobalamin metabolism with a focus on cobalamin absorption and malabsorption. As described above, the main mechanisms implicated in this absorption have been clinically characterized and the main actors on the molecular level have been identified. Nevertheless, other actors and/or cofactors of this cobalamin malabsorption may be currently still uncovered, including mutations in genes encoding important proteins of the cobalamin metabolic pathway. Moreover, many clinically diagnosed cobalamin deficiencies remain unexplained and molecular tools aimed at targeting genes involved in cobalamin absorption and cellular uptake signaling pathways will pave the way for new therapeutic approaches to efficiently treat all cobalamin deficiency.

Acknowledgments

We are indebted to Professor Marc Imler and Jean-Louis Schlienger who initiated our work on cobalamin in humans. The research on cobalamin deficiency was supported by a grant of the Fondation de France (Prix Robert et Jacqueline Zittoun 2004).

Take Home Messages

- Cobalamin (vitamin B12) deficiency is particularly common whatever the age of the patient, but may be unrecognized because of its subtle clinical manifestations, although they can be potentially serious, particularly from a neuropsychiatric and hematological perspective.
- Cobalamin metabolism is complex and requires many processes and steps, any one of which, if not present, may lead to cobalamin deficiency.
- In the setting of cobalamin malabsorption, the two main diseases are Biermer's disease and the syndrome of food–cobalamin malabsorption.
- Biermer's disease is an autoimmune disease characterized by the destruction of the gastric mucosa, especially fundal, associated with a primarily cell-mediated autoimmune process.
- The food–cobalamin malabsorption, which has only recently been well-identified, is a disorder characterized by the inability to release cobalamin from food or its binding proteins. This syndrome is usually caused by atrophic gastritis, related or unrelated to *H. pylori* infection, and long-term ingestion of antacids and biguanides.
- At present, cobalamin deficiencies related to gastric or intestinal resection or damages have become rare.
- Besides these disorders, mutations in genes encoding endocytic receptors involved in the ileal absorption and cellular uptake of cobalamin (CUBN, AMN, and TC II) have been recently uncovered and explain, at least in part, the hereditary component of megaloblastic anemia and of Imerslund–Gräsbeck.

References

Ahuja, R., Yammani, R., Bauer, J.A., Kalra, S., Seetharam, S., Seetharam, B., 2008. Interactions of cubilin with megalin and the product of the amnionless gene (AMN): effect on its stability. Biochem. J. 410, 301–308.

Aimone-Gastin, I., Pierson, H., Jeandel, C., Bronowicki, J.P., Plénat, F., Lambert, D., et al., 1997. Prospective evaluation of protein bound vitamin B12 (cobalamin) malabsorption in the elderly using trout flesh labelled in vivo with 57Co-cobalamin. Gut 41, 475–479.

Aminoff, M., Carter, J.E., Chadwick, R.B., Johnson, C., Gräsbeck, R., Abdelaal, M. A., et al., 1999. Mutations in CUBN, encoding the intrinsic factor-vitamin B12 receptor, cubilin, cause hereditary megaloblastic anaemia 1. Nat. Genet. 21, 309–313.

Andrès, E., Goichot, B., Schlienger, J.L., 2000. Food–cobalamin malabsorption: a usual cause of vitamin B12 deficiency. Arch. Intern. Med. 160, 2061–2062.
Andrès, E., Goichot, B., Perrin, A.E., Vinzio, S., Demangeat, C., Schlienger, J.L., 2001a. Sjögren's syndrome: a potential new aetiology of mild cobalamin deficiency. Rheumatology (Oxford) 40, 1196–1197.
Andrès, E., Kurtz, J.E., Perrin, A.E., Maloisel, F., Demangeat, C., Goichot, B., et al., 2001b. Oral cobalamin therapy for the treatment of patients with food–cobalamin malabsorption. Am. J. Med. 111, 126–129.
Andrès, E., Noel, E., Goichot, B., 2002. Metformin-associated vitamin B12 deficiency. Arch. Intern. Med. 162, 2251–2252.
Andrès, E., Noel, E., Kaltenbach, G., Perrin, A.E., Vinzio, S., Goichot, B., et al., 2003. Vitamin B12 deficiency with normal Schilling test or non-dissociation of vitamin B12 and its carrier proteins in elderly patients. A study of 60 patients. Rev. Med. Interne. 24, 218–223.
Andrès, E., Loukili, N.H., Noel, E., Kaltenbach, G., Abdelgheni, M.B., Perrin, A.E., et al., 2004. Vitamin B12 (cobalamin) deficiency in elderly patients. CMAJ 171, 251–254.
Andrès, E., Affenberger, S., Vinzio, S., Kurtz, J.E., Noel, E., Kaltenbach, G., et al., 2005a. Food–cobalamin malabsorption in elderly patients: clinical manifestations and treatment. Am. J. Med. 118, 1154–1159.
Andrès, E., Loukili, N.H., Noel, E., Maloisel, F., Vinzio, S., Kaltenbach, G., et al., 2005b. Oral cobalamin (daily dose of 1000 μg) therapy for the treatment of patients with pernicious anemia. An open label study of 10 patients. Curr. Ther. Res. 66, 13–22.
Andrès, E., Federici, L., Kaltenbach, G., 2008. Hematological manifestations related to cobalamin deficiency in elderly patients. Eur. J. Intern. Med. 19, 149–150.
Andrès, E., Zulfiqar, A., Vogel, T., Kaltenbach, G., 2018. Systematic review and pragmatic clinical approach to oral and nasal vitamin B12 (cobalamin) treatment in patients with vitamin B12 deficiency related to gastrointestinal disorders. J. Clin. Med. (10), pii: E304.
Bauman, W.A., Shaw, S., Jayatilleke, E., Spungen, A.M., Herbert, V., 2000. Increased intake of calcium reverses vitamin B12 malabsorption induced by metformin. Diabetes Care 23, 1227–1231.
Birn, H., 2006. The kidney in vitamin B12 and folate homeostasis: characterization of receptors for tubular uptake of vitamins and carrier proteins. Am. J. Physiol. Renal Physiol. 291, F22–F36.
Birn, H., Verroust, P.J., Nexo, E., Hager, H., Jacobsen, C., Christensen, E.I., et al., 1997. Characterization of an epithelial approximately 460-kDa protein that facilitates endocytosis of intrinsic factor-vitamin B12 and binds receptor-associated protein. J. Biol. Chem. 272, 26497–26504.
Carmel, R., 1995. Malabsorption of food cobalamin. Baillieres Clin. Haematol. 8, 639–655.
Carmel, R., 2000. Current concepts in cobalamin deficiency. Annu. Rev. Med. 51, 357–375.
Carmel, R., 2003. Mild transcobalamin I (haptocorrin) deficiency and low serum cobalamin concentrations. Clin. Chem. 49, 1367–1374.
Cavalcoli, F., Zilli, A., Conte, D., Massironi, S., 2017. Micronutrient deficiencies in patients with chronic atrophic autoimmune gastritis: a review. World J. Gastroenterol. 23, 563–572.
Christensen, E.I., Birn, H., 2002. Megalin and cubilin: multifunctional endocytic receptors. Nat. Rev. Mol. Cell Biol. 3, 256–266.
Christensen, E.I., Gliemann, J., Moestrup, S.K., 1992. Renal tubule gp330 is a calcium binding receptor for endocytic uptake of protein. J. Histochem. Cytochem. 40, 1481–1490.

Dali-Youcef, N., Andrès, E., 2009. An update on cobalamin deficiency in adults. QJM 102, 17–28.
Fyfe, J.C., Madsen, M., Hojrup, P., Christensen, E.I., Tanner, S.M., de la Chapelle, A., et al., 2004. The functional cobalamin (vitamin B12)-intrinsic factor receptor is a novel complex of cubilin and amnionless. Blood 103, 1573–1579.
Gräsbeck, R., 2006. Imerslund–Gräsbeck syndrome (selective vitamin B(12) malabsorption with proteinuria). Orphanet J. Rare Dis. 1, 17.
Green, R., Allen, L.H., Bjørke-Monsen, A.L., Brito, A., Guéant, J.L., Miller, J.W., et al., 2017. Vitamin B12 deficiency. Nat. Rev. Dis. Primers 3, 17040.
Guéant, J.L., Champigneulle, B., Gaucher, P., Nicolas, J.P., 1990. Malabsorption of vitamin B12 in pancreatic insufficiency of the adult and of the child. Pancreas 5, 559–567.
He, Q., Madsen, M., Kilkenney, A., Gregory, B., Christensen, E.I., Vorum, H., et al., 2005. Amnionless function is required for cubilin brush-border expression and intrinsic factor-cobalamin (vitamin B12) absorption in vivo. Blood 106, 1447–1453.
Healton, E.B., Savage, D.G., Brust, J.C., Garrett, T.J., Lindenbaum, J., 1991. Neurologic aspects of cobalamin deficiency. Medicine (Baltimore) 70, 229–245.
Herrmann, W., Obeid, R., 2012. Cobalamin deficiency. Subcell. Biochem. 56, 301–322.
Herrmann, W., Obeid, R., 2013. Utility and limitations of biochemical markers of vitamin B12 deficiency. Eur. J. Clin. Invest. 43, 231–237.
Herrmann, W., Obeid, R., Schorr, H., Geisel, J., 2005. The usefulness of holotranscobalamin in predicting vitamin B12 status in different clinical settings. Curr. Drug. Metab. 6, 47–53.
Holt, P.R., 2007. Intestinal malabsorption in the elderly. Dig. Dis. 25, 144–150.
Imerslund, O., 1960. Idiopathic chronic megaloblastic anemia in children. Acta Paediatr. Suppl. 49 (Suppl 119), 1–115.
Institute of Medicine, 1998. Dietary Reference Intake of Thiamin, Riboflavin, Niacin, Vitamin B6, Folate, Vitamin B12, Panthotenic Acid, Biotin and Choline Food and Nutrition Board. National Academies Press, Washington DC.
Jung, S.B., Nagaraja, V., Kapur, A., Eslick, G.D., 2015. Association between vitamin B12 deficiency and long-term use of acid-lowering agents: a systematic review and meta-analysis. Intern. Med. J. 45, 409–416.
Kalantry, S., Manning, S., Haub, O., Tomihara-Newberger, C., Lee, H.G., Fangman, J., et al., 2001. The amnionless gene, essential for mouse gastrulation, encodes a visceral-endoderm-specific protein with an extracellular cysteine-rich domain. Nat. Genet. 27, 412–416.
Kaptan, K., Beyan, C., Ural, A.U., Cetin, T., Avcu, F., Gulsen, M., et al., 2000. *Helicobacter pylori*—is it a novel causative agent in vitamin B12 deficiency? Arch. Intern. Med. 160, 1349–1353.
Korenberg, J.R., Argraves, K.M., Chen, X.N., Tran, H., Strickland, D.K., Argraves, W. S., 1994. Chromosomal localization of human genes for the LDL receptor family member glycoprotein 330 (LRP2) and its associated protein RAP (LRPAP1). Genomics 22, 88–93.
Kozyraki, R., Kristiansen, M., Silahtaroglu, A., Hansen, C., Jacobsen, C., Tommerup, N., et al., 1998. The human intrinsic factor-vitamin B12 receptor, cubilin: molecular characterization and chromosomal mapping of the gene to 10p within the autosomal recessive megaloblastic anemia (MGA1) region. Blood 91, 3593–3600.
Kristiansen, M., Kozyraki, R., Jacobsen, C., Nexo, E., Verroust, P.J., Moestrup, S.K., 1999. Molecular dissection of the intrinsic factor-vitamin B12 receptor, cubilin, discloses regions important for membrane association and ligand binding. J. Biol. Chem. 274, 20540–20544.

Kristiansen, M., Aminoff, M., Jacobsen, C., de La Chapelle, A., Krahe, R., Verroust, P.J., et al., 2000. Cubilin P1297L mutation associated with hereditary megaloblastic anemia 1 causes impaired recognition of intrinsic factor-vitamin B(12) by cubilin. Blood 96, 405–409.
Kuzminski, A.M., Del Giacco, E.J., Allen, R.H., Stabler, S.P., Lindenbaum, J., 1998. Effective treatment of cobalamin deficiency with oral cobalamin. Blood 9, 1191–1198.
Li, N., Rosenblatt, D.S., Kamen, B.A., Seetharam, S., Seetharam, B., 1994. Identification of two mutant alleles of transcobalamin II in an affected family. Hum. Mol. Genet. 3, 1835–1840.
Li, Y., Xia, R., Zhang, B., Li, C., 2018. Chronic atrophic gastritis: a review. J. Environ. Pathol. Toxicol. Oncol. 37, 241–259.
Lindenbaum, J., Rosenberg, I.H., Wilson, P.W., Stabler, S.P., Allen, R.H., 1994. Prevalence of cobalamin deficiency in the Framingham elderly population. Am. J. Clin. Nutr. 60, 2–11.
Maes, M.L., Fixen, D.R., Linnebur, S.A., 2017. Adverse effects of proton-pump inhibitor use in older adults: a review of the evidence. Ther. Adv. Drug Saf. 8, 273–297.
Markle, H.V., 1996. Cobalamin. Crit. Rev. Clin. Lab. Sci. 33, 247–356.
Matthews, J.H., 1995. Cobalamin and folate deficiency in the elderly. Baillieres Clin. Haematol. 8, 679–697.
Miles, L.M., Allen, E., Mills, K., Clarke, R., Uauy, R., Dangour, A.D., 2016. Vitamin B-12 status and neurologic function in older people: a cross-sectional analysis of baseline trial data from the older people and enhanced neurological function (OPEN) study. Am. J. Clin. Nutr. 104, 790–796.
Miller, J.W., 2018. Proton pump inhibitors, H2receptor antagonists, metformin, and vitamin B-12 deficiency: clinical implications. Adv. Nutr. 9, 511S–518S.
Moestrup, S.K., Birn, H., Fischer, P.B., Petersen, C.M., Verroust, P.J., Sim, R.B., et al., 1996. Megalin-mediated endocytosis of transcobalamin–vitamin–B12 complexes suggests a role of the receptor in vitamin-B12 homeostasis. Proc. Natl. Acad. Sci. U.S.A. 93, 8612–8617.
Nexo, E., Hoffmann-Lücke, E., 2011. Holotranscobalamin, a marker of vitamin B-12 status: analytical aspects and clinical utility. Am. J. Clin. Nutr. 94, 359S–365S.
Nicolas, J.P., Gueant, J.L., 1994. Absorption, distribution and excretion of vitamin B12. Ann. Gastroenterol. Hepatol. (Paris) 30, 270–276. 81; discussion 81–82.
Okuda, K., 1962a. Starvation and renal uptake of vitamin B12. Nature 195, 292–293.
Okuda, K., 1962b. Relationship between intake of vitamin B12 and its storage by the kidney in the rat J. Nutr. 77, 131–136.
O'Leary, F., Samman, S., 2010. Vitamin B12 in health and disease. Nutrients 2, 299–316.
Orlando, R.A., Exner, M., Czekay, R.P., Yamazaki, H., Saito, A., Ullrich, R., et al., 1997. Identification of the second cluster of ligand-binding repeats in megalin as a site for receptor–ligand interactions. Proc. Natl. Acad. Sci. U.S.A. 94, 2368–2373.
Out, M., Top, W.M.C., Lehert, P., Schalkwijk, C.A., Stehouwer, C.D.A., Kooy, A., 2018. Long-term treatment with metformin in type 2 diabetes and vitamin D levels: a post-hoc analysis of a randomized placebo-controlled trial. Diabetes Obes. Metab. 20, 1951–1956.
Pruthi, R.K., Tefferi, A., 1994. Pernicious anemia revisited. Mayo Clin. Proc. 69, 144–150.
Quadros, E.V., 2010. Advances in the understanding of cobalamin assimilation and metabolism. Br. J. Haematol. 148, 195–204.
Rizzo, G., Laganà, A.S., Rapisarda, A.M., La Ferrera, G.M., Buscema, M., Rossetti, P., et al., 2016. Vitamin B12 among vegetarians: status, assessment and supplementation. Nutrients 8, pii: E767.

Saito, A., Pietromonaco, S., Loo, A.K., Farquhar, M.G., 1994. Complete cloning and sequencing of rat gp330/"megalin," a distinctive member of the low density lipoprotein receptor gene family. Proc. Natl. Acad. Sci. U.S.A. 91, 9725–9729.

Scott, J.S., Treston, A.M., Bowman, E.P., Owens, J.A., Cooksley, W.G., 1984. The regulatory roles of liver and kidney in cobalamin (vitamin B12) metabolism in the rat: the uptake and intracellular binding of cobalamin and the activity of the cobalamin-dependent enzymes in response to varying cobalamin supply. Clin. Sci. (Lond.) 67, 299–306.

Stabler, S.P., Allen, R.H., Savage, D.G., Lindenbaum, J., 1990. Clinical spectrum and diagnosis of cobalamin deficiency. Blood 76, 871–881.

Surendran, S., Adaikalakoteswari, A., Saravanan, P., Shatwaan, I.A., Lovegrove, J.A., Vimaleswaran, K.S., 2018. An update on vitamin B12-related gene polymorphisms and B12 status. Genes Nutr. 13, 2.

Tanner, S.M., Aminoff, M., Wright, F.A., Liyanarachchi, S., Kuronen, M., Saarinen, A., et al., 2003. Amnionless, essential for mouse gastrulation, is mutated in recessive hereditary megaloblastic anemia. Nat. Genet. 33, 426–429.

Tanner, S.M., Li, Z., Perko, J.D., Oner, C., Cetin, M., Altay, C., et al., 2005. Hereditary juvenile cobalamin deficiency caused by mutations in the intrinsic factor gene. Proc. Natl. Acad. Sci. U.S.A. 102, 4130–4133.

Teplitsky, V., Huminer, D., Zoldan, J., Pitlik, S., Shohat, M., Mittelman, M., 2003. Hereditary partial transcobalamin II deficiency with neurologic, mental and hematologic abnormalities in children and adults. Isr. Med. Assoc. J. 5, 868–872.

Termanini, B., Gibril, F., Sutliff, V.E., Yu, F., Venzon, D.J., Jensen, R.T., 1998. Effect of long-term gastric acid suppressive therapy on serum vitamin B12 levels in patients with Zollinger–Ellison syndrome. Am. J. Med. 104, 422–430.

Toh, B.H., van Driel, I.R., Gleeson, P.A., 1997. Pernicious anemia. N. Engl. J. Med. 337, 1441–1448.

van Asselt, D.Z., Merkus, F.W., Russel, F.G., Hoefnagels, W.H., 1998. Nasal absorption of hydroxocobalamin in healthy elderly adults. Br. J. Clin. Pharmacol. 45, 83–86.

van Asselt, D.Z., Blom, H.J., Zuiderent, R., Wevers, R.A., Jakobs, C., van den Broek, W.J., et al., 2000. Clinical significance of low cobalamin levels in older hospital patients. Neth. J. Med. 57, 41–49.

Wang, H., Li, L., Qin, L.L., Song, Y., Vidal–Alaball, J., Liu, T.H., 2018. Oral vitamin B12 versus intramuscular vitamin B12 for vitamin B12 deficiency. Cochrane Database Syst. Rev. 3.

Watanabe, F., Yabuta, Y., Bito, T., Teng, F., 2014. Vitamin B12–containing plant food sources for vegetarians. Nutrients 6, 1861–1873.

Wickramasinghe, S.N., 2006. Diagnosis of megaloblastic anaemias. Blood Rev. 20, 299–318.

Wong, C.W., Leung, C.S., Leung, C.P., Cheng, J.N., 2018. Association of metformin use with vitamin B12 deficiency in the institutionalized elderly. Arch. Gerontol. Geriatr. 79, 57–62.

Yammani, R.R., Seetharam, S., Dahms, N.M., Seetharam, B., 2003. Transcobalamin II receptor interacts with megalin in the renal apical brush border membrane. J. Membr. Biol. 193, 57–66.

CHAPTER 20

γ-Tocotrienol reversal of the Warburg effect in breast cancer cells is associated with 5′-AMP-activated kinase activation

Paul William Sylvester and Venkateshwara Dronamraju
College of Pharmacy, University of Louisiana at Monroe, Monroe, LA, United States

Contents

Summary points

- This chapter focuses on the antibreast cancer mechanism of action of γ-tocotrienol, a rare natural form of vitamin E.
- One of the characteristic features of cancer cell metabolism is aerobic glycolysis, also known as the "Warburg effect."
- The adenosine triphosphate produced during glycolysis is used to meet the energy demands, while metabolite intermediates of glycolysis

Molecular Nutrition
DOI: https://doi.org/10.1016/B978-0-12-811907-5.00007-5

provide for biomass end products, all of which are required for sustained and rapid cell proliferation.

- 5′-AMP-activated kinase (AMPK) is an enzyme that acts as a metabolic sensor in cells and helps maintain energy balance, and AMPK appears to provide protective benefits against a variety of metabolic disorders, particularly cancer.
- γ-Tocotrienols' inhibition of human breast cancer cell proliferation is associated with a significant reduction in glucose consumption and intracellular expression of glycolytic enzymes.
- Furthermore, γ-tocotrienol treatment significantly decreased the levels of phosphorylated (activated) Akt and FoxO3 levels, and induced a corresponding increase in phosphorylated (activated) AMPK levels in these cells.
- Since activated Akt and FoxO3 promote aerobic glycolysis and AMPK blocks this effect, these findings indicate that γ-tocotrienol-induced reversal of the Warburg effect in breast cancer cells is directly associated with an increase in AMPK activation.
- These findings suggest that γ-tocotrienol may provide significant benefits in the treatment of highly malignant cancers that characteristically metabolize glucose by aerobic glycolysis.

Definitions of words and terms

Vitamin E: Vitamin E represents a family of eight naturally occurring compounds that are structurally very similar. All forms of vitamin E have a chemical structure that consists of a chromanol ring structure with a phytyl tail attached at the 8 position. The vitamin E family is further divided into two subgroups called tocopherols and tocotrienols.

Tocotrienols: Tocotrienols, along with tocopherols, are a subgroup within the vitamin E family of compounds. Although very similar in chemical structure, tocotrienols differ from tocopherols in that they contain an unsaturated isoprenoid tail, whereas tocopherols contain a saturated phytyl tail. The various isoforms of tocotrienols and tocopherols (α, β, γ, and δ) differ from one another based on their methylation patterns on the chromanol ring.

Adenosine triphosphate (ATP): ATP is a phosphorylate molecule that supplies energy for biochemical processes within living cells.

Glycolysis: Glycolysis is an oxygen-independent metabolic process that converts glucose into pyruvate and free energy (ATP).

Oxidative phosphorylation: Oxidative phosphorylation is an oxygen-dependent metabolic pathway that converts various nutrients to produce large amounts of free energy (ATP).

Anaerobic glycolysis: Anaerobic glycolysis is a metabolic process that occurs when adequate oxygen is not available for oxidative phosphorylation, so that energy is produced by the conversion of glucose to lactate. It is a far less efficient process for producing ATP than oxidative phosphorylation.

Warburg effect: The Warburg effect, also called aerobic glycolysis, is a metabolic process by which cancer cells produce cellular energy by metabolizing glucose to lactate, even in the presence of adequate oxygen. Although the Warburg effect is an inefficient means to generate ATP, it provides macromolecular precursors that are necessary for cancer cells to maintain their rapid rate of growth and proliferation.

5′-AMP activate protein kinase (AMPK): AMPK is a serine/threonine/ kinase that acts as a metabolic sensor in cells. During conditions of metabolic stress, AMPK becomes activated and subsequently acts to shut down energy-consuming pathways and turn on energy-producing pathways. It also functions to shift cellular metabolism from using glucose to using lipids as a primary source of cellular energy.

20.1 γ-Tocotrienol and cancer

Vitamin E is the general term to describe a family of eight naturally occurring compounds, that is further divided into two subgroups called tocopherols and tocotrienols. Tocotrienols are relatively rare and only found in limited sources such as palm, rice bran, and annatto bean oil (Ong, 1993). All vitamin E isoforms consist of a chromanol ring structure with a long tail attached at the 2 position. However, tocopherols have a saturated phytyl, whereas tocotrienols have an unsaturated isoprenoid tail. Fig. 20.1 shows how the various isoforms of tocotrienol differ in their methylation patterns at the 5, 7, and 8 positions of the chromanol ring to form alpha (α)-, beta (β)-, gamma (γ)-, and delta (δ)-isomers (Behery et al., 2010; Elnagar et al., 2010). Initial experiments characterized the differential antiproliferative and apoptotic effects of individual tocopherols and tocotrienols, and determined that tocotrienols were significantly more potent in suppressing cancer cell growth and inducing programmed cell death than tocopherols (McIntyre et al., 2000a,b).

Isomer	R_1	R_2
α	CH_3	CH_3
β	CH_3	H
γ	H	CH_3
δ	H	H

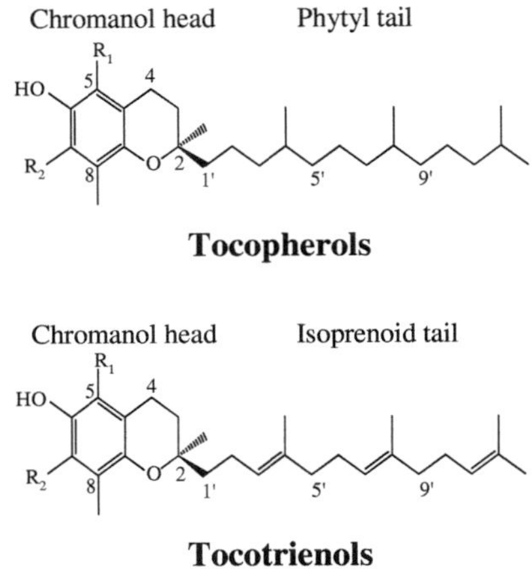

Figure 20.1 ***Chemical structure of tocopherols and tocotrienols.*** Vitamin E is the general term to describe a family of eight naturally occurring compounds that is further divided into two subgroups called tocopherols and tocotrienols. All vitamin E isoforms consist of a chromanol ring structure with a long tail attached at the 2 position. However, tocopherols have a saturated phytyl, whereas tocotrienols have an unsaturated isoprenoid tail. The various isoforms of tocotrienol differ in their methylation patterns at the 5, 7, and 8 positions of the chromanol ring to form α-, β-, γ-, δ-isomers.

The anticancer effects of tocotrienols were initially discovered while investigating high dietary fat intake on mammary tumorigenesis in laboratory animals. Results showed that high dietary intake of palm oil inhibited carcinogen-induced mammary carcinogenesis in rats (Sylvester, 1986), while palm oil diets stripped of tocotrienols had no protective effect (Nesaretnam et al., 1992). The relative anticancer potency of the different vitamin isoforms was characterized as δ-tocotrienol $\geq$ γ-tocotrienol $>$ α-tocotrienol $>> >$ α-tocopherol (McIntyre et al., 2000a,b). Experimental evidence also showed that tocotrienols are preferentially and selectively taken up into mammary tumor cells as compared to tocopherols (McIntyre et al., 2000a,b).

Many of the early in vitro studies characterizing the anticancer effects of tocotrienols were conducted used serum-free defined media containing endothelial growth factor (EGF) as a mitogen (Sylvester and Shah, 2005). Since tocotrienols were found to inhibit EGF-dependent mitogenesis in normal and neoplastic mammary epithelial cells, it was hypothesized that tocotrienol may act to inhibit EGF-dependent EGF-receptor activation and/or signal transduction (Sylvester et al., 2001). Numerous downstream signaling cascades can be initiated following ligand-induced ErbB/HER receptor activation, including the mitogen-activated protein kinase (MAPK), phosphatidylinositol 3-kinase (PI3K)/Akt, and protein kinase C (PKC) pathways (Sylvester et al., 2001). Studies showed that EGF-dependent proliferation in mammary epithelial cells is associated with a large increase in PKCα activity (Birkenfeld et al., 1996a). Tocotrienols have been shown to inhibit PKC activation and the antiproliferative effects of tocotrienols in mammary epithelial cells was associated with a suppression in PKCα activation and translocation to the plasma membrane (Birkenfeld et al., 1996b). Other studies showed that tocotrienols' inhibition of EGF-dependent proliferation of preneoplastic CL-S1 mouse mammary epithelial cells resulted from an inhibition of G-protein-mediated activation of adenylyl cyclase and cAMP production (Sylvester et al., 2002).

The inhibitory effects of tocotrienols on PI3K/Akt and NFκB signaling were first demonstrated by Shah et al. (2003). Results showed that tocotrienol treatment induced a dose- and time-dependent inhibition of EGF-dependent Akt phosphorylation (activation) in mammary tumor cells, and these effects were not found to be associated with an increase in either phosphatase and tensin homolog (PTEN) or protein phosphatase 2A (PP2A) phosphatase activity (Shah et al., 2003). Tocotrienol treatment was also shown to decrease NFκB transcriptional activity, apparently by suppressing the activation of IKK-α/β, an enzyme associated with inducing NFκB activation (Shah and Sylvester, 2005). Although, tocotrienol treatment was found to inhibit EGF-dependent activation of several mitogenic pathways, there was no evidence that tocotrienols directly targeted these signaling molecules (Shah and Sylvester, 2005). Therefore it was hypothesized that tocotrienols must be acting upstream of these pathways to attenuate ErbB/HER receptor activation and mitogenic signaling.

Cell proliferation is a complex process that involves cell cycle progression. This progression is an ordered chain of events that involves the preparation for DNA replication called the Gap 1 phase (G1), followed by DNA synthesis called the S phase (S), followed by the preparation for cell division called the Gap 2 phase (G) phase, and finally cell division, mitosis (M). Entry into each phase is highly regulated by cyclins and cyclin-dependent kinases (CDKs) that specifically act as regulatory binding proteins. Activation of the cyclin/CDK complex leads to the phosphorylation and inactivation of various inhibitors of cell cycle progression including retinoblastoma protein (Rb), such as p15, p27, and p21. Studies have shown that γ-tocotrienol significantly reduced cyclin D1, cyclin-dependent kinases CDK4, CDK2, and CDK6 levels between 4 and 24 hours after EGF exposure in mammary cancer cells (Samant et al., 2010). Tocotrienol treatment was also found to significantly increase CDK inhibitor (CKI) p27 prior to and after EGF exposure (Samant et al., 2010). Further, tocotrienol treatment also induced a significant reduction in retinoblastoma (Rb) protein phosphorylation at ser780 and ser807/811 and demonstrated that the antiproliferative effects of γ-tocotrienol are partly mediated by the blockade of cell cycle progression (Samant et al., 2010).

Lipid raft microdomains within the plasma membrane are enriched with sphingolipids and cholesterol, and are very stable and rigid structures as compared to the surrounding more fluid plasma membrane (Chamberlain, 2004; Pike, 2003). A ligand binding to its receptor results in the translocation and dimerization of the receptor within the lipid raft microdomain. Following dimerization, the cytoplasmic domain of the receptor undergoes tyrosine phosphorylation (Park and Han, 2009; Pike, 2005, 2009). These tyrosine autophosphorylation sites are required for the interaction and activation of the downstream substrates involved in mediating intracellular second messenger signal transduction. Studies have shown that γ-tocotrienol treatment caused a disruption in lipid raft microdomain integrity in cancer cells, which subsequently resulted in a disruption in receptor tyrosine kinase dimerization, activation, and signaling, and at least partially explains the wide range of inhibitory effects tocotrienols display on numerous signal transduction pathways (Alawin et al., 2017; Alawin et al., 2016).

20.1.1 Key facts of vitamin E

- The term "vitamin E" represents a family of eight naturally occurring compounds.
- The vitamin E family is further divided into two subgroups called tocopherols and tocotrienols.
- While tocopherol are very abundant and are abundantly found in most dietary fats and oils, tocotrienols are rare and found in limited sources, particularly palm oil.
- All isoforms of vitamin E contain a cyclic ring structure with a long tail attached at the 2 position.

- The major difference between the two subgroups of vitamin E is that tocopherols have a saturated phytyl tail, whereas tocotrienols have an unsaturated isoprenoid tail.
- Different isoforms within each vitamin E subgroup differ in the methylation patterns on their ring structure.
- While tocopherols display little or no anticancer activity, tocotrienols display potent anticancer effects against a wide range of tumor cell types.
- The anticancer activity of tocotrienols is mediated by its action to inhibit specific growth-promoting signaling pathways that are overactive or unregulated in cancer cells.

20.2 Cancer metabolism and aerobic glycolysis

Most nonproliferating differentiated cells depend on the efficiency of ATP production through oxidative phosphorylation to maintain metabolic homeostasis. As a result, such cells metabolize glucose to pyruvate through glycolysis, and then completely oxidize pyruvate to CO_2 through the oxidative phosphorylation in the mitochondria, where oxygen is the final acceptor in an electron transport chain that generates ATP (Ward and Thompson, 2012). It is only under anaerobic conditions that nonproliferating differentiated cells convert pyruvate to lactate. In contrast, most cancer cells produce large amounts of lactate regardless of the availability of oxygen and this form of metabolism is referred to as aerobic glycolysis or the "Warburg effect" (DeBerardinis et al., 2008; Vander Heiden et al., 2009). In mammalian cells, glucose and glutamate are the primary fuels that are catabolized to maintain cellular functions, and are also the primary source of carbon, nitrogen, free energy, and the reducing equivalents necessary to support cell growth and division (Vander Heiden et al., 2009). If cancer cells catabolize all of the glucose to carbon dioxide through oxidative phosphorylation in mitochondria in order to maximize ATP production, these cells will not produce sufficient macromolecular precursors such as acetyl-CoA for fatty acids, glycolytic intermediates for nonessential amino acids for protein, and ribose for nucleotides synthesis (Vander Heiden et al., 2009). However, the requirement for macromolecule precursors is easily obtained in cancer cells through aerobic glycolysis, which occurs even in the presence of adequate oxygen (DeBerardinis et al., 2008; Vander Heiden et al., 2009). Cancer cells can also change their metabolism in response to growth factor signaling (Ward and Thompson, 2012). In contrast to the catabolic metabolism that is observed in normal cells, aerobic glycolysis is fundamental to cell growth and proliferation, and occurs independently of ATP demand (Ward and Thompson, 2012; Vander Heiden et al., 2009). These findings are further evidenced by studies that showed glioblastoma cells in culture convert as much as 90% of the glucose and 60% of the glutamine they acquire into lactate or alanine when measured by ^{13}C-nuclear magnetic resonance spectroscopy (DeBerardinis et al., 2008).

Activation of the PI3K/Akt pathway is one of the common events in human cancers. The activation of the PI3K/Akt pathway leads to increased glucose uptake and glycolysis by enhancing the membrane localization of glucose transporters, activating hexokinase-II, and activating phosphofructokinase to commit glucose to glycolytic metabolism (Ward and Thompson, 2012; Vander Heiden et al., 2009; Elstrom et al., 2004). In normal nonproliferating cells, fatty acid synthesis occurs at low rates as lipids are obtained through the circulation, whereas in proliferating cancer cells the majority of fatty acids are derived from de novo synthesis, despite a sufficient supply of extracellular lipids (Hatzivassiliou et al., 2005). A key enzyme linking glucose metabolism to lipid synthesis is ATP citrate lyase (ACL), which catalyzes the conversion of citrate to cytosolic acetyl-CoA (Hatzivassiliou et al., 2005). Furthermore, Akt promotes the shunting of mitochondrial citrate from the tricarboxylic acid cycle to acetyl-CoA production by phosphorylating and activating ACL. Since citrate is a negative allosteric regulator of glycolysis, the breakdown of cytosolic citrate by ACL is a critical step in PI3K/Akt-induced reprogramming of a cancer cell's metabolism (Ward and Thompson, 2012). Studies have shown that gene silencing or pharmacological inhibition of ACL limits in vitro proliferation and in vivo tumor growth of tumor cells, resulting from a suppression of aerobic glycolysis (Hatzivassiliou et al., 2005). Furthermore, the activation of PI3K/Akt results in the activation of mTOR, and mTOR promotes protein synthesis by increasing the translation of transcription factors c-Myc and hypoxia-inducible factor α (HIF-1α) (Cantor and Sabatini, 2012). HIF-1α facilitates aerobic glycolysis by inducing the expression of pyruvate dehydrogenase kinase 1 which inhibits the activity of pyruvate dehydrogenase (Cantor and Sabatini, 2012). The inhibition of pyruvate dehydrogenase prevents the entry of pyruvate into the mitochondria and thereby facilitates the conversion of pyruvate into lactate (Cantor and Sabatini, 2012). The increased expression of c-Myc stimulates lactate dehydrogenase A (LDHA) activity, which catalyzes the conversion of pyruvate to lactate (Dang et al., 2009). Fig. 20.2 summarizes the role of various mediators in regulating metabolism in cancer cells.

Cancer cells preferentially produce isoforms of metabolic enzymes that support metabolic diversions during tumorigenesis (Ward and Thompson, 2012). Studies have shown that cancer cells preferentially express pyruvate kinase M2 (PKM2), an embryonic form of pyruvate kinase over the adult form pyruvate kinase M1 (Christofk et al., 2008). It is interesting that PKM2 has lower enzymatic activity than PKM1 and unlike PKM1, PKM2 can be inhibited by tyrosine kinase signaling (Vander Heiden et al., 2009; Christofk et al., 2008). It is hypothesized that the expression of spliced variant PKM2 is elevated in proliferating cancer cells and acts to facilitate aerobic glycolysis (Ward and Thompson, 2012). Since PKM2 has decreased enzymatic activity as compared to PKM1, there is a slower conversion of phosphoenol pyruvate to pyruvate in cancer cells, and this leads to the accumulation of upstream glycolytic intermediates. These metabolites are diverted into various anabolic pathways, such as pyrimidine, serine/glycine, and glycerol biosynthesis pathways, eventually resulting in altered cancer cell metabolism (Ward and Thompson, 2012).

Studies were conducted to determine the effects of γ-tocotrienol on oncogenic c-Myc activity and degradation in human Michigan Cancer Foundation-7 (MCF-7) breast cancer cells. Treatment with 0–8 μM γ-tocotrienol resulted in a dose-responsive inhibition of MCF-7 cancer cell growth, and these effects were associated with a decrease in total c-Myc, phosphorylated-S62-c-Myc, and a corresponding increase in p-T58-c-Myc (Parajuli et al., 2015a). γ-Tocotrienol treatment also caused a decrease in PI3K, phosphorylated (activated) Akt, phosphorylated (inactive) GSK-3β, phosphorylated (activated) mTOR, and phosphorylated (activated) Erk 1/2 levels, but had no effect on MYC mRNA levels in these cells (Parajuli et al., 2015a). Furthermore, these antiproliferative effects were also associated with a decrease in cyclin D1 and cyclin-dependent kinase 4 (CDK4), and a corresponding increase in p27 (Parajuli et al., 2015a). Additional studies showed that similar treatment with γ-tocotrienol resulted in an increase in FBW7 levels, an E3 ligase that

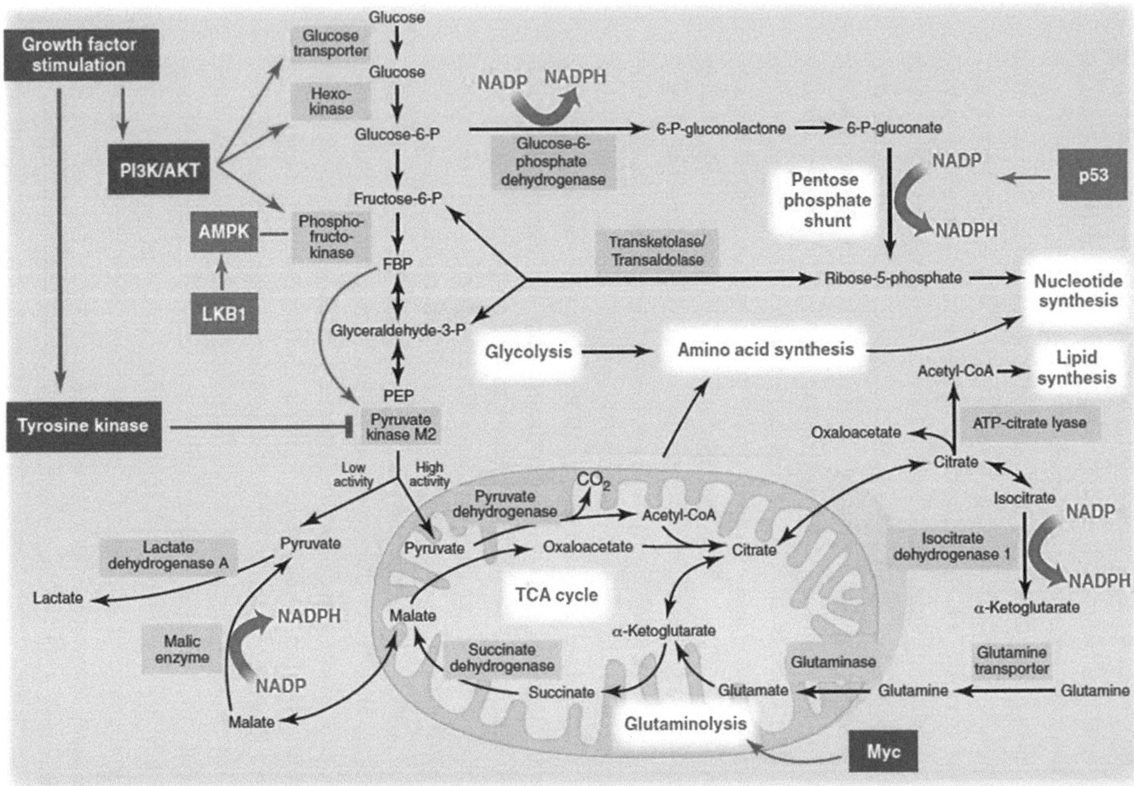

Figure 20.2 ***Various mediators involved in regulating metabolism in cancer cells.*** A primary source of energy adenosine triphosphate (ATP) in all cells is produced from the metabolism of glucose. During glycolysis glucose is converted to pyruvate through a series of enzymatic reactions, which result in the production of relatively low amounts of ATP. Pyruvate then enters the mitochondria and through the process of oxidative phosphorylation mediated by enzymes in the tricarboxylic acid cycle (TCA cycle), nutrients are efficiently metabolized to produce high levels of ATP. However, in cancer cells, oncogenic growth factors stimulate glycolytic enzyme activity and inhibit oxidative phosphorylation resulting in aerobic glycolysis or the Warburg effect. The activation of AMPK inhibits the expression and activity of glycolytic enzymes and ultimately suppresses the Warburg effect in cancer cells. *Adapted from Vander Heiden, M.G., Cantley, L.C., Thompson, C.B., 2009. Understanding the Warburg effect: the metabolic requirements of cell proliferation. Science 324, 1029–1033.*

initiates ubiquitination of c-Myc, but had no effect on PP2A and Pin 1 propyl isomerase levels in these tumor cells (Parajuli et al., 2015a). γ-Tocotrienol-induced c-Myc degradation was also found to be associated with GSK-3β activation and proteasomal function.

Furthermore, cancer cells display increased glucose consumption and a corresponding increase in lactate production even in the presence of oxygen compared to the normal cells, a hallmark of the Warburg effect or aerobic glycolysis (Parajuli et al., 2015b). Aerobic glycolysis is regulated by the activation of the PI3K/Akt/mTOR pathway and oncogenic transcription factors, such as c-Myc and the HIF-1α. Studies conducted to determine the effects of γ-tocotrienol on aerobic glycolysis in human MCF-7 breast cancer cells showed that treatment with 0−10 μM γ-tocotrienol resulted in a dose-responsive inhibition of MCF-7 cell growth (Parajuli et al., 2015b). This treatment was also found to result in a relatively large reduction in glucose utilization and a corresponding decrease in intracellular ATP production and extracellular lactate excretion by MCF-7 mammary tumor cells (Parajuli et al., 2015b). Fig. 20.3 shows Western blot analysis of γ-tocotrienol anticancer effects showing that these effects are also associated with a large decrease in the expression of intracellular enzymes involved in regulating aerobic glycolysis, including hexokinase-II, phosphofructokinase, pyruvate kinase M2, and LDHA, in MCF-7 human breast cancer cells (Parajuli et al., 2015b). In addition, these γ-tocotrienol-induced effects were associated with a corresponding reduction in signaling proteins associated with the regulation of aerobic glycolysis, particularly phosphorylated (active) Akt, phosphorylated (active) mTOR, and c-Myc, but had no effect on the protein expression of HIF-1α or glucose transporter-1 (GLUT-1) (Parajuli et al., 2015b). Taken together, these findings demonstrate that the antiproliferative effects of γ-tocotrienol are associated with a reduction in oncogenic c-Myc (S62) levels, PI3K/Akt/mTOR and RAS/MEK/MAPK mitogenic signaling, and a corresponding increase in GSK-3β-dependent ubiquitination and degradation of c-Myc. These findings also demonstrate that the antiproliferative effects of γ-tocotrienol are also associated with concurrent inhibition of aerobic glycolysis and PI3K/Akt/mTOR and c-Myc signaling (Parajuli et al., 2015b), and suggest that γ-tocotrienol treatment might be beneficial in breast cancer with aberrant c-Myc signaling and altered metabolic changes.

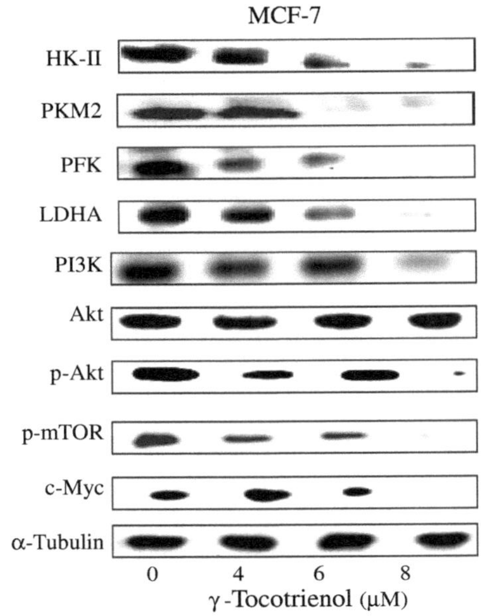

Figure 20.3 ***Western blot analysis of γ-tocotrienol effects on the relative protein levels of key aerobic glycolytic proteins, glucose and lactate transporters, and PI3K, Akt, mTOR, c-Myc, and HIF-1α in human MCF-7 breast cancer cells.*** Treatment with γ-tocotrienol resulted in a dose-responsive reduction in glycolytic enzyme expression including hexokinase-II (HK-II), phosphofructokinase (PFK), pyruvate kinase M2 (PKM2), and lactate dehydrogenase A (LDHA). γ-Tocotrienol treatment was also associated with a corresponding reduction in the levels of phosphorylated (active) Akt, phosphorylated (active) mTOR, and c-Myc. These findings demonstrate that γ-tocotrienol treatment inhibits Akt/mTOR signaling, c-Myc expression, and aerobic glycolysis. *Adapted from Parajuli, P., Tiwari, R.V., Sylvester, P.W., 2015a. Antiproliferative effects of γ-tocotrienol are associated with a suppression in c-Myc expression in mammary tumor cells. Cell Prolif. 48(11), 421–432 and Parajuli, P., Tiwari, R.V., Sylvester, P.W., 2015b. Anticancer effects of gamma-tocotrienol are associated with a suppression in aerobic glycolysis. Biol. Pharm. Bull. 38, 1352–1360.*

20.2.1 Key facts of cancer metabolism and the Warburg effect

- During aerobic conditions, normal cells metabolize glucose to pyruvate through glycolysis and then completely oxidize pyruvate to CO_2 through oxidative phosphorylation to generate large amounts of ATP.
- However, during anaerobic conditions, glucose is converted to pyruvate and then pyruvate is converted to lactate, and as such very little ATP is produced as compared to aerobic metabolism.

- In contrast, most cancer cells produce large amounts of lactate regardless of the availability of oxygen and this form of metabolism is referred to as aerobic glycolysis or the "Warburg effect."
- Aerobic glycolysis is less efficient for producing ATP, but it also produces large amounts of macromolecules that are necessary for cancer cell growth and survival.
- As such, cancer cells characteristically have a high expression of numerous enzymes that are involved in mediating aerobic glycolysis.

20.3 5′-AMP-activated protein kinase structure and function

AMPK is a serine/threonine kinase enzyme that acts as a metabolic sensor in mammalian cells. It is a heterotrimeric enzyme that is made up of α, β, and γ subunits. The α and β subunits have two isoforms each (α1, α2; β1, β2), while the γ subunit has three isoforms (γ1, γ2, γ3) (Hardie, 2003; Steinberg and Kemp, 2009). The α subunit has serine and threonine kinase domains and is responsible for the catalytic activity of AMPK. The β subunit has binding sites for glycogen, although its function remains unclear. However, the β subunit does bind to both α and γ subunits and may function as a linker subunit. The γ subunit has two Bateman domains, which have binding sites for AMP and ATP. Binding to AMP causes allosteric activation of the enzyme, while binding to ATP inhibits its activity (Hardie, 2003; Steinberg and Kemp, 2009). Therefore the γ subunit functions as a regulatory subunit of the enzyme.

The activation of AMPK involves a multistep process that is initiated by a perceived energy imbalance in the cell. The ratio of the phosphate-rich molecule AMP versus ATP acts as a cellular indicator for the regulation of energy balance by AMPK. When energy consumption exceeds the energy production in the cells, AMP accumulates in the cell. The γ subunit binds the excess AMP molecules and the AMPK enzyme undergoes conformational changes that allow the α subunit to be phosphorylated by an upstream kinase on threonine residue 172 (Thr-172). This allosteric activation by AMP and phosphorylation by an upstream kinase are essential for complete activation of the AMPK enzyme (Hardie, 2003). There are three reported upstream activating kinases for AMPK. These are calmodulin-dependent kinase-β (CAMKK-β), liver kinase B1 (LKB1), and transforming growth factor β-activated kinase (TAK1) (Woods et al., 2003; Hawley et al., 2003). CAMKK-β is reported to activate AMPK in neurons and T-cells, whereas LKB1 is widely distributed in many tissues and acts as the primary activator for AMPK. The exact role of TAK1-dependent AMPK activation is not clearly understood (Hawley et al., 2003). In addition, it has been reported that protein phosphatase-2Cα (PP-2Cα) acts as a phosphatase that inactivates AMPK. Various xenobiotics like metformin, AICAR, and tocotrienols are also known to activate AMPK (Kim et al., 2016). While metformin activation of AMPK is LKB1-dependent, AICAR acts as an AMP mimetic and promotes the allosteric activation of AMPK. The role of xenobiotics in modulating AMPK activity is shown in Fig. 20.4.

Following activation, AMPK acts as a metabolic regulator that shuts down energy-consuming pathways and turns on energy-producing pathways, thereby switching the cell's metabolism from a catabolic to an anabolic state. Since AMPK activation is sensitive to cellular levels of AMP, it acts as a metabolic switch in regulating cellular energy homeostasis and plays an important role in modulating various cellular processes, such as lipid metabolism, glucose homeostasis, and mitochondrial biogenesis (Steinberg and Kemp, 2009).

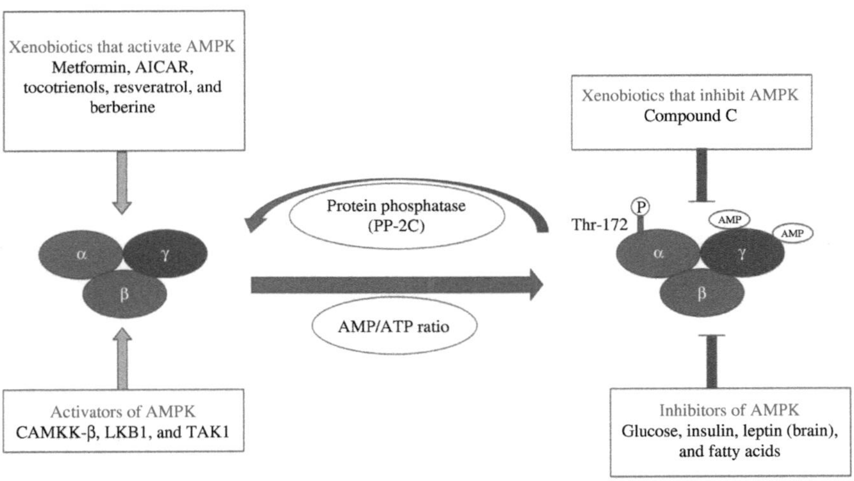

Figure 20.4 ***Role of xenobiotics in modulating AMPK activity.*** Binding of AMP to the γ subunit and the phosphorylation of Thr-172 are essential for activation of AMPK. Various agents and drugs can function as activators (or inhibitors) of AMPK. Similarly, various physiological conditions can also induce a change in hormone levels and the expression of cellular enzymes, which then act to modulate AMPK activity. Protein phosphatases such as PP-2C also play a role in modulating AMPK activity.

The role of AMPK activation on lipid metabolism is also well established. Activated AMPK is a known inhibitor of acetyl-CoA carboxylase (ACC). Activated ACC converts acetyl-CoA to malonyl CoA, which is an early step in fatty acid synthesis (Steinberg and Kemp, 2009). Phosphorylation of ACC by AMPK reduces the formation of malonyl CoA, which also acts as an allosteric inhibitor of fatty acid oxidation in the mitochondria. In addition, AMPK also inhibits the action of fatty acid synthase, which is critical for the synthesis of palmitate (Steinberg and Kemp, 2009). It has also been reported that AMPK inhibits the activity of hydroxy-methyl-3-glutaryl-coA (HMG-CoA) and reduces the synthesis of cholesterol through its regulation of ACC and HMG-CoA (Steinberg and Kemp, 2009). In addition, AMPK has been shown to promote lipolysis in adipose tissue. Therefore the activation of AMPK promotes energy production through lipid breakdown while simultaneously preventing processes that promote lipid synthesis (Steinberg and Kemp, 2009).

AMPK also plays an important role in regulating glucose homeostasis during conditions of metabolic stress. Glucose homeostasis is the balance between glucose consumption and the production of glucose equivalents by glycogenolysis and gluconeogenesis in the muscle and liver. In skeletal muscle, AMPK is activated during exercise and acts to stimulate glucose uptake through increased activity of glucose transporters like GLUT4 (Derave et al., 2000). Similarly, the liver increases circulating glucose levels by stimulating the breakdown of glycogen by glycogenolysis, and by generating glucose equivalents by the breakdown of noncarbohydrate sources by gluconeogenesis (Derave et al., 2000). AMPK has been reported to inhibit gluconeogenesis in the liver by suppressing the activity of gluconeogenesis enzymes such as phosphoenol pyruvate carboxy kinase and glucose-6-phosphatase (Lee et al., 2010). Mice lacking liver LKB1 show little or no AMPK activity and characteristically display severe glucose intolerance (Sakamoto et al., 2005). Taken together, these findings demonstrate the important role of AMPK in regulating glucose production by the liver.

20.3.1 Key facts of 5′-AMP-activated kinase and metabolic function

- AMPK is a serine/threonine kinase enzyme that acts as a metabolic sensor in mammalian cells.
- AMPK binding to AMP causes allosteric activation of the enzyme, while binding to ATP inhibits its activity.

- Following AMP-induced activation, AMPK acts as a metabolic regulator that shuts down energy-consuming pathways and turns on energy-producing pathways, thereby switching the cell's metabolism from a catabolic to an anabolic state.
- Specifically, AMPK activation results in a shift in metabolism from using glucose to using lipids as a primary source of cellular energy.

20.4 γ-Tocotrienol effects on 5′-AMP-activated kinase activation and aerobic glycolysis

Previous experimental findings showed that the treatment of mammary tumor cells with γ-tocotrienol is associated with a decrease in glycolytic enzymes and glycolysis-promoting pathways that could impair the cancer cell metabolism (Parajuli et al., 2015b). Additional studies focused on determining the direct effects of γ-tocotrienol on AMPK activity in human breast cancer. In these studies, γ-tocotrienol induced a dose-responsive inhibition in human MCF-7 and MDA-MB-231 breast cancer cell growth, as compared to cells in their respective vehicle-treated control groups, while higher doses of γ-tocotrienol had no effect on the growth or viability of normal human MCF-10A mammary epithelial cells. Furthermore, MCF-7 cells and MDA-MB-231 cells treated with 0–6 μM γ-tocotrienol displayed a dose-responsive increase in glucose metabolism as compared to cells in their respective vehicle-treated control groups. These same treatments also induced a corresponding dose-dependent decrease in the glycolytic enzymes, hexokinase-II, phosphofructokinase, pyruvate kinase, and pyruvate dehydrogenase in MCF-7 and MDA-MB-231 breast cancer cells, as compared to cells in their respective vehicle-treated control groups.

Experimental findings also showed that treatment of MCF-7 cells with 3–7 μM γ-tocotrienol or MDA-MB-231 cells with 2–6 μM γ-tocotrienol displayed no differences in total Akt levels, as compared to cells in their respective vehicle-treated control groups. However, MCF-7 and MDA-MB-231 cells treated with γ-tocotrienol displayed a relatively large dose-dependent decrease in phosphorylated-Akt (activated) levels, as compared to cells in their respective vehicle-treated control groups. Immunocytochemical staining studies showed that vehicle-treated MCF-7 and MDA-MB-231 cells display positive phosphorylated-Akt staining in nearly 75% and 90% of their cells, respectively, whereas treatment of these cells with γ-tocotrienol showed relatively large reductions in positive phosphorylated-Akt immunofluorescent staining.

MCF-7 or MDA-MB-231 cells with γ-tocotrienol had little effect or no effect on the total intracellular levels of AMPKα, AMPKβ, or LKB1, as compared to cells in their respective vehicle-treated control groups. In contrast, these same treatments with γ-tocotrienol induced a dose-responsive increase in the relative levels of phosphorylated-AMPKα (activated) and phosphorylated-AMPKβ (activated) in MCF-7 and MDA-MB-231 cells, as compared to cells in the respective vehicle-treated control groups. Additional studies showed that MCF-7 cells or MDA-MB-231 cells treated with γ-tocotrienol had little effect or no effect on the total intracellular levels of FoxO3a, whereas γ-tocotrienol treatment resulted in a large reduction in phosphorylated (activated) FoxO3, as compared to cells in their respective vehicle-treated control groups. Similarly, immunocytochemical staining showed that MCF-7 and MDA-MB-231 cells in their respective control groups displayed positive FoxO3 staining primarily in the cytoplasm. In contrast, MCF-7 cells treated with 5 μM γ-tocotrienol or MDA-MB-231 cells treated with 4 μM γ-tocotrienol show the majority of positive FoxO3a staining appearing in the nuclei of MCF-7 and MDA-MB-231 breast cancer cells. Follow-up studies showed that coimmunoprecipitation demonstrated an intimate protein—protein interaction between AMPK and FoxO3a in these same breast cancer cells treated with γ-tocotrienol, as compared to cells in their respective vehicle-treated control groups. Fig. 20.5 summarizes Western blot analysis of γ-tocotrienol treatment effects on glycolytic enzyme, Akt, AMPK, and FoxO3 signaling proteins in MCF-7 human breast cancer cells.

20.4.1 Key facts of γ-tocotrienol-induced 5′-AMP-activated kinase activation and inhibition of the Warburg effect in breast cancer cells

- γ-Tocotrienol treatment inhibits oxygen and glucose consumption in human breast cancer cells.
- Similarly, treatment with γ-tocotrienol induces a dose-responsive increase in AMPK activation and a corresponding decrease in glycolytic enzyme expression.
- γ-Tocotrienol-induced AMPK activation is also associated with a large decrease in Akt and FoxO3 activity.

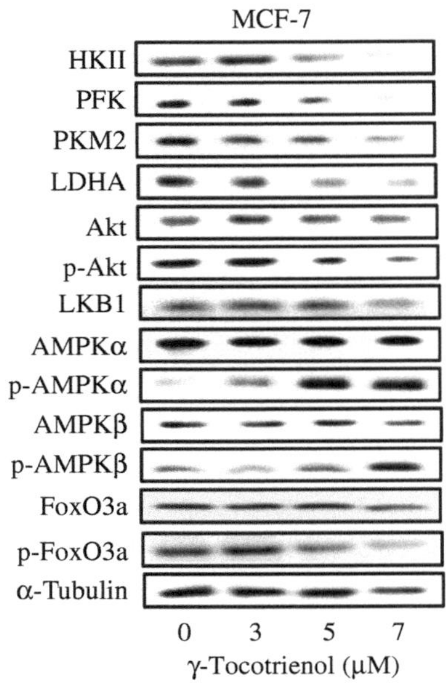

Figure 20.5 ***Western blot analysis of γ-tocotrienol effects on the relative protein levels of key aerobic glycolytic proteins, glucose and lactate transporters, and various signaling proteins.*** Treatment with γ-tocotrienol resulted in a dose-responsive reduction in glycolytic enzyme expression including hexokinase-II (HK-II), phosphofructokinase (PFK), pyruvate kinase M2 (PKM2), and lactate dehydrogenase A (LDHA), and a corresponding decrease in phosphorylated (active) Akt and phosphorylated (active) mTOR. These effects were also associated with a corresponding increase in phosphorylated AMPKα and AMPKβ (active) and a decrease in phosphorylated (active) FoxO3a (p-FoxO3a). Since activated Akt and FoxO3 promote aerobic glycolysis and AMPK blocks this effect, these findings indicate that γ-tocotrienol-induced reversal of the Warburg effect in breast cancer cells is directly associated with an increase in AMPK activation.

- These findings demonstrate that γ-tocotrienol significantly attenuates the Warburg effect in human breast cancer cells and this action is associated with a significant reduction in cancer cell growth and survival.

20.5 Conclusion

These findings demonstrate that the antiproliferative effects of γ-tocotrienol are mediated, at least in part, by a reversal of the Warburg effect in breast cancer cells grown in culture. Treatment with γ-tocotrienol resulted in a dose-dependent reduction in glucose consumption and expression in glycolytic enzymes in MCF-7 and MDA-MB-231 breast cancer cells. Furthermore, γ-tocotrienol treatment significantly decreased the levels of phosphorylate (activated) Akt and FoxO3 levels, and induced a corresponding increase in phosphorylated (activated) AMPK levels in these cells. Since activated Akt and FoxO3 promote aerobic glycolysis and AMPK blocks this effect, these finding indicate that γ-tocotrienol-induced reversal of the Warburg effect in breast cancer cells is directly associated with an increase in AMPK activation. These findings suggest that γ-tocotrienol may provide significant benefits in the treatment of highly malignant cancers that characteristically metabolize glucose by aerobic glycolysis.

References

Alawin, O.A., Ahmed, R.A., Ibrahim, B.A., Briski, K.P., Sylvester, P.W., 2016. Antiproliferative effects of gamma-tocotrienol are associated with lipid raft disruption in HER2-positive human breast cancer cells. J. Nutr. Biochem. 27, 266–277.

Alawin, O.A., Ahmed, R.A., Dronamraju, V., Briski, K.P., Sylvester, P.W., 2017. -Tocotrienol-induced disruption of lipid rafts in human breast cancer cells is associated with a reduction in exosome heregulin content. J. Nutr. Biochem. 48, 83–93.

Behery, F.A., Elnagar, A.Y., Akl, M.R., Wali, V.B., Abuasal, B., Kaddoumi, A., et al., 2010. Redox-silent tocotrienol esters as breast cancer proliferation and migration inhibitors. Bioorg. Med. Chem. 18, 8066–8075.

Birkenfeld, H.P., McIntyre, B.S., Briski, K.P., Sylvester, P.W., 1996a. Protein kinase C isoenzyme expression in normal mouse mammary epithelial cells grown in primary culture. Proc. Soc. Exp. Biol. Med. 213, 65–70.

Birkenfeld, H.P., McInntyre, B.S., Briski, K.P., Sylvester, P.W., 1996b. Role of protein kinase C in modulating epidermal growth factor- and phorbol ester-induced mammary epithelial cell growth in vitro. Exp. Cell Res. 223, 183–191.

Cantor, J.R., Sabatini, D.M., 2012. Cancer cell metabolism: one hallmark, many faces. Cancer Discov. 2, 881–898.

Chamberlain, L.H., 2004. Detergents as tools for the purification and classification of lipid rafts. FEBS Lett. 559, 1–5.

Christofk, H.R., Vander Heiden, M.G., Harris, M.H., Ramanathan, A., Gerszten, R.E., Wei, R., et al., 2008. The M2 splice isoform of pyruvate kinase is important for cancer metabolism and tumour growth. Nature 452, 230–233.

Dang, C.V., Le, A., Gao, P., 2009. MYC-induced cancer cell energy metabolism and therapeutic opportunities. Clin. Cancer Res. 15, 6479–6483.

DeBerardinis, R.J., Lum, J.J., Hatzivassiliou, G., Thompson, C.B., 2008. The biology of cancer: metabolic reprogramming fuels cell growth and proliferation. Cell Metab. 7, 11–20.

Derave, W., Ai, H., Ihlemann, J., Witters, L.A., Kristiansen, S., Richter, E.A., et al., 2000. Dissociation of AMP-activated protein kinase activation and glucose transport in contracting slow-twitch muscle. Diabetes 49, 1281–1287.

Elnagar, A.Y., Wali, V.B., Sylvester, P.W., El Sayed, K.A., 2010. Design and preliminary structure–activity relationship of redox-silent semisynthetic tocotrienol analogues as inhibitors for breast cancer proliferation and invasion. Bioorg. Med. Chem. 18, 755–768.

Elstrom, R.L., Bauer, D.E., Buzzai, M., Karnauskas, R., Harris, M.H., Plas, D.R., et al., 2004. Akt stimulates aerobic glycolysis in cancer cells. Cancer Res 64, 3892–3899.
Hardie, D.G., 2003. Minireview: the AMP-activated protein kinase cascade: the key sensor of cellular energy status. Endocrinology 144, 5179–5183.
Hatzivassiliou, G., Zhao, F., Bauer, D.E., Andreadis, C., Shaw, A.N., Dhanak, D., et al., 2005. ATP citrate lyase inhibition can suppress tumor cell growth. Cancer Cell 8, 311–321.
Hawley, S.A., Boudeau, J., Reid, J.L., Mustard, K.J., Udd, L., Makela, T.P., et al., 2003. Complexes between the LKB1 tumor suppressor, STRAD alpha/beta and MO25 alpha/beta are upstream kinases in the AMP-activated protein kinase cascade. J. Biol. 2, 28.
Kim, J., Yang, G., Kim, Y., Kim, J., Ha, J., 2016. AMPK activators: mechanisms of action and physiological activities. Exp. Mol. Med. 48, e224.
Lee, J.-M., Seo, W.-Y., Song, K.-H., Chanda, D., Kim, Y.D., Kim, D.-K., et al., 2010. AMPK-dependent repression of hepatic gluconeogenesis via disruption of CREB · CRTC2 complex by orphan nuclear receptor small heterodimer partner. J. Biol. Chem. 285, 32182–32191.
McIntyre, B.S., Briski, K.P., Gapor, A., Sylvester, P.W., 2000a. Antiproliferative and apoptotic effects of tocopherols and tocotrienols on preneoplastic and neoplastic mouse mammary epithelial cells. Proc. Soc. Exp. Biol. Med. 224, 292–301.
McIntyre, B.S., Briski, K.P., Tirmenstein, M.A., Fariss, M.W., Gapor, A., Sylvester, P.W., 2000b. Antiproliferative and apoptotic effects of tocopherols and tocotrienols on normal mouse mammary epithelial cells. Lipids 35, 171–180.
Nesaretnam, K., Khor, H.T., Ganeson, J., Chong, Y.H., Sundram, K., Gapor, A., 1992. The effects of vitamin E tocotrienols from palm oil on chemically induced mammary carcinogenesis in female rats. Nutr. Res. 12, 879–892.
Ong, A.S.H., 1993. Natural sources of tocotrienols. In: Packer, L., Fuchs, P.J. (Eds.), Vitamin E in Health and Disease. Jarcel Dekker, New York, pp. 3–8.
Parajuli, P., Tiwari, R.V., Sylvester, P.W., 2015a. Antiproliferative effects of γ-tocotrienol are associated with a suppression in c-Myc expression in mammary tumor cells. Cell Prolif. 48 (11), 421–432.
Parajuli, P., Tiwari, R.V., Sylvester, P.W., 2015b. Anticancer effects of gamma-tocotrienol are associated with a suppression in aerobic glycolysis. Biol. Pharm. Bull. 38, 1352–1360.
Park, J.H., Han, H.J., 2009. Caveolin-1 plays important role in EGF-induced migration and proliferation of mouse embryonic stem cells: involvement of PI3K/Akt and ERK. Am. J. Physiol. Cell Physiol. 297, C935–C944.
Pike, L.J., 2003. Lipid rafts: bringing order to chaos. J. Lipid Res. 44, 655–667.
Pike, L.J., 2005. Growth factor receptors, lipid rafts and caveolae: an evolving story. Biochim. Biophys. Acta 1746, 260–273.
Pike, L.J., 2009. The challenge of lipid rafts. J. Lipid Res. 50 (Suppl.), S323–S328.
Sakamoto, K., McCarthy, A., Smith, D., Green, K.A., Grahame Hardie, D., Ashworth, A., et al., 2005. Deficiency of LKB1 in skeletal muscle prevents AMPK activation and glucose uptake during contraction. EMBO J. 24, 1810–1820.
Samant, G.V., Wali, V.B., Sylvester, P.W., 2010. Anti-proliferative effects of gamma-tocotrienol on mammary tumour cells are associated with suppression of cell cycle progression. Cell Prolif. 43, 77–83.
Shah, S.J., Sylvester, P.W., 2005. Gamma-tocotrienol inhibits neoplastic mammary epithelial cell proliferation by decreasing Akt and nuclear factor kappaB activity. Exp. Biol. Med. (Maywood) 230, 235–241.

Shah, S., Gapor, A., Sylvester, P.W., 2003. Role of caspase-8 activation in mediating vitamin E-induced apoptosis in murine mammary cancer cells. Nutr. Cancer 45, 236–246.
Steinberg, G.R., Kemp, B.E., 2009. AMPK in health and disease. Physiol. Rev. 89, 1025–1078.
Sylvester, P.W., 1986. Role of acute caloric-restriction in murine tumorigenesis. Prog. Clin. Biol. Res. 222, 517–528.
Sylvester, P.W., Shah, S.J., 2005. Mechanisms mediating the antiproliferative and apoptotic effects of vitamin E in mammary cancer cells. Front. Biosci. 10, 699–709.
Sylvester, P.W., McIntyre, B.S., Gapor, A., Briski, K.P., 2001. Vitamin E inhibition of normal mammary epithelial cell growth is associated with a reduction in protein kinase C(alpha) activation. Cell Prolif. 34, 347–357.
Sylvester, P.W., Nachnani, A., Shah, S., Briski, K.P., 2002. Role of GTP-binding proteins in reversing the antiproliferative effects of tocotrienols in preneoplastic mammary epithelial cells. Asia Pac. J. Clin. Nutr. 11 (Suppl. 7), S452–S459.
Vander Heiden, M.G., Cantley, L.C., Thompson, C.B., 2009. Understanding the Warburg effect: the metabolic requirements of cell proliferation. Science 324, 1029–1033.
Ward, P.S., Thompson, C.B., 2012. Metabolic reprogramming: a cancer hallmark even warburg did not anticipate. Cancer Cell 21, 297–308.
Woods, A., Johnstone, S.R., Dickerson, K., Leiper, F.C., Fryer, L.G.D., Neumann, D., et al., 2003. LKB1 is the upstream kinase in the AMP-activated protein kinase cascade. Curr. Biol. 13, 2004–2008.

CHAPTER 21

Vitamin D receptor activation and prevention of arterial aging

Andrea Stucchi[1], Ferruccio Conte[1], Andrea Galassi[1], Paola Ciceri[2] and Mario Cozzolino[1]

[1]Renal Division, Renal Division and Laboratory of Experimental Nephrology, ASST Santi Paolo e Carlo, Dipartimento di Scienze della Salute, S. Paolo Hospital, Department of Health Sciences, University of Milan, Milan, Italy

[2]Renal Research Laboratory, Department of Nephrology, Dialysis and Renal Transplant, Fondazione Ca' Granda IRCCS, Ospedale Maggiore Policlinico, Milan, Italy

Contents

Key facts

- The insight to modulate the gut microbiota was proposed more than a thousand years ago and gave rise to the spectrum of therapeutic tools and the provision of growth substrates for resident microorganisms (the concept of prebiotics).
- Prebiotic food research has also been limited in recent years, following a ruling from the European regulatory bodies that does not recommend the labeling of food products as prebiotics and their inherent health claims.

Molecular Nutrition
DOI: https://doi.org/10.1016/B978-0-12-811907-5.00006-3

- The compounds such as vitamins, antibiotics, minerals, and bacteriophages could alter the composition of the host's microorganisms but their acceptability as prebiotics is still under debate. In recent years, soy milk has emerged from being considered as a "poor man's meat" to become a value-added food with a promising future in native food markets.
- The versatility of lactic acid bacteria encourages researchers to obtain new insights in their search for novel compounds for the ever-growing competitive functional food market.

Summary points

- The current chapter emphasizes the inclusion of riboflavin (B_2) in soy milk and its role in redox-mediated gut modulation.
- Soy contains a negligible amount of B_2 which is directly related to oxidative stress and various health complications.
- B_2 is recognized as a substance that can affect the microbiome on the basis of its redox-mediated prebiotic potential, but its underlying mechanism has not yet been elucidated.
- The design of soybean-based functional B_2-biofortified milk as part of a normal diet could make up an interesting alternative to the existing fortification methods.
- The consideration of B_2 in the prebiotic category can afford a more rational basis for the credentials of novel prebiotic compounds for modulating the gut microbiota.

21.1 Background

Patients with chronic kidney disease (CKD) have a high risk of premature arterial aging and cardiovascular disease (CVD). In particular, the risk of cardiovascular death is 10 times higher in CKD patients than in the general population (Moody et al., 2013). The progressive decrease of renal function is associated with an increased risk of major vascular events and all-cause mortality (Mafham et al., 2011).

Premature aging and early vascular modifications are the main features of arterial change in end-stage renal disease (Kooman et al., 2014). Arterial aging may represent the underlying cause of most CVD in the general population and in some chronic diseases (hypertension, CKD, diabetes mellitus), as the consequence of complex structural and functional modifications occurring in arterial vessels with increasing age (Tesauro et al., 2017). Mechanisms involved in arterial aging are numerous and not all of them are well recognized yet. Clinical studies have established that the main vascular modifications that occur in aging are endothelial dysfunction and arterial stiffness (Donato et al., 2007). Arterial stiffness may be considered as the adaptive mechanism of arterial vessels to changes in the stroke volume. During systolic contraction a portion of the stroke volume is stored in the large central arteries, mainly the aorta, with the elastic distention of their walls. This elastic force subsequently returns the blood previously stored to the peripheral circulation (Gerard, 2018). The gold standard for measuring arterial stiffness is considered to be the carotid–femoral pulse wave velocity (PWV), which demonstrates an association of arterial stiffness with morbidity and mortality for CVD (Pannier et al., 2005). Endothelial dysfunction and arterial stiffness are closely interconnected mediators of age-dependent vascular dysfunction. The stiffer the artery, the greater will be the exposure of the endothelium to hemodynamic load, promoting endothelial activation, inflammation, and damage (Janic et al., 2014). With increasing age, structural alterations can observed in the endothelium of arterial vessels, due to many factors like insulin resistance, decline in growth hormone, and finally cellular senescence (Paneni et al., 2017). Increasing deposits of advanced glycosylated end products (AGEs) in the basement membrane and interstitial space are observed and involve an increase in the glycated structure in the basement membrane, which becomes stiffened and fractured. These modifications in the basement membrane promote endothelial inflammation and dysfunction in vascular smooth muscle cells (VSMC). At the same time an increase in angiotensin II activity stimulates the transformation of VSMC into fibroblasts with a further increase in the stiffness of the vessel's walls (Rodríguez et al., 2016). So the inflammatory condition may constitute the signal that drives cellular changes in the remodeling of the arterial wall (Harvey et al., 2015).

Nowadays there are many studies demonstrating a clear association between vitamin D deficiency and the prevalence of chronic diseases including CVD. These studies showed an inverse relationship between vitamin D_3 levels and hypertension, insulin resistance, type 2 diabetes mellitus, and dyslipidemia. All of these alterations are actually considered as assessed risk factors for developing hypertrophic and dilative cardiomyopathy (Vimaleswaran et al., 2014). Moreover the alterations in vascular structure and function observed in hypertension are quite similar to the changes observed in vascular aging (Harvey et al., 2015). Epidemiological reports concerning vitamin D deficiency and CV risk have also been supported by experimental studies. Vitamin D receptors (VDRs) and 1-α-hydroxylase are expressed in cardiovascular tissues, and in VDRs knockout rats an increased ventricular mass and an evolution toward promoting fibrotic extracellular matrix formation, left ventricular dilation, and finally electromechanical dysfunction has been observed (Mancuso et al., 2008). VDRs are also expressed in endothelial cells, and their activation seems to affect vascular tone in hypertensive models and modulate calcium influx across the cell membrane and the contraction of endothelium-related muscular smooth cells (Al Mheid and Quyyumi, 2017). As demonstrated by Li et al. (2002) 1,25-OH_3 vitamin D has an important role in negatively regulating the renin–angiotensin–aldosterone system (RAAS) with consequences regarding the control of hypertension (Vimaleswaran et al., 2014). An inverse relationship between vitamin D and plasma renin activity were revealed in hypertensive subjects and thus there is an excessive increase in blood pressure as a result of salt intake in hypertensive patients with vitamin D deficiency (Vaidya and Williams, 2012). Impaired vitamin D metabolism is known to be involved in the worsening of the atherogenesis process and in the hastening arterial of calcification (Beveridge et al., 2015).

21.2 Vascular calcifications mechanisms

Vascular calcifications (VCs) in the CKD population show not only a different genesis and localization, but also an earlier onset than in the general population.

It seems impossible to explain the high incidence of cardiovascular (CV) disease in CKD patients only by common risk factors—such as hypertension, aging, smoking, diabetes, and dyslipidemia—suggesting the presence of other different pathological pathways (London et al., 2003). VC is characterized by the development of two pathologies: atherosclerosis and arteriosclerosis. VSMC calcification may be considered a typical and pathognomonic lesion in CKD vascular disease and it is a specific hallmark of vascular aging. In patients with CKD, the alteration in the metabolism of calcium and phosphate finally leads to vascular smooth muscle calcification, while endothelial dysfunction and atherosclerosis are due to other CKD pathophysiologic alterations, such as RAAS activation or insulin resistance. Both pathologies contribute to the VC process during CKD progression.

21.3 Vitamin D deficiency

Vitamin D insufficiency or deficiency is common in patients with CKD and is associated with overall and cardiovascular mortality (Pilz et al., 2016). Vitamin D reduction in CKD is caused by different pathogenetic mechanisms, such as:

Glomerular filtration rate decline, which is caused by decreased delivery of 25(OH)D to renal tubules, elevation of phosphatonine FGF-23 that inhibits 1-alfa-hydroxylase and stimulates 24-hydroxylase, the inhibition of parathyroid hormone effects caused by metabolic acidosis and uremic toxins (Christakos et al., 2012).

Proteinuria, which is caused by decreased tubular uptake of 25(OH)D by megalin (Gonzalez et al., 2004) and renal loss of vitamin D binding protein (DBP) (Melamed et al., 2006).

Tubular dysfunction, which causes the decrease and inhibition of 1-α-hydroxylase activity because of tubular damage (Bukoski et al., 1989) and tubular acidosis (Wong et al., 2014).

Therapeutic 1,25(OH)2D3 usage, which induces the inhibition of 1-α-hydroxylase and 25-hydroxylase in extrarenal tissue.

21.4 Vitamin D receptors

According to recent reports, vitamin D receptor activators (VDRAs) play an important role in the prevention of premature vascular aging (Marangella et al., 2009; Franczyk et al., 2014). The large distribution of VDRs suggests that vitamin D does not have an effect just on calcium—phosphorus metabolism, but that it is really involved in different organ functions including the cardiovascular, immune, gastrointestinal, and endocrine systems. Thus vitamin D may have a lot of pleiotropic effects, most of them independent of calcium—phosphorus metabolism (Cozzolino et al., 2009a). The impact of the "nonclassical effects" of vitamin D therapy and its mechanisms, in particular related to the cardiovascular system, are evaluated in preclinical and clinical studies. Several studies conducted both in animals and humans have investigated the role of VDRs in premature arterial aging and the association of low vitamin D and CVD, suggesting that the supplementation of vitamin D could improve survival rates in CKD patients.

21.5 Vitamin D/vitamin D receptor activator physiology

Vitamin D is the term generally used to indicate vitamin D2 (or ergocalciferol) and vitamin D3 (or cholecalciferol). These precursors are transported into the liver by a DBP and are transformed by 25-hydroxylase; then the 1α-hydroxylase in the kidney produces the active form, calcitriol, which exerts its function on the VDR in many different tissues (Zittermann, 2003). Table 21.1 shows the different types of VDRAs according to Kidney Disease: Improving Global Outcomes (KDIGO) (Kidney Disease: Improving Global Outcomes KDIGO CKD-MBD Update Work Group, 2017). VDRAs are classified as selective or nonselective forms. It is well known that there are different types of vitamin D: the natural form of calcitriol, and synthetic analogs of vitamin D2 and D3 such as alfacalcidol, doxercalciferol, falecalcitriol, maxacalcitol, and paricalcitol. Calcitriol is the naturally active form of vitamin D, while paricalcitol and maxacalcitol are considered as selective VDR activators (sVDRAs) (Bover et al., 2014), (Cozzolino et al., 2011)].

The affinity to circulating DBP is one of the factors that allows for the differentiation of selective and nonselective activators. In fact maxacalcitol has about 400–500 times less binding affinity to DBP than calcitriol, with also a shorter half-life and a more rapid removal from the circulation (Kobayashi et al., 1991).

The synthesis of sVDRAs has come about due to a clinical need to widen the therapeutic approaches and to try to reduce the risk of hypercalcemia and hyperphosphatemia related to the use of VDRAs. Moreover, sVDRAs more efficiently inhibit the synthesis and secretion of parathormone with a minor intestinal absorption of calcium and phosphate. Therefore sVDRAs reduce the risk of extra skeletal deposition of calcium and phosphate, such as vascular or valvular calcifications.

Most of the nutritional requirements of vitamin D are derived from cutaneous solar ultraviolet radiation (approximately 80%) (Kimlin, 2008) and the rest comes from the diet or supplementation (Holick, 2007a). For these reasons vitamin D could be considered a prohormone and not classified only as a vitamin. The best measurement for vitamin D status is its metabolite 25-hydroxyvitamin D (25(OH)D) level (Zittermann, 2003;

Table 21.1 The different types of native vitamin D and vitamin D receptor activators.

Type of components	Description	Name	Molecule	Standardized nomenclature
Vitamin D	Native or dietary	Cholecalciferol	Vitamin D3	Native vitamin D
	Vitamin D	Ergocalciferol	Vitamin D2	
	Result of the first hydroxylation of vitamin D in the liver	Calcidiol	25-Hydroxyvitamin D2/D3	25D
Active vitamin D	Product of the second hydroxylation of vitamin D in the kidneys. Binds to VDR directly	Calcitriol	1,25-Hydroxyvitamin D3	1.25D
	A synthetic calcitriol analog that transforms into calcitriol in the liver before binding to the VDR	Alfacalcidol	1α-Hydroxyvitamin D3	1-α
Selective VDR activator	Synthetic VDR agonist. Selectively activates the subsequent metabolic routes	Paricalcitol	19-Nor-1α	Selective VDR
			Dihydroxyvitamin D2,25	activator
		Maxacalcitol	22-Oxa-1,25-dihydroxyvitamin D3	Selective VDR activator

Table 21.2 Plasma levels of 25(OH)D and nutritional status ((Kennel et al., 2010; Norman, 2008)).

Vit D nutritional status	25(OH)D plasma level (ng/mL)
Severe deficiency	<5
Deficiency	5–12
Insufficiency	12–20
Sufficiency	20–49
High	>50
Possible toxicity	>80

Holick, 2004). Table 21.2 presents the plasma levels of 25(OH)D and vitamin D nutritional status (Kennel et al., 2010). Vitamin D deficiency has been linked to several health outcomes (Basit, 2013), including musculoskeletal (rickets, bone fractures, osteomalacia, osteopenia, osteoporosis, and muscle weakness) (Holick, 2007b) and nonskeletal complications (Judd and Tangpricha, 2010). Nonskeletal complications include CVD and risk factors (Kendrick et al., 2009; Kim et al., 2008) such as congestive heart failure (Zittermann et al., 2006), impaired systolic and diastolic function (Pekkanen et al., 2015), myocardial infarction (Giovannucci et al., 2008), peripheral vascular disease (McGreevy and Williams, 2011), abdominal aortic aneurysm in older men (Wong et al., 2013), nonvalvular atrial fibrillation (Demir et al., 2014; Ozcan et al., 2015), and hypertension (Pavlovic et al., 2011). Calcitriol is the active form of vitamin D and must bind to the VDR to perform its functions. Cholecalciferol also, but only at a high concentration, has the capacity to bind to the VDR. The VDR is a nuclear receptor and it is a member of a nuclear steroid receptor family acting as a factor of ligand-dependent transcription of many genes related to the synthesis and secretion of PTH and other proteins related to mineral metabolism, cell growth, and cell differentiation. VDRs are not present only in skeletal tissue, but also in several other sites, such as cardiac tissue, VSMC, endothelial cells, renal tissue, and the immune system (Valdivielso, 2009), as shown in Table 21.3. The generation of a VDR–vitamin D complex induces a conformational change in a particular domain of the receptor (AF-2 domain). This activation step appears to be required for the recruitment of VDR-interacting proteins, known as coactivators and corepressors (Ebert et al., 2006). It has been recognized in both "classical" and "nonclassical" genomic vitamin D/VDR actions; nevertheless, calcitriol can exert rapid "nongenomic" actions that occur

Table 21.3 VDRs body distributions.

Tissue
Brain
Parotid glands
Parathyroid glands
Lungs
Heart
Immune system
Muscles
Liver
GI system: stomach, intestine
Pancreas
Kidney
Reproductive system
Skin
Bone
Arteries

within minutes of exposure to calcitriol. These rapid actions regulate intracellular calcium fluxes, the degree of protein phosphorylation, acetylation, and subcellular localization, which could also modify genomic signals (Dusso, 2005).

21.6 Vitamin D receptor activation and cardiovascular disease

Cardiovascular calcification is a common health problem that affects CKD patients. The alteration of vitamin D metabolism contributes not only to the development of mineral and bone disorders, considered a classical biological effect of vitamin D, but has also several "nonclassical" effects, as shown in Table 21.4.

Several studies, both preclinical and clinical, showed that abnormally low and high vitamin D levels promote cardiovascular calcifications in CKD patients. For this reason, the choice and monitoring of the right vitamin D plays a major role in the prevention and treatment of CVD in CKD patients.

21.7 Preclinical studies

The evidence from preclinical studies seems to indicate the existence of a particular relationship between vitamin D levels and VC: both low

Table 21.4 Classical and nonclassical effect of vitamin D.

Classical effects	
Intestine	Increases calcium and phosphate absorption
Bone	Induces FGF-23 production, bone remodeling
	Improves bone mineralization
	Increases bone release in hypocalcemia
Parathyroid	Inhibits PTH synthesis and secretion
Nonclassical effects	
Kidney	Antiproteinuric effect
	Decreases magnesium absorption
	Stimulates calcium and phosphate absorption
	Suppression of RAA system
	Increases nephrin expression
	Decreases NF-kB activation
Cardiovascular	Inhibition of RAA system
	Suppression of ANP
	Inhibition of smooth muscle cells proliferation
	Decreases the risk of hypertension and CV diseases
Immune system	Stimulates innate immunity
	Inhibition of tH1 cells and promotion of Th2 cells
	Repression of INF, IL-2, and GMCSF
Pancreas	Increases insulin secretion and sensitivity
	Expression of insulin receptor
	Increases glucose uptake
Cancer	Regulation of apoptosis and antitumor activity

vitamin D blood levels and toxic vitamin D blood levels seem to cause similar damage to the cardiovascular system (Grübler et al., 2017).

One of the first studies showed that the supplementation of rats with toxic doses of vitamins D2 or D3 induced massive calcifications (Takeo et al., 1989). In a more recent study in 2008 with male white rabbits, the effects of an 8-week treatment of vitamin D_2 alone at 25,000 IU/4 days weekly were evaluated on the development of aortic valve stenosis (AVS) and function. Changes in valves were compared with those in endothelial function and in valvular measurement of thioredoxin-interacting protein (TXNIP), a marker/mediator of reactive oxygen species-induced oxidative stress. Vitamin D_2-treated rabbits developed AVS with increased aortic valve backscattering AV_{BS} (17.6 ± 1.4 vs 6.7 ± 0.8 dB, $P < .0001$), increased transvalvular velocity, and transvalvular pressure gradient (both $P < .01$ via two-way ANOVA) compared to the control group. There was associated valve calcification, lipid deposition, and macrophage infiltration. Endothelial function was markedly impaired, and intravalvular TXNIP concentration increased. Vitamin D_2 supplementation induces the development of aortic stenosis in rabbits: interactions with endothelial function and TXNIP (Ngo et al., 2008). Moreover, in uremic rats, non-toxic doses of calcitriol were able to favor VCs (Becker et al., 2011). Despite this evidence, several studies showed that vitamin D deficiency could lead to similar cardiovascular calcifications. As shown in experimental research (Mathew et al., 2008), the administration of low doses of calcitriol is able to shield the aortic intima, in a murine model of adynamic bone disorder, from the CKD-induced calcification. In an important study from Lau et al. (2012), calcitriol or paricalcitol administration in a murine CKD model fed with a dietary phosphate load induced aortic medial calcification, VDRA therapy was associated with increased serum and urine klotho levels, increased phosphaturia, correction of hyperphosphatemia, and lowering of serum fibroblast growth factor-23. There was no effect on elastin remodeling or inflammation; however, the expression of the anticalcification factor, osteopontin, in aortic medial cells was increased.

21.8 Clinical studies

CVD is the commonest cause of death in CKD patients and vitamin D deficiency has been associated with several cardiovascular risk factors (Lavie et al., 2011), as described in Fig. 21.1.

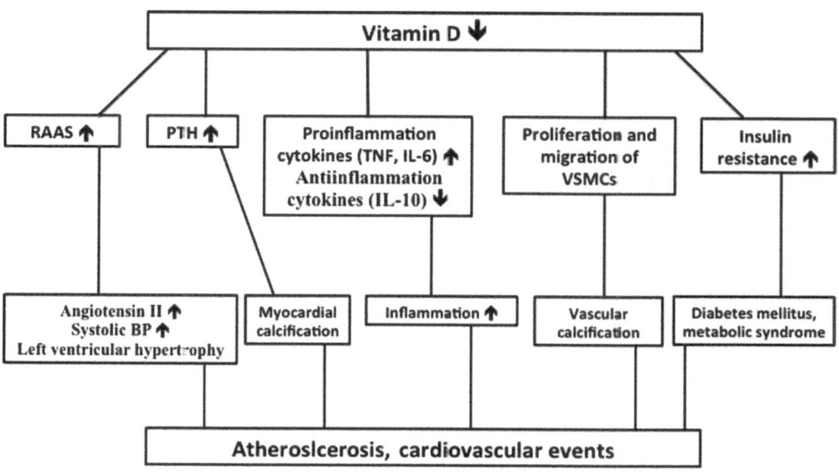

Figure 21.1 Potential mechanisms for cardiovascular effects of vitamin D deficiency.

The lack of vitamin D promotes the development of secondary hyperparathyroidism and reduces VDR activation contributing to an increase of CV morbidity and mortality in CKD patients (Berl and Henrich, 2006). The pathological CV effects comprise hypertension, VC, smooth muscle cell proliferation, and fibrosis. These are pathological CV effects linked to vitamin D deficiency that lead to myocardial and arterial thickening, and left ventricular hypertrophy (LVH) (Andress, 2006). Several observational studies highlighted that the risk of CV mortality in the general population and especially in patients affected by renal failure could be reduced by systemic activation of VDRs (Cozzolino et al., 2009b). Furthermore, a meta-analysis by Autier et al. Autier and Gandini (2007), with some randomized trials analyzing the impact of vitamin D among patients with different health conditions, showed that vitamin D intake could reduce the all-cause mortality rates.

Analysis from National Health and Nutrition Examination Survey III (NHANES III) showed low vitamin D was associated with CVD and CVD risk factors including diabetes mellitus (Kendrick et al., 2009). Moreover, in a subsequent case–control study with 18,225 US men, the risk of myocardial infarction was higher with low vitamin D in comparison to sufficient values. Lastly, further analysis exploiting data from NHANES highlighted a high prevalence of hypovitaminosis D in cardiovascular patients (Kim et al., 2008).

A study from Luo et al. (2016) reported that in patients with CKD not undergoing hemodialysis, arterial stiffness increases inversely with the lowering of vitamin D. Vitamin D deficiency is found also to be associated with an increased PWV and arterial stiffness along with increased LVH and CV mortality in dialysis patients (Thadhani et al., 2011). A randomized, double blind, placebo-controlled trial reported favorable effects of vitamin D supplementation on vascular endothelial function and inflammatory biomarkers in vitamin D–deficient patients with nondiabetic stage 3–4 CKD, confirming the beneficial effects of the correction of vitamin D deficiency on vascular function. This data showed that serum 25(OH)D and 1,25(OH)2D increased and flow-mediated dilation (FMD) significantly improved after cholecalciferol supplementation [mean change in FMD%: 5.8% (95% CI: 4.0%–7.5%, $P < .001$)]. Endothelium independent nitroglycerine-mediated dilatation, PWV, iPTH, iFGF-23, and interlukin-6 also showed favorable changes [(Kumar et al., 2017)].

Hypertension is strictly related to vitamin D deficiency. It seems that the lack of vitamin D increases blood pressure activating the renin–angiotensin system, as suggested in a prospective cohort study performed on 3316 patients; plasma renin and angiotensin II concentrations had a constant increase with decreasing levels of 25(OH)D and 1,25(OH)D (Tomaschitz et al., 2010). Vimaleswaran et al. (2014) reported the result of a Mendelian randomization study with data from 146,581 subjects suggesting that people with genetic variants associated with low endogenous production of 25(OH)D present an increased risk of hypertension. Moreover, a study including about 500 hypertensive and normotensive individuals showed a link between 25(OH)D levels and the Fok1 polymorphism of the VDR gene in the regulation of plasma renin activity in hypertension. These data confirmed the important role of the vitamin D–VDR complex in the regulation of plasma renin in humans and suggested the administration of vitamin D analogs as renin inhibitors, like ACE inhibitor (ACE-i) or angiotensinogen receptor blockers (ARBs), in patients with hyperreninemia (Vaidya et al., 2011).

21.9 Conclusion

Vitamin D should be considered as a hormone with the presence of specific receptors in almost all cells of the body both on the plasma and nuclear membranes (Norman, 2008). Receptor activation is the mechanism by which vitamin D exercises both the specific activity and the so-called pleiotropic actions. There are numerous literature reports on the associations between a vitamin D deficit and increases in CVD. In CKD patients the role of alterations in the metabolism of vitamin D in the increased CV risk is well documented, through the mechanisms of aggravation of arterial stiffness and endothelial dysfunction. VC, especially in CKD patients, is a critical point in the expression of arterial stiffness and alteration of endothelial functions. Vitamin D deficiency is one of the main factors exacerbating VC in CKD patients together with a complex interaction between increasing factors favoring and reducing the inhibition factors of the calcification process. Vitamin D deficiency is common in patients with CKD because of GFR decline, renal tubular dysfunction, and proteinuria. Several factors, including vitamin D deficiency, exacerbate VC in patients with CKD. Nutritional vitamin D and VDRAs supplements facilitate the alleviation of vitamin D–dependent or vitamin D–independent VC. Nonselective VDRAs may increase VC by inducing hyperphosphatemia and hypercalcemia. Nutritional vitamin D supplements may provide an ancillary role for ameliorating uremic VC. Despite a large amount of observational and experimental studies suggesting the role of vitamin D deficiency in the genesis of arterial senescence and of CVD development, the causality of this relationship remains to be established. Most large trials of vitamin D therapy with CV need well-established end points to support vitamin D therapy for cardiovascular protection.

References

Al Mheid, I., Quyyumi, A.A., 2017. Vit D and cardiovascular disease. J. Am. Coll. Cardiol. 70 (1), 89–100.

Andress, D.L., 2006. Vitamin D in chronic kidney disease: a systemic role for selective vitamin D receptor activation. Kidney Int. 69 (1), 33–43.

Autier, P., Gandini, S., 2007. Vitamin D supplementation and total mortality: a meta-analysis of randomized controlled trials. Arch. Intern. Med. 167, 1730–1737.

Basit, S., 2013. Vitamin D in health and disease: a literature review. Br. J. Biomed. Sci. 70, 161–172.

Becker, L.E., Koleganova, N., Piecha, G., Noronha, I.L., Zeier, M., Geldyyev, A., et al., 2011. Effect of paricalcitol and calcitriol on aortic wall remodeling in uninephrectomized ApoE knockout mice. Am. J. Physiol. Renal Physiol. 300 (3), F772–F782. Available from: https://doi.org/10.1152/ajprenal.00042.2010 (Epub December 15, 2010).

Berl, T., Henrich, W., 2006. Kidney-heart interactions: epidemiology, pathogenesis, and treatment. Clin. J. Am. Soc. Nephrol. 1, 8–18.

Beveridge, L.A., Struthers, A.D., Khan, F., D-PRESSURE Collaboration, et al., 2015. Effect of vitamin D supplementation on blood pressure: a systematic review and meta-analysis incorporating individual patient data. JAMA Intern. Med. 175, 745–754.

Bover, J., DaSilva, I., Furlano, M., Lloret, M.J., Diaz-Encarnacion, M.M., Ballarin, J., et al., 2014. Clinical uses of 1,25-dihydroxy-19-nor-vitamin D(2) (paricalcitol). Curr. Vasc. Pharmacol. 12 (2), 313–323.

Bukoski, R.D., DeWan, P., McCarron, D.A., 1989. 1,25 (OH)2 vitamin D3 modifies growth and contractile function of vascular smooth muscle of spontaneously hypertensive rats. Am. J. Hypertens. 2 (7), 553–556.

Christakos, S., Ajibade, D.V., Dhawan, P., Fechner, A.J., Mady, L.J., 2012. Vitamin D: metabolism. Rheum. Dis. Clin. N. Am. 38 (1), 1–11. Available from: https://doi.org/10.1016/j.rdc.2012.03.003. vii.

Cozzolino, M., Ciceri, P., Volpi, E.M., Olivi, L., Messa, P.G., 2009a. Pathophysiology of calcium and phosphate metabolism impairment in chronic kidney disease. Blood Purif. 27 (4), 338–344.

Cozzolino, M., Fallabrino, G., Pasho, S., Olivi, L., Ciceri, P., Volpi, E., et al., 2009b. Importance of vitamin D receptor activation in clinical practice. Contrib. Nephrol. 163, 213–218.

Cozzolino, M., Bover, J., Vervloet, M., Brandenburg, V.M., 2011. A multidisciplinary review of the science of vitamin D receptor activation. Kidney Int. Suppl. 1, 107–110.

Demir, M., Uyan, U., Melek, M., 2014. The effects of vitamin D deficiency on atrial fibrillation. Clin. Appl. Thromb. Hemost. 20, 98–103.

Donato, A.J., Eskurza, I., Silver, A.E., et al., 2007. Direct evidence of endothelial oxidative stress with aging in humans: relation to impaired endothelium dependent dilation and up regulation of nuclear factor-kB. Circ. Res. 100, 1659–1666.
Dusso, A., 2005. Vitamin D. Am. J. Physiol. Renal Physiol. 289, F8–F28.
Ebert, R., Schütze, N., Adamski, J., Jakob, F., 2006. Vitamin D signaling is modulated on multiple levels in health and disease. Mol. Cell Endocrinol. 248, 149e59.
Franczyk, A., Stolarz-Skrzypek, K., Wesołowska, A., Czarnecka, D., 2014. Vitamin D and vitamin D receptor activators in treatment of hypertension and cardiovascular disease. Cardiovasc. Haematol. Disord. Drug Targets 14, 34–44.
Gerard, M., 2018. London arterial stiffness in chronic kidney disease and end-stage renal disease. Blood Purif. 45, 154–158.
Giovannucci, E., Liu, Y., Hollis, B., Rimm, E., 2008. 25-Hydroxyvitamin D and risk of myocardial infarction in men: a prospective study. Arch. Intern. Med. 168, 1174–1180.
Gonzalez, E.A., Sachdeva, A., Oliver, D.A., Martin, K.J., 2004. Vitamin D insufficiency and deficiency in chronic kidney disease: a single center observational study. Am. J. Nephrol. 24 (5), 503–510.
Grübler, M.R., März, W., Pilz, S., Grammer, T.B., Trummer, C., Müllner, C., et al., 2017. Vitamin-D concentrations, cardiovascular risk and events—a review of epidemiological evidence. Rev. Endocr. Metab. Disord. 18 (2), 259–272. Available from: https://doi.org/10.1007/s11154-017-9417-0.
Harvey, A., Montezano, A.C., Touyz, R.M., 2015. Vascular biology of aging—implications in hypertension. J. Mol. Cell. Cardiol. 83, 112–121.
Holick, M.F., 2004. Vitamin D: importance in the prevention of cancers, type 1 diabetes, heart disease, and osteoporosis. Am. J. Clin. Nutr. 79, 362–371.
Holick, M.F., 2007a. Optimal vitamin D status for the prevention and treatment of osteoporosis. Drugs Aging 24 (12), 1017–1029.
Holick, M.F., 2007b. Vitamin D deficiency. N. Engl. J. Med. 357, 266–281.
Janic, M., Lunder, M., Sabovic, M., 2014. Arterial stiffness and cardiovascular therapy. Biomed. Res. Int. 2014, 621437.
Judd, S.E., Tangpricha, V., 2010. Vitamin D deficiency and risk for cardiovascular disease. Am. J. Med. Sci. 117, 503–511.
Kendrick, J., Targher, G., Smits, G., Chonchol, M., 2009. 25-Hydroxyvitamin D deficiency is independently associated with cardiovascular disease in the third National Health and nutrition examination survey. Atherosclerosis. 205, 255–260.
Kennel, K.A., Drake, M.T., Hurley, D.L., 2010. Vitamin D deficiency in adults: when to test and how to treat. Mayo Clin Proc. 85 (8), 752–758.
Kidney Disease: Improving Global Outcomes (KDIGO) CKD-MBD Update Work Group, 2017. KDIGO 2017 clinical practice guideline update for the diagnosis, evaluation, prevention, and treatment of Chronic Kidney Disease–Mineral and Bone Disorder (CKD-MBD). Kidney Int. Suppl. 7, 1–59.
Kim, D., Sabour, S., Sagar, U., Adams, S., Whellan, D., 2008. Prevalence of hypovitaminosis D in cardiovascular diseases (from the National Health and nutrition examination survey 2001 to 2004). Am. J. Cardiol. 102, 1540–1544.
Kimlin, M.G., 2008. Geographic location and vitamin D synthesis. Mol. Aspects Med. 29, 453–461.
Kobayashi, T., Okano, T., Tsugawa, N., Masuda, S., Takeuchi, A., Nishii, Y., 1991. Metabolism and transporting system of 22-oxacalcitriol. Contrib. Nephrol. 91, 129–133.
Kooman, J.P., Kotanko, P., Schols, A.M., et al., 2014. Chronic kidney disease and premature aging. Nat. Rev. Nephrol. 10, 732–742.

Kumar, V., Yadav, A.K., Lal, A., Kumar, V., Singhal, M., Billot, L., et al., 2017. A randomized trial of vitamin D supplementation on vascular function in CKD. J. Am. Soc. Nephrol. 28, 3100–3108.

Lau, W.L., Leaf, E.M., Hu, M.C., Takeno, M.M., Kuro-o, M., Moe, O.W., et al., 2012. Vitamin D receptor agonists increase klotho and osteopontin while decreasing aortic calcification in mice with chronic kidney disease fed a high phosphate diet. Kidney Int. 82 (12), 1261–1270. Available from: https://doi.org/10.1038/ki.2012.322 (Epub August 29, 2012).

Lavie, C.J., Lee, J.H., Milani, R.V., 2011. Vitamin D and Cardiovascular disease: will it live up to its hype? J. Am. Coll. Cardiol. 58, 1547–1556.

Li, Y.C., Kong, J., Wei, M., Chen, Z.F., Liu, S.Q., Cao, L.P., 2002. 1, 25-Dihydroxyvitamin D3 is a negative endocrine regulator of the renin-angiotensin system. J. Clin. Invest. 110, 229–238.

London, G.M., Guerin, A.P., Marchais, S., Metivier, F., Pannier, B., Adda, H., 2003. Arterial media calcification in end-stage renal disease: impact on all-cause and cardiovascular mortality. Nephrol. Dial Transplant 18, 1731–1740.

Luo, Q., Wang, L.L., Gao, Y.H., 2016. Association between serum 25-hydroxyvitamin D and arterial stiffness in non-dialysis dependent CKD. Eur. J. Clin. Nutr. 70 (2), 274–276.

Mafham, M., Emberson, J., Landray, M.J., Wen, C.-P., Baigent, C., 2011. Estimated glomerular filtration rate and the risk of major vascular events and all-cause mortality: a meta-analysis. PLoS One 6 (10), article e25920.

Mancuso, P., Rahman, A., Hershey, S.D., Dandu, L., Nibbelink, K.A., Simpson, R.U., 2008. 1,25-Dihydroxyvitamin-D3 treatment reduces cardiac hypertrophy and left ventricular diameter in spontaneously hypertensive heart failure-prone (cp/þ) rats independent of changes in serum leptin. J. Cardiovasc. Pharmacol. 51, 559–564.

Marangella, M., Berutti, S., Fabbrini, L., 2009. Selective vitamin D receptor activation: effect on renal physiopathology. G. Ital. Nefrol. 26 (Suppl. 49), S23e9.

Mathew, S., Lund, R.J., Chaudhary, L.R., Geurs, T., Hruska, K.A., 2008. Vitamin D receptor activators can protect against vascular calcification. J. Am. Soc. Nephrol. 19 (8), 1509–1519. Available from: https://doi.org/10.1681/ASN.2007080902 (Epub April 30, 2008).

McGreevy, C., Williams, D., 2011. New insights about vitamin D and cardiovascular disease: a narrative review. Ann. Intern. Med. 155, 820–826.

Melamed, M.L., Eustace, J.A., Plantinga, L., et al., 2006. Changes in serum calcium, phosphate, and PTH and the risk of death in incident dialysis patients: a longitudinal study. Kidney Int. 70 (2), 351–357.

Moody, W.E., Edwards, N.C., Chue, C.D., Ferro, C.J., Townend, J.N., 2013. Arterial disease in chronic kidney disease. Heart 99 (6), 365–372.

Ngo, D.T.M., Stafford, I., Kelly, D.J., Sverdlov, A.L., Wuttke, R.D., et al., 2008. Vitamin D2 supplementation induces the development of aortic stenosis in rabbits: Interactions with endothelial function and thioredoxin-interacting protein. Eur. J. Pharmacol. 590 (1–3, 20), 290–296.

Norman, A.W., 2008. From vitamin D to hormone D: fundamentals of the vitamin D endocrine system essential for good health. Am. J. Clin. Nutr. 88 (Suppl.), 491S–499SS.

Ozcan, O.U., Gurlek, A., Gursoy, E., Gerede, D.M., Erol, C., 2015. Relation of vitamin D deficiency and new-onset atrial fibrillation among hypertensive patients. J. Am. Soc. Hypertens. 9, 307–312.

Paneni, F., Cañestro, C.D., Libby, P., Lüscher, T.F., Camici, G.G., 2017. The aging cardiovascular system understanding it at the cellular and clinical levels. Am. Coll. Cardiol. 69, 1952–1967.

Pannier, B., Guérin, A.P., Marchais, S.J., et al., 2005. Stiffness of capacitive and conduit arteries: prognostic significance for end-stage renal disease patients. Hypertension 45, 592–596.
Pavlovic, D., Josipovic, J., Pavlovic, N., 2011. Vitamin D and hypertension. Period. Biol. 113, 299–302.
Pekkanen, M.P., Ukkola, O., Hedberg, P., Piira, O.P., Lepojärvi, S., Lumme, J., et al., 2015. Serum 25-hydroxyvitamin D is associated with major cardiovascular risk factors and cardiac structure and function in patients with coronary artery disease. Nutr. Metab. Cardiovasc. Dis. 25, 471–478.
Pilz, S., Verheyen, N., Grübler, M.R., Tomaschitz, A., März, W., 2016. Vitamin D and cardiovascular disease prevention. Nat. Rev. Cardiol. 13 (7), 404–417.
Rodríguez, A.J., Scott, D., Srikanth, V., Ebeling, P., 2016. Effect of vitamin D supplementation on measures of arterial stiffness: a systematic review and metaanalysis of randomized controlled trials. Clin. Endocrinol. (Oxf.) 84, 645–657.
Takeo, S., Anan, M., Fujioka, K., Kajihara, T., Hiraga, S., Miyake, K., et al., 1989. Functional changes of aorta with massive accumulation of calcium. Atherosclerosis. 77 (2–3), 175–181.
Tesauro, M., Mauriello, A., Rovella, V., Annicchiarico-Petruzzelli, M., Cardillo, C., Melino, G., et al., 2017. Arterial aging: from endothelial dysfunction to vascular calcification. J. Intern. Med. 281, 471–482.
Thadhani, R., Appelbaum, E., Chang, Y., Pritchett, Y., Bhan, I., Agarwal, R., et al., 2011. Vitamin D receptor activation and left ventricular hypertrophy in advanced kidney disease. Am. J. Nephrol. 33 (2), 139–149.
Tomaschitz, A., Pilz, S., Ritz, E., Grammer, T., Drechsler, C., Boehm, B.O., et al., 2010. Independent association between 1,25-dihydroxyvitamin D, 25-hydroxyvitamin D and the renin-angiotensin system: the Ludwigshafen Risk and Cardiovascular Health (LURIC) study. Clin. Chim. Acta 411, 1354–1360.
Vaidya, A., Williams, J.S., 2012. The relationship between vitamin D and the renin-angiotensin system in the pathophysiology of hypertension, kidney disease and diabetes. Metabolism 61, 450–458.
Vaidya, A., Sun, B., Forman, J.P., Hopkins, P.N., Brown, N.J., Kolatkar, N.S., et al., 2011. The Fok1 vitamin D receptor gene polymorphism is associated with plasma renin activity in Caucasians. Clin. Endocrinol. (Oxf.) 74, 783–790.
Valdivielso, J.M., 2009. The physiology of vitamin D receptor activation. Contrib. Nephrol. 163, 206e12.
Vimaleswaran, K.S., et al., 2014. Association of vitamin D status with arterial blood pressure and hypertension risk: a Mendelian randomisation study. Lancet Diabetes Endocrinol. 2, 719–729.
Wong, M.S.K., Leisegang, M.S., Kruse, C., et al., 2014. Vitamin D promotes vascular regeneration. Circulation 130 (12), 976–986.
Wong, Y.Y.E., Flicker, L., Yeap, B.B., McCaul, K.A., Hankey, G.J., Norman, P.E., 2013. Is hypovitaminosis D associated with abdominal aortic aneurysm, and is there a dose-response relationship? Eur. J. Vasc. Endovasc. Surg. 45, 657–664.
Zittermann, A., 2003. Vitamin D in preventive medicine: are we ignoring the evidence? Br. J. Nutr. 89, 552–572.
Zittermann, A., Schleithoff, S.S., Koerfer, R., 2006. Vitamin D insufficiency in congestive heart failure: why and what to do about it? Heart Fail. Rev. 11, 25–33.

CHAPTER 22

Vitamin D in immune regulation and diabetes mellitus

Ihor Shymanskyi, Olha Lisakovska, Dmytro Labudzinskyi, Anna Mazanova and Mykola Veliky
Department of Biochemistry of Vitamins and Coenzymes, Palladin Institute of Biochemistry of National Academy of Sciences of Ukraine, Kyiv, Ukraine

Contents

Definition of words and terms

Autoimmunity: An aberrant systemic immune response of an organism against its own healthy cells and tissues, that manifests in various autoimmune diseases.

Calcidiol (25-hydroxyvitamin D): A precursor for calcitriol and the major circulating metabolite of vitamin D_3. This prohormone is synthesized in the liver from cholecalciferol by its hydroxylation in the 25 position by the enzyme cholecalciferol-25-hydroxylase.

Calcitriol (1,25-dihydroxycholecalciferol): The hormonally active form of vitamin D, which is formed in the kidney tissue from 25OHD by the renal 25-hydroxyvitamin D_3-1-(alpha)-hydroxylase.

Cholecalciferol (vitamin D_3): A steroid hormone and one of the most common forms of the vitamin D group, which is synthesized in the skin of animals from 7-dehydrocholesterol under the influence of UV-radiation or may be absorbed from dietary sources in the intestine.

Molecular Nutrition
DOI: https://doi.org/10.1016/B978-0-12-811907-5.00013-0

***Cytokines*:** A broad category of small secreted proteins that are involved in interactions and communications between cells during immune responses and promote the recruitment of specific cells toward the sites of inflammation. Cytokines are produced by a broad range of cell populations, including immune cells (macrophages, B and T lymphocytes, mast cells), endothelial cells, fibroblasts, stromal cells, Schwann cells, etc.

***Diabetes mellitus*:** A group of chronic, metabolic, polyethiologic, and endocrine-related disorders caused by inherited or acquired deficiency in insulin production (type 1 diabetes, insulin-dependent) by the pancreas, or by the ineffectiveness of the insulin produced, when cells fail to respond to insulin properly (type 2 diabetes, noninsulin-dependent).

***Vitamin D receptor*:** A member of the nuclear hormone receptor superfamily that acts as a ligand-inducible transcription factor. Intracellular vitamin D receptor mediates the action of 1,25-dihydroxycholecalciferol and regulates the expression of a wide variety of genes.

***Immune response*:** A versatile set of adaptive processes to form specifically reactive cells and proteins directed against antigenes. It occurs through consecutive interactions between antigen-presenting cell and various types of T and B cells.

22.1 Introduction

Studies that began with the identification of calcitriol and vitamin D receptor (VDR) in the early 1970s and have continued to the present day have significantly expanded our knowledge of the biological role of vitamin D (VD) in living organisms. The unfading interest concerning the metabolism and properties of VD can be explained by two main reasons: (1) the world trend toward VD deficiency among the population, which is confirmed to be associated with a variety of common human pathologies; and (2) this interest is fueled by new ideas about the pleiotropic extraskeletal effects (para- and autocrine) of VD's hormonally active form (Christakos et al., 2016). Multiple lines of evidence suggest that VD can be involved in inflammatory response in norm and immune-regulated disorders (e.g., infectious diseases, cancers, autoimmunity, and diabetes). This chapter summarizes the data on the immunomodulatory function of calcitriol and analyzes the association of the VD—auto/paracrine system disturbances with chronic inflammation and diabetes mellitus.

22.2 Vitamin D synthesis and activation

Vitamin D (VD) (calciferol) belongs to the group of secosteroids that can be absorbed from dietary sources in the form of cholecalciferol (VD3) or ergocalciferol (VD2), although it is mainly synthesized in the lower layers of the epidermis from 7-dehydrocholesterol (7DHC) in response to the action of ultraviolet B radiation, (Fig. 22.1) (Hoseinzadeh et al., 2018). 7DHC forms a thermodynamically unstable previtamin D3 followed by

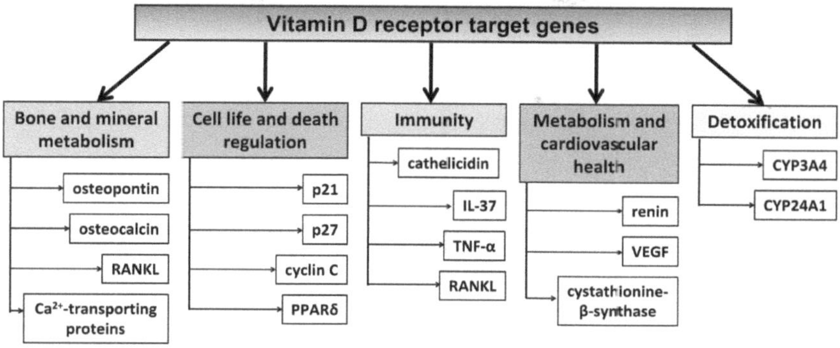

Figure 22.1 Vitamin D receptor target genes.

Key facts of vitamin D receptor target genes

- Vitamin D receptor (VDR) is a member of the nuclear hormone receptor superfamily, and acts as a ligand-inducible transcription factor.
- Intracellular VDR mediates the action of 1,25-dihydroxycholecalciferol (1,25 $(OH)_2D$) and regulates the expression of a wide variety of genes.
- 1,25$(OH)_2D$ directly binds to the VDR. This complex recruits the RXR and interacts with the specific DNA sequences (vitamin D response elements, —VDREs) for activation of vitamin D target genes.
- The highest VDR expression is found in metabolic tissues, such as the intestine, kidney, skin, and the thyroid gland, yet moderate VDR expression occurs in nearly all tissues.
- VDR modulates a variety of biological processes, including calcium and phosphorus homeostasis, cell proliferation, differentiation, migration and apoptosis, angiogenesis, and immune response.
- Mutations in the VDR gene are associated with type 2 vitamin D-resistant rickets.
- Some of the differences between individuals may be related to genetic variations of VDR (polymorphism), affecting VD signaling via VDR.

CYP, Cytochrome P450; *ILs*, interleukins; *PPARδ*, peroxisome proliferator-activated receptor δ; *RANKL*, receptor activator of nuclear factor kappa B ligand; *TNF-α*, tumor necrosis factor-α; *VEGF*, vascular endothelial growth factor.

thermal isomerization to VD3. Vitamin D3 and its metabolites, as lipophilic substances, are transported by the VD-binding protein (VDBP). In the liver, VD3 undergoes hydroxylation by vitamin D 25-hydroxylase (CYP2R1 and CYP27A1 isoforms) to produce 25-hydroxyvitamin D (25OHD3, or calcidiol), the major circulating VD3 metabolite that is largely biologically inactive. Further hydroxylation of 25OHD3 is catalyzed by 1α-hydroxylase (CYP27B1) in the kidney or in extrarenal tissues and leads to the formation of the biologically active 1,25(OH)2D3 (calcitriol). Metabolic inactivation of 25OHD3 and 1,25(OH)2D3 occurs through their hydroxylation by 24-hydroxylase (CYP24A1) (Bikle, 2014).

Two multiligand endocytic receptors, megalin and cubulin, provide the internalization of $1{,}25(OH)_2D_3$ bound to the VDBP into cells. Intracellularly, the interaction of $1{,}25(OH)_2D_3$ with the VDR initiates a complex cascade of molecular events culminating in gene transactivation or transrepression (Lu et al., 2018). In general the known VDR-regulated genes can be grouped as shown in Fig. 22.2. $1{,}25(OH)_2D_3$ synthesized in the kidney mainly fulfils the endocrine function shown in Fig. 22.1.

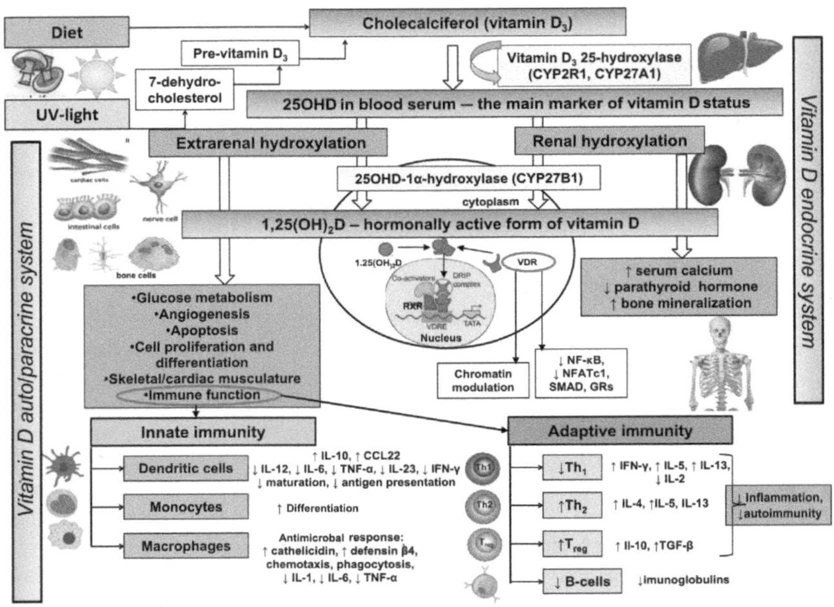

Figure 22.2 Vitamin D—auto/paracrine system in immune regulation
For the manifestation of biological activities VD undergoes two-stage hydroxylation by the enzymes of the cytochrome P450 family. This pathway involves the formation of the main circulating metabolite, calcidiol, produced by CYP2R1 and the hormonally active form, calcitriol, synthesized by CYP27B1. Calcitriol, via VD receptors, modulates transcription of various genes, involved in mineral metabolism and in noncalcemic functions, including innate and adaptive immunity. In brief, vitamin D immunomodulation includes the attenuation of Th1 and stimulation of Th2 cells proliferation. Similarly, vitamin D induces the synthesis, secretion, and release of antiinflammatory cytokines, while inhibiting proinflammatory cytokines. *$1{,}25(OH)_2D$*, 1,25-Dihydroxycholecalciferol; *25OHD*, 25-hydroxyvitamin D; *CYP*, cytochrome P450; *GRs*, glucocorticoid receptors; *IFN-γ*, interferon-γ; *ILs*, interleukins; *NFATc1*, nuclear factor of activated T cells 1; *NF-κB*, nuclear factor kappa B; *RXR*, retinoid X receptor; *TGF-β*, transforming growth factor β; *Th1*, type 1 T helper; *Th2*, type 2 T helper; *TNF-α*, tumor necrosis factor-α; *Treg*, regulatory T cells; *VDR*, vitamin D receptor; *VDRE*, vitamin D response element.

Calcitriol was most commonly reported to stimulate the absorption of phosphate and calcium in the intestine, regulate bone tissue remodeling, suppress the synthesis of parathyroid hormone (PTH), and enhance the expression of fibroblast growth factor 23 (FGF23), which inhibits CYP27B1 activity in the kidney (Fleet, 2017). Apart from the fact that renal synthesis is the main source of circulatory 1,25$(OH)_2D_3$, in extrarenal tissues (brain, vessels, skin, large intestine, placenta, prostate, and immune cells, etc.). Calcitriol also regulates local molecular and biochemical processes, showing potential to induce nonclassical auto/paracrine responses (Bikle, 2016).

The level of circulating 25OHD is generally accepted as a biomarker for VD status. 25OHD values lower than 25 nmol/L are related to rickets and osteomalacia, and hereafter are designated as severe deficiency. The emerging data highlighting the association of low VD levels with nonskeletal pathologies raises the question as to the optimal levels necessary for general health and well-being. At present most experts agree that plasma 25OHD levels <50 nmol/L may sustain long-term adverse health consequences and are classified as "deficiency." As the 75 nmol/L of 25OHD is the level above which there is no further stimulation of PTH, it is therefore considered as "sufficiency." Table 22.1 summarizes the criteria proposed by the US Endocrine Society for VD status, intended for normal healthy populations to ensure not only skeletal health (Pramyothin and Holick, 2012).

Table 22.1 Vitamin D status guidelines.

Vitamin D status	25OHD (nmol/L)	25OHD (ng/mL)
Deficiency	<50	<20
Insufficiency	50–75	20–30
Sufficiency	75–100	30–44
Toxicity	>250	>100

Key facts of vitamin D status

- Circulating 25OHD is a robust and reliable marker of vitamin D status.
- Vitamin D deficiency is associated with an increased risk of several diseases such as diabetes, cancer, autoimmune, cardiovascular, and infectious diseases, depression, dementia, and musculoskeletal **decline**.
- Clinical risk factors for vitamin D deficiency are inadequate sun exposure, limited oral intake, impaired intestinal absorption, long-term use of medications (glucocorticoids, antiepileptic drugs) and aging.
- The concept of the personal vitamin D response index (via measuring vitamin D sensitive molecular parameters) can better describe the efficiency of the molecular response to supplementation with vitamin D and should be provided for an optimized vitamin D supplementation.

22.3 Role of vitamin D in immune regulation and inflammatory responses

In retrospect, the finding that $1,25(OH)_2D_3$ could interfere with the formation of interleukins (ILs) was the first discovery that expanded the VD research field far beyond the limits of calcium homeostasis and the regulation of bone metabolism. The ILs are a large group of cytokines that mediate the interactions between immune and inflammatory cells by modulating cell growth, differentiation, and functional activation. Besides being produced in the leukocytes at different stages of their differentiation, further cell types involved in specific organ-related diseases with confirmed inflammatory components (keratinocytes, trophoblasts, adipocytes, and endothelial cells) are capable of synthesizing ILs and VD-hormone was shown to strongly influence the expression of both ILs and their receptors. Further cytokines, such as tumor necrosis factor alpha (TNF-α) and interferon gamma (IFN-γ), as well as growth factors, such as toll-like receptors, C-reactive protein (CRP), and enzymes, which generate inflammation mediators (cyclooxygenase, 5-lipoxygenase) have also been identified as calcitriol targets (Skrobot et al., 2018).

By influencing various cell types related to the immune system (monocytes/macrophages, dendritic, T and B cells), VD exerts the cell-type specific regulation of genes involved in the inflammatory processes shown in Table 22.1 and provides interaction between VD signaling and other signaling cascades that promote inflammation (Bivona et al., 2017). Two main observations underscore the immune modulatory effect of VD: (1) the presence of VDR in immune cells and their ability to produce VD-hormone locally, which acts on immune cells either in an autocrine, paracrine, or intracrine fashion; and (2) regulates multiple pathways of innate and adaptive segments of the immune system.

22.3.1 Vitamin D and innate immunity

Dendritic cells (DCs), which are the most potent antigen-presenting cells (APCs) of the innate immune system that stimulate the lymphocytes of adaptive immunity to remove the invaders through antigen presentation, are major targets of VD (Barragan et al., 2015). Calcitriol, by inhibiting the secretion of the immune-stimulating cytokine IL-12 and enhancing the production of the immunosuppressive cytokine IL-10 in DCs, decreases the antigen presentation and maintains immature phenotype and tolerogenic properties of these cells (Corripio-Miyar et al., 2017).

Accordingly, $1,25(OH)_2D_3$ prevents activation of costimulatory molecules (CD40, CD80, CD83, and CD86) and major histocompatibility complex (MHC) class II protein expression in DCs resulting in their inability to activate alloreactive T cells (Penna and Adorini, 2000; Brosbøl-Ravnborg et al., 2013). The inhibitory action of calcitriol on DCs differentiation and maturation as well as the modulation of their activation and survival account for reduced T helper 1 (Th1) cell response, which thoroughly explains the immunosuppressive activity of $1,25(OH)_2D_3$.

Other differentiated members of the monocytic lineage, that is, macrophages as well as monocytes themselves, have also been investigated, but the effects of $1,25(OH)_2D_3$ in these cells remain controversial. VD suppresses the proliferation and stimulatory properties of monocytes (Brosbøl-Ravnborg et al., 2013). For several members of the interleukin family (e.g., IL-1, IL-6, and IL-8) as well as TNF-α, both positive and negative regulation by calcitriol has been found (Bhalla et al., 1991; Di Rosa et al., 2012). These effects seem to depend on the time of cells' stimulation, the degree of their maturation, the stimulus that is employed, and other factors.

Furthermore, VD affects innate immunity through its direct stimulatory action on the synthesis of cathelicidin and defensin induced by the activation of toll-like receptors. These low molecular weight host defense antimicrobial peptides possess a broad spectrum of activity against bacteria, viruses, and fungi in the immune cells (Sato et al., 2013).

22.3.2 Vitamin D and adaptive immunity

VD modulates adaptive immunity, which is based on an antigen-specific immune response, involving the interaction of T and B cells. These cells, especially in an immunologically active state, can express VDR (Szymczak and Pawliczak, 2016). Calcitriol may act indirectly on lymphocytes through paracrine signaling by APCs or directly through VDR. Early studies indicated that $1,25(OH)_2D_3$ suppresses T lymphocyte proliferation most probably by reducing IL-2 transcription (Chambers et al., 2014). The CD4 + subset of T cells, also referred to as T helper (Th) cells, is known to assist other leukocytes in immune processes, including the maturation of B cells into plasma cells and the activation of cytotoxic T cells and macrophages. CD4 + Th cells recognize peptides presented by MHC II molecules of APCs. They can differentiate into one of several subtypes, such as Th1, Th2, Th17, Th22, and Treg cells, which secrete various cytokines to facilitate different types of immune responses. Recently, over 100 target genes have been identified in mature CD4 + Th cells with 57 genes being repressed and 45 genes being upregulated by VD-hormone (Mahon et al., 2003).

In vitro studies revealed the ability of 1,25$(OH)_2D_3$ to inhibit IFN-γ secretion by CD4 + Th1 cells (Jeffery et al., 2009). Accordingly, VD was indicated to stimulate the formation of Th2 cells by increasing IL-4 synthesis (Mahon et al., 2003). The resulting effect supports a shift of T cell responses from a Th1 type toward Th2 reactions with concomitant suppression of Th17 that promotes the development of tolerogenic phenotype. 1,25$(OH)_2D_3$ inhibited the differentiation of Th17 cells through its suppressive effect on IL-17 and RANKL (receptor activator of NF-κB ligand) synthesis (Sun et al., 2018). Previous in vitro and in vivo studies have revealed that the RANKL signals favor the survival of DCs, thereby activating the immune response (Akiyama et al., 2012). In addition, 1,25$(OH)_2D_3$ activates Treg cells, which suppress the immune response and mediate immune tolerance by inducing IL-10 formation (Barrat et al., 2002).

Cytotoxic (killer) T cells, also known as CD8 + T cells, destroy virus-infected and tumor cells, and are also implicated in proinflammatory responses and autoimmunity. It was shown that VD reduces the proliferation of CD8 + T cells, which recognize their targets by binding to antigen associated with MHC I molecules present on the surface of all nucleated cells. They express VDR at the highest level compared to other immune cells. VDR-knockout CD8 + T cells exhibit an increased proliferation without antigen stimulation due to an increased production of IL-2 (Chen et al., 2014). Several studies have also demonstrated the regulatory role of VD on the expression of some other cytokines secreted by CD8 + T cells, such as IL-6, IL-12, TNF-α, IL-5, and TGF-β.

22.3.3 Cytokines in regulation of vitamin D-metabolizing enzymes

Renal CYP27B1 is mainly regulated by PTH (produced in response to low calcium status), FGF23 (produced in the bone to inhibit CYP27B1 in response to elevated serum phosphates), and calcitriol itself (Kägi et al., 2018). Regarding the regulation of extrarenal CYP27B1 synthesis, it was established to be tissue-specific and strongly dependent on cytokines. This is the case for INF-γ and TNF-α, for which it has been shown that they stimulate CYP27B1 production in monocytes and macrophages without

PTH involvement. Moreover, CYP27B1 in immune cells is not negatively regulated by $1,25(OH)_2D_3$ and the role for CYP24A1 is also negligible. Importantly, the key limiting factor for efficient calcitriol synthesis in immune cells is the availability of $25OHD_3$ (Overbergh et al., 2006). Similarly as in immune cells, keratinocytes also demonstrated the stimulatory potential of INF-γ and TNF-α on CYP27B1 expression. Calcitriol was not active to directly inhibit this gene. However, calcitriol can restrict its own abundance in the epidermis by inducing the catabolizing enzyme CYP24A1. $1,25(OH)_2D_3$-induced transcription of CYP24A1 is readily implementable due to the presence of multiple VD response elements (VDRE) within its gene promoter (Xie et al., 2002).

These findings suggest that increased CYP24A1 expression and activity elicited by cytokines, along with insufficient substrate accessibility could be important limiting factors for calcitriol synthesis that might lead to impaired VD signaling in immune and other extrarenal cells and contribute to inflammation. A closer look at whether other proinflammatory cytokines could determine the abnormal outcome of calcitriol action in the immune system, affecting the enzymes that metabolize VD, is warranted. The overall effect of VD on the immune system is summarized in Fig. 22.1.

22.4 Vitamin D and diabetes mellitus

22.4.1 Vitamin D modulates β-cell function

The term "diabetes mellitus" describes multifactorial metabolic disease characterized by hyperglycemia as the result of defects in insulin secretion (type 1 diabetes, T1D) and/or the obstruction of insulin function in target tissues (type 2 diabetes, T2D). T1D is an autoimmune disease caused by the progressive T cell-mediated destruction of insulin-producing β cells in the pancreas. The triggers for the autoimmune attack have not been fully elucidated, but it is now widely accepted that both environmental and genetic factors are important contributors. The discovery of *VDR* and *CYP27B1* coexpression in pancreatic islet cells along with their expression in activated CD4+ and CD8+ T lymphocytes, B cells, granulocytes, and antigen-presenting cells (macrophages and DCs) supports the putative role of an impaired vitamin D pathway in autoimmune diabetes.

Variations at genes within the MHC (in humans, also referred to as the HLA complex) can be the key genetic determinants of T1D development. The most recognized is the association of T1D with polymorphisms of HLA II genes encoding DQ and DR (3). The DR–DQ haplotypes conferring the highest risk are HLA-DRB1*03 (DR3), typically present in haplotypic association with DQA1*05:01-DQB1*02:01 (DQ2), and HLA-DRB1*04 (DR4) observed in haplotypic association with DQA1*03-DQB1*03:02 (DQ8). It is precisely in conjunction with these variants of HLA II on APCs that the autoantigens are presented to Ths in the thymus and peripheral tissues, particularly in the lymph nodes surrounding the pancreas (Sharp et al., 2018). The most well-known autoantigens include preproinsulin, insulinoma-associated antigen from the family of transmembrane tyrosine protein phosphatases 2, glutamate decarboxylase, and zinc transporter (ZnT8). Upon the action of the stimulus, CD4 + Th1 cells induce pancreatic β cell destruction by stimulating CD8 + killer T cells to attack the Langerhans islets. VD deficiency causes an increased formation of CD4 + Th1 cells and the propagation of proinflammatory cytokines occurs. 1,25$(OH)_2D_3$ was indicated to suppress the proliferation of Th1 cells and their ability to produce cytokines. As a consequence of reduced secretion of IL-2 and IFN-γ by CD4 + cells and the stimulation of IL-5 and IL-10 secretion, the immune system switches from the Th1 to tolerogenic Th2 cell response (Alfonso et al, 2009).

In addition to immunomodulating properties, VD seems to play a role in the regulation of insulin secretion from β cells. VD deficiency in rodents negatively affects glucose-stimulated insulin secretion and human epidemiological studies also link poor VD status with T1D and T2D. Preincubation of mouse and human islets with 1,25$(OH)_2D_3$ enhances glucose-stimulated insulin secretion and increases glucose-stimulated calcium influx. The R-type voltage-gated calcium channel gene, *Cacna1e* (genetic variability of the major subunit), which contains a conserved VDRE in intron 7, was shown to be highly upregulated by 1,25$(OH)_2D_3$ in human and mouse islets (Kjalarsdottir et al., 2018). Evidence from in vitro studies has demonstrated that pancreatic islets, similar to immune cells, express VDR and 25-hydroxyvitamin D-1α-hydroxylase, suggesting that local production of 1,25$(OH)_2D_3$ is vital for normal islets functioning. Pancreas can also respond to circulating levels of calcitriol (Wolden-Kirk et al., 2013). However, while an in vitro trial revealed stimulatory action on preproinsulin mRNA in cultured islets isolated from fed rats, there was no effect of calcitriol in vivo. Nevertheless, vitamin D restored insulin secretion in vitamin D-deficient animals (Bourlon et al., 1999).

More recently, dedifferentiation has been identified as one of the mechanisms of β cell failure associated with T2D. In a study on mouse insulinoma cell line cultured in a high-glucose environment, treatment with VD normalized decreased VDR activity and enhanced the expression of essential transcription factors, such as Pdx1 and MafA, subsequently increasing Ins1 and Ins2 expression and protecting β cells against pathological dedifferentiation (Neelankal John et al., 2018).

22.4.2 Vitamin D—auto/paracrine system in diabetes mellitus

VD insufficiency/deficiency is common in subjects with T1D and T2D; however whether this association is causal remains largely undefined. Regarding the mechanisms of vitamin deficiency in T1D, the interplay of genetic, nutrition, and environmental factors seems to affect the circulating level of the VD status marker, 25OHD. As VD biosynthesis and its signaling are regulated by genes encoding the VDR and enzymes for calciferol activation, their polymorphisms may significantly alter the bioavailability and specific effects of VD metabolites. The increased risk for T1D was shown to be closely related to low 25OHD resulting from VD pathway polymorphisms (e.g., *VDR*, *CYP2R1*, *CYP27B1*, *VDBP*, and *cubulin*). For a comprehensive review please see Penna-Martinez and Badenhoop (2017). Available data, however, indicate variable genetic predispositions to T1D that depend on the ethnic origin of the populations studied.

As VD deficiency was shown to enhance the risk for T1D, it provided the rationale for vitamin D supplementation to manage this disease. The therapeutic benefits from VD treatment on T1D were found in some clinical trials (Grammatiki et al., 2017). Significant positive effects of vitamin D supplementation in the form of alphacalcidole and cholecalciferol on daily insulin dose, fasting, and stimulated C-peptide levels were observed in patients newly diagnosed with T1D, whereas supplementation with calcitriol had no effect (Gregoriou et al., 2017). Intervention trials and meta-analyses demonstrated vitamin D's potential to prevent the development of T1D in infants (Hypponen et al., 2001). Intervention trials also proved the specific requirements of adequate VD doses to achieve VD sufficiency. Treg cells of patients with T1D who received cholecalciferol at a dose of 4000 IU daily for 3 months demonstrated a differential response to VD action according to VDR single nucleotide polymorphisms (Moran-Auth et al., 2015). These data suggest that doses may need to be personalized to achieve targeted effects due to pharmacogenomic variations in T1D.

Moreover, many human observational studies have associated low VD status with the incidence of metabolic syndrome and T2D. Similar to T1D genetic analysis, several polymorphisms have been described in VDR genes that are capable of altering VDR protein activity and can be ascribed to the development of metabolic syndrome and T2D (Karonova et al., 2018; Han et al., 2017). However, the results of VD intervention trials have been inconsistent. Some observations found that VD supplementation significantly improved the glycemic control and the metabolic parameters in patients with prediabetes and diabetes. Several other meta-analyses showed that VD had no significant effects on fasting glucose, glycated hemoglobin, and insulin resistance in T2D patients.

Only a limited number of experimental trials address the diabetes-associated disturbances in the VD pathway and their prevention by VD supplementation using animal models. In our prior experiments conducted in STZ-induced diabetic male rats, we investigated the role of vitamin D in the regulation of CYP27B1 and VDR expression at transcriptional and translational levels in different tissues of T1D rats (Mazanova et al., 2018). It was shown that T1D caused a decrease in blood 25OHD that correlated with downregulation of CYP27A1 and CYP2R1 expression. VD deficiency was accompanied by elevated synthesis of renal CYP27B1 and VDR. Conversely, CYP27B1 and VDR expression decreased in the liver, bone tissue, and bone marrow. We also revealed a strong increase (interim data) in the expression of the mRNA of the main VD catabolic enzyme CYP24A1 in the liver and kidneys that could be one of the likely mechanisms explaining VD deficiency and the impairment of its signaling in the experimental T1D. Cholecalciferol supplementation at a dose of 1000 IU/per kg of body weight for 30 days was effective in correcting impaired VD—endo/para/autocrine systems in the kidneys and extrarenal tissues of diabetic rats.

22.4.3 Antiinflammatory effect of vitamin D in diabetes mellitus

Some of the previously mentioned mechanisms linking VD to the regulation of the immune response support a role for the VD—endo/para/autocrine system disorders in the pathogenesis of inflammatory and autoimmune diseases, including diabetes mellitus. Accordingly T1D has been associated with VD deficiency and the onset of autoimmunity in diabetes was established to be preceded by a proinflammatory cytokine profile in serum (Grammatiki et al., 2017). However, the existing observational data are still scarce as to whether there is any causal link between VD deficiency and proinflammatory processes in the manifestation of autoimmune diabetes.

Several clinical investigations have shown that VD either preserved the function of β cells from autoimmune destruction, or made it difficult to reduce the residual β cell function in children and adults with T1D, yet a few trials did not find any role for VD supplementation (Shih et al., 2016). A study of VD effect on Treg cells in TD1 patients revealed an improved suppressive capacity of Treg cells after the treatment as compared with placebo control (Treiber et al., 2015) (Fig. 22.3). Calcitriol has been shown to increase phospho-STAT6, IL-4, and IL-10 levels, as well as arginase activity, and lowers phospho-STAT4, IFN-γ, and IL-17 levels in recent-onset human T1D (Ysmail-Dahlouk et al., 2016). In accordance with these data, calcitriol supplementation decreased serum and urinary levels of inflammatory markers, such as IL-6, TNF-α, and ICAM-1, in diabetic patients (Mao et al., 2014).

It has been previously shown that the treatment of nonobese diabetic (NOD) mice with a vitamin D analog arrests the progression of insulitis,

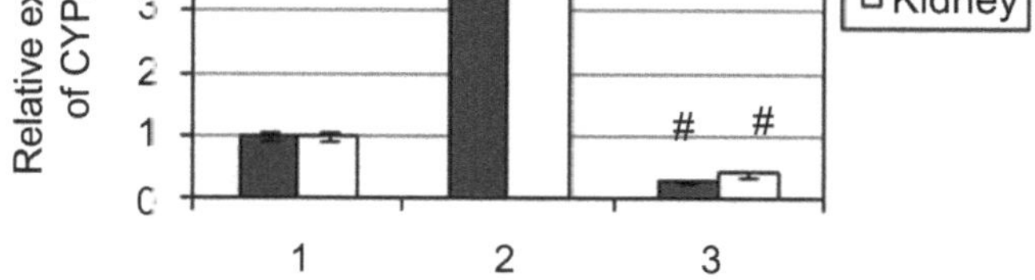

Figure 22.3 mRNA level of CYP24A1 in liver and kidney of diabetic rats and after vitamin D_3 treatment.
Transcript level (mRNA) of CYP24A1 was determined by real-time quantitative polymerase chain reaction (RT-PCR): 1, control group; 2, T1D group; 3, T1D + 100 IU of vitamin D_3 group. Data were normalized to glyceraldehyde 3-phosphate dehydrogenase, pooled from three independent experiments ($n = 6$ rats/group) and calculated using the ΔΔCt method. Results are expressed as mean ± SEM.*$P \leq .05$ versus control group; $^{\#}P \leq .05$ versus diabetes group.

blocks Th1 cell infiltration into the pancreas, and markedly reduces T1D development (Giarratana et al., 2004). Along with the established increase in insulin secretion and suppression of the demise of pancreatic β cells after cholecalciferol administration, animal models also confirmed that the beneficial effect of VD may be due to its antiinflammatory effect. VD decreased interferon γ-positive CD8 + T cells and elevated CD4 + CD25 + FoxP3 + T cells in pancreatic lymph nodes of NOD mice (Takiishi et al., 2014). Moreover, $1{,}25(OH)_2D_3$ administration to nonobese and nondiabetic mice strongly modulated chemokine and cytokine profiles and prevented diabetes, however, calcitriol elicited unwanted calcemic side effects (Gysemans et al., 2005).

The effect of VD on the T cell segment of the immune system has been the subject of a recent study conducted by our research group on a mouse model of autoimmune diabetes. As is known, the ratio of CD4 + to CD8 + lymphocyte subsets can partially reflect proinflammatory and autoimmune processes in the body (Chen et al., 2014). Consistent with this view, we, in turn, showed that T1D mellitus was accompanied by a shift in the ratio of subsets of peripheral blood lymphocytes as well as spleen lymphocytes toward the prevalence of CD4 + T cells, and these changes were observed under conditions of pronounced deficiency in serum 25OHD (Labudzynskyi et al., 2016a,b). Altered CD4 + /CD8 + ratio can be attributed, at least partially, to an increase in the number of Th1 and Th17 cells, which, unlike Th2, secrete proinflammatory cytokines and are involved in autoimmune reactions (Alfonso et al., 2009). T lymphocytes isolated from the spleen of diabetic animals showed a higher level of inflammatory markers, such as the NF-κB p65 subunit phosphorylated at Serine 311. It was also found that the phytohemagglutinin-induced proliferative activity of the whole fraction of spleen T lymphocyte decreases almost twofold in T1D. Cholecalciferol treatment revealed its significant normalizing effect on the ratio of CD4 + to CD8 + T cells both in the blood and in the spleen. Additionally, VD increased proliferative activity of spleen lymphocytes and diminished the level of activated phospho-p65/NF-kB and its nuclear translocation in spleen T cells.

In line with numerous studies that have found that chronic inflammation is one of the hallmark mechanisms of diabetes-associated complications, we further confirmed the antiinflammatory effects of VD in liver injury related to experimental T1D. Our findings have shown a possible link (Fig. 22.4) between VD deficiency in T1D and increased hepatic levels of IL-6 and osteopontin mRNA (Labudzynskyi et al., 2016a,b), and

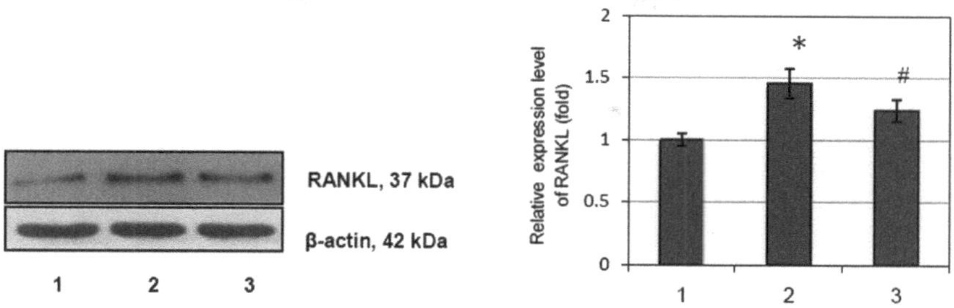

Figure 22.4 Protein level of RANKL in liver tissue of diabetic rats and after vitamin D_3 treatment.
Protein level of RANKL was determined by western-blot analysis: 1, control group; 2, T1D group; 3, T1D + 100 IU of vitamin D_3 group. Representative immunoblots are quantified using β-actin as a loading control. The bar graphs of RANKL are presented as mean ± SEM.*$P \leq .05$ versus control group; $^{\#}P \leq .05$ versus diabetes group.

protein levels of RANKL (unpublished data). Enhanced RANKL content may have either a protective or deteriorating role in inflammation-associated liver injury induced by diabetes. VD supplementation exerted a beneficial effect on inflammatory processes in liver tissue related to T1D.

T2D is characterized by hyperglycemia as a result of a combination of insulin resistance in peripheral tissues and insufficient insulin secretion from pancreatic islet β-cells. There is accumulating evidence that the activation of inflammatory pathways interferes with the metabolism of insulin and impairs its signaling. In turn, insulin resistance results in an enhanced expression of proinflammatory cytokines that cause inflammatory response and low-intensity chronic inflammation, further exacerbating insulin resistance. Meta-analysis of prospective studies have shown that elevated levels of inflammatory cytokines (IL-1β, IL-6, IL-18, and CRP), TNF-α, and low levels of adiponectin strongly correlate with T2D risk (Liu et al., 2016). Only a few clinical trials have been conducted to test the efficacy of VD supplementation on inflammatory markers in T2D, with controversial results. A recent meta-analysis of randomized controlled trials indicates VD's ability to enhance leptin levels with a reducing effect on CRP and TNF-α levels that improved the chronic low-grade inflammation in diabetic patients (Mousa et al., 2018). Nevertheless, in several other studies VD supplementation did not have any positive influence on TNF-α and IL-6 levels, β-cell function, insulin sensitivity, or glycemic control in T2D subjects (Wagner et al., 2016).

T2D animal studies showed that VD administration improved the glycemic index and insulin resistance by decreasing the levels of

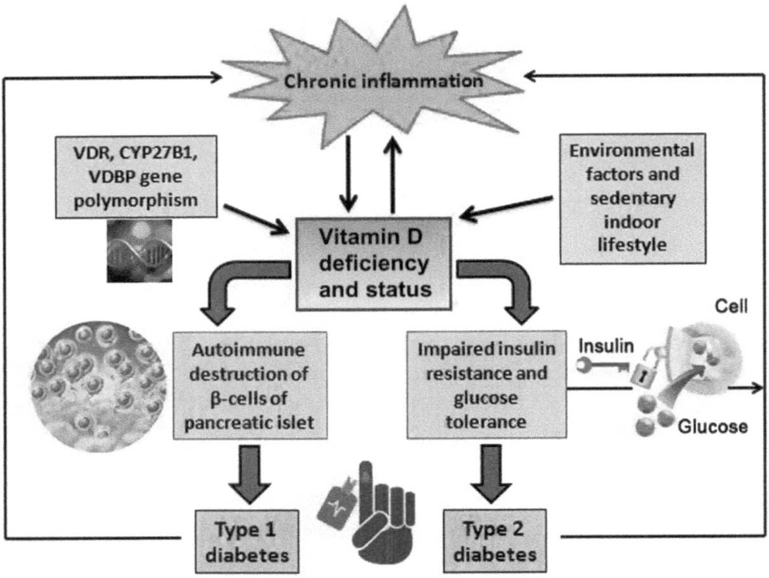

Figure 22.5 Proposed scheme linking vitamin D deficiency to inflammation and diabetes mellitus.

insulin-degrading enzymes and activating the phosphorylation of insulin receptors. The VDR agonist paricalcitol was shown to modulate the markers of pancreatic oxidative stress (catalase, syperoxide dismutase, and glutathione peroxidase) and inflammation (C-peptide, adiponectin, IL-2, and TNF-α) in T2D rats, significantly lowering blood glucose and insulin resistance (Ali et al., 2018) (Fig. 22.5).

22.5 Conclusions

Calcitriol modulates the transcription of various genes, particularly those involved in mineral metabolism and in noncalcemic functions, including immune regulation. Changes in cytochrome activities responsible for the formation of hydroxylated metabolites of cholecalciferol can play a crucial role in disturbing the bioavailability of VD and VDR-mediated cellular signaling linked to the development of widespread chronic diseases. Epidemiological and observational studies have reported an association between low plasma levels of 25OHD and the risk of type 1 and 2 diabetes mellitus. Several studies have shown that inherited variation in VD genes is associated with diabetes, supporting a genetic etiological role for VD deficiency related to the disease.

VD deficiency may predispose to altered insulin secretion and hyperglycemia either through direct action via VDR activation, or indirectly through augmented inflammatory processes and autoimmunity. VD supplementation prevents the inflammation by downregulating proinflammatory and upregulating antiinflammatory factors. The antiinflammatory effect of VD has been proven to counteract the initiation and progression of diabetes. On the other hand, there is growing evidence that low-intensity chronic inflammation may, in turn, interfere with the normal metabolism of VD, resulting in exacerbated proinflammatory cytokines expression (Fig. 22.5). Some of the current conflicting results regarding insignificant effects of VD supplementation or the lack of an association between VD status and diabetes may be related to a predisposing role for VDR polymorphisms and those of the VD metabolism genes. Future directions may address the relevance of these polymorphisms to immune regulation in diabetes mellitus and other immune-mediated diseases.

References

Akiyama, T., Shinzawa, M., Akiyama, N., 2012. RANKL–RANK interaction in immune regulatory systems. World J. Orthop. 3, 142–150.

Alfonso, B., Liao, E., Busta, A., Poretsky, L., 2009. Vitamin D in diabetes mellitus—a new field of knowledge poised for D-velopment. Diabetes Metabol. Res. Rev. 25, 417–419.

Ali, T., El Esawy, B., Elaskary, A., 2018. Effect of paricalcitol on pancreatic oxidative stress, inflammatory markers, and glycemic status in diabetic rats. Ir. J. Med. Sci. 187, 75–84.

Barragan, M., Good, M., Kolls, J., 2015. Regulation of dendritic cell function by vitamin D. Nutrients 7, 8127–8151.

Barrat, F., Cua, D., Boonstra, A., Richards, D., Crain, C., Savelkoul, H., et al., 2002. In vitro generation of interleukin 10-producing regulatory CD4+ T cells is induced by immunosuppressive drugs and inhibited by T helper type 1 (Th1)- and Th2-inducing cytokines. J.Exp. Med. 195, 603–616.

Bhalla, A.K., Paavonen, T., Williams, M., Delves, P., Lydyard, P., 1991. Regulation of interleukin-1 and tumour necrosis factor gene expression in myelomonocytic cell lines by 1,25-dihydroxyvitamin D_3. Immunology 72, 61–64.

Bikle, D., 2014. Vitamin D metabolism, mechanism of action, and clinical applications. Chem. Biol. 21, 319–329.

Bikle, D., 2016. Extraskeletal actions of vitamin D. Ann. N. Y. Acad. Sci. 1376, 29–52.

Bivona, G., Agnello, L., Ciaccio, M., 2017. Vitamin D and immunomodulation: is it time to change the reference values? Ann. Clin. Lab. Sci. 47, 508–510.

Bourlon, P., Billaudel, B., Faure-Dussert, A., 1999. Influence of vitamin D_3 deficiency and 1,25 dihydroxyvitamin D3 on de novo insulin biosynthesis in the islets of the rat endocrine pancreas. J. Endocrinol. 160, 87–95.

Brosbøl-Ravnborg, A., Bundgaard, B., Höllsberg, P., 2013. Synergy between vitamin D_3 and Toll-like receptor agonists regulates human dendritic cell response during maturation. Clin. Dev. Immunol. 2013, 807971.

Chambers, E., Suwannasaen, D., Mann, E., Urry, Z., Richards, D., Lertmemongkolchai, G., et al., 2014. 1α,25-Dihydroxyvitamin D_3 in combination with transforming growth factor-β increases the frequency of Foxp3 + regulatory T cells through preferential expansion and usage of interleukin-2. Immunology 143, 52–60.

Chen, J., Bruce, D., Cantorna, M., 2014. Vitamin D receptor expression controls proliferation of naive $CD8^+$ T cells and development of CD8 mediated gastrointestinal inflammation. BMC Immunol. 15, 6.

Christakos, S., Dhawan, P., Verstuyf, A., Verlinden, L., Carmeliet, G., 2016. Vitamin D: metabolism, molecular mechanism of action, and pleiotropic effects. Physiol. Rev. 96, 365–408.

Corripio-Miyar, Y., Mellanby, R., Morrison, K., McNeilly, T., 2017. 1,25-Dihydroxyvitamin D_3 modulates the phenotype and function of monocyte derived dendritic cells in cattle. BMC Vet. Res. 13, 390.

Di Rosa, M., Malaguarnera, G., De Gregorio, C., Palumbo, M., Nunnari, G., Malaguarnera, L., 2012. Immuno-modulatory effects of vitamin D_3 in human monocyte and macrophages. Cell. Immunol. 280, 36–43.

Fleet, J., 2017. The role of vitamin D in the endocrinology controlling calcium homeostasis. Mol. Cell. Endocrinol. 453, 36–45.

Giarratana, N., Penna, G., Amuchastegui, S., Mariani, R., Daniel, K., Adorini, L., 2004. A vitamin D analog down-regulates proinflammatory chemokine production by pancreatic islets inhibiting T cell recruitment and type 1 diabetes development. J. Immunol. 173, 2280–2287.

Grammatiki, M., Rapti, E., Karras, S., Ajjan, R., Kotsa, K., 2017. Vitamin D and diabetes mellitus: causal or casual association? Rev. Endocr. Metab. Disord. 18, 227–241.

Gregoriou, E., Mamais, I., Tzanetakou, I., Lavranos, G., Chrysostomou, S., 2017. The effects of vitamin D supplementation in newly diagnosed type 1 dabetes patients: systematic review of randomized controlled trials. Rev. Diabet. Stud. 14, 260–268.

Gysemans, C., Cardozo, A., Callewaert, H., Giulietti, A., Hulshagen, L., Bouillon, R., et al., 2005. 1,25-Dihydroxyvitamin D_3 modulates expression of chemokines and cytokines in pancreatic islets: implications for prevention of diabetes in nonobese diabetic mice. Endocrinology 146, 1956–1964.

Han, F., Lv, Y., Gong, L., Liu, H., Wan, Z., Liu, L., 2017. VDR Gene variation and insulin resistance related diseases. Lipids Health Dis. 16, 157.

Hoseinzadeh, E., Taha, P., Wei, C., Godini, H., Ashraf, G.M., Taghavi, M., et al., 2018. The impact of air pollutants, UV exposure and geographic location on vitamin D deficiency. Food Chem. Toxicol. 113, 241–254.

Hypponen, E., Laara, E., Reunanen, A., Jarvelin, M., Virtanen, S., 2001. Intake of vitamin D and risk of type 1 diabetes: a birth-cohort study. Lancet 358, 1500–1503.

Jeffery, L., Burke, F., Mura, M., Zheng, Y., Qureshi, O., Hewison, M., et al., 2009. 1,25-Dihydroxyvitamin D_3 and IL-2 combine to inhibit T cell production of inflammatory cytokines and promote development of regulatory T cells expressing CTLA-4 and FoxP3. J. Immunol. 183, 5458–5467.

Kägi, L., Bettoni, C., Pastor-Arroyo, E., Schnitzbauer, U., Hernando, N., Wagner, C., 2018. Regulation of vitamin D metabolizing enzymes in murine renal and extrarenal tissues by dietary phosphate, FGF23, and $1,25(OH)_2D_3$. PLoS One 13, e0195427.

Karonova, T., Grineva, E., Belyaeva, O., Bystrova, A., Jude, E., Andreeva, A., et al., 2018. Relationship between vitamin D status and vitamin D receptor gene polymorphisms with markers of metabolic syndrome among adults. Front. Endocrinol. (Lausanne) 9, 448.

Kjalarsdottir, L., Tersey, S., Vishwanath, M., Chuang, J., Posner, B., Mirmira, R., et al., 2018. 1,25-Dihydroxyvitamin D_3 enhances glucose-stimulated insulin secretion in mouse and human islets: a role for transcriptional regulation of voltage-gated calcium channels by the vitamin D receptor. J. Steroid Biochem. Mol. Biol. 185, 17–26 (ahead of print).

Labudzynskyi, D., Manoylov, K., Shymansky, I., Veliky, M., 2016a. Immunoregulatory effects of vitamin D_3 in experimentally induced type 1 diabetes. Cytol. Genet. 50, 231–240.

Labudzynskyi, D., Shymanskyy, I., Veliky, M., 2016b. Role of vitamin D_3 in regulation of interleukin-6 and osteopontin expression in liver of diabetic mice. Eur. Rev. Med. Pharmacol. Sci. 20, 2916–2919.

Liu, C., Feng, X., Li, Q., Wang, Y., Li, Q., Hua, M., 2016. Adiponectin, TNF-α and inflammatory cytokines and risk of type 2 diabetes: a systematic review and meta-analysis. Cytokine 86, 100–109.

Lu, M., Taylor, B., Körner, H., 2018. Genomic effects of the vitamin D receptor: potentially the link between vitamin D, immune cells, and multiple sclerosis. Front. Immunol. 9, 477.

Mahon, B., Wittke, A., Weaver, V., Cantorna, M., 2003. The targets of vitamin D depend on the differentiation and activation status of CD4 positive T cells. J. Cell. Biochem. 89, 922–932.

Mao, L., Ji, F., Liu, Y., Zhang, W., Ma, X., 2014. Calcitriol plays a protective role in diabetic nephropathy through anti-inflammatory effects. Int. J. Clin. Exp. Med. 7, 5437–5444.

Mazanova, A., Shymanskyi, I., Lisakovska, O., Hajiyeva, L., Komisarenko, Y., Veliky, M., 2018. Effects of cholecalciferol on key components of vitamin D-endo/para/autocrine system in experimental type 1 diabetes. Int. J. Endocrinol. 2018, 2494016.

Moran-Auth, Y., Penna-Martinez, M., Badenhoop, K., 2015. VDR FokI polymorphism is associated with a reduced T-helper cell population under vitamin D stimulation in type 1 diabetes patients. J. Steroid Biochem. Mol. Biol. 148, 184–186.

Mousa, A., Naderpoor, N., Teede, H., Scragg, R., de Courten, B., 2018. Vitamin D supplementation for improvement of chronic low-grade inflammation in patients with type 2 diabetes: a systematic review and meta-analysis of randomized controlled trials. Nutr. Rev. 76, 380–394.

Neelankal John, A., Iqbal, Z., Colley, S., Morahan, G., Makishima, M., Jiang, F., 2018. Vitamin D receptor-targeted treatment to prevent pathological dedifferentiation of pancreatic β cells under hyperglycaemic stress. Diabetes Metab. 44, 269–280.

Overbergh, L., Stoffels, K., Waer, M., Verstuyf, A., Bouillon, R., Mathieu, C., 2006. Immune regulation of 25-hydroxyvitamin D-1alpha-hydroxylase in human monocytic THP1 cells: mechanisms of interferon-gamma-mediated induction. J. Clin. Endocrinol. Metab. 91, 3566-3374.

Penna, G., Adorini, L., 2000. 1-alpha-25-dihydroxyvitamin D_3 inhibits differentiation, maturation, activation, and survival of dendritic cells leading to impaired alloreactive T cell activation. J. Immunol. 164, 2405–2411.

Penna-Martinez, M., Badenhoop, K., 2017. Inherited variation in vitamin D genes and type 1 diabetes predisposition, Genes (Basel), 8. p. E125.

Pramyothin, P., Holick, M., 2012. Vitamin D supplementation: guidelines and evidence for subclinical deficiency. Curr. Opin. Gastroenterol. 28, 139–150.

Sato, E., Imafuku, S., Ishii, K., Itoh, R., Chou, B., Soejima, T., et al., 2013. Vitamin D-dependent cathelicidin inhibits mycobacterium marinum infection in human monocytic cells. J. Dermatol. Sci. 70, 166–172.

Sharp, S., Weedon, M., Hagopian, W., Oram, R., 2018. Clinical and research uses of genetic risk scores in type 1 diabetes. Curr. Opin. Genet. Dev. 50, 96–102.

Shih, E., Mittelman, S., Pitukcheewanont, P., Azen, C., Monzavi, R., 2016. Effects of vitamin D repletion on glycemic control and inflammatory cytokines in adolescents with type 1 diabetes. Pediatr. Diabetes 17, 36–43.
Skrobot, A., Demkow, U., Wachowska, M., 2018. Immunomodulatory role of vitamin D: a review. Adv. Exp. Med. Biol. 1108, 13–23.
Sun, D., Luo, F., Xing, J., Zhang, F., Xu, J., Zhang, Z., 2018. 1,25$(OH)_2D_3$ inhibited Th17 cells differentiation via regulating the NF-κB activity and expression of IL-17. Cell Prolif. 51, e12461.
Szymczak, I., Pawliczak, R., 2016. The active metabolite of vitamin D_3 as a potential immunomodulator. Scand. J. Immunol. 83, 83–91.
Takiishi, T., Ding, L., Baeke, F., Spagnuolo, I., Sebastiani, G., Laureys, J., et al., 2014. Dietary supplementation with high doses of regular vitamin D_3 safely reduces diabetes incidence in NOD mice when given early and long term. Diabetes 63, 2026–2036.
Treiber, G., Prietl, B., Frohlich-Reiterer, E., Lechner, E., Ribitsch, A., Fritsch, M., et al., 2015. Cholecalciferol supplementation improves suppressive capacity of regulatory T-cells in young patients with new-onset type 1 diabetes mellitus—a randomized clinical trial. Clin. Immunol. 161, 217–224.
Wagner, H., Alvarsson, M., Mannheimer, B., Degerblad, M., Ostenson, C., 2016. No effect of high-dose vitamin D treatment on β-cell function, insulin sensitivity, or glucose homeostasis in subjects with abnormal glucose tolerance: a randomized clinical trial. Diabetes Care 39, 345–352.
Wolden-Kirk, H., Overbergh, L., Gysemans, C., Brusgaard, K., Naamane, N., Van Lommel, L., et al., 2013. Unraveling the effects of 1,25OH2D3 on global gene expression in pancreatic islets. J. Steroid Biochem. Mol. Biol. 136, 68–79.
Xie, Z., Munson, S., Huang, N., Portale, A., Miller, W., Bikle, D., 2002. The mechanism of 1,25-dihydroxyvitamin D_3 autoregulation in keratinocytes. J. Biol. Chem. 277, 36987–36990.
Ysmail-Dahlouk, L., Nouari, W., Aribi, M., 2016. 1,25-Dihydroxyvitamin D_3 down-modulates the production of proinflammatory cytokines and nitric oxide and enhances the phosphorylation of monocyte-expressed STAT6 at the recent-onset type 1 diabetes. Immunol. Lett. 179, 122–130.

CHAPTER 23

Vitamin E: nutritional aspects

Pierangelo Torquato, Rita Marinelli, Desirée Bartolini and Francesco Galli
Departement of Pharmaceutical Science, University of Perugia, Laboratory of Clinical Biochemistry and Nutrition, Perugia, Italy

Contents

Key facts of vitamin E

- Vitamin E is an essential micronutrient represented by a group of molecules (four tocopherols and four tocotrienols).
- α-Tocopherol is the most important form of this vitamin.
- Fat-rich food is the main dietary source of vitamin E, especially edible oils and seeds.
- Vitamin E is a fat-soluble antioxidant used to preserve oxidizable lipids in food products as well as in cosmetics and pharmaceuticals (it prevents rancidity of fats and oils).
- The same antioxidant function is important to protect lipids in cells and body fluids, thus representing a natural antiaging component of human tissues.
- Vitamin E also influences the expression of groups of genes with physiological roles in the central nervous system, liver, blood, and immune system.

Molecular Nutrition
DOI: https://doi.org/10.1016/B978-0-12-811907-5.00019-1

- A deficiency of vitamin E is often a mild and benign condition obtained after a prolonged exposure to a reduced intake of the vitamin. Alternatively, it occurs secondarily to defects of the gastrointestinal tract associated with fat malabsorption and/or altered lipid metabolism.
- Severe deficiency occurs in the case of a genetic disorder known as ataxia with vitamin E deficiency (a defect in the hepatic binding protein of this vitamin associated with major neurological abnormalities)
- The liver controls the uptake and distribution of this vitamin to peripheral tissues and organs (illustrated in the accompanying Chapter 24, Vitamin E: metabolism and molecular aspects).
- The liver also prevents the accumulation of this vitamin by means of specific mechanisms of excretion and degradation (products of these processes are eliminated with feces and urine).
- Some physiological metabolites of vitamin E have been proposed to provide important biological functions alternative to the vitamin precursors.

Summary points

- This chapter focuses on the micronutrient vitamin E, a plant-derived family of molecules (four tocopherols and four tocotrienols).
- Edible oils and seeds are the main dietary sources of this vitamin, and in general it is abundantly represented in fat-rich food products.
- Often vitamin E is utilized as an antioxidant ingredient to preserve oxidizable lipids of food, cosmetics and pharmaceutical products.
- α-Tocopherol is the most represented and active form of vitamin E in human tissues.
- This is the main lipid antioxidant (H atom donor) of cellular membranes and possibly of intracellular fats (endosomes and vacuoles) and circulating lipoproteins.
- Vitamin E also binds to, and influences the activity of, specific cellular proteins includeing nuclear receptors, transcription factors, transporters, and enzyme proteins.
- Defects in the antioxidant and gene regulation function of this vitamin have been described and have been associated with alterations in physiological processes of the central nervous system (especially the cerebellum and hippocampus), liver tissue, immune system, and blood cells.
- Vitamin E deficiency is usually a low-grade and relatively benign condition (reversible with dietary or nutritional interventions). It is often

secondary to a lower intake of the vitamin or to a disease state, such as a defect of the gastrointestinal tract and malabsorption, liver and lipid metabolism disorders, etc.

- Severe deficiency is observed in a rare genetic disorder known as ataxia with vitamin E deficiency, this is a defect of the α-TOH binding protein gene that encodes for a hepatic protein responsible for vitamin E binding and distribution with the circulating lipoproteins to all extrahepatic tissues.
- The liver controls the metabolism of this vitamin through its vitamer-selective uptake and lipoprotein-mediated distribution to peripheral tissues, and elimination of vitamin excess by means of specific mechanisms of catabolism and excretion (essentially with bile).
- Some of the metabolites produced during its catabolism are potent modulators of inflammatory and lipid metabolism pathways, compatible with a provitamin mechanism already described for other fat-soluble vitamins, such as vitamin A and D (described in the accompanying Chapter 24, Vitamin E: metabolism and molecular aspects).

23.1 General concepts and historical steps in vitamin E research

We write this chapter in a time of renewed interest toward one of the most studied and marketed vitamins ever. Scientific investigation into vitamin E has been very extensive for nearly a century of history from its discovery in 1922 (Evans and Bishop, 1922), with about 50,000 items retrieved in PubMed and a trend in publication time-course (Fig. 23.1) showing steady growth of interest up to 2005 that has been identified as "*Annus Horribilis*" of vitamin E due to the publication of negative results coming from a meta-analysis of clinical trials.[1] Recent projections however demonstrate that the bad moments are over. From 2008 onward, the number of publications started again to rise with a wealth of studies on different aspects that include

[1] In 2005 Miller et al. (2005) published a dose-response meta-analysis showing that high-dosage (≥400 IU/d, corresponding to 268 mg/d of α-tocopherol) vitamin E supplementation was associated with a small, but statistically significant, increased risk of mortality (relative risk, 1.04 [95% CI, 1.01−1.07]). In this study the authors concluded that "high-dosage vitamin E supplementation was likely to be harmful. Even in the best case, it offered no benefit in prolonging life." These findings however were highly controversial, and other studies criticized the methodology and conclusion of this meta-analysis (recently reviewed in Galli et al., 2017). However, since then concerns have been expressed by several authors in recommending dosages higher than that dose, especially in subjects at a higher risk of cardiovascular disease.

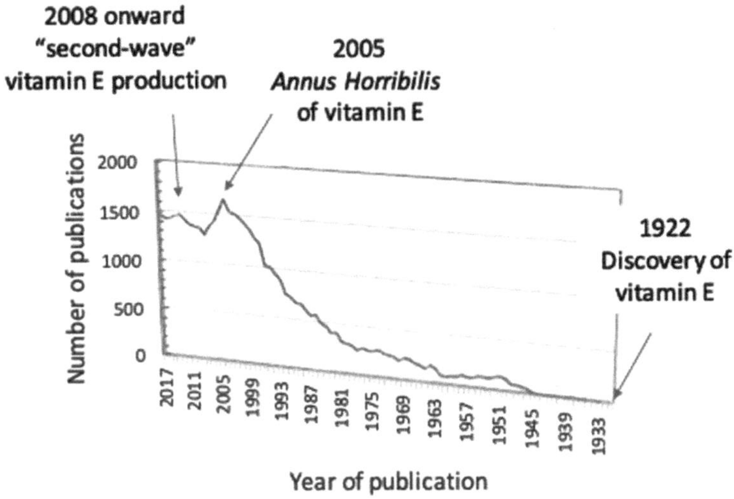

Figure 23.1 PubMed search on vitamin E publications. Retrieved items (all type) at October 2018 are shown together with three moments of the publication curve highlighted that are discussed in the text as relevant for the evolution of this field; search terms were: vitamin E OR tocopherol OR tocotrienol OR tocopheryl.

emerging functions and already established health-promoting effects of vitamin E. Several of these studies are still pursuing the so far frustrating aim of defining the precise role of essential nutrient (discussed in section 23.3.1).

Natural and synthetic forms of vitamin E are among the most important and widespread ingredients of food products and the cosmetics industry (essentially as antioxidants and stabilizers of unsaturated lipids) and health-promoting effects are claimed for functional food and nutraceuticals that contain this vitamin in its different forms as the major active principle or coingredient. The demand of natural forms of this vitamin for all these applications is now increasing, as it is for many other ingredients of the food, cosmetics, and pharmaceutical industry.

The main steps in vitamin E's scientific history are summarized in Table 23.1. It was discovered in 1922 by Evans and Bishop as an unknown fat-soluble factor essential for rat fertility, that is, a compound capable of preventing fetal resorption in female rats (Evans and Bishop, 1922). A few years later Sure (1927) obtained the same results after performing similar experiments and called the substance "vitamin E" since vitamins A, B, C, and D were already known at that time. α-Tocopherol (α-TOH) was the first form of the vitamin to be isolated in pure form from

Table 23.1 The main steps of vitamin E history over a century of research.

1922	Discovery of vitamin E (terms coined by Sure in 1927) by Evans and Bishop as the X compound present in plants and essential for female rats' fertility	Evans and Bishop (1922) and Sure (1927)
1930	Isolation of in pure form from wheat germ	Evans et al. (1936)
	Identification of α-TOH structure	Fernholz (1938)
	Synthesis in racemic (*all*-rac) forms	Karrer et al. (1938)
1940	Identification of vitamin E as a fat-soluble chain-breaking antioxidant, followed by first studies defining differences between vitamers in terms of biological and antioxidant activity	Mattill (1947) and Tappel (1953)
1950	Discovery of urinary metabolites of vitamin E oxidation, the Simon's metabolites	Eisengart et al. (1956) and Gross et al. (1956)
1960	First isolation and characterization of tocotrienols	Schudel et al. (1963)
	Correlation between deficiency of vitamin E and pathological situations, such as anemia due to hemolysis caused by erythrocyte fragility and fat malabsorption syndrome	Kayden et al. (1965)
1970	Synthesis of tocotrienols by Scott	Scott et al. (1976)
	Identification of the gene defect of α-TTP causing an inherited disorder responsible for severe vitamin E deficiency	Catignani and Bieri (1977)
	Studies on the synergistic interaction of vitamin E with coantioxidants, such as vitamin C	Packer et al. (1979)
1980	Vitamin E identified as main fat-soluble antioxidant of human plasma	Burton et al. (1982)
	Identification in urine of short-chain metabolite of α-TOH synthesized in response to vitamin E excess	Chiku et al. (1984)
	First studies of vitamin E's influence on signal transduction and gene transcription pathways	Mahoney and Azzi (1988)

(*Continued*)

Table 23.1 (Continued)

1990	Vitamin E supplementation leads to relief of symptoms caused by different α-TTP mutations	Traber et al. (1990)
	First identification of CEHC in human serum	Stahl et al. (1999)
	Findings on vitamin E as a prooxidant in the absence of ascorbate	Bowry et al. (1992)
	Antioxidant effects associated with preventing liver lipid peroxidation and hepatotoxicity in CCl_4-treated animals	Parola et al. (1992)
	Murray et al. isolated from human urine a mild potency natriuretic factor the structure of which coincided with γ-CEH	Murray et al. (1995) and Kantoci et al. (1997)
	First identification of CEHC in human serum	Stahl et al. (1999)
2000	Identification of PXR nuclear receptor and CYP3A4 as key players of vitamin E metabolism	Birringer et al. (2001), Birringer et al. (2002), and Landes et al. (2003)
	Description of cytochrome P450-dependent tocopherol ω-hydroxylation pathway by Sontag And Parker	Sontag and Parker (2002)
	CEHCs measured in human blood and urine as biomarkers of physiological and disease-related metabolism of vitamin E	Galli et al. (2002, 2004c) and Himmelfarb et al. (2003)
	Demethyl CEHCs identified as modulators of cyclooxygenase-2 (COX-2) in inflammatory cells and cell cycle checkpoints of cancer cells	Jiang et al. (2000) and Galli et al. (2004a)
	α-Tocopheryl phosphate demonstrated to form as a physiological metabolite in different tissues and organisms	Munteanu et al. (2004) and Ogru et al. (2003)
	A function of vitamin E metabolism as an alternative to catabolism was proposed for the first time, vitamin E was suggested to behave as a provitamin and hormonal substance	Galli et al. (2007)

(*Continued*)

Table 23.1 (Continued)

	Demethyl LCMs as COX-2 inhibitors	Jiang et al. (2008)
	Setting up of a semisynthesis procedure to produce LCMs from garcinoic acid and first demonstration of anticancer activity of LCMs	Mazzini et al. (2009)
2010	13′-LCMs were demonstrated to be potent 5-lipoxygenase inhibitors with in vivo antiinflammatory activity	Jiang et al. (2011) and Pein et al. (2018)
	α-13′-LCMs first identified in human blood of healthy subjects	Ciffolilli et al. (2015) and Wallert et al. (2014)
	Vitamin E therapy introduced in clinical guidelines of NASH	Watanabe et al. (2015)
	13′-LCMs identified as PXR agonists	Podszun et al. (2017)
	α-13-LCMs and α-TQ quantified in healthy subjects and in chronic kidney disease and NAFLD patients	Giusepponi et al. (2017) and Torquato et al. (2019a)
Today	The aim of today's research remains that of providing a conclusive definition of essentiality for this "orphan" vitamin	

wheat germ (WG) in 1936 (Evans et al., 1936), and then in the unsaponifiable lipid fraction of different plants, of which the first to be investigated were lettuce, cottonseeds, and palm oil (Evans et al., 1936 and references therein). Its structure was determined by Fernholz (1938) together with its synthesis in the racemic (*all*-rac) form (Karrer et al., 1938).

Other forms of this vitamin have been identified as natural components of plant organisms and then of food products (Fig. 23.2). These include eight members (or vitamers) divided into two subfamilies: four TOHs and four tocotrienols (T3s). The latter are characterized by the presence of three double bonds on the side chain of the molecule, and were isolated for the first time in 1963 by Schudel et al. (1963) and synthesized by Scott et al. (1976). The number of methyl group substituents on the chroman ring identifies the four vitamers in each subfamily (designated the Greek letters α, β, γ, and δ), with the α form as the fully methylated

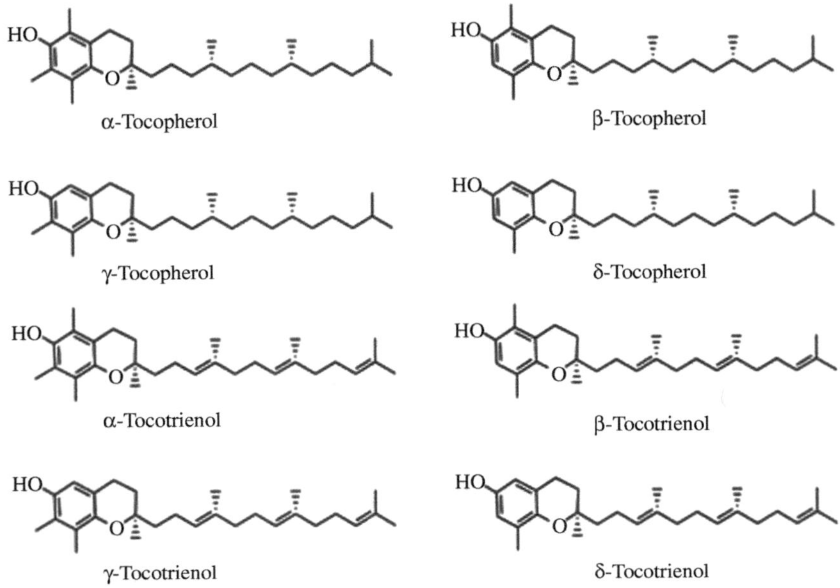

Figure 23.2 Chemical structures of tocopherols (TOHs) and tocotrienols (T3).

and the gamma as the dimethyl counterpart (Fig. 23.2). The identification of multiple TOHs and T3s forms stimulated comparative studies that demonstrated differences between the vitamers in terms of both the biological function (fertility test) and antioxidant activity. For example, TOHs were found to be increasingly effective as antioxidants in the order of magnitude $\alpha > \beta > \gamma > \delta$ as assessed by an oxidation test on lard (Mattill, 1947) and the same potency order was observed for the animal fertility test and other biological assays, some of which have been utilized to establish the adequate or recommended intake of this vitamin in humans, such as hydrogen peroxide-induced lysis of red blood cells or plasma lipid peroxidation (recently reviewed in Galli et al., 2017; Schmolz et al., 2016).

Soon after its discovery, the rat fertility effects of wheat germ oil (WGO) vitamin E were speculated to find support from the "antioxygenic" properties of this oil (Olcott and Mattill, 1931), and these pioneering studies paved the way to the identification of vitamin E as a fat-soluble antioxidant (originally reviewed in Mattill, 1947). That step of vitamin E history was boosted by the increasing interest on free radicals and their role in the oxidation chemistry of unsaturated lipids that in those years stimulated a number of studies on this chain reaction process and its inhibition by antioxidants. The latter became important subjects of basic and translational studies at the end of 1940s (Mattill, 1947; Tappel, 1953) and starting from that point, the definition of vitamin E as a "chain-breaking" antioxidant arose. Other steps that stimulated the attention of the scientific community on the antioxidant role of vitamin E were the identification of endogenous metabolites derived from its oxidation in animal and human urine, also known as Simon's metabolites (Eisengart et al., 1956; Gross et al., 1956), and then the demonstration in the 1980s that this vitamin is the main lipid-soluble antioxidant of human plasma (Burton et al., 1982). Further studies in the same years demonstrated the synergistic interaction of vitamin E with coantioxidants, essentially the water-soluble molecule ascorbate (vitamin C) identified by Packer et al. (1979).

The importance of such synergy was further confirmed by the evidence that in the absence of ascorbate, vitamin E can behave as a prooxidant leading to "TOH-mediated peroxidation" (Bowry et al., 1992). One of the strongest and clinically relevant pieces of evidence in support of the antioxidant role of this vitamin in vivo was the demonstration that vitamin E prevented lipid peroxidation and hepatotoxicity upon exposure of animal models to the free radical-generating agent CCl_4 (Parola et al., 1992). Later on, other antioxidants, such as ubiquinol ($Q_{10}H_2$) and various polyphenolics (Bowry et al., 1995), were demonstrated to be effective in inhibiting lipid peroxidation, not only in homogeneous solution, but also in heterogeneous systems such as membranes and lipoproteins (Niki and Noguchi, 2004), but their biological relevance as chain breakers of cell membranes and plasma lipids was demonstrated to be much lower in comparison with that of α-TOH, that is, the main fat-soluble H atom donor of human tissues (reviewed elsewhere in Forman et al., 2014; Traber and Atkinson, 2007).

In the 1960s, reports of vitamin E deficiency in humans with various fat malabsorption syndromes began to appear. Anemia due to hemolysis caused by erythrocyte fragility was reported as a common symptom in vitamin E-deficient humans (Kayden et al., 1965). The most relevant inherited disorder responsible for severe vitamin E deficiency was identified as a gene defect of hepatic α-TOH binding protein (α-TTP) (Catignani and Bieri, 1977) associated with impaired lipoprotein metabolism of α-TOH and severe neurologic symptomatology (Gotoda et al., 1995; Ouahchi et al., 1995). This disease was referred to as to "ataxia with vitamin E deficiency" (AVED; OMIM No. 277460). More than 20 different α-TTP mutations have been described in AVED subjects (Di Donato et al., 2010) and the symptomatology can be efficiently cured by vitamin E supplementation (Traber et al., 1990). In the 1980s vitamin E was identified as modulating signal transduction and gene transcription pathways of different cell models and tissues and this regulatory function was suggested to be independent from the antioxidant function of this vitamin.

In the same years, Chiku et al. (1984) reported on a urinary metabolite of δ-TOH that was not a free radical-generated oxidation product (as in the case of the Simon's metabolites mentioned before), but rather a tail-shortened, water-soluble compound synthesized in response to vitamin E excess and defined as a short-chain metabolite (SCM).

In 2002 Sontang and Parker described for the first time in hepatocyte maintained in culture the pathway involving the cytochrome P450-mediated omega-hydroxylation of the carbon ending of the TOH side chain to form the long-chain metabolite (LCM) "α-13′-OH" (Sontag and Parker, 2002). In those years, some molecular players of this metabolism had tentatively been identified and were proposed to include the nuclear receptor PXR as a main regulation hub for the series of detoxification/drug metabolizing genes that govern the different steps of vitamin E catabolism and excretion (Birringer et al., 2001, 2002; Landes et al., 2003). Then the importance, but not the exclusive role, of the liver in this metabolism was demonstrated (Parker et al., 2004).

Murray et al. (1995) isolated from human urine a mild potency natriuretic factor of which the structure was demonstrated to coincide with that of SCM γ-carboxyethyl hydroxychromanol (γ-CEHC) (Kantoci et al., 1997), and Jiang et al. (2000) described a modulation effect of desmethyl SCMs on cyclooxygenase-2 (COX-2) activity of inflammatory cells; soon after our laboratories described the inhibitory activity of these SCM on cell cycle checkpoints associated with cancer cell proliferation and apoptotic cell death (Galli et al., 2004a), respectively. After these pioneering studies, the hypothesis of a biological role for this metabolism alternative to vitamin E catabolism was suggested (Galli et al., 2007). In those years the possibility to prepare LCMs with a semisynthesis procedure based on a natural precursor of these metabolites purified from Garcinia kola (GK) seeds, that is, glutaric aciduria (Mazzini et al., 2009), provided an important opportunity to develop analytical strategies to assess their levels and formation mechanisms in humans, and then to test biological functions in different experimental contexts (recently reviewed in Schubert et al., 2018). A few years later Jiang and coworkers found that δ-TOH-derived 13′-LCMs are potent inhibitors of 5-lipoxygenase and possess in vivo antiinflammatory activity (Jiang et al., 2011 and references therein).

In the last three decades the formation process and levels of SCMs, MCMs, and LCMs have been investigated in different cell models as well as in liver and other solid tissues, in bile, feces, and urine of animal models and humans, as either free or conjugated forms (reviewed in Birringer, 2010; Torquato et al., 2016, 2019b). Recently, new analytical procedures (Russo et al., 2017; Torquato et al., 2018a, 2019b) have been developed to evaluate the complete series of enzymatic and free radical-derived metabolites of α-TOH in cell culture and tissue samples, and importantly in human blood. Applications of these studies in our laboratories and in other centers included the characterization of the human metabolome of vitamin E during supplementation studies in healthy subjects and in nutritional assessment of pathologies, such as chronic kidney disease, nonalcoholic fatty liver disease and steatohepatitis (NAFLD and NASH, respectively) and metabolic syndrome (Bartolini et al., 2017; Ciffolilli et al., 2015; Galli et al., 2004b; Russo et al., 2017; Traber et al., 2017).

In recent years an increasing number of investigations have demonstrated different biological effects for the LCMs formed by the ω-hydroxylase activity of cytochrome P450 and also for α-tocopheryl phosphate (recently reviewed in Galli et al., 2017; Schubert et al., 2018). Gene regulation and homeostatic effects of these metabolites have been demonstrated in different experimental models, such as inflammatory, neuronal, and hepatic cells, and in vivo in animal models of acute inflammation (Pein et al., 2018; Schmolz et al., 2014), and the molecular mechanisms underlying these responses are now under investigation in several laboratories. Such recent achievements conclude this excursus through the main steps of this almost 100-year history with new and intriguing perspectives on the biological and nutritional role(s) of this "orphan vitamin" (i.e., a vitamin that is still waiting to be assigned a specific vitamin function).

23.2 Antioxidant activity

Vitamin E is a fat-soluble antioxidant, one of the most important and widely employed in the preservation of autooxidizable lipid components in the food industry as well as in cosmetics.

In the characteristic reaction mechanism, tocochromanol directly reacts with a lipoperoxyl radical (LOO$^•$) through an H atom donation mechanism producing less reactive species, that is, a lipid peroxide (LOOH) and a tocopheryl radical (TO$^•$) (Fig. 23.3).

The H donating properties of vitamin E proposed in this reaction mechanism identify a Type I or chain-breaking antioxidant (Chaiyasit et al., 2007). This is distinct from secondary (Type II or preventive) antioxidants because the latter do not directly interact with FR, but prevent their formation by means of different processes that include, for example, metal chelation, repair of primary antioxidants, UV absorption, decomposition of reactive intermediates. In addition, there are tertiary (Type III or fixer) antioxidants that repair oxidatively damaged biomolecules,

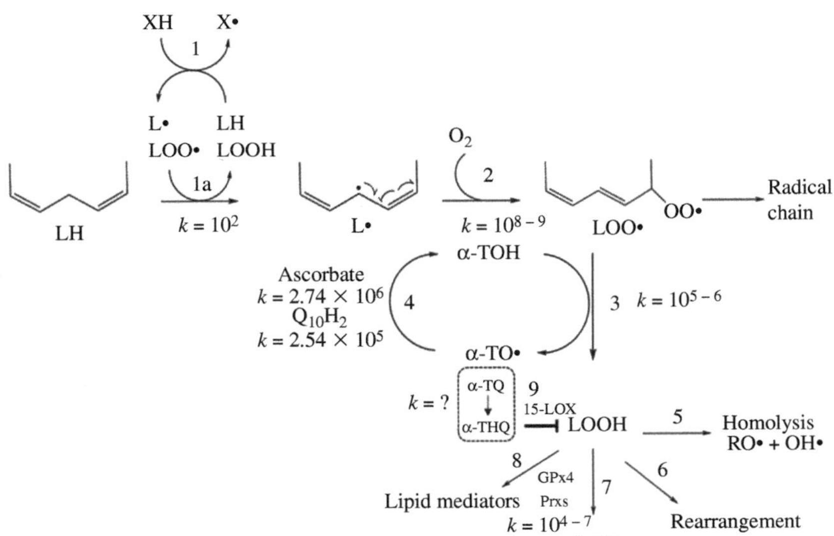

Figure 23.3 Lipid peroxidation and the antioxidant reaction of α-tocopherol (α-TOH). *LH*, polyunsaturated lipid; *L*$^•$, lipid radical; *LOO*$^•$, lipoperoxyl radical; *LOOH*, lipid hydroperoxide; *LOH*, lipid alcohol; α-*TO*$^•$, α-tocopheryl radical; α-*TQ*, α-tocopheryl quinone; α-*THQ*, α-tocopheryl hydroquinone. *k*, rate constants in M^{-1} s^{-1}. Steps 1–9 are discussed in the text. *Modified from Brigelius-Flohe, R., 2009. Vitamin E: the shrew waiting to be tamed. Free Radic. Biol. Med. 46, 543–554.*

essentially by H atom or electron transfer mechanism. All forms of vitamin E could be defined also as multifunctional antioxidants in that their activity includes more than one of these mechanisms (i.e., Type 1 + Type 3), and also affects enzymatic processes that cause lipid oxidation as well as enzymatic protection and repair pathways with transcriptional and kinetics effects. α-TOH can definitely not compete with cellular molecules (proteins, DNA, or even lipids) for the highly reactive hydroxyl or alkoxyl radicals, simply due to its much lower concentration and by its absence in soluble fractions. An antioxidant action for this vitamin, however, becomes conceivable if only lipid phases are considered (reviewed in Brigelius-Flohe, 2009).

The formation of the initiating radical ($X^{\bullet}$), which abstracts an H radical from unsaturated lipids, can be triggered by light, heat, traces of transition metal ion, and, of course, by other radicals or radical-producing chemicals such as azodyes (Fig. 23.3, reaction 1). Rate constants for the reaction of a lipoperoxyl radical ($LOO^{\bullet}$) or a lipid radical ($L^{\bullet}$) with lipids (LH) are about $10^2\ M^{-1}\ s^{-1}$ (Fig. 23.3, reaction 1a). The subsequent reaction of $L^{\bullet}$ with oxygen leading to $LOO^{\bullet}$ is almost diffusion controlled ($k = 10^8 - 10^9\ M^{-1}\ s^{-1}$) (Fig. 23.3, reaction 2). The resulting $LOO^{\bullet}$ propagates the radical chain if not scavenged, for example, by α-TOH (Fig. 23.3, reaction 3). The reaction rate between $LOO^{\bullet}$ and α-TOH is much faster ($k = 10^5 - 10^6\ M^{-1}\ s^{-1}$) than the reaction rate between $LOO^{\bullet}$ and an unsaturated fatty acid (Fig. 23.3, reaction 1a), which suggests that α-TOH always prevents lipid peroxidation by interfering with the propagation of the free radical chain at this particular site. A preferential reaction of $LOO^{\bullet}$ and α-TOH would, however, only occur if lipids and α-TOH were present in similar concentrations. The concentration of α-TOH in membranes, however, is about one molecule for every 100−1000 molecules of phospholipids. The ratio varies with the nature of the fatty acid species present in phospholipids and with the cellular organelle' structure, with the highest α-TOH content observed in lysosomes (Atkinson et al., 2008). Thus lipids and α-TOH react with $LOO^{\bullet}$ at best with comparable velocity (Brigelius-Flohe, 2009).

A reaction of α-TOH with $L^{\bullet}$ is possible in principle in view of the high rate constant ($k = 10^6\ M^{-1}\ s^{-1}$) (not shown in Fig. 23.3), but should be physiologically hard given the higher oxygen concentration compared with the α-TOH levels (Brigelius-Flohe, 2009). $\alpha TO^{\bullet}$ regeneration to α-TOH may occur through ascorbate-mediated H atom transfer (Fig. 23.3, reaction 4), a typical Type II or coantioxidant reaction

(Chaiyasit et al., 2007) occurring at the water interface of the lipid layer in that ascorbate is a hydrosoluble molecule. This coantioxidant reaction, however, is debated and in vivo evidence for an interplay between vitamin E and vitamin C is limited (Brigelius-Flohe, 2009).

Apart from ascorbate, $Q_{10}H_2$ can act as a coantioxidant by scavenging the $\alpha TO^{\bullet}$ (Bowry et al., 1995). The rate constant for the reaction between $\alpha TO^{\bullet}$ and $Q_{10}H_2$ in isopropanol/water is $2.54 \times 10^5\ M^{-1}\ s^{-1}$ (Mukai et al., 1992), which appears to be kinetically less efficient compared with ascorbate reaction ($k = 2.74 \times 10^6\ M^{-1}\ s^{-1}$); nevertheless, that rate could be high enough to let $Q_{10}H_2$ work as a TOH-regenerating system under physiological conditions and in specific membrane microenvironments (Itoh et al., 2008). For example, in mitochondria $Q_{10}H_2$ concentrations are high enough to allow an efficient recycling of α-TOH via the $Q_{10}H_2$ pool, which is continuously restored by the respiratory chain (Kagan et al., 1990; Maguire et al., 1992). However, $Q_{10}H_2$ levels are usually too low to allow any relevant turnover on the plasmalemma and other subcellular membranes (Upston et al., 1999), and this represents a major limit in figuring out an in vivo relevance of α-TOH regeneration by cellular quinols, which in fact remains to be proven of most tissues.

The intriguing question of whether the antioxidant potential of vitamin E, which is easily demonstrated in vitro, is actually available in vivo for protection against oxidative damage is still waiting for a conclusive answer. Currently, available markers of oxidative damage are unsuitable to solve this puzzle. Plasma malondialdehyde levels, pentane exhalation, plasma lipid hydroperoxide, F2-isoprostane or carbonyl concentrations, glutathione, and glutathione peroxidase 1 levels in erythrocytes, under various conditions have not consistently been changed by vitamin E supplementation (Dragsted, 2008). Also estimation of 8-oxo-7,8-dihydroguanine yielded equivocal conclusions (Loft et al., 2008). Metabolic products that selectively form during the free radical-mediated transformation of vitamin E (Fig. 23.4) are presumed to more reliably disclose its antioxidant action. The analysis of these oxidation compounds has been used to give a measure of lipid peroxidation in cellular membranes (Jain et al., 1996; Liebler et al., 1996; Terentis et al., 2002) and α-tocopheryl quinone (α-TQ) appears to represent the main product of this reaction scheme in human tissues and biological fluids (Mottier et al., 2002; Torquato et al., 2019a). This metabolite appertains to one of the two groups of unstable primary autooxidation products of α-TOH (recently reviewed in Torquato et al., 2019b). The first group consists of eight substituted tocopherones (hydroxy- or alkyldioxy-tocopherones) which are formed by one-electron donation of α-TOH or

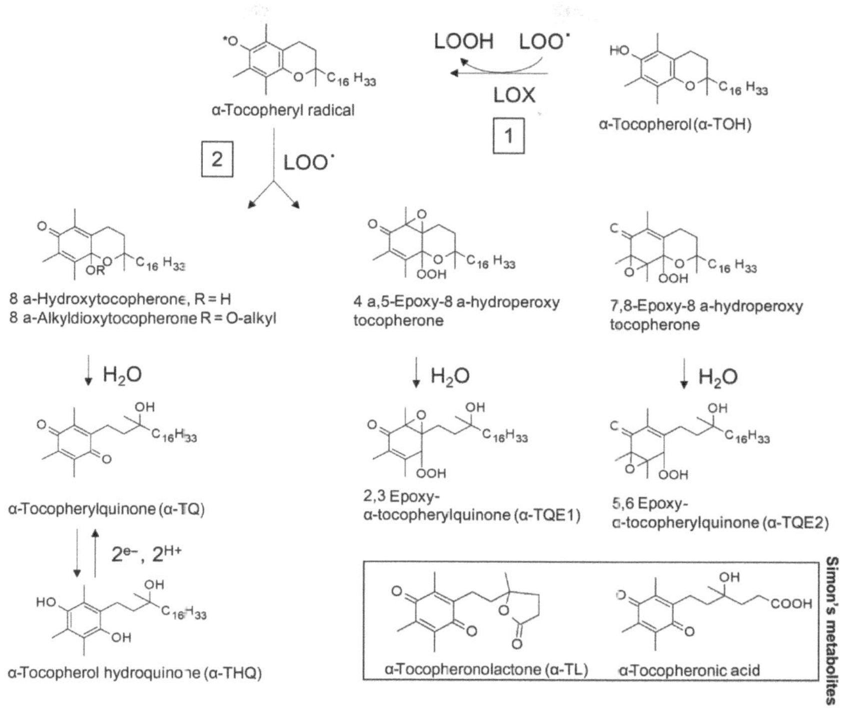

Figure 23.4 Nonenzymatic (free radical-dependent) pathway of vitamin E (α-TOH) oxidation. Main steps of reaction occurring during the lipoperoxyl radical scavenging activity of α-TOH are described. α-TOH scavenges lipid peroxyl radicals (LOO•) formed by spontaneous of LOX-mediated processes to yield lipid hydroperoxides (LOOH) (reaction 1). α-Tocopheryl radical can scavenge a second LOO• molecule forming nonradical products through different steps of molecular rearrangement (reaction 2). Some of these products are physiologic metabolites that can be measured in body fluids and tissues as biomarkers of the in vivo free radical-mediated oxidation of vitamin E. *Modified from Torquato, P., Giusepponi, D., Galarini, R., Bartolini, D., Piroddi, M., Galli, F., 2019b. Analysis of vitamin E metabolites. In: Niki, E. (Ed.), Vitamin E: Chemistry and Nutritional Benefits. The Royal Society of Chemistry.*

tocopherone cation hydrolysis that readily hydrolyzes to α-TQ. The two-electron reduction of α-TQ yields α-tocopheryl hydroquinone, α-THQ (Liebler et al., 1996) (Fig. 23.4). Under appropriate reducing conditions, α-TQ can coexist with its hydroquinone derivative to form a redox couple of possible physiological relevance in lipid signaling (reviewed elsewhere in Galli et al., 2007; Hinman et al., 2018) (Fig. 23.4).

The second group consists of isomeric epoxy (hydroperoxy)-tocopherones, which are formed by an unknown mechanism to spontaneously arrange to epoxyquinones (α-TQE1 and α-TQE2) (Fig. 23.4). These latter molecules are precursors of the Simon's metabolites (Eisengart et al., 1956), α-tocopheronic acid and α-tocopheronolactone (α-TL). Sharma et al. (2013) recently demonstrated that conjugates of α-TL are a biomarker of oxidative stress in children with type 1 diabetes. Downstream of the vitamin E redox node, lipid hydroperoxides (LOOH) are formed. These are reactive oxygen species (ROS), since their homolytic cleavage leads to the two most reactive radicals, that is, $HO^{\bullet}$ and $LO^{\bullet}$ (Fig. 23.3, reaction 5), thereby causing branching of the radical chain and other potentially harmful reactions with biomolecules (Maiorino et al., 1989). Under physiological conditions, LOOH are metabolized, for example, by glutathione peroxidase (GPx4) or certain peroxiredoxins, forming stable lipid alcohol products (LOH) (Fig. 23.3, reaction 7) (Hofmann et al., 2002; Maiorino et al., 1989).

However, LOOHs are not only dangerous chain-branching ROS. They also have activity as signal transduction molecules and are a source of lipid mediators. Because of their hydrophilic -OOH group they can cause a rearrangement of lipids in the membrane (Fig. 23.3, reaction 6) which might affect membrane-associated enzymes as it is deduced from the preferential cleavage of oxidized fatty acids from membrane phospholipids by the activity of phospholipase A2 (PLA2) (Kambayashi et al., 1998). These effects discussed in detail elsewhere (Hermann et al. (2014)). Include in the model of neuronal cell membrane peroxidation and PLA2 activation, alterations of the membrane microarchitecture and ion channel activity, interfering with cell excitability and other aspects of neuronal cell integrity and function. Other events that conspire with these structural and functional changes include the release of lipid mediators of inflammatory and synaptic pathways (extracellular effects), metabolic and mitochondrial pathways (intracellular effects), and cell death programs (Hermann et al., 2014). Hydroperoxy fatty acids (LOOH) (Fig. 23.3, reaction 7) are released by the activity of PLA2 to generate a number of bioactive metabolites, such as hydroxy fatty acids, epoxides, diols, or are further peroxidized to generate lipoxins and short-chain reactive carbonyls (reviewed in Murphy and Gijon, 2007) (Fig. 23.3, reaction 8). Epoxy and hydroxyl lipids, such as leukotriene A4 and B4 and their downstream derivatives, are potent and physiological mediators, formed through the arachidonic acid cascade, which is initiated by the α-TOH-regulated enzyme 5-lipoxygenase (5-LOX) (Mousley et al., 2007; Pein et al., 2018). Other oxidized fatty acids such as HPODEs (hydroperoxyoctadecadienoic acids), HODEs (hydroxyoctadecadienoic acids), HPETEs (hydroperoxyeicosatetraenoic acids), and HETEs (hydroxyeicosatetraenoic acids), which can be formed enzymatically or by spontaneous oxidations, have been shown to exert various signaling functions (Droge, 2002; Finkel, 2003). In this context, the primary function of α-TOH should be preventing the oxidative damage and destruction of biomembranes by means of its antioxidant function. However, several pieces of evidence, such as the aforementioned modulation of 5-LOX activity, suggest for this vitamin form a broader role as homeostatic agent of cellular membranes and more in general of lipid structures (such as intracellular lipid stores and lipoproteins). In keeping with this, the concerted radical scavenging activity of vitamin E and cellular peroxidases and their cytoprotection function, support a role for this vitamin on the lipoxygenase-dependent control of cell death programs (reviewed in Carlson et al., 2016). Examples of this role were first described in "oxytosis", a death mechanism investigated in neuronal cells that appears to involve in a concerted fashion the PLA2 and 12-LOX-dependent formation of LOOH that functions as a death messenger (Khanna et al., 2003, 2010). This role was then confirmed in the more recently identified "ferroptosis". This is a specific and iron-dependent death program sustained by the LOOH generating activity of 15-LOX (Kagan et al., 2017). Intriguingly both enzymatic (cytochrome P450 derived long-chain forms) and redox-dependent (i.e., α-THQ) metabolites of α-TOH have the potential to control some of these pathways (Fig. 23.3, reaction 9) (Hinman et al., 2018; Pein et al., 2018; Schmolz et al., 2018) consistent with other and possibly more articulated mechanisms of modulation of peroxide signaling for this vitamin (further discussed in Chapter 24).

23.3 Nutritional aspects

Vitamin forms of the TOH and T3 subfamilies (Fig. 23.2) are synthesized in photosynthetic organisms as a group of molecules with a polar chromanol ring and a lipophilic polyprenyl side chain (Mene-Saffrane and Pellaud, 2017). Several intermediates are generated during this biosynthesis process, many of which are of some interest as plant bioactives and medicinal products. A comprehensive and systematic review on the structurally diverse tocochromanols and chromenols found in photosynthetic organisms, including marine organisms, and as metabolic intermediates in animals, has recently been published by Birringer et al. (2018).

Oily plants are natural sources of this vitamin in nature; usually seeds serve as raw matter to produce edible oils with considerable contents of TOHs and T3s (the main ones are reported in Table 23.2), but also other plant food processing products can be used with this aim (Shahidi and de Camargo, 2016).

Table 23.2 Content of tocopherols and tocotrienols (mg/100 g of oil) in some common edible oils.

Oil	α-TOH	β-TOH	γ-TOH	δ-TOH	α-T3	β-T3	γ-T3	δ-T3	References
Barley	14.2–20.1	0.60–1.90	3.50–15.1	0.90–4.60	46.5–76.1	nd–12.4	8.50–18.6	0.50–2.60	Moreau et al. (2007)
Coconut	0.20–1.82	tr–0.25	tr–0.12	nd–0.39	1.09–3.00	nd–0.17	0.33–0.64	nd–0.10	Schwartz et al. (2008) and Syväoja et al. (1986)
Corn	18.0–25.7	0.95–1.10	44.0–75.2	2.20–3.25	0.94–1.50	nd	1.30–2.00	nd–0.26	Schwartz et al. (2008) and Syväoja et al. (1986)
Cottonseed	30.5–57.3	0.04–0.30	10.5–31.7	tr	nr	nr	nr	nr	Desai et al. (1988)
Linseed	0.54–1.20	nd–tr	52.0–57.3	0.75–0.95	nd	nd	nd	nd	Schwartz et al. (2008) and Syväoja et al. (1986)
Olive	11.9–17.0	nd–0.27	0.89–1.34	nd–tr	nd–tr	nd	nd	nd–tr	Schwartz et al. (2008) and Syväoja et al. (1986)
Palm	6.05–42.0	nd–0.42	tr–0.02	nd–0.02	5.70–26.0	nr–0.82	11.3–36.0	3.33–8.00	Ng et al. (2004)
Peanut	8.86–30.4	nd–0.38	3.50–19.2	0.85–3.10	nd	nd	nd	nd	Carpenter (1979) and Syväoja et al. (1986)
Rapeseed	18.9–24.0	nd–tr	37.0–51.0	0.98–1.90	nd	nd	nd	nd	Schwartz et al. (2008) and Syväoja et al. (1986)
Rice bran	0.73–15.9	0.19–2.50	0.26–8.00	0.03–2.70	0.84–13.8	tr–2.6	1.74–23.1	0.14–2.53	Goufo and Trindade (2014)
Safflower	36.7–47.7	nd–1.20	tr–2.56	tr–0.65	nd	nd	nd	nd	Carpenter (1979) and Syväoja et al. (1986)
Sesame	0.24–36.0	0.28–0.80	16.0–57.0	0.17–13.0	tr	nd	0.34	nr	Schwartz et al. (2008)
Soybean	9.53–12.0	1.00–1.31	61.0–69.9	23.9–26.00	nd	nd	nd	nd	Warner and Mounts (1990)
Sunflower	32.7–59.0	tr–2.40	1.40–4.50	0.27–0.50	0.11–nd	nd	tr	tr	Desai et al. (1988) and Schwartz et al. (2008)
Wheat germ	133–256	31.2–65.0	tr–52.3	nd–0.55	2.5–3.6	nd–8.2	nd–1.85	nd–0.24	Eisenmenger and Dunford (2008) and Hassanien et al. (2014)

nd, Not detected; *nr*, not reported; *tr*, trace.

Source: Modified from Shahidi, F., de Camargo, A.C., 2016. Tocopherols and tocotrienols in common and emerging dietary sources: occurrence, applications, and health benefits. Int. J. Mol. Sci. 17, E1745.

Almonds, hazelnuts, germ oil, and sunflower oil contain high amounts of α-TOH, while walnuts, palm oil, and soybeans predominantly contain γ-TOH (Cardenas and Ghosh, 2013). T3 are widely found in some cereals, palm oil, and rice bran oil (Wong and Radhakrishnan, 2012). Coconut oil, cocoa butter, soybeans, barley, and wheat germ (WG) are also naturally occurring sources of T3s (Dutta and Dutta, 2003), whereas vegetables and fruits, with the exception of dried apricots, some legumes, avocado, and green olives, contain lower levels of vitamin E forms (Shahidi and de Camargo, 2016). The concentration of vitamin E forms contained in food depends on several factors, such as growing, harvesting, and any further processing (refining or cooking) (Dutta and Dutta, 2003; Shahidi and de Camargo, 2016).

Palm oil has overtaken soybean oil as the world's leading vegetable oil (Carter et al., 2007). Although α-TOH is present in palm oil, γ-T3 is the major compound among other homologs. It is worth mentioning that palm oil has been reported to be the only edible oil with γ-T3 as the major lipophilic antioxidant among the common castor, coconut, corn, linseed, olive, peanut, soybean, sunflower, WG, and cod liver oils (Syväoja et al., 1986). Soybean oil is also very important due to its high global production, especially in Brazil, China, Argentina, and the United States (Shahidi and de Camargo, 2016). The content of γ-TOH in soybean oil has been reported to be seven times higher than that of α-TOH, which is the most common form in human tissues (discussed later). Similar to soybean oil, α-TOH is not the most prominent tocol in canola or rapeseed oil, in which the content of γ-TOH was up to 2.7-fold higher compared to that of α-TOH (Schwartz et al., 2008). Furthermore, none of the previous oils had α-TOH as the main tocol; therefore the assumption that α-TOH is the most common form should be made with caution because, at least in terms of vegetable oil production, this information may not be representative. Conversely, α-TOH comprises more than 93% of the tocols in sunflower oil, and predominates over the other forms of vitamin E in safflower, canola, WGO, cottonseed, and olive oil.

In fact the four most consumed edible oils are palm oil, soybean oil, canola oil, and sunflower oil in order of global consumption. γ-T3 is the most prominent tocol in the first (palm oil), while γ-TOH is the most prominent one in the second (soybean oil). α-TOH is the main TOH only in the third (canola oil) and fourth most consumed oil (sunflower oil), but canola concentrations of vitamin E are relatively low (about 30 mg/100 g, with 65%–80% α-TOH) and oils from sunflower cultivars obtained by mutagenesis and genetic recombination (Velasco et al., 2004) had 77% and 68% of β- and δ-TOHs, respectively.

The Mediterranean diet has been in the spotlight due to its association with a lower incidence of cancer, cardiovascular disease, and Parkinson and Alzheimer disease (Sofi et al., 2014). Olive oil is the characteristic lipid source of the Mediterranean diet (Piroddi et al., 2017). The most important differences between extra virgin and traditional olive oils are due to differences in their manufacturing processes. The industrial process of extra virgin olive oil (EVOO) includes pressing of the olive fruit in a solvent-free process; moreover, no heat is applied, which is beneficial for the retention of its bioactive phenolic compounds, including tocols (Piroddi et al., 2017). EVOO has α-TOH as its major tocol form (Table 23.2). A recent study (Caporaso et al., 2015) demonstrated that the content of α-TOH varies greatly in commercial olive oils. The same study suggested that considering a daily intake of 30 g of EVOO, this could supply on average 50% of the recommended intake (RDI) for α-TOH [i.e., 12−15 mg/d of vitamin E (IOM, 2000)]. A food product can be considered a source of vitamin E as long as its consumption offers a supplement of at least 15% of the vitamin E RDI (EFSA, 2010); therefore the commercial EVOO producers are allowed to use this health claim.

23.3.1 "Essentiality" of vitamin E

Vitamin E belongs to the group of fat-soluble vitamins. As such it should be recommended on the bases of its essentiality, but after almost a century on from its discovery, a definition of essential nutrient by the identification of a specific deficiency phenotype still remains problematic, at least in the general population.

Dietary recommendations proposed in the late 1990s (IOM, 2000) provided adequate intake (AI) levels of essential nutrients. In the case of vitamin E (as α-TOH) these corresponded to 15 mg/d for healthy adults and 19 mg/d during breast-feeding. Notwithstanding, there is no generally accepted definition of what is an "adequate" intake of this vitamin. The actual amount of vitamin E that ensures the absence of deficiency symptoms is difficult to establish in the general population, or at the individual level, since developing a condition of clinically relevant deficiency is extremely rare under physiological conditions or rather impossible due to the reserve of this vitamin stored in adipose tissue (approximately 90%

of the body's vitamin E content). Apparently, this is sufficient to buffer the interorgan metabolism of the vitamin for years (Handelman et al., 1994) and to delay symptoms of vitamin E undersupply for a long time, usually decades (Ulatowski and Manor, 2015). In contrast, serious (primary or secondary) vitamin E deficiency can present with acute symptoms, such as neuropathy and myopathy, consistent with the assumption that vitamin E is essential for the development and maintenance of the central nervous system. But even this view on vitamin E essentiality is problematic. In more detail, Ulatowski and Manor (2015) recently described clinical and metabolic features of primary and secondary deficiencies. Familial isolated vitamin E deficiency, which is also known as ataxia with isolated vitamin E deficiency (AVED, OMIM #277460), is categorized as a primary vitamin E deficiency. It is produced by mutations in the gene coding for the TOH transfer protein (α-TTP) (Arita et al., 1997; Catignani and Bieri, 1977), a protein that is considered to be the "gatekeeper" of vitamin E status in that it mediates high-affinity binding of RRR-α-TOH (natural form of α-TOH) in liver cells, facilitating its selective incorporation in nascent VLDL and secretion in the circulation for the distribution to extrahepatic tissues (Ulatowski and Manor, 2015).

As a consequence of this gene defect, AVED patients have the capacity to absorb vitamin E in the intestine, but have an extremely poor ability to retain it in the different tissues (Arita et al., 1997; Ouahchi et al., 1995; Sokol et al., 1988). The heterogeneity of mutations in AVED patients is linked to large variations of the clinical presentation of the disease (Manor and Morley, 2007; Martinello et al., 1998). The disease generally appears between ages 5 and 15 years and its symptoms include, in addition to extremely low vitamin E levels (below 2 μM, while normal levels are between 20 and 35 μM (Hensley et al., 2004)), progressive ataxia, clumsiness of the hands, loss of proprioception, and areflexia (Harding et al., 1985; Schuelke, 1993).

According to the pathological findings by Yokota et al. (2000), in a postmortem case with α-TTP mutation the major anomalies were retinal atrophy, severe dying back-type degeneration of the posterior column, and massive accumulation of lipofuscin in neurons including dorsal root ganglion (DRG) cells, which were almost identical to those in vitamin E-deficient animals and patients with fat malabsorption. Also mild loss of Purkinje cells was noted. The mild Purkinje cell loss might be related to the mutant α-TTP in the cerebellum. By contrast in the DRG, thought to be mainly responsible for ataxia, no expression of α-TTP was detected, and the tissue concentration of vitamin E increased to normal after supplementation. It is therefore considered that oral supplementation of vitamin E should effectively counteract the progression of ataxia (Yokota et al., 2000). In other studies however, after supplementation in α-TTP$^{-/-}$ mice, vitamin E became normal in plasma, but not in the cerebellum, which has been suggested to sustain the loss of cerebellar Purkinje cells as a major pathogenic event of the disease (Ulatowski et al., 2014).

The secondary deficiencies include disorders of lipid absorption and transport as well as impaired lipoprotein metabolism (Hentati et al., 2012). Due to its fat solubility, vitamin E requires dietary lipids for its absorption in the gastrointestinal tract (GI). Consequently, the diminution of plasma vitamin E is associated with situations present in patients with fat malabsorption (premature and very low birth weight infants; cystic fibrosis; gastric bypass; Crohn's disease; liver disease or pancreatic insufficiency; abetalipoproteinemia) (Hentati et al., 2012; Muller et al., 1983). These secondary states of deficiency are in general suboptimal conditions of the vitamin E status, that is, vitamin E levels in blood are lowered, but not absent, to the point that signs of damage to plasma or blood cell lipids can occur at least in some subjects, as observed for instance in cystic fibrosis patients (Iuliano et al., 2009).

Although attempts have been made to unify the symptoms of secondary and primary deficiency states in terms of oxidative damage (Elkamil et al., 2015; Farrell et al., 1977; Martinello et al., 1998; Schuelke, 1993), a closer analysis of available data indicates a large heterogeneity in the clinical presentation of the different diseases and in the capability to respond to vitamin E therapy. In these studies oxidative stress was not conclusively demonstrated to represent a major pathogenic event of the peripheral and central nervous system, and also of peripheral blood cells. The same lack of evidence about a causal association between vitamin E deficiency and oxidative stress has emerged from animal studies carried out in *α-TTP*-deficient mice fed a vitamin E-deficient diet (Gohil et al., 2003; Ulatowski et al., 2014; Yokota et al., 2001). Therefore these studies clearly demonstrate the complexity of the human phenotype of AVED as well as of *α-TTP*-manipulated animals and the difficulty to identify a prevailing deficiency phenotype. This remains a major obstacle to conclusively defining the essentiality of vitamin E.

23.3.2 Dietary intake and recommendations

The difficulty to detect overt symptoms of deficiency in the general population also limits the possibility of providing "evidence-based" recommendations on the dietary intake of vitamin E. This is also the main reason for the disparities between nutritional guidelines and recommendations of different regions. Nutritional assessment strategies are affected by this lack of knowledge as well, the relevance of which is highly questionable. For example, the correlation of hydrogen peroxide-induced erythrocyte lysis and plasma α-TOH concentrations is used as an indicator of vitamin E status in US, while in Germany lipid peroxidation is the corresponding indicator (recently reviewed in Schmolz et al., 2016). In keeping with this approach, the Institute of Medicine (IOM) definition of AI of this vitamin takes into account the relationship with the intake of polyunsaturated fatty acids (PUFA) (IOM, 2000) as actual substrate of its antioxidant activity. In this case the recommended intake of vitamin E should correlate with the amount of PUFA in food in the proportion of 0.5 mg *RRR*-α-TOH/g of diene fatty acid, or rather diene equivalents. Obviously the approach to suggest such an intake ratio implies too many approximations and lacks the support of a specific verification strategy of nutritional outcomes (e.g., this could include the investigation of tissue's PUFA levels and antioxidant protection, or other indicators of their metabolism and function as lipid components of the cell membrane and mediators of signal transduction pathways). Again, demonstrated health benefits of vitamin E go beyond the generic concept of essentiality and antioxidant function proposed so far in nutritional guidelines and even in health claim resolutions of the European Food Safety Authority (EFSA) (2010). In fact its depletion and repletion affect gene expression in vitro and in vivo, indicating broader effects than just PUFA's protection from oxidation, that are further described below and in the next chapter of this book. Such molecular indicators could help to identify differences in recommended dosages in subpopulations of subjects and the relationship with changes in physiological states or during pathological conditions. As a clear example of this, previous nutritional guidelines reported that the required amount of vitamin E increases with age for infants and children and decreases in the elderly independent of gender (IOM, 2000). Expert opinion, however, recently suggested a different view, with vitamin E intake recommendations that should increase in older adults based on specific requirements, some of which are associated with age-dependent decline of immune cell function and control of specific molecular (gene-related) processes across inflammatory pathways that are potentially important, but yet ignored, indicators of the dietary requirement for this vitamin (Meydani et al., 2018). Although these limits remain a main obstacle to improving nutritional strategies and health policies, the recent work of EFSA started to consider these aspects. The present recommended daily allowance (RDA) for vitamin E have been replaced by this organism with newly defined AI levels that are as follows: men 13 mg/d, women 11 mg/d, infants/children 5–13 mg/d (depending on age) (Peter et al., 2015). Although several foods contain naturally occurring sources of vitamin E, such intake recommendations are not frequently achieved in the general population (Schmolz et al., 2016). In fact, the intake of vitamin E is generally low and very similar across all regions. According to a recent systematic review, the intakes of α-TOH and other vitamin E forms are below the RDA for the major part of the population, or even below the estimated average requirement of 12 mg/d, in both developing and industrialized countries (Peter et al., 2015). More than 90% of US Americans are reported to consume insufficient amounts of vitamin E (Traber, 2014). Vitamin E intake is also considered low in other countries such as the United Kingdom, Germany, and the Netherlands (Troesch et al., 2012).

Dietary habits also play a significant role to determine which vitamin E form is primarily consumed; a Mediterranean diet, for example, contains a significant amount of leafy greens, which contain high levels of α-TOH (Jiang et al., 2001), while the US diet is rich in γ-TOH (Jiang et al., 2001). Nutritional assessment is another critical point that embraces aspects that include the choice of appropriate specimens and analytical strategies, the identification of reference values in the different populations, the effect of different diseases, and other interfering variables, such as medications, lifestyle-related factors, etc. The determination of vitamin E levels in serum or plasma is the main form of assessment for the vitamin status (Galli et al., 2007). An increasing number of studies reported serum concentrations at which beneficial effects may occur and this type of evaluation could have more relevance than other aspects in determining the optimal intake and vitamin status in the general population and even in specific subgroups. Using this rationale, a recent revision of the literature concluded that α-TOH concentrations in serum below 9 μmol/L for men or below 12 μmol/L for women are considered as deficient and only marginal for healthy adults, respectively (Traber, 2014). Prospective observational studies suggested that a serum α-TOH concentration of 30 μmol/L or above has beneficial effects on human health, with alleged applications including the prevention of cardiovascular disease and different types of cancer (Biesalski et al., 1997; Mangialasche et al., 2012). The relevance of this α-TOH concentration target is further supported by pentane concentration in exhaled air, a marker of oxidative damage, which is very low at and above this α-TOH serum concentrations (Lemoyne et al., 1987). In the α-TOH, β-Carotene Cancer Prevention Study, higher baseline serum concentrations of α-TOH were associated with lower total and cause-specific mortality; the lowest total mortality was observed at 30 μmol/L serum α-TOH (Wright et al., 2006).

When supplements are used to improve the vitamin E status, toxicity and other safety concerns must be considered (Schmolz et al., 2016). Apparently vitamin E intake can be increased up to 300 mg/d (450 IU/d) without any complication (Yap et al., 2001). Even short-term high-dose administration of vitamin E was not reported to have adverse effects (Zondlo Fiume, 2002). Although controversial, vitamin E supplementation may have no effect on all-cause mortality even at supranutritional doses (Berry et al., 2009; Curtis et al., 2014; Jiang et al., 2014). However, the risk of developing side effects during vitamin E supplementation in some groups of patients cannot be ruled out and may deserve further investigation (Galli et al., 2017). Specific groups at risk of cardiovascular disease, especially subjects with increased thrombotic risk, should be considered with some precaution during vitamin E supplementation (Zondlo Fiume, 2002). In this context the Miller's meta-analysis of vitamin E prevention trials and its conclusions (introduced in the footnote of Section 23.1), had the merit of stimulating attention to this risk, and it was an occasion for the scientific community to ponder more cautious approaches to the generic measures of prevention based on high-dose vitamin supplementation protocols. On the other hand, a scientific statement from the American Heart Association Nutrition Committee, that remains valid so far, supports the view that an optimal intake of natural vitamin E, introduced with a well-balanced diet, appears to be the best way to obtain prevention effects, if any, on myocardial infarction, stroke, and other atherothrombotic conditions and such a health recommendation should be extended to all natural antioxidants in food (American Heart Association Nutrition Committee et al., 2006).

Unfortunately, at present there is no consensus on which level of supranutritional intake of vitamin E may avoid the risk of side effects in the long term, if any. But it is quite obvious that even an intake of a few times the RDA for this vitamin—that is far below the threshold level of increased risk for cancer and all-cause mortality reported for patients with cardiovascular disease in the Miller's study (400 IU/d)—is sufficient to produce a saturation effect on plasma vitamin E concentrations of healthy individuals. Therefore increasing the dosage of supplements to hundreds of milligrams per day will sustain just the catabolism and excretion of the vitamin excess. To assume a beneficial effect from this excess we should assume that the mechanisms behind this metabolism or the produced metabolites may affect health-promoting biological processes of the GI and also of other organs and tissues, such as arteries and the myocardium, some brain areas, immune cells, etc. Such a vision is compatible with the proposed role of α-TOC as a provitamin (originally postulated in Galli et al., 2007) and further described in the next chapter.

23.3.3 Vitamin E in the secondary prevention of human diseases

Vitamin E has been speculated to exert health-promoting effects in a number of epidemiology, preclinical, and observational studies. Positive effects were reported on cancer, age-related immune dysfunction, skin problems, liver pathologies, and neurodegenerative diseases, and above all on atherosclerosis and associated cardiovascular complications, such as stroke and myocardial infarction (recently reviewed in Azzi, 2018; Galli and Azzi, 2010; Galli et al., 2017). Unluckily, the largest and well-designed/conducted secondary prevention trials have produced conflicting and even negative outcomes. Available results and their systematic assessment in review papers and meta-analysis studies demonstrate how most of the promising findings obtained at the preclinical and observational level cannot be confirmed in large clinical trials, thus frustrating most of the proposed clinical applications. Emblematic are the prevention trials on atherosclerotic cardiovascular disease and cancer (reviewed in Bjelakovic et al., 2012; Galli et al., 2017). Rather, some studies already presented in the previous sections provided negative results, suggesting an increased risk of adverse events and all-cause mortality. In the recent meta-analysis of Bjelakovic et al. (2012) evaluating vitamin E trials together with studies on other antioxidant supplements, such as the provitamin A compound β-carotene, the authors concluded that: "We found no evidence to support antioxidant supplements for primary or secondary prevention. β-Carotene and vitamin E seem to increase mortality, and so may higher doses of vitamin A. Antioxidant supplements need to be considered as medicinal products and should undergo sufficient evaluation before marketing."

Absence of evidence on the efficacy of α-TOC in the prevention of Alzheimer's dementia and mild cognitive impairment was recently reported in another meta-analysis study by Farina et al. (2017). These authors, however, reported on the absence of an increased risk of adverse effects and mortality in the evaluated trials.

The reasons behind the negative results of several vitamin E prevention studies could be many, such as biased selections of the study populations, disease type and stage of progression, differences in sample size and treatment duration, form and dosages of vitamin E utilized in the different studies, outcome measurements and duration of the observation that is surely a critical issue in chronic diseases, etc. Alternatively it could be considered that vitamin E could not efficiently interfere with the multifaceted pathogenic mechanisms of most of the investigated diseases, even if these mechanisms include oxidative stress as a supposed unifying underlying event and vitamin E can act as a fat-soluble antioxidant. The possibility that, and the reasons way, vitamin E could not behave as a therapeutic antioxidant in vivo are worth investigating further and as discussed in a recent review article by Azzi (2018); these may include the fact that age-related diseases are not primarily sustained by oxidative stress, or again, that oxidative stress is not a modifiable causal risk factor of these pathologies.

Therefore with regards to what we know, at present there is no reason to recommend supranutritional doses of vitamin E to the general population with the aim of preventing risk factors of chronic and age-related diseases unless specific conditions of (primary or secondary) vitamin E deficiency are diagnosed (discussed before in Section 23.3.1 and in Ulatowski and Manor, 2015). These include for instance specific cases such as some gastrointestinal conditions associated with malabsorption and lipid metabolism disorders, such as cystic fibrosis, some liver diseases, such as NAFLD and NASH, and chronic kidney disease (recently described in Galli et al., 2004c, 2017; Giusepponi et al., 2017; Torquato et al., 2018b). These cases however require accurate/personalized nutritional and clinical evaluation before and during the intervention. Taking into consideration NAFLD and NASH patients, improved liver histology and hepatometabolic cues of the disease have been reported by daily intakes of 400–800 mg α-TOC in both children and adults (Lavine et al., 2011; Pacana and Sanyal, 2012; Sanyal et al., 2010) and vitamin E supplementation has now been included in clinical guidelines of some regions as a first intervention measure for nondiabetic NASH patients (reviewed in Galli et al., 2017), but the appropriateness and efficacy of vitamin E therapy administered to these patients alone or in combination with other micronutrient vitamins (the most common are the ω-3 DHA and vitamin D) have not been investigated so far. Only recently nutritional and lipidomics biomarkers have been proposed for an application in clinical trials to evaluate these aspects (Giusepponi et al., 2017; Torquato et al., 2018b,c).

23.4 Conclusions

This chapter presents the most relevant information on the antioxidant, nutritional, and health-promoting properties of vitamin E. After a century of studies some of these aspects are still far from being completely elucidated, especially the definition of the clinical and molecular consequences of its deficiency states, and consequently of validated nutritional recommendations and disease prevention and curative applications. All these aspects are now the subject of an intense research in several laboratories, keeping high the interesest for this vitamin in the scientific community.

References

American Heart Association Nutrition Committee, Lichtenstein, A.H., Appel, L.J., Brands, M., Carnethon, M., Daniels, S., et al., 2006. Diet and lifestyle recommendations revision 2006: a scientific statement from the American Heart Association Nutrition Committee. Circulation 114, 82–96.

Arita, M., Nomura, K., Arai, H., Inoue, K., 1997. Alpha-tocopherol transfer protein stimulates the secretion of alpha-tocopherol from a cultured liver cell line through a brefeldin A-insensitive pathway. Proc. Natl. Acad. Sci. U.S.A. 94, 12437–12441.

Atkinson, J., Epand, R.F., Epand, R.M., 2008. Tocopherols and tocotrienols in membranes: a critical review. Free Radic. Biol. Med. 44, 739–764.

Azzi, A., 2018. Many tocopherols, one vitamin E. Mol. Asp. Med. 61, 92–103.

Bartolini, D., Torquato, P., Barola, C., Russo, A., Rychlicki, C., Giusepponi, D., et al., 2017. Nonalcoholic fatty liver disease impairs the cytochrome P-450-dependent metabolism of alpha-tocopherol (vitamin E). J. Nutr. Biochem. 47, 120–131.

Berry, D., Wathen, J.K., Newell, M., 2009. Bayesian model averaging in meta-analysis: vitamin E supplementation and mortality. Clin. Trials 6, 28–41.

Biesalski, H.K., Bohles, H., Esterbauer, H., Furst, P., Gey, F., Hundsdorfer, G., et al., 1997. Antioxidant vitamins in prevention. Clin. Nutr. 16, 151–155.

Birringer, M., 2010. Analysis of vitamin E metabolites in biological specimen. Mol. Nutr. Food. Res. 54, 588–598.

Birringer, M., Drogan, D., Brigelius-Flohe, R., 2001. Tocopherols are metabolized in HepG2 cells by side chain omega-oxidation and consecutive beta-oxidation. Free Radic. Biol. Med. 31, 226–232.

Birringer, M., Pfluger, P., Kluth, D., Landes, N., Brigelius-Flohe, R., 2002. Identities and differences in the metabolism of tocotrienols and tocopherols in HepG2 cells. J. Nutr. 132, 3113–3118.

Birringer, M., Siems, K., Maxones, A., Frank, J., Lorkowski, S., 2018. Natural 6-hydroxychromanols and -chromenols: structural diversity, biosynthetic pathways and health implications. RSC Adv. 8, 4803–4841.

Bjelakovic, G., Nikolova, D., Gluud, L.L., Simonetti, R.G., Gluud, C., 2012. Antioxidant supplements for prevention of mortality in healthy participants and patients with various diseases. Cochrane Database Syst. Rev. (3), CD007176.

Bowry, V.W., Ingold, K.U., Stocker, R., 1992. Vitamin E in human low-density lipoprotein. When and how this antioxidant becomes a pro-oxidant. Biochem. J. 288 (Pt 2), 341–344.

Bowry, V.W., Mohr, D., Cleary, J., Stocker, R., 1995. Prevention of tocopherol-mediated peroxidation in ubiquinol-10-free human low density lipoprotein. J. Biol. Chem. 270, 5756–5763.

Brigelius-Flohe, R., 2009. Vitamin E: the shrew waiting to be tamed. Free Radic. Biol. Med. 46, 543–554.

Burton, G.W., Joyce, A., Ingold, K.U., 1982. First proof that vitamin E is major lipid-soluble, chain-breaking antioxidant in human blood plasma. Lancet 2, 327.

Caporaso, N., Savarese, M., Paduano, A., Guidone, G., De Marco, E., Sacchi, R., 2015. Nutritional quality assessment of extra virgin olive oil from the Italian retail market: do natural antioxidants satisfy EFSA health claims? J. Food Compos. Anal. 40, 154–162.

Cardenas, E., Ghosh, R., 2013. Vitamin E: a dark horse at the crossroad of cancer management. Biochem. Pharmacol. 86, 845–852.

Carlson, B.A., Tobe, R., Yefremova, E., Tsuji, P.A., Hoffmann, V.J., Schweizer, U., et al., 2016. Glutathione peroxidase 4 and vitamin E cooperatively prevent hepatocellular degeneration. Redox Biol. 9, 22–31.

Carpenter, A.P., 1979. Determination of tocopherols in vegetable oils. J. Am. Oil Chem. Soc. 56, 668–671.

Carter, C., Finley, W., Fry, J., Jackson, D., Willis, L., 2007. Palm oil markets and future supply. Eur. J. Lipid Sci. Technol. 109, 307–314.

Catignani, G.L., Bieri, J.G., 1977. Rat liver alpha-tocopherol binding protein. Biochim. Biophys. Acta 497, 349–357.

Chaiyasit, W., Elias, R.J., McClements, D.J., Decker, E.A., 2007. Role of physical structures in bulk oils on lipid oxidation. Crit. Rev. Food Sci. Nutr. 47, 299–317.

Chiku, S., Hamamura, K., Nakamura, T., 1984. Novel urinary metabolite of d-delta-tocopherol in rats. J. Lipid Res. 25, 40–48.

Ciffolilli, S., Wallert, M., Bartolini, D., Krauth, V., Werz, O., Piroddi, M., et al., 2015. Human serum determination and in vitro anti-inflammatory activity of the vitamin E metabolite alpha-(13′-hydroxy)-6-hydroxychroman. Free Radic. Biol. Med. 89, 952–962.

Curtis, A.J., Bullen, M., Piccenna, L., McNeil, J.J., 2014. Vitamin E supplementation and mortality in healthy people: a meta-analysis of randomised controlled trials. Cardiovasc. Drugs Ther. 28, 563–573.

Desai, I.D., Bhagavan, H., Salkeld, R., Dutra de Oliveira, J.E., 1988. Vitamin E content of crude and refined vegetable oils in Southern Brazil. J. Food Compos. Anal. 1, 231–238.

Di Donato, I., Bianchi, S., Federico, A., 2010. Ataxia with vitamin E deficiency: update of molecular diagnosis. Neurol. Sci. 31, 511–515.

Dragsted, L.O., 2008. Biomarkers of exposure to vitamins A, C, and E and their relation to lipid and protein oxidation markers. Eur. J. Nutr. 47 (Suppl. 2), 3–18.

Droge, W., 2002. Free radicals in the physiological control of cell function. Physiol. Rev. 82, 47–95.

Dutta, A., Dutta, S.K., 2003. Vitamin E and its role in the prevention of atherosclerosis and carcinogenesis: a review. J. Am. Coll. Nutr. 22, 258–268.

EFSA, 2010. EFSA Scientific Opinion on the substantiation of health claims related to vitamin E and protection of DNA, proteins and lipids from oxidative damage (ID

160, 162, 1947), maintenance of the normal function of the immune system (ID 161, 163), maintenance of normal bone (ID 164), maintenance of normal teeth (ID 164), maintenance of normal hair (ID 164), maintenance of normal skin (ID 164), maintenance of normal nails (ID 164), maintenance of normal cardiac function (ID 166), maintenance of normal vision by protection of the lens of the eye (ID 167), contribution to normal cognitive function (ID 182, 183), regeneration of the reduced form of vitamin C (ID 203), maintenance of normal blood circulation (ID 216) and maintenance of normal a scalp (ID 2873) pursuant to Article 13(1) of Regulation (EC) No. 1924/2006. EFSA J. 8 (10), 1816.

Eisengart, A., Milhorat, A.T., Simon, E.J., Sundheim, L., 1956. The metabolism of vitamin E. II. Purification and characterization of urinary metabolites of alpha-tocopherol. J. Biol. Chem. 221, 807–817.

Eisenmenger, M., Dunford, N.T., 2008. Bioactive components of commercial and supercritical carbon dioxide processed wheat germ oil. J. Am. Oil Chem. Soc. 85, 55–61.

Elkamil, A., Johansen, K.K., Aasly, J., 2015. Ataxia with vitamin E deficiency in Norway. J. Mov. Disord. 8, 33–36.

Evans, H.M., Bishop, K.S., 1922. On the existence of a hitherto unrecognized dietary factor essential for reproduction. Science 56, 650–651.

Evans, H.M., Emerson, O.H., Emerson, G.A., 1936. The isolation from wheat germ oil of an alcohol, α-tocopherol, having the properties of vitamin E. J. Biol. Chem. 133, 319–322.

Farina, N., Llewellyn, D., Isaac, M., Tabet, N., 2017. Vitamin E for Alzheimer's dementia and mild cognitive impairment. Cochrane Database Syst. Rev. 4, CD002854.

Farrell, P.M., Bieri, J.G., Fratantoni, J.F., Wood, R.E., di Sant'Agnese, P.A., 1977. The occurrence and effects of human vitamin E deficiency. A study in patients with cystic fibrosis. J. Clin. Invest. 60, 233–241.

Fernholz, E., 1938. On the constitution of α-tocopherol. J. Am. Chem. Soc. 60, 700–705.

Finkel, T., 2003. Oxidant signals and oxidative stress. Curr. Opin. Cell Biol. 15, 247–254.

Forman, H.J., Davies, K.J., Ursini, F., 2014. How do nutritional antioxidants really work: nucleophilic tone and para-hormesis versus free radical scavenging in vivo. Free Radic. Biol. Med. 66, 24–35.

Galli, F., Azzi, A., 2010. Present trends in vitamin E research. Biofactors 36, 33–42.

Galli, F., Lee, R., Dunster, C., Kelly, F.J., 2002. Gas chromatography mass spectrometry analysis of carboxyethyl-hydroxychroman metabolites of alpha- and gamma-tocopherol in human plasma. Free Radic. Biol. Med. 32, 333–340.

Galli, F., Stabile, A.M., Betti, M., Conte, C., Pistilli, A., Rende, M., et al., 2004a. The effect of alpha- and gamma-tocopherol and their carboxyethyl hydroxychroman metabolites on prostate cancer cell proliferation. Arch. Biochem. Biophys. 423, 97–102.

Galli, F., Buoncristiani, U., Conte, C., Aisa, C., Floridi, A., 2004b. Vitamin E in uremia and dialysis patients. Ann. N. Y. Acad. Sci. 1031, 348–351.

Galli, F., Floridi, A.G., Floridi, A., Buoncristiani, U., 2004c. Accumulation of vitamin E metabolites in the blood of renal failure patients. Clin. Nutr. 23, 205–212.

Galli, F., Polidori, M.C., Stahl, W., Mecocci, P., Kelly, F.J., 2007. Vitamin E biotransformation in humans. Vitam. Horm. 76, 263–280.

Galli, F., Azzi, A., Birringer, M., Cook-Mills, J.M., Eggersdorfer, M., Frank, J., et al., 2017. Vitamin E: emerging aspects and new directions. Free Radic. Biol. Med. 102, 16–36.

Giusepponi, D., Torquato, P., Bartolini, D., Piroddi, M., Birringer, M., Lorkowski, S., et al., 2017. Determination of tocopherols and their metabolites by liquid-chromatography coupled with tandem mass spectrometry in human plasma and serum. Talanta 170, 552–561.

Gohil, K., Schock, B.C., Chakraborty, A.A., Terasawa, Y., Raber, J., Farese Jr., R.V., et al., 2003. Gene expression profile of oxidant stress and neurodegeneration in transgenic mice deficient in alpha-tocopherol transfer protein. Free Radic. Biol. Med. 35, 1343–1354.

Gotoda, T., Arita, M., Arai, H., Inoue, K., Yokota, T., Fukuo, Y., et al., 1995. Adult-onset spinocerebellar dysfunction caused by a mutation in the gene for the alpha-tocopherol-transfer protein. N. Engl. J. Med. 333, 1313–1318.

Goufo, P., Trindade, H., 2014. Rice antioxidants: phenolic acids, flavonoids, anthocyanins, proanthocyanidins, tocopherols, tocotrienols, γ-oryzanol, and phytic acid. Food Sci. Nutr. 2, 75–104.

Gross, C.S., Milhorat, A.T., Simon, E.J., 1956. The metabolism of vitamin E. I. The absorption and excretion of D-alpha-tocopheryl-5-methyl-C14-succinate. J. Biol. Chem. 221, 797–805.

Handelman, G.J., Epstein, W.L., Peerson, J., Spiegelman, D., Machlin, L.J., Dratz, E.A., 1994. Human adipose alpha-tocopherol and gamma-tocopherol kinetics during and after 1 y of alpha-tocopherol supplementation. Am. J. Clin. Nutr. 59, 1025–1032.

Harding, A.E., Matthews, S., Jones, S., Ellis, C.J., Booth, I.W., Muller, D.P., 1985. Spinocerebellar degeneration associated with a selective defect of vitamin E absorption. N. Engl. J. Med. 313, 32–35.

Hassanien, M.M.M., Abdel-Razek, A.G., Rudzińska, M., Siger, A., Ratusz, K., Przybylski, R., 2014. Phytochemical contents and oxidative stability of oils from non-traditional sources. Eur. J. Lipid Sci. Technol. 116, 1563–1571.

Hensley, K., Benaksas, E.J., Bolli, R., Comp, P., Grammas, P., Hamdheydari, L., et al., 2004. New perspectives on vitamin E: γ-tocopherol and carboxyethylhydroxychroman metabolites in biology and medicine. Free Radic. Biol. Med. 36, 1–15.

Hentati, F., El-Euch, G., Bouhlal, Y., Amouri, R., 2012. Ataxia with vitamin E deficiency and abetalipoproteinemia. Handb. Clin. Neurol. 103, 295–305.

Hermann, P.M., Watson, S.N., Wildering, W.C., 2014. Phospholipase A2 – nexus of aging, oxidative stress, neuronal excitability, and functional decline of the aging nervous system? Insights from a snail model system of neuronal aging and age-associated memory impairment. Front. Genet. 5, 419.

Himmelfarb, J., Kane, J., McMonagle, E., Zaltas, E., Bobzin, S., Boddupalli, S., et al., 2003. Alpha and gamma tocopherol metabolism in healthy subjects and patients with end-stage renal disease. Kidney Int. 64, 978–991.

Hinman, A., Holst, C.R., Latham, J.C., Bruegger, J.J., Ulas, G., McCusker, K.P., et al., 2018. Vitamin E hydroquinone is an endogenous regulator of ferroptosis via redox control of 15-lipoxygenase. PLoS ONE 13, e0201369.

Hofmann, B., Hecht, H.J., Flohe, L., 2002. Peroxiredoxins. Biol. Chem. 383, 347–364.

IOM, 2000. Dietary Reference Intakes for Vitamin C, Vitamin E, Selenium, and Carotenoids. National Academies Press, Washington, DC.

Itoh, S., Nagaoka, S., Mukai, K., 2008. Kinetic study of the tocopherol regeneration reaction by biological hydroquinones in micellar solution. J. Phys. Chem. A 112, 448–456.

Iuliano, L., Monticolo, R., Straface, G., Zullo, S., Galli, F., Boaz, M., et al., 2009. Association of cholesterol oxidation and abnormalities in fatty acid metabolism in cystic fibrosis. Am. J. Clin. Nutr. 90, 477–484.

Jain, S.K., Wise, R., Bocchini Jr., J.J., 1996. Vitamin E and vitamin E-quinone levels in red blood cells and plasma of newborn infants and their mothers. J. Am. Coll. Nutr. 15, 44–48.

Jiang, Q., Elson-Schwab, I., Courtemanche, C., Ames, B.N., 2000. Gamma-tocopherol and its major metabolite, in contrast to alpha-tocopherol, inhibit cyclooxygenase activity in macrophages and epithelial cells. Proc. Natl. Acad. Sci. U.S.A. 97, 11494–11499.

Jiang, Q., Christen, S., Shigenaga, M.K., Ames, B.N., 2001. Gamma-tocopherol, the major form of vitamin E in the US diet, deserves more attention. Am. J. Clin. Nutr. 74, 714–722.

Jiang, Q., Yin, X., Lill, M.A., Danielson, M.L., Freiser, H., Huang, J., 2008. Long-chain carboxychromanols, metabolites of vitamin E, are potent inhibitors of cyclooxygenases. Proc. Natl. Acad. Sci. U.S.A. 105, 20464–20469.

Jiang, Z., Yin, X., Jiang, Q., 2011. Natural forms of vitamin E and 13′-carboxychromanol, a long-chain vitamin E metabolite, inhibit leukotriene generation from stimulated neutrophils by blocking calcium influx and suppressing 5-lipoxygenase activity, respectively. J. Immunol. 186, 1173–1179.

Jiang, S., Pan, Z., Li, H., Li, F., Song, Y., Qiu, Y., 2014. Meta-analysis: low-dose intake of vitamin E combined with other vitamins or minerals may decrease all-cause mortality. J. Nutr. Sci. Vitaminol. (Tokyo) 60, 194–205.

Kagan, V., Serbinova, E., Packer, L., 1990. Antioxidant effects of ubiquinones in microsomes and mitochondria are mediated by tocopherol recycling. Biochem. Biophys. Res. Commun. 169, 851–857.

Kagan, V.E., Mao, G., Qu, F., Angeli, J.P., Doll, S., Croix, C.S., et al., 2017. Oxidized arachidonic and adrenic PEs navigate cells to ferroptosis. Nat. Chem. Biol. 13, 81–90.

Kambayashi, Y., Yamamoto, Y., Nakano, M., 1998. Preferential hydrolysis of oxidized phosphatidylcholine in cholesterol-containing phosphatidylcholine liposome by phospholipase A2. Biochem. Biophys. Res. Commun. 245, 705–708.

Kantoci, D., Wechter, W.J., Murray Jr., E.D., Dewind, S.A., Borchardt, D., Khan, S.I., 1997. Endogenous natriuretic factors 6: the stereochemistry of a natriuretic gamma-tocopherol metabolite LLU-alpha. J. Pharmacol. Exp. Ther. 282, 648–656.

Karrer, P., Fritzsche, H., Ringier, B.H., Salomon, H., 1938. Synthese des α-tocopherols. Helv. Chim. Acta 21, 820–825.

Kayden, H.J., Silber, R., Kossmann, C.E., 1965. The role of vitamin E deficiency in the abnormal autohemolysis of acanthocytosis. Trans. Assoc. Am. Physicians 78, 334–342.

Khanna, S., Roy, S., Ryu, H., Bahadduri, P., Swaan, P.W., Ratan, R.R., et al., 2003. Molecular basis of vitamin E action: tocotrienol modulates 12-lipoxygenase, a key mediator of glutamate-induced neurodegeneration. J. Biol. Chem. 278, 43508–43515.

Khanna, S., Parinandi, N.L., Kotha, S.R., Roy, S., Rink, C., Bibus, D., et al., 2010. Nanomolar vitamin E α-tocotrienol inhibits glutamate-induced activation of phospholipase A2 and causes neuroprotection. J. Neurochem. 112, 1249–1260.

Landes, N., Pfluger, P., Kluth, D., Birringer, M., Ruhl, R., Bol, G.F., et al., 2003. Vitamin E activates gene expression via the pregnane X receptor. Biochem. Pharmacol. 65, 269–273.

Lavine, J.E., Schwimmer, J.B., Van Natta, M.L., Molleston, J.P., Murray, K.F., Rosenthal, P., et al., 2011. Effect of vitamin E or metformin for treatment of nonalcoholic fatty liver disease in children and adolescents: the TONIC randomized controlled trial. JAMA 305, 1659–1668.

Lemoyne, M., Van Gossum, A., Kurian, R., Ostro, M., Axler, J., Jeejeebhoy, K.N., 1987. Breath pentane analysis as an index of lipid peroxidation: a functional test of vitamin E status. Am. J. Clin. Nutr. 46, 267–272.

Liebler, D.C., Burr, J.A., Philips, L., Ham, A.J., 1996. Gas chromatography-mass spectrometry analysis of vitamin E and its oxidation products. Anal. Biochem. 236, 27–34.

Loft, S., Moller, P., Cooke, M.S., Rozalski, R., Olinski, R., 2008. Antioxidant vitamins and cancer risk: is oxidative damage to DNA a relevant biomarker? Eur. J. Nutr. 47 (Suppl. 2), 19–28.

Maguire, J.J., Kagan, V., Ackrell, B.A., Serbinova, E., Packer, L., 1992. Succinate-ubiquinone reductase linked recycling of alpha-tocopherol in reconstituted systems and mitochondria: requirement for reduced ubiquinone. Arch. Biochem. Biophys. 292, 47–53.
Mahoney, C.W., Azzi, A., 1988. Vitamin E inhibits protein kinase C activity. Biochem. Biophys. Res. Commun. 154, 694–697.
Maiorino, M., Coassin, M., Roveri, A., Ursini, F., 1989. Microsomal lipid peroxidation: effect of vitamin E and its functional interaction with phospholipid hydroperoxide glutathione peroxidase. Lipids 24, 721–726.
Mangialasche, F., Xu, W., Kivipelto, M., Costanzi, E., Ercolani, S., Pigliautile, M., et al., 2012. Tocopherols and tocotrienols plasma levels are associated with cognitive impairment. Neurobiol. Aging 33, 2282–2290.
Manor, D., Morley, S., 2007. The alpha-tocopherol transfer protein. Vitam. Horm. 76, 45–65.
Martinello, F., Fardin, P., Ottina, M., Ricchieri, G.L., Koenig, M., Cavalier, L., et al., 1998. Supplemental therapy in isolated vitamin E deficiency improves the peripheral neuropathy and prevents the progression of ataxia. J. Neurol. Sci. 156, 177–179.
Mattill, H.A., 1947. Antioxidants. Annu. Rev. Biochem. 16, 177–192.
Mazzini, F., Betti, M., Netscher, T., Galli, F., Salvadori, P., 2009. Configuration of the vitamin E analogue garcinoic acid extracted from Garcinia kola seeds. Chirality 21, 519–524.
Mene-Saffrane, L., Pellaud, S., 2017. Current strategies for vitamin E biofortification of crops. Curr. Opin. Biotechnol. 44, 189–197.
Meydani, S.N., Lewis, E.D., Wu, D., 2018. Perspective: should vitamin E recommendations for older adults be increased? Adv. Nutr. 9, 533–543.
Miller 3rd, E.R., Pastor-Barriuso, R., Dalal, D., Riemersma, R.A., Appel, L.J., Guallar, E., 2005. Meta-analysis: high-dosage vitamin E supplementation may increase all-cause mortality. Ann. Intern. Med. 142, 37–46.
Moreau, R.A., Wayns, K.E., Flores, R.A., Hicks, K.B., 2007. Tocopherols and tocotrienols in barley oil prepared from germ and other fractions from scarification and sieving of hulless barley. Cereal Chem. 84, 587–592.
Mottier, P., Gremaud, E., Guy, P.A., Turesky, R.J., 2002. Comparison of gas chromatography-mass spectrometry and liquid chromatography-tandem mass spectrometry methods to quantify alpha-tocopherol and alpha-tocopherolquinone levels in human plasma. Anal. Biochem. 301, 128–135.
Mousley, C.J., Tyeryar, K.R., Vincent-Pope, P., Bankaitis, V.A., 2007. The Sec14-superfamily and the regulatory interface between phospholipid metabolism and membrane trafficking. Biochim. Biophys. Acta 1771, 727–736.
Mukai, K., Itoh, S., Morimoto, H., 1992. Stopped-flow kinetic study of vitamin E regeneration reaction with biological hydroquinones (reduced forms of ubiquinone, vitamin K, and tocopherolquinone) in solution. J. Biol. Chem. 267, 22277–22281.
Muller, D.P., Lloyd, J.K., Wolff, O.H., 1983. Vitamin E and neurological function. Lancet 1, 225–228.
Munteanu, A., Zingg, J.M., Ogru, E., Libinaki, R., Gianello, R., West, S., et al., 2004. Modulation of cell proliferation and gene expression by alpha-tocopheryl phosphates: relevance to atherosclerosis and inflammation. Biochem. Biophys. Res. Commun. 318, 311–316.
Murphy, R.C., Gijon, M.A., 2007. Biosynthesis and metabolism of leukotrienes. Biochem. J. 405, 379–395.
Murray Jr., E.D., Kantoci, D., DeWind, S.A., Bigornia, A.E., D'Amico, D.C., King Jr., J. G., et al., 1995. Endogenous natriuretic factors 3: isolation and characterization of human natriuretic factors LLU-alpha, LLU-beta 1, and LLU-gamma. Life Sci. 57, 2145–2161.

Ng, M.H., Choo, Y.M., Ma, A.N., Chuah, C.H., Hashim, M.A., 2004. Separation of vitamin E (tocopherol, tocotrienol, and tocomonoenol) in palm oil. Lipids 39, 1031–1035.

Niki, E., Noguchi, N., 2004. Dynamics of antioxidant action of vitamin E. Acc. Chem. Res. 37, 45–51.

Ogru, E., Gianello, R., Libinaki, R., Smallridge, A., Bak, R., Geytenbeek, S., et al., 2003. Vitamin E Phosphate: An Endogenous Form of Vitamin E. Medimond Med. Pub, Englewood, pp. 127–132.

Olcott, H.S., Mattill, H.A., 1931. The unsaponifiable lipids of lettuce. J. Biol. Chem. 93, 65–70.

Ouahchi, K., Arita, M., Kayden, H., Hentati, F., Ben Hamida, M., Sokol, R., et al., 1995. Ataxia with isolated vitamin E deficiency is caused by mutations in the alpha-tocopherol transfer protein. Nat. Genet. 9, 141–145.

Pacana, T., Sanyal, A.J., 2012. Vitamin E and nonalcoholic fatty liver disease. Curr. Opin. Clin. Nutr. Metab. Care 15, 641–648.

Packer, J.E., Slater, T.F., Willson, R.L., 1979. Direct observation of a free radical interaction between vitamin E and vitamin C. Nature 278, 737–738.

Parker, R.S., Sontag, T.J., Swanson, J.E., McCormick, C.C., 2004. Discovery, characterization, and significance of the cytochrome P450 ω-hydroxylase pathway of vitamin E catabolism. Ann. N. Y. Acad. Sci. 1031, 13–21.

Parola, M., Leonarduzzi, G., Biasi, F., Albano, E., Biocca, M.E., Poli, G., et al., 1992. Vitamin E dietary supplementation protects against carbon tetrachloride-induced chronic liver damage and cirrhosis. Hepatology 16, 1014–1021.

Pein, H., Ville, A., Pace, S., Temml, V., Garscha, U., Raasch, M., et al., 2018. Endogenous metabolites of vitamin E limit inflammation by targeting 5-lipoxygenase. Nat. Commun. 9, 3834.

Peter, S., Friedel, A., Roos, F.F., Wyss, A., Eggersdorfer, M., Hoffmann, K., et al., 2015. A systematic review of global alpha-tocopherol status as assessed by nutritional intake levels and blood serum concentrations. Int. J. Vitam. Nutr. Res. 85, 261–281.

Piroddi, M., Albini, A., Fabiani, R., Giovannelli, L., Luceri, C., Natella, F., et al., 2017. Nutrigenomics of extra-virgin olive oil: a review. Biofactors 43, 17–41.

Podszun, M.C., Jakobi, M., Birringer, M., Weiss, J., Frank, J., 2017. The long chain alpha-tocopherol metabolite alpha-13′-COOH and gamma-tocotrienol induce P-glycoprotein expression and activity by activation of the pregnane X receptor in the intestinal cell line LS 180. Mol. Nutr. Food. Res. 61.

Russo, A., Bartolini, D., Torquato, P., Giusepponi, D., Barola, C., Galarini, R., et al., 2017. CYP4F2 repression and a modified alpha-tocopherol (vitamin E) metabolism are two independent consequences of ethanol toxicity in human hepatocytes. Toxicol. In Vitro 40, 124–133.

Sanyal, A.J., Chalasani, N., Kowdley, K.V., McCullough, A., Diehl, A.M., Bass, N.M., et al., 2010. Pioglitazone, vitamin E, or placebo for nonalcoholic steatohepatitis. N. Engl. J. Med. 362, 1675–1685.

Schmolz, L., Wallert, M., Heise, J., Galli, F., Werz, O., Birringer, M., et al., 2014. Regulation of inflammatory pathways by an a-tocopherol long-chain metabolite and a d-tocotrienol-related natural compound. Free Radic. Biol. Med. 75 (Suppl. 1), S48.

Schmolz, L., Birringer, M., Lorkowski, S., Wallert, M., 2016. Complexity of vitamin E metabolism. World J. Biol. Chem. 7, 14–43.

Schmolz, L., Schubert, M., Kirschner, J., Kluge, S., Galli, F., Birringer, M., et al., 2018. Long-chain metabolites of vitamin E: interference with lipotoxicity via lipid droplet associated protein PLIN2. Biochim. Biophys. Acta Mol. Cell. Biol. Lipids 1863, 919–927.

Schubert, M., Kluge, S., Schmolz, L., Wallert, M., Galli, F., Birringer, M., et al., 2018. Long-chain metabolites of vitamin E: metabolic activation as a general concept for lipid-soluble vitamins? Antioxidants (Basel), 7. p. E10.

Schudel, P., Mayer, H., Metzger, J., Rüegg, R., Isler, O., 1963. Über die chemie des vitamins E. 5. Mitteilung. Die synthese von rac. all-trans-ζ1- und-ε-Tocopherol. Helv. Chim. Acta 46, 2517–2526.

Schuelke, M., 1993. Ataxia with vitamin E deficiency. In: Adam, M.P., Ardinger, H.H., Pagon, R.A., Wallace, S.E., Bean, L.J.H., Stephens, K., Amemiya, A. (Eds.), GeneReviews. University of Washington, Seattle, WA.

Schwartz, H., Ollilainen, V., Piironen, V., Lampi, A.-M., 2008. Tocopherol, tocotrienol and plant sterol contents of vegetable oils and industrial fats. J. Food Compos. Anal. 21, 152–161.

Scott, J.W., Bizzarro, F.T., Parrish, D.R., Saucy, G., 1976. Syntheses of (2R, 4′R, 8′R)-α-tocopherol and (2R, 3′E, 7′E)-α-tocotrienol. Helv. Chim. Acta 59, 290–306.

Shahidi, F., de Camargo, A.C., 2016. Tocopherols and tocotrienols in common and emerging dietary sources: occurrence, applications, and health benefits. Int. J. Mol. Sci. 17, E1745.

Sharma, G., Muller, D.P., O'Riordan, S.M., Bryan, S., Dattani, M.T., Hindmarsh, P.C., et al., 2013. Urinary conjugated alpha-tocopheronolactone—a biomarker of oxidative stress in children with type 1 diabetes. Free Radic. Biol. Med. 55, 54–62.

Sofi, F., Macchi, C., Abbate, R., Gensini, G.F., Casini, A., 2014. Mediterranean diet and health status: an updated meta-analysis and a proposal for a literature-based adherence score. Public Health Nutr. 17, 2769–2782.

Sokol, R.J., Kayden, H.J., Bettis, D.B., Traber, M.G., Neville, H., Ringel, S., et al., 1988. Isolated vitamin E deficiency in the absence of fat malabsorption--familial and sporadic cases: characterization and investigation of causes. J. Lab. Clin. Med. 111, 548–559.

Sontag, T.J., Parker, R.S., 2002. Cytochrome P450 omega-hydroxylase pathway of tocopherol catabolism. Novel mechanism of regulation of vitamin E status. J. Biol. Chem. 277, 25290–25296.

Stahl, W., Graf, P., Brigelius-Flohe, R., Wechter, W., Sies, H., 1999. Quantification of the alpha- and gamma-tocopherol metabolites 2,5,7,8-tetramethyl-2-(2′-carboxyethyl)-6-hydroxychroman and 2,7,8-trimethyl-2-(2′-carboxyethyl)-6-hydroxychroman in human serum. Anal. Biochem. 275, 254–259.

Sure, B., 1927. Dietary requirements for reproduction. Science 66, 265–266.

Syväoja, E.-L., Piironen, V., Varo, P., Koivistoinen, P., Salminen, K., 1986. Tocopherols and tocotrienols in Finnish foods: oils and fats. J. Am. Oil Chem. Soc. 63, 328–329.

Tappel, A.L., 1953. The inhibition of hematin-catalyzed oxidations by alpha-tocopherol. Arch. Biochem. Biophys. 47, 223–225.

Terentis, A.C., Thomas, S.R., Burr, J.A., Liebler, D.C., Stocker, R., 2002. Vitamin E oxidation in human atherosclerotic lesions. Circ. Res. 90, 333–339.

Torquato, P., Ripa, O., Giusepponi, D., Galarini, R., Bartolini, D., Wallert, M., et al., 2016. Analytical strategies to assess the functional metabolome of vitamin E. J. Pharm. Biomed. Anal. 124, 399–412.

Torquato, P., Bartolini, D., Giusepponi, D., Piroddi, M., Galarini, R., Galli, F., 2018a. Increased levels of alpha-tocopherylquinone (alpha-TQ) demonstrate a higher vitamin E oxidation rate in non-alcoholic fatty liver disease (NAFLD) patients. Free Radic. Biol. Med. 120, S122.

Torquato, P., Bartolini, D., Giusepponi, D., Piroddi, M., Sebastiani, B., Saluti, G., et al., 2018b. Increased plasma levels of the lipoperoxyl radical-derived vitamin E metabolite alpha-tocopheryl quinone are an early indicator of lipotoxicity in fatty liver subjects. Free Radic. Biol. Med. 131, 115–125.

Torquato, P., Giusepponi, D., Alisi, A., Galarini, R., Bartolini, D., Piroddi, M., et al., 2018c. Nutritional biomarkers of docosahexaenoic acid-based multivitamin therapy in pediatric NASH. Sci. Rep. 9 (1), 2045.
Torquato, P., Bartolini, D., Giusepponi, D., Piroddi, M., Galarini, R., Galli, F., 2019a. Increased plasma levels of the free radical-derived vitamin E oxidation metabolite α-tocopheryl quinone are an early indicator of lipotoxicity in fatty liver subjects. Free Radic. Biol. Med. 131, 115–125.
Torquato, P., Giusepponi, D., Galarini, R., Bartolini, D., Piroddi, M., Galli, F., 2019b. Analysis of vitamin E metabolites. In: Niki, E. (Ed.), Vitamin E: Chemistry and Nutritional Benefits. The Royal Society of Chemistry.
Traber, M.G., 2014. Vitamin E inadequacy in humans: causes and consequences. Adv. Nutr. 5, 503–514.
Traber, M.G., Atkinson, J., 2007. Vitamin E, antioxidant and nothing more. Free Radic. Biol. Med. 43, 4–15.
Traber, M.G., Sokol, R.J., Burton, G.W., Ingold, K.U., Papas, A.M., Huffaker, J.E., et al., 1990. Impaired ability of patients with familial isolated vitamin E deficiency to incorporate alpha-tocopherol into lipoproteins secreted by the liver. J. Clin. Invest. 85, 397–407.
Traber, M.G., Mah, E., Leonard, S.W., Bobe, G., Bruno, R.S., 2017. Metabolic syndrome increases dietary alpha-tocopherol requirements as assessed using urinary and plasma vitamin E catabolites: a double-blind, crossover clinical trial. Am. J. Clin. Nutr. 105, 571–579.
Troesch, B., Hoeft, B., McBurney, M., Eggersdorfer, M., Weber, P., 2012. Dietary surveys indicate vitamin intakes below recommendations are common in representative Western countries. Br. J. Nutr. 108, 692–698.
Ulatowski, L.M., Manor, D., 2015. Vitamin E and neurodegeneration. Neurobiol. Dis. 84, 78–83.
Ulatowski, L., Parker, R., Warrier, G., Sultana, R., Butterfield, D.A., Manor, D., 2014. Vitamin E is essential for purkinje neuron integrity. Neuroscience 260, 120–129.
Upston, J.M., Terentis, A.C., Stocker, R., 1999. Tocopherol-mediated peroxidation of lipoproteins: implications for vitamin E as a potential antiatherogenic supplement. FASEB J. 13, 977–994.
Velasco, L., Pérez-Vich, B., Fernández-Martínez, J.M., 2004. Novel variation for the tocopherol profile in a sunflower created by mutagenesis and recombination. Plant Breed. 123, 490–492.
Wallert, M., Mosig, S., Rennert, K., Funke, H., Ristow, M., Pellegrino, R.M., et al., 2014. Long-chain metabolites of alpha-tocopherol occur in human serum and inhibit macrophage foam cell formation in vitro. Free Radic. Biol. Med. 68, 43–51.
Warner, K., Mounts, T.L., 1990. Analysis of tocopherols and phytosterols in vegetable oils by HPLC with evaporative light-scattering detection. J. Am. Oil Chem. Soc. 67, 827.
Watanabe, S., Hashimoto, E., Ikejima, K., Uto, H., Ono, M., Sumida, Y., et al., 2015. Evidence-based clinical practice guidelines for nonalcoholic fatty liver disease/nonalcoholic steatohepatitis. Hepatol. Res. 45, 363–377.
Wong, R.S., Radhakrishnan, A.K., 2012. Tocotrienol research: past into present. Nutr. Rev. 70, 483–490.
Wright, M.E., Lawson, K.A., Weinstein, S.J., Pietinen, P., Taylor, P.R., Virtamo, J., et al., 2006. Higher baseline serum concentrations of vitamin E are associated with lower total and cause-specific mortality in the alpha-tocopherol, beta-carotene cancer prevention study. Am. J. Clin. Nutr. 84, 1200–1207.
Yap, S.P., Yuen, K.H., Wong, J.W., 2001. Pharmacokinetics and bioavailability of alpha-, gamma- and delta-tocotrienols under different food status. J. Pharm. Pharmacol. 53, 67–71.

Yokota, T., Uchihara, T., Kumagai, J., Shiojiri, T., Pang, J.J., Arita, M., et al., 2000. Postmortem study of ataxia with retinitis pigmentosa by mutation of the alpha-tocopherol transfer protein gene. J. Neurol. Neurosurg. Psychiatry 68, 521–525.
Yokota, T., Igarashi, K., Uchihara, T., Jishage, K., Tomita, H., Inaba, A., et al., 2001. Delayed-onset ataxia in mice lacking alpha-tocopherol transfer protein: model for neuronal degeneration caused by chronic oxidative stress. Proc. Natl. Acad. Sci. U.S. A. 98, 15185–15190.
Zondlo Fiume, M., 2002. Final report on the safety assessment of tocopherol, tocopheryl acetate, tocopheryl linoleate, tocopheryl linoleate/oleate, tocopheryl nicotinate, tocopheryl succinate, dioleyl tocopheryl methylsilanol, potassium ascorbyl tocopheryl phosphate, and tocophersolan. Int. J. Toxicol. 21 (Suppl. 3), 51–116.

Further reading

Abe, C., Uchida, T., Ohta, M., Ichikawa, T., Yamashita, K., Ikeda, S., 2007. Cytochrome P450-dependent metabolism of vitamin E isoforms is a critical determinant of their tissue concentrations in rats. Lipids 42, 637–645.
Bardowell, S.A., Duan, F., Manor, D., Swanson, J.E., Parker, R.S., 2012. Disruption of mouse cytochrome p450 4f14 (Cyp4f14 gene) causes severe perturbations in vitamin E metabolism. J. Biol. Chem. 287, 26077–26086.
Behrens, W.A., Thompson, J.N., Madere, R., 1982. Distribution of alpha-tocopherol in human plasma lipoproteins. Am. J. Clin. Nutr. 35, 691–696.
Burton, G.W., Traber, M.G., Acuff, R.V., Walters, D.N., Kayden, H., Hughes, L., et al., 1998. Human plasma and tissue alpha-tocopherol concentrations in response to supplementation with deuterated natural and synthetic vitamin E. Am. J. Clin. Nutr. 67, 669–684.
Cho, J.Y., Kang, D.W., Ma, X., Ahn, S.H., Krausz, K.W., Luecke, H., et al., 2009. Metabolomics reveals a novel vitamin E metabolite and attenuated vitamin E metabolism upon PXR activation. J. Lipid Res. 50, 924–937.
Chung, S., Ghelfi, M., Atkinson, J., Parker, R., Qian, J., Carlin, C., et al., 2016. Vitamin E and phosphoinositides regulate the intracellular localization of the hepatic alpha-tocopherol transfer protein. J. Biol. Chem. 291, 17028–17039.
Clevidence, B.A., Lehmann, J., 1989. Alpha- and gamma-tocopherol levels in lipoproteins fractionated by affinity chromatography. Lipids 24, 137–140.
Cohn, W., Goss-Sampson, M.A., Grun, H., Muller, D.P., 1992. Plasma clearance and net uptake of alpha-tocopherol and low-density lipoprotein by tissues in WHHL and control rabbits. Biochem. J. 287 (Pt 1), 247–254.
Drevon, C.A., 1991. Absorption, transport and metabolism of vitamin E. Free Radic. Res. Commun. 14, 229–246.
Freiser, H., Jiang, Q., 2009. Optimization of the enzymatic hydrolysis and analysis of plasma conjugated gamma-CEHC and sulfated long-chain carboxychromanols, metabolites of vitamin E. Anal. Biochem. 388, 260–265.
Grebenstein, N., Schumacher, M., Graeve, L., Frank, J., 2014. Alpha-tocopherol transfer protein is not required for the discrimination against gamma-tocopherol in vivo but protects it from side-chain degradation in vitro. Mol. Nutr. Food Res. 58, 1052–1060.
Hacquebard, M., Carpentier, Y.A., 2005. Vitamin E: absorption, plasma transport and cell uptake. Curr. Opin. Clin. Nutr. Metab. Care 8, 133–138.
Horiguchi, M., Arita, M., Kaempf-Rotzoll, D.E., Tsujimoto, M., Inoue, K., Arai, H., 2003. pH-dependent translocation of alpha-tocopherol transfer protein (alpha-TTP) between hepatic cytosol and late endosomes. Genes Cells 8, 789–800.

Hosomi, A., Arita, M., Sato, Y., Kiyose, C., Ueda, T., Igarashi, O., et al., 1997. Affinity for α-tocopherol transfer protein as a determinant of the biological activities of vitamin E analogs. FEBS Lett. 409, 105–108.

Ikeda, S., Tohyama, T., Yamashita, K., 2002. Dietary sesame seed and its lignans inhibit 2,7,8-trimethyl-2(2′-carboxyethyl)-6-hydroxychroman excretion into urine of rats fed gamma-tocopherol. J. Nutr. 132, 961–966.

Jiang, Q., Freiser, H., Wood, K.V., Yin, X., 2007. Identification and quantitation of novel vitamin E metabolites, sulfated long-chain carboxychromanols, in human A549 cells and in rats. J. Lipid Res. 48, 1221–1230.

Johnson, C.H., Slanar, O., Krausz, K.W., Kang, D.W., Patterson, A.D., Kim, J.H., et al., 2012. Novel metabolites and roles for alpha-tocopherol in humans and mice discovered by mass spectrometry-based metabolomics. Am. J. Clin. Nutr. 96, 818–830.

Kamal-Eldin, A., Frank, J., Razdan, A., Tengblad, S., Basu, S., Vessby, B., 2000. Effects of dietary phenolic compounds on tocopherol, cholesterol, and fatty acids in rats. Lipids 35, 427–435.

Kluth, D., Landes, N., Pfluger, P., Muller-Schmehl, K., Weiss, K., Bumke-Vogt, C., et al., 2005. Modulation of Cyp3a11 mRNA expression by alpha-tocopherol but not gamma-tocotrienol in mice. Free Radic. Biol. Med. 38, 507–514.

Kolleck, I., Schlame, M., Fechner, H., Looman, A.C., Wissel, H., Rustow, B., 1999. HDL is the major source of vitamin E for type II pneumocytes. Free Radic. Biol. Med. 27, 882–890.

Kono, N., Arai, H., 2015. Intracellular transport of fat-soluble vitamins A and E. Traffic 16, 19–34.

Kostner, G.M., Oettl, K., Jauhiainen, M., Ehnholm, C., Esterbauer, H., Dieplinger, H., 1995. Human plasma phospholipid transfer protein accelerates exchange/transfer of alpha-tocopherol between lipoproteins and cells. Biochem. J. 305 (Pt 2), 659–667.

Lemaire-Ewing, S., Desrumaux, C., Neel, D., Lagrost, L., 2010. Vitamin E transport, membrane incorporation and cell metabolism: is alpha-tocopherol in lipid rafts an oar in the lifeboat? Mol. Nutr. Food Res. 54, 631–640.

Mardones, P., Strobel, P., Miranda, S., Leighton, F., Quinones, V., Amigo, L., et al., 2002. Alpha-tocopherol metabolism is abnormal in scavenger receptor class B type I (SR-BI)-deficient mice. J. Nutr. 132, 443–449.

Mustacich, D.J., Leonard, S.W., Devereaux, M.W., Sokol, R.J., Traber, M.G., 2006. Alpha-tocopherol regulation of hepatic cytochrome P450s and ABC transporters in rats. Free Radic. Biol. Med. 41, 1069–1078.

Parker, R.S., Sontag, T.J., Swanson, J.E., 2000. Cytochrome P4503A-dependent metabolism of tocopherols and inhibition by sesamin. Biochem. Biophys. Res. Commun. 277, 531–534.

Qian, J., Morley, S., Wilson, K., Nava, P., Atkinson, J., Manor, D., 2005. Intracellular trafficking of vitamin E in hepatocytes: the role of tocopherol transfer protein. J. Lipid Res. 46, 2072–2082.

Roager, H.M., Sulek, K., Skov, K., Frandsen, H.L., Smedsgaard, J., Wilcks, A., et al., 2014. *Lactobacillus acidophilus* NCFM affects vitamin E acetate metabolism and intestinal bile acid signature in monocolonized mice. Gut Microbes 5, 296–303.

Ross, A.B., Chen, Y., Frank, J., Swanson, J.E., Parker, R.S., Kozubek, A., et al., 2004. Cereal alkylresorcinols elevate gamma-tocopherol levels in rats and inhibit gamma-tocopherol metabolism in vitro. J. Nutr. 134, 506–510.

Sevrioukova, I.F., Poulos, T.L., 2013. Understanding the mechanism of cytochrome P450 3A4: recent advances and remaining problems. Dalton Trans. 42, 3116–3126.

Sontag, T.J., Parker, R.S., 2007. Influence of major structural features of tocopherols and tocotrienols on their omega-oxidation by tocopherol-omega-hydroxylase. J. Lipid Res. 48, 1090–1098.

Stahl, W., van den Berg, H., Arthur, J., Bast, A., Dainty, J., Faulks, R.M., et al., 2002. Bioavailability and metabolism. Mol. Asp. Med. 23, 39–100.

Tanabe, M., Fukushima, T., Usui, N., Aoyama, N., Tsunoda, M., Imai, K., 2004. Intravenous administration of 2,7,8-trimethyl-2-(beta-carboxyethyl)-6-hydroxy chroman (gamma-CEHC) to rats and determination of its plasma concentration and urinary sodium excretion. Biomed. Chromatogr. 18, 727–734.

Taylor, L., Krueger, N., Malysheva, O., Atkinson, J., Parker, R.S., 2018. ω-Hydroxylation of α-tocopheryl quinone reveals a dual function for cytochrome P450-4F2 in vitamin E metabolism. Bioorg. Med. Chem. 26 (20), 5555–5565.

Torquato, P., Bartolini, D., Giusepponi, D., Saluti, G., Russo, A., Barola, C., et al., 2016b. Alpha-13′-OH is the main product of α-tocopherol metabolism and influences CYP4F2 and PPAR gamma gene expression in HepG2 human hepatocarcinoma cells. Free Radic. Biol. Med. 96, S19–S20.

Traber, M.G., Kayden, H.J., 1984. Vitamin E is delivered to cells via the high affinity receptor for low-density lipoprotein. Am. J. Clin. Nutr. 40, 747–751.

Traber, M.G., Lane, J.C., Lagmay, N.R., Kayden, H.J., 1992. Studies on the transfer of tocopherol between lipoproteins. Lipids 27, 657–663.

Traber, M.G., Ramakrishnan, R., Kayden, H.J., 1994. Human plasma vitamin E kinetics demonstrate rapid recycling of plasma RRR-alpha-tocopherol. Proc. Natl. Acad. Sci. U.S.A. 91, 10005–10008.

Traber, M.G., Burton, G.W., Hamilton, R.L., 2004. Vitamin E trafficking. Ann. N. Y. Acad. Sci. 1031, 1–12.

Zhang, W.X., Thakur, V., Lomize, A., Pogozheva, I., Panagabko, C., Cecchini, M., et al., 2011. The contribution of surface residues to membrane binding and ligand transfer by the alpha-tocopherol transfer protein (alpha-TTP). J. Mol. Biol. 405, 972–988.

CHAPTER 24

Vitamin E: metabolism and molecular aspects

Pierangelo Torquato[1], Rita Marinelli[1], Desirée Bartolini[1], Danilo Giusepponi[2], Gabriele Cruciani[3], Lydia Siragusa[4], Roberta Galarini[2], Bartolomeo Sebastiani[3], Antimo Gioiello[1] and Francesco Galli[1]
[1]Department of Pharmaceutical Science, University of Perugia, Laboratory of Clinical Biochemistry and Nutrition, Perugia, Italy
[2]Istituto Zooprofilattico Sperimentale dell'Umbria e delle Marche "Togo Rosati", Perugia, Italy
[3]Department of Chemistry, Biology and Biotechnology, University of Perugia, Perugia, Italy
[4]Molecular Horizon, Perugia, Italy

Contents

24.1 Introduction

The vitamin E family of molecules encompasses eight fat-soluble vitamers (described in Chapter 23: Vitamin E: nutritional aspects), the metabolism of which is a complex and highly regulated process intimately connected with lipoprotein metabolism. Key steps of this metabolism include uptake, distribution, and catabolism of the different vitamers introduced with the diet. In this respect, differences exist when the metabolism of alpha-tocopherol (α-TOH) is compared with that of

Molecular Nutrition
DOI: https://doi.org/10.1016/B978-0-12-811907-5.00020-8

all other vitamin forms, involving different signal transduction and gene transcription mechanisms, and enzymatic functions. Importantly, these mechanistic aspects of vitamin E metabolism have recently been identified to play a role in the health-promoting effects of this vitamin, affecting lipid metabolism and detoxification processes, immune cell modulation, and cardiovascular protection mechanisms. Only in the last years has it been proposed that vitamin E transforms to a series of bioactive metabolites which play important roles that are alternative or synergic to the classical functions of vitamin E. These aspects are presented in the following sections of this chapter.

24.2 Metabolism

24.2.1 Intestinal absorption and tissue distribution

The intestinal absorption of TOHs and tocotrienols (T3s) is generally assumed to follow that of cholesterol and other fat-soluble vitamins (recently reviewed elsewhere in Galli et al., 2017; Schubert et al., 2018). It is therefore dependent on processes that include the formation of mixed micelles with the aid of bile acids, the activity of pancreatic lipases and esterases for hydrolysis of triglycerides, and the cleavage of tocopheryl esters, as well as the synthesis of vitamin E-containing chylomicrons in the intestinal mucosa with subsequent chylomicron secretion into the lymph (Drevon, 1991). Following chylomicron catabolism, some of the newly absorbed vitamin E is released and transferred to other lipoproteins and then into tissues (Stahl et al., 2002) and some remains with the chylomicron remnants. After uptake by the liver, RRR-α-TOH and the other 2R-stereoisomers are differentiated from the other forms of vitamin E and secreted by the liver into the circulation via very-low-density lipoproteins (VLDL) (Galli et al., 2007). Subsequently about half of the VLDL are catabolized via lipoprotein lipase (LPL) and transformed to low-density lipoproteins (LDL), with LDL being the major carrier for α-TOH in blood (Galli et al., 2007).

The α-tocopherol transfer protein (α-TTP) has long been considered to represent the main protein with the function of discriminating between different TOHs for the selective enrichment of nascent VLDL. The affinity of α-TTP for TOHs is the highest in the case of α-TOH and varies in the following order of magnitude: natural α-TOH = 100%; β-TOH = 38%; γ-TOH = 9%, and δ-TOH = 2%. At least for α-TOH and γ-TOH, such affinity order correlates with their abundance in plasma, compatible with a role for this protein as a main vitamin-binding and lipoprotein distribution factor of liver cells (Hosomi et al., 1997). This notion, however, was contradicted by the observation that in rats the discrimination of α-TTP against γ-TOH [which is about 2%–20% of total vitamin E with significant variation in the different human tissues (Burton et al., 1998)] can be reduced by the simultaneous ingestion of phytochemicals that interact with other components of vitamin E metabolism (Ikeda et al., 2002; Kamal-Eldin et al., 2000; Ross et al., 2004). These studies and others in the literature suggested an alternative explanation to the selective binding of α-TTP for α-TOH as the reason behind its preferential retention in the liver and other tissues. These studies included the discovery that vitamin E is degraded (or transformed) to side chain-shortened carboxyethyl hydroxychromanol (CEHC) metabolites by the sequential intervention of cytochrome P450 (CYP)-mediated ω-hydroxylation and β-oxidation-like enzymatic reactions, a pathway that in liver cells preferentially metabolizes the non-α congeners of TOH and T3 (Birringer et al., 2002; Sontag and Parker, 2002, 2007). Notwithstanding, other authors are keeping with the notion that α-TTP's main function is that of maintaining normal α-TOH concentrations in the plasma and extrahepatic tissues (Traber et al., 2004) by facilitating the transport of α-TOH from the lysosomes to the plasma membranes (Qian et al., 2005), followed by the continuous export of α-TOH from the liver to the plasma (Traber et al., 2004). The mechanisms that govern this latter step are however largely elusive. The enrichment of plasma in RRR-α-TOH does not seem to correspond linearly with the enrichment of nascent VLDL precursors from either the endoplasmic reticulum or the Golgi apparatus. Arita et al. (1997) demonstrated that the suppression of the endoplasmic reticulum/Golgi secretory pathway using "brefeldin A", did not affect the release of α-TOH, indicating that the VLDL enrichment with α-TOH may probably occur as a post-VLDL secretory process. However, it was proposed that α-TTP transfers α-TOH into nascent VLDL from the endosome, multivesicular bodies, and lysosome (Traber et al., 2004). Further, Kono and Arai (2015) suggest that α-TTP translocates from the cytosol to late endosomes/lysosomes to acquire α-TOH, which has been taken up by endocytosis or released from lipoproteins. The outer membrane of the endocytic vesicles is enriched with both *RRR*-α-TOH and *SRR*-α-TOH by ATP-binding cassette transporter (ABCA1), followed by the selective uptake of *RRR*-α-TOH via α-TTP

(Traber et al., 2004). Non-α-TOH forms are not protected against ω-hydroxylation after endocytosis and are further transported to the endoplasmic reticulum and the late endosomal compartment (Grebenstein et al., 2014). The α-TTP/α-TOH complex moves to the plasma membrane where it is targeted by phosphatidylinositol bisphosphates (PIP2), which are essential interaction partners of α-TTP (Kono and Arai, 2015), suggesting a protein−membrane transport mechanism (Zhang et al., 2011) in which α-TTP acts as an α-TOH/PIP2 exchanger (Kono and Arai, 2015). A "flippase" has been suggested to be involved in the transfer of α-TOH to the outer leaflet of the plasma membrane (Horiguchi et al., 2003) followed by a spontaneous transfer of α-TOH to nascent VLDL particles in the perisinusoidal space (Traber et al., 2004). Similar to chylomicrons, triglycerides in VLDL particles are enzymatically hydrolyzed by LPL resulting in the stepwise formation of LDL. The LDL particles carry the major portion of plasma α-TOH and that low-density lipoprotein receptor (LDLR)-mediated endocytosis contributes significantly to the uptake of α-TOH into cells (Traber and Kayden, 1984). However, α-TOH can be taken up by tissue via other pathways, including LDLR-independent mechanisms (Cohn et al., 1992), and other intracellular transport proteins may be involved (reviewed elsewhere in Schmolz et al., 2016).

High-density lipoprotein particles (HDL) provide a means for α-TOH to be secreted out of the extrahepatic tissues in order to be transported through the circulation back to the liver. HDL contain the lowest concentration of vitamin E per particle and their levels in plasma are lower compared to LDL; notwithstanding, HDL are the most potent donors of vitamin E to several target tissues (Kolleck et al., 1999; Traber et al., 1992). One possible explanation for this role was given by Clevidence and Lehmann (1989) who speculated that HDL contain more components for binding α-TOH besides serum apolipoprotein AI and ApoE (Behrens et al., 1982). Furthermore, it has been suggested that the supply of vitamin E by HDL could be more important under pathophysiological conditions, such as oxidative stress, most likely independent from the HDL-mediated uptake of cholesterol (Kolleck et al., 1999).

The HDL-interacting scavenger receptor SR-B1 controls the uptake and accumulation of α-TOH in specific tissues (Mardones et al., 2002) and in vitro experiments identified SR-B1 as a potential player of α-TOH uptake (Kolleck et al., 1999). Vitamin E, or rather α-TOH, has been shown to actively move between lipoproteins of different density classes (Traber et al., 1992). During the LPL-mediated lipolysis step, vitamin E remains incorporated either in chylomicron remnants (in the case of chylomicrons) or in LDL (in the case of VLDL). phospholipid transfer protein (PLTP) mediates the transfer of α-TOH between the different classes of lipoproteins and also the exchange of α-TOH between HDL and cell membranes (Kostner et al., 1995). Another member of the group of lipid transfer proteins, the cholesteryl ester transfer protein, has also been suggested as having a role in vitamin E transport and metabolism (Lemaire-Ewing et al., 2010).

Another important aspect of vitamin E metabolism to consider is that between 30% and 70% of the vitamin E introduced with the diet is not absorbed and distributed to the tissues, being directly excreted in the feces. Factors affecting intestinal absorption are many and may include food composition (food lipids promote the vitamin absorption) and the functioning of lipid digestion and absorption mechanisms. Other aspects of vitamin E metabolism that may affect the vitamin status include the elimination throughout enzymatic catabolism and biliary excretion of metabolic products into the ileum (Galli et al., 2007); some of these compounds are reabsorbed systemically through the enterohepatic recirculation and are excreted as urinary metabolites, the rest of them are excreted with the feces.

The role of the gut microbes in the degradation of TOHs and T3s, and their effect on the bioavailability of these forms, have not been elucidated. Some pieces of information revealed that *Lactobacillus acidophilus* (L-NCFM) affected vitamin E acetate metabolism and the intestinal bile acid signature in monocolonized mice. In fact, L-NCFM unconjugates taurocholic acid to cholic acid; the latter is an activator of the pancreatic bile acid-dependent carboxyl-ester hydrolase, which may increase the conversion of α-TOH-acetate into α-TOH, the form of vitamin E taken up by the enterocyte through the absorption of micelles (Roager et al., 2014). A recent study in mice demonstrated that treatment with antibiotics affects the CYP450-dependent catabolism of vitamin E thus influencing the vitamin levels in the liver and blood (Ran et al., 2019). This study also demonstrated that drug-induced dysbiosis mainly affects the availability of the less retained vitamers(desmethyl and T3 forms) and the tissue levels of their metabolites, some of which have been identified to be potent bioactives (Section 24.4).

24.2.2 Enzymatic metabolism and excretion

The CYP-dependent metabolism of vitamin E was described in the early 1980s thanks to the pioneering observation made by Nakamura's group (Chiku et al., 1984) of a short-chain urinary metabolite in rats fed a diet rich in δ-TOH, the origin of which was independent from that of free radical-derived metabolites. All vitamers are degraded to vitamer-specific physiological metabolites; these maintain an intact chromanol ring, while changes occur in the side-chain essentially aimed at shortening it (Galli et al., 2007). In the liver tissue this arm of vitamin E metabolism is essentially associated with the catabolism and excretion of the dietary vitamin exceeding the physiological needs, that is, the quota of vitamer overcoming the capability of specialized liver proteins to bind and transfer it to nascent VLDL (Chung et al., 2016; Hacquebard and Carpentier, 2005). The catabolism of TOHs and T3s begins with an ω-hydroxylation of the side-chain which is catalyzed by CYP enzymes. This oxidation is the rate-limiting step in vitamin E metabolism (Bardowell et al., 2012). Using reporter-gene assays combined with a systematical screening of CYP enzymes, Sontag and Parker proposed CYP4F2 as one of the main isoforms involved in the enzymatic metabolism of vitamin E (Sontag and Parker, 2002). This isoform exhibited higher specificity for the unsubstituted carbon at position C5 of the chromanol ring so that γ-TOH and δ-TOH are metabolized more efficiently than α-TOH, which in turn stimulates the metabolism of other vitamin E forms. Moreover, the authors found higher Vmax values for T3s than for their corresponding TOHs, suggesting that CYP4F2 contributes to the preferential physiological retention of α-TOH compared to other vitamin E forms that are thus preferentially metabolized. This finding supports the view of a central role for this pathway in modulating the biopotency of the different forms of vitamin E, that is, TOH and T3 vitamers (Sontag and Parker, 2002, 2007). CYP4F2 has recently been suggested to catalyze terminal carbon ω-hydroxylation of α-tocopheryl quinone (α-TQ), that is, the antioxidant activity-derived metabolite of α-TOH. As expected from α-TOH metabolism, this reaction process, besides producing the ω-HO metabolite α-13-OH-α-TQ, leads on to the formation of the carboxylic acid derivative of α-tocopheryl quinone, that is, α-13-COOH-α-TQ (Taylor et al., 2018). The CYP3A4 isoform is the most important CYP enzyme in humans with wide substrate promiscuity (Sevrioukova and Poulos, 2013). Parker et al. suggested that this is the main isoform involved in vitamin E metabolism (Parker et al., 2000), demonstrating that the incubation with

1 μmol/L ketoconazole and sesamin for 48 hours (these are natural CYP3A4 inhibitors) can block the metabolism of TOHs [α-TOH and γ-TOH in primary rat hepatocytes or γ- and δ-TOH in HepG2/C3A cells (25 μmol/L each)] to their corresponding short-chain metabolites (SCMs) by approximately 90%. Similar results were observed in rats after oral gavage of 50 mg/kg body weight ketoconazole (Abe et al., 2007). Conversely, rifampicin, an inducer of CYP3A4 activity, markedly stimulates *all-rac*-α-TOH degradation in HepG2 cells (Birringer et al., 2001). Again, feeding mice with 200 mg/day of α-TOH for 9 months resulted in 1.7-fold higher mRNA expression of *Cyp3a11* (this is the murine orthologue of human *CYP3A4*) levels compared to after 3 months (Kluth et al., 2005) and similar effects were observed after subcutaneous injection of 0.1 mg/g body weight α-TOH in rats (Mustacich et al., 2006). It is worth noting that Landes et al. (2003) showed that vitamin E may act as an agonist of pregnane X receptor (PXR). It is known that expression and activity of several CYP isoforms, including CYP3A4, are modulated by structurally diverse xenobiotics via PXR. In fact, this nuclear receptor is a master regulator of enzymes and transporters involved in the metabolism of xenobiotics and endobiotics (Cho et al., 2009). Moreover, recent studies described that liver cells exposed to conditions of lipotoxicity, for example, by the treatment with ethanol (Russo et al., 2017) or fatty acids to generate a steatogenic phenotype (Bartolini et al., 2017), show a sustained α-TOH catabolism. This type of response was found to occurr in the presence of a transient repression of *CYP4F2* and marked overexpression of other CYP isoforms, including *CYP3A4*. These findings further support a role for this latter CYP isoform, but not for CYP4F2, in the hepatic metabolism of vitamin E. Furthermore, these studies demonstrated for the first time that lipotoxicity can interfere with the hepatic metabolism of vitamin E leading to CYP gene pattern reprogramming (Bartolini et al., 2017; Russo et al., 2017 and references therein). The participation of other transcription factors and gene-regulation proteins in the modulation of inducible and repressible forms of CYP450 beside PXR may include PPARγ (Torquato et al., 2016) as a main player at the interface of vitamin E and long-chain fatty acid metabolism (discussed in Chapter 4: Vitamin E: structure and forms).

The main steps and compounds associated with the enzymatic metabolism of TOHs and T3s are summarized in Fig. 24.1. Table 24.1 shows the conjugated forms of enzymatic metabolites produced by the activity of hepatic transferases that have been identified in biological fluids and feces (mainly as sulfated and glucuronidated species).

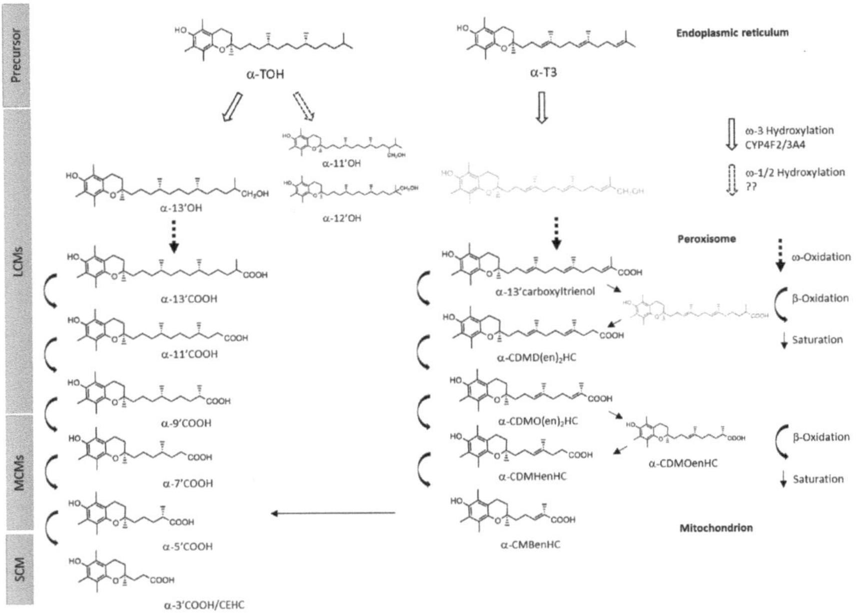

Figure 24.1 Metabolism of vitamin E. This metabolism starts with one cycle of CYP4F2/3A4-mediated ω-hydroxylation, followed by five cycles of β-oxidation. Recent evidence demonstrated the existence of alterative ω-1 and 2 hydroxylation in Cyp4f14$^{-/-}$ mice (Bardowell et al., 2012). The structures without names are molecules or steps which fit into the general concept but need further experimental confirmation and molecular characterization.
α-TOH, α-Tocopherols; *α-T3,* α-tocotrienols; *13′-OH,* 13′-hydroxychromanol; *13′-COOH,* 13′-carboxychromanol; *LCMs,* long-chain metabolites; *MCMs,* medium-chain metabolites; *SCM,* short-chain metabolites; *CDMD(en)2HC,* carboxydimethyldecadienylhydroxychromanol; *CDMOenHC,* carbodimethyloctenylhydroxychromanol; *CDMHenHC,* carboxymethylhexenylhydroxychromanol; *CMBenHC,* carboxymethylbutadienylhydroxychromanol; *CDMOHC,* carboxymethyloctylhydroxychromanol; *CDMHHC,* carboxymethylhexylhydroxychromanol; *CMBHC,* carboxymethylbutylhydroxychromanol; *CEHC,* carboxyethylhydroxychromanols. *Modified from Schmolz, L., Birringer, M., Lorkowski, S., Wallert, M., 2016. Complexity of vitamin E metabolism. World J. Biol. Chem. 7, 14–43*

24.3 Receptors/sensors, signal transduction and gene modulation effects

24.3.1 Role of vitamin E in signal transduction and transcriptional mechanisms

The gene response to vitamin E varies in a cell- and tissue-specific manner, as well as being species specific. Protein interactions responsible for

Table 24.1 Conjugates of vitamin E metabolites and their excretion.

Metabolite	Conjugate	Organism	Excretion	
LCM	Sulfates	Rats and in vitro	Feces	Freiser and Jiang (2009), Jiang et al. (2007)
MCM	Ether glucuronides	Human and mouse	Urine/feces	Johnson et al. (2012)
	Sulfates	Human		
SCM	Glucosides, glutamine	Mouse	Urine/feces	Cho et al. (2009), Johnson et al. (2012)
	Taurine, glycine, or glycine glucuronides	Human and mouse	Urine	Johnson et al. (2012)
	Sulfates	Rats		Tanabe et al. (2004)

Source: Modified from Schmolz, L., Birringer, M., Lorkowski, S., Wallert, M., 2016. Complexity of vitamin E metabolism. World J. Biol. Chem. 7, 14–43.

Table 24.2 Nuclear receptors and transcription factors identified to respond to vitamin E administration in cells and animal models.

Pregnane X receptor (PXR)
Constitutive androstane receptor (CAR)
RAR-related orphan receptor alpha (RORα)
Peroxisome proliferator-activated receptor γ (PPARγ)
Estrogen receptor beta (ERβ)
Nuclear factor erythroid-derived 2-like 2 (Nrf2)
Hypoxia-inducible factor 1 alpha (Hif1-α)
Nuclear factor kappa B (NFkB)

this response include nuclear receptors and some transcriptional nodes of energy metabolism, redox homeostasis, and inflammatory pathways, some of which are summarized in Table 24.2 (recently reviewed elsewhere in Azzi, 2018; Zingg, 2015).

At the same time TOHs and T3s influence distinct signal transduction pathways that directly or indirectly modulate gene-regulation mechanisms at different levels. It is apparent that such a regulatory function of this family of vitamers occurs by means of different, essentially low-to-mild affinity and transient, protein interactions, the nature of which remain poorly characterized. These may include the interaction with α-TTP that is believed to mediate vitamin E uptake and trafficking in the cell systems via a PIP-regulated process (Chung et al., 2016; Kono et al., 2013), and tocopherol-associated proteins (TAPs) that are also important in regulating PI3K activity and gene response of normal and tumoral cells (reviewed in Zingg, 2015). The latter group of proteins include TAP1, 2, and 3 isoforms, which correspond to the members of the SEC14L family identified as SEC14L2, 3, and 4, respectively. In this family, TAP1 has been reported to bind with high-affinity α-TOH, but not other forms of vitamin E, and to translocate into the nucleus to promote gene transcription in a α-TOH-dependent manner (Yamauchi et al., 2001; Zimmer et al., 2000). Other vitamin E-binding proteins are located on the extracellular environment and cell surface, and include PLTP, afamin, albumin, scavenger receptors and membrane transporters, such as the SR class B type I (SR-BI) and CD36, and some members of the ATP-binding cassette transporter family (ABCA1 and ABCG1) (Zingg, 2015).

Single-gene and microarray gene expression studies carried out in the last decades have explored signal transduction and transcriptional effects of vitamin E in several experimental models, such as rodents fed with

Table 24.3 Some gene response systems under the influence of tocopherol (TOH) or tocotrienol molecules in different experimental systems.

Tocopherol effect (up↑ or down↓ regulation)	Gene systems	References
Vitamin E acetate ↓	Immune response: NFkB	Flohe et al. (1997), Suzuki and Packer (1993)
γ and α-TOH ↑α-TOH↓	Cholesterol homeostasis: PPARγ LXR (including receptors LXR-regulated: CD36, ABCA1, and ABCG1)	De Pascale et al. (2006) Rode et al. (2008)
γ and α-TOH ↑Garcinoic acid and α-LCMs ↑	Lipid metabolism and inflammation: PPARα, PPARγ	Poynter and Daynes (1998) Torquato et al. (2016)
α-TOH ↑	Steroidogenesis: AP-1 and Ref-1	Abidi et al. (2004)
α-TOH↓	Platelet aggregation: GP IIb	Chang et al. (2000)
T3 ↑ LCMs ↑ (?)	Xenobiotic detoxification: PXR, including PXR-regulated genes: CYP3A4, Pgp	Landes et al. (2003) Podszun et al. (2017)
T3 ↑	Estrogen receptor: ERβ (including genes Erβ-regulated MIC-1, ECR-1, and cathepsin D)	Comitato et al. (2010)

NFκB, Nuclear factor kappa-light-chain-enhancer of activated B cells; *PPARγ*, peroxisome proliferator-activated receptor gamma; *LXR*, liver X receptor; *CD36*, cluster of differentiation 36; *ABCA1*, ATP-binding cassette transporter; *ABCG1*, ATP-binding cassette G1 transporter; *PPARα*, Peroxisome proliferator-activated receptor alpha; *AP-1*, activator protein-1; *Ref-1*, redox-regulated protein; *GP IIP*, glycoprotein IIb; *PXR*, pregnane X receptor; *CYP3A4*, cytochrome P3A4; *ERβ*, estrogen receptor beta; *MIC-1*, macrophage inhibitory cytokine 1; *ECR-1*, estrogen receptor 1.

different types of diets or α-TTP-deficient mice, as well as in human cells and tissues (recently discussed in Brigelius-Flohe, 2009; Galli et al., 2017). For example, microarray data demonstrated that changes in vitamin E intake produce permanent stimulation or depletion of specific gene clusters, such as those for vesicular transport, or neuronal and muscular functions, respectively (reviewed in Brigelius-Flohe and Galli, 2010 and references therein); other examples of gene-regulation systems under the influence of vitamin E molecules are reported in Table 24.3. These studies suggest the view that vitamin E produces direct and specific gene-regulation effects, influencing the activity of receptors and transcription factors, but as a matter of fact, no vitamin E-specific receptor has conclusively been identified so far, as known for instance in the case of the other fat-soluble vitamins A and D (Galli et al., 2017; Schubert et al., 2018).

It is worth noting that the only genes responding to high doses of α-TOH in vivo, in a relatively short time, are those involved in vitamin E elimination, that is, hepatic CYP and ABC transporters. Induction of these genes appears to depend on PXR activation, a nuclear receptor that responds to lipophilic xenobiotics, such as several steroids and drugs (Landes et al., 2003; Podszun et al., 2017). However, direct binding to PXR could only be demonstrated for T3s, apparently not for TOHs (Zhou et al., 2004), and the in vivo induction of the CYP gene response, assessed by Cyp3a11 expression (the murine orthologue of human CYP3A4), required supranutritional amounts of α-TOH (Kluth et al., 2005; Mustacich et al., 2006). Thus the regulation of xenobiotic metabolism has been suggested to be the main, and possible the only, gene response effect of α-TOH, the meaning of which was proposed to be that of self-regulating its own metabolism to prevent accumulation (Traber, 2010). Compatible with this reductionist view, recent evidence in the literature has demonstrated that long-chain metabolites (LCMs) with α and non-α configuration are much stronger activators of PXR as well as of PPARγ nuclear receptor compared to their TOH and T3 precursors (Podszun et al., 2017; Torquato et al., 2016; Galli F., Gioiello A., Mani S., unpublished data), suggesting a potent feed-forward mechanism for the catabolism and elimination of the vitamin excess. Other authors are now pointing to a different ("nonreductionist") view, compatible with a role of vitamin E as a provitamin. This view, originally proposed in Galli et al. (2007), is now supported by further convincing evidence on the biological role of LCMs. This role appears to occur through the direct modulation of enzymatic activities, such as 5-LOX-dependent production of inflammatory eicosanoids (described in Jiang et al., 2011; Pein et al., 2018 and further discussed later in this section), and transcriptional function of nuclear receptors influencing long-chain fatty acid availability/ metabolism (e.g., by CYP3A4 and Pgp upregulation). Intriguingly, other gene responses are now emerging to indicate that most of these provitamin-derived effects could be particularly important for the control of the metabolism and toxicity (lipotoxicity) of cellular lipids. Beside PPARγ protein modulation (Torquato et al., 2016), these include the transcriptional regulation and activity of the lipid droplet-associated protein PLIN2 (Schmolz et al., 2018) that responds to α-LCMs, but not to α-TOH, to promote cytoprotection under conditions of lipotoxicity.

However, if PXR or another functionally equivalent receptor or sensor could regulate in a specific way the gene response to vitamin E, all forms of this vitamin should result in the same gene response pattern, but this does not appear to be the case. For example, T3 regulates expression and activity of genes differently from those regulated by α-TOH (Comitato et al., 2010; Viola et al., 2012). The finding that T3s, but not TOHs, can bind to estrogen receptor β (ERβ) and initiate the expression of estrogen-dependent genes (for example, MIC-1, ECR-1, and cathepsin D) in ERβ-expressing breast cancer cells, appears to confirm such a discrepancy, highlighting the presence of different molecular targets for the different forms of this vitamin. These findings and other differences among the molecular and cellular responses to TOHs and T3s (reviewed in Khanna et al., 2010; Viola et al., 2012) also resulted in the provocative question of whether T3 should still be grouped in the vitamin E family of molecules (Brigelius-Flohe and Galli, 2010).

Besides a role in side-chain unsaturation (i.e., TOH vs T3), other epitopes of vitamin E molecule appear to play a key role in producing vitamer and metabolite-specific gene responses (discussed in Schmolz et al., 2017; Viola et al., 2012, 2013). These appear to include both the methylation pattern of chromanols and the availability of the hydroxyl group in position 6 of the ring for reaction (assessed after either reversible or irreversible derivatization). This demonstrates that different portions of the vitamin E molecule intervene in the physical and functional interaction with receptors and transcription factors, thus influencing the catabolism and/or the provitamin activity of the vitamin forms.

24.3.2 Vitamin E as enzyme activity regulator

The first enzyme found to be regulated by vitamin E was protein kinase C (PKC) which is specifically inhibited by the α-TOH form (Mahoney and Azzi, 1988). Since then, a number of additional enzymes have been identified as inhibition targets of this vitamin, some of which were introduced earlier in this Chapter and in Chapter 23. These include nicotinamide adenine dinucleotide phosphate (NADPH) oxidase (Cachia et al., 1998; Egger et al., 2001), phospholipase A2 (Egger et al., 2001), PKB/Akt (Kempna et al., 2004), 5-LOX (Kempna et al., 2004; Pein et al., 2018), 12-LOX and 15-LOX (Kagan et al., 2017; Khanna et al., 2003), and cyclooxygenase-2 (COX-2) (Jiang et al., 2000; Wu et al., 1998). Enzymes activated by α-TOH include protein phosphatase 2A (PP2A) (Ricciarelli et al., 1998)—the mechanism of this activation remains elusive after 20 years from its discovery—diacylglycerol kinase (DGK) (McNally and Anderson, 2003; Tran et al., 1994), and dose-dependently HMG-CoA reductase (Khor and Ng, 2000).

PKC inhibition was demonstrated to occur by preventing its phosphorylation-dependent activation via enhanced PP2A activity (Ricciarelli et al., 1998). Moreover, translocation of PKC to the membrane, which is required for activity, is also prevented (Boscoboinik et al., 1991). Activation of NADPH oxidase is attenuated by the inhibition of the PP2A- and PKC-dependent translocation of p67phox (Egger et al., 2001) or p47phox (Cachia et al., 1998) to the membrane. Inhibition of 5-LOX by α-TOH, similarly to PKC, appears to involve complex recruitment processes. Lipopolysaccharide (LPS)-stimulated release of tumor necrosis factor (TNF) is decreased by α-TOH and other 5-LOX inhibitors. Upon Ca^{2+}-triggered activation, 5-LOX and PLA2 translocate to the perinuclear envelope where they assemble with the 5-LOX-activating protein (FLAP) (reviewed in Murphy and Gijon, 2007). The role of FLAP is not fully understood yet. It might be a scaffolding protein that facilitates assembly of both cytosolic proteins at the nuclear membrane or it might bind arachidonic acid (AA) released by PLA2 and present this substrate to 5-LOX. Inhibition of 12-LOX and 15-LOX has also been demonstrated, whereby the effectiveness of T3s was overall markedly higher than that of TOHs (Kagan et al., 2017; Khanna et al., 2003). Mechanistic aspects of this inhibition are still elusive, but compelling evidence suggests that tocochromanols can at the same time strongly suppress nonregiospecific free radical components of LOX-catalyzed phospholipid peroxidation (Arai et al., 1995) and compete for the polyunsaturated fatty acid (PUFA) substrates binding sites (via a "corking" mechanism). Similar inhibitory mechanisms appear to occur in the case of PLA2, that provides LOXs of PUFA substrates. Competition of vitamin E with phospholipid substrates at the catalytic site of PLA2 has been consistently demonstrated by cocrystallization experiments carried out on snake venom enzyme in which α-TOH was demonstrated to bind the catalytic pocket of one of the two enzyme monomers (Chandra et al., 2002). Kinetics and inhibition studies agreed with the crystallographic results. Further crystallization experiments suggested also the effects of α-TOH binding on the stability of the dimeric form of the enzyme (Takeda et al., 2004).

PLA2 activity was inhibited in platelets (Douglas et al., 1986), macrophages (Douglas et al., 1986), and liposomes (Grau and Ortiz, 1998), but surprisingly it was enhanced in endothelial cells (Wu et al., 2005), and thus the effect of vitamin E appears to be stimulation specific. PLA2 enzymes consist of a large and diverse superfamily of at least 14 separate groups. Subgroups I, II, III, V, and IX–XIV require Ca^{2+} for activity and are, although not generally, associated with membrane trafficking events. Subgroups IV, VI, VII, and VIII are serine esterases and mainly involved in Ca^{2+}-independent membrane trafficking, tubule formation, and membrane fusion (reviewed in Brown et al., 2003). By the formation of lysophospholipids, PLA2 enzymes induce changes in the membrane curvature (Hermann et al., 2014). Therefore PLA2 not only releases AA to provide the precursor for lipid mediators, but it can also influence the activity of membrane-bound or membrane-incorporated proteins. As introduced earlier in this section, inhibition of PLA2 activity by vitamin E has been attributed to an interference with the accessibility of the substrate to PLA2 in the membrane (Grau and Ortiz, 1998). This "corking effect" produces the highest inhibition in the case of α-TOH that compared with other TOHs, less deeply penetrates into the membrane possibly by the fully-methylated structure of the chroman group. Which of the various forms of PLA2 is preferentially inhibited by this vitamin has not yet been described and this could be the reason for the discrepancies in the activity modulation (inhibition/activation) patterns described so far in literature.

LPS- or interleukin1-β (1IL-1β)-stimulated COX-2 activity was preferentially decreased by γ-TOH and its metabolite γ-CEHC (Jiang et al., 2000), whereas higher concentrations of α-TOH were required for inhibition. γ-TOH was suggested to compete with AA for the active site of COX-2. Finally, vitamin E inhibited phosphorylation of PKB/Akt (Kempna et al., 2004). δ-TOH was the most effective form in producing this effect and, worthy of note, the activation of the enzyme requires translocation to the membrane and subsequent phosphorylation by phosphoinositide-dependent kinase 1, indicating that also here vitamin E may influence translocation processes and lipid–protein interactions within the PI3K/Akt pathway, important for several cellular processes and as targets of anticancer therapies (Thillai et al., 2017). A transient translocation to the membrane is also reported to influence PP2A and the PKC-dependent control of DGK activity that might be related to the proposed functions of α-TOH in vesicular transport and in several aspects of immune and cancer cell biology (reviewed in Zingg, 2007, 2015).

24.4 Vitamin E metabolites as bioactive molecules

24.4.1 On the origin of the bioactivation hypothesis of vitamin E

Catabolic steps in the metabolism of vitamin E have always been seen as a process to eliminate an excess of this micronutrient (Schmolz et al., 2016). Accordingly, it has been suggested that the urinary SCM α-CEHC is an indicator of an adequate vitamin E supply (Schultz et al., 1995), and is only excreted at a certain threshold level of the hepatic vitamin (Traber, 2013). The same could be proposed for γ-TOH metabolism, the second most abundant form of vitamin E in human tissues (Galli et al., 2002, 2003).

It was 1995 when Murray et al. (1995) isolated from human urine a mild potency natriuretic factor, the structure of which was demonstrated to coincide with that of SCM γ-CEHC (Kantoci et al., 1997), and at the beginning of the 2000s some pioneering studies provided the first pieces of evidence on the activity of desmethyl SCMs on COX-2 activity of inflammatory cells and cell cycle checkpoints of cancer cells (Galli et al., 2004a; Jiang et al., 2000).

The demonstration that SCMs, and even more so LCMs (discussed later), of α-TOH are bioactive molecules, stimulated the hypothesis that besides the "excess/elimination route" there could be an even more important "activation route" of this vitamin. In keeping with this hypothesis originally proposed in Galli et al. (2007), other studies confirmed the preliminary data obtained on SCMs and went on to identify LCMs as more potent bioactives formed throughout the enzymatic and nonenzymatic routes of vitamin E metabolism (described in the next section and in Table 24.4).

In this respect, vitamin E appears to follow the same mechanism described for other fat-soluble vitamins that promote their gene regulation function by means of their metabolites (recently reviewed elsewhere in Galli et al., 2017; Podszun et al., 2017; Schubert et al., 2018). When looking at vitamin A and D, for example, metabolism transforms alimentary or endogenous precursors into the active forms that exhibit the

Table 24.4 Main biological functions of vitamin E metabolites.

Vitamin E metabolites	Biological effects	Targets	References
Long-chain metabolites (LCMs)			
α-13'-OH; δ-13'-COOH	Antiproliferative effect		Mazzini et al. (2009)
α- and δ-13'-COOH	Proapoptotic effect	Caspase-3 and 9, PARP-1	Birringer et al. (2010)
α-13'-COOH	Antiatherogenic effect	CD36	Wallert et al. (2014)
	Immune regulation and antiinflammatory function	5-LOX	Pein et al. (2018)
	Xenobiotic metabolism	Pgp	Podszun et al. (2017)
	Antilipotoxic effect	PLIN2	Schmolz et al. (2018)
α-13'-OH; α-13'-COOH; δ-T3-13'-COOH	Lipid homeostasis	PPARγ, CYP4F2	Torquato et al. (2016)
δ-13'-COOH	Antiinflammatory effect	COX-2, PGE_2	Jiang et al. (2008)
δ-T3-13'-COOH; α-13'-COOH		Il1β, Il6, and TNFα	Schmolz et al. (2014)
α-TQ/α-THQ	Antiferroptotic activity	15-LOX	Taylor et al. (2018)
α-TOH phosphate	Angiogenic and vasculogenic effects	VEGF	Zingg et al. (2010)
Short-chain metabolites (SCMs)			
γ-CEHC	Natriuretic properties	70 pS K + channel	Wechter et al. (1996)
γ-CEHC	Antiproliferative and antioxidant effects	Cyclin D1	Galli et al. (2004b)
γ-CEHC		NO_x scavenging	Galli et al. (2004b)
α-CEHC; γ-CEHC	Antiinflammatory effects	PGE_2	Grammas et al. (2004)

TNFα, Tumor necrosis factor alpha; *PGE_2*, prostaglandin E_2; *CD36*, cluster of differentiation 36; *PPARγ*, peroxisome proliferator-activated receptor gamma; *CYP4F2*, cytochrome P4F2; *PLIN2*, perilipin 2; *COX-2*, cyclooxygenase-2; *Il1β*, interleukin 1 beta; *Il 6*, interleukin 6; *VEGF*, vascular endothelial growth factor; *Pgp*, P-glycoprotein.

underlying vitamin properties. However, crucial data are still missing to conclusively confirm a provitamin mechanism of action for vitamin E in animal organisms. So far, in fact, no specific binding protein, cellular transporter, or cellular receptor have been identified for the metabolites that discriminate the vitamin precursors. This is keeping the role and mechanism of the action of vitamin E still enigmatic (Blaner, 2013; Brigelius-Flohe, 2009; Brigelius-Flohe and Galli, 2010).

A possible explanation for this lack of evidence on a specific receptor is that the biological activity of the vitamin E-related molecules (that can be identified with the definition of "vitamin E metabolome") may depend on multiple and highly variable lipid—protein interactions occurring at the same time on several protein cavities (identified as the "vitamin E interactome") of the cell. Together these interactions may produce the underlying biological response even in the absence of a specific high-affinity interaction. This type of scenario compatible with a "fluid receptor" model based on the formation of a series of transient and low-affinity interactions, may help to explain, for example, the multiple effects that vitamin E and other cellular lipids produce on apparently unrelated and even divergent cell pathways.

Different from high-affinity interactions, which include those with α-TTP and TAP1 described before, many of these low-affinity interactions are difficult to capture with the available lipidomics and proteomics methods because of their fugacity and promiscuity (disrupting cell structures, fractionating cellular components and isolating/extracting lipids or protein fractions, are all processes that conceivably interfere with the physiological interactome of vitamin E and with that of many other cellular lipids). However, some of them can be predicted, for instance, by the in silico exploration of cellular interactomes; then, the results of such explorative studies can be verified at the functional and molecular level. As an example of this approach, we utilized the bioinformatics procedure previously described in Siragusa et al. (2014) to comparatively explore the interactome of α-TOH and that of its LCMs α-13′-OH and α-13′-COOH, which should differ on the bases of available biological and molecular results (described in the next section). This procedure is based on a semiautomated method for comparing and clustering protein pockets, called BioGPS, that combines the GRID molecular interactions fields (MIFs) with FLAP pharmacophoric fingerprints. With this procedure about 700K potential cavities detected on protein structures available for

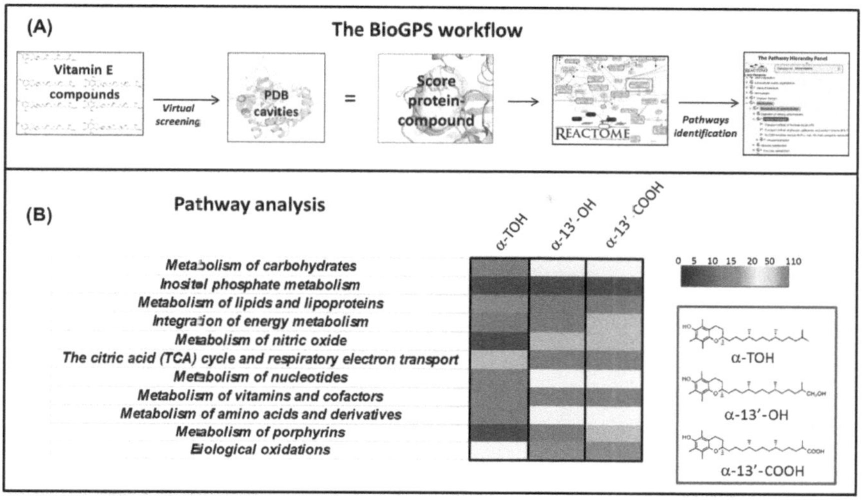

Figure 24.2 In silico strategy to explore the vitamin E interactome. (A) Workflow of BioGPS analysis method utilized to identify potential interaction cavities for vitamin E on human proteins. The BioGPS platform combines the GRID molecular interactions fields (MIFs) with FLAP pharmacophoric fingerprints. (B) Reactome pathway analysis of BioGPS data on the protein interactions identified for α-tocopherol (α-TOH) and its long-chain metabolites (LCMs) α-13′-OH and α-13′-COOH (data were from a partial exploration of the interaction field database: 70K cavities over 700K).

consultation on public databases can be interrogated to identify potential interactions with small molecules and their localization in cellular pathways and biological functions. This latter step is implemented assessing BioGPS results with the Reactome pathway analysis tool (https://reactome.org). The workflow and output representation of this bioinformatics analysis are reported in Fig. 24.2. The aim of identifying different interaction patterns for α-TOH and its LCMs was already achieved after exploration of about 70K cavities (Fig. 24.2B), and interestingly enough, interaction scores of both α-TOH and LCMs were the highest on pathways that nicely fit with the biological context of vitamin E, such as the metabolism of lipids and lipoproteins and biological oxidations. Protein hits identified in these pathways (Table 24.5) included nuclear receptors, proteins associated with endogenous sterols and bile acid metabolism, and CYP450 isoenzymes, such as CYP2E1. All these hits are reported to have a role in the hepatic metabolism of vitamin E (reviewed in Russo et al., 2017; Traber, 2004).

Table 24.5 Possible protein interactions of α-tocopherol (α-TOH) and its long-chain metabolites (LCMs) α-13′-OH and α-13′-COOH identified with the in silico analysis method of Fig. 24.1 (the first 10 protein hits are shown).

Rank	Uniprot	Protein name	Organism	Reactome-higher levels	Reactome-lower levels
1	P10826	Retinoic acid receptor beta	*Homo sapiens* (human)	Gene expression, signal transduction, transmembrane transport of	Nuclear receptor transcription pathway, orphan transporters, and signaling by retinoic acid
2	P62483	Voltage-gated potassium channel subunit beta-2	*Rattus norvegicus* (rat)	Neuronal system	Voltage-gated potassium channels
3	P80188	Neutrophil gelatinase-associated lipocalin	*Homo sapiens* (human)	Transmembrane transport of small molecules	Iron uptake and transport, Orphan transporters
4	P97612	Fatty acid amide hydrolase 1	*Rattus norvegicus* (rat)	–	Fatty acid catabolic process
5	P11509	Cytochrome P450 2A6	*Homo sapiens* (human)	Metabolism	CYP2E1 reactions, xenobiotics
6	P05181	Cytochrome P450 2E1	*Homo sapiens* (human)	Metabolism	CYP2E1 reactions, xenobiotics
7	P04040	Catalase	*Homo sapiens* (human)	Cellular responses to stress, Metabolism	Detoxification of reactive oxygen species, purine catabolism
8	Q02127	Dihydroorotate dehydrogenase	*Homo sapiens* (human)	Metabolism	Pyrimidine biosynthesis
9	Q9Y6A2	Cholesterol 24-hydroxylase	*Homo sapiens* (human)	Metabolism	Endogenous sterols, synthesis of bile acids, and bile salts via 24-hydroxycholesterol
10	Q9NTG7	NAD-dependent protein deacetylase sirtuin-3	*Homo sapiens* (human)	Organelle biogenesis and maintenance	Transcriptional activation of mitochondrial biogenesis

24.4.2 Proposed physiological functions of long-chain metabolites

An increasing number of studies are now reporting on biological activity of LCMs of vitamin E, suggesting physiological functions for these molecules (Table 24.4).

The first biological studies on these metabolites were performed by Mazzini et al. (2009) who developed a semisynthesis procedure to produce the RRR form of α-LCMs (α-13′-OH and α-13′-COOH) starting from garcinoic acid (GA), a plant analogue of the physiological LCM *trans*-13′-carboxy-δ-T3. GA was isolated from the African bitternut of *Garcinia kola* according to the original procedure published by Terashima et al. (1997). α-13′-COOH was synthesized from GA by the hydrogenation of aliphatic side-chain double bounds and the subsequent methylation of the chroman ring. Then α-13′-OH was obtained by LiAlH4-mediated reduction of α-13′-COOH acid function (Mazzini et al., 2009). These semisynthesis protocols and the resulting pure compounds have represented a major breakthrough in the field allowing the first analytical and biological/functional studies. Using GA-derived α-LCMs in vitro, convincing data were obtained on activities that are specific for these LCM and distinct from those observed for the metabolic precursor α-TOH (Birringer et al., 2010; Ciffolilli et al., 2015; Wallert et al., 2014, 2015).

For example, in human macrophages α-LCMs decreased uptake of oxidized LDL (oxLDL) and oxLDL-induced lipid accumulation, likely due to reduced phagocytic activity. At the same time, α-LCMs induced the expression of the scavenger receptor CD36, which is the major receptor for oxLDL uptake. Further studies provided evidence that α-LCMs influence oxLDL uptake independent of CD36. A key finding of these studies (Wallert et al., 2014) was that α-LCMs promote their effects at lower concentrations and with a mechanism that was different from that of α-TOH. Furthermore, α-LCMs exhibit antiinflammatory activity blocking the LPS-induced release of proinflammatory mediators and nitric oxide production (Ciffolilli et al., 2015; Wallert et al., 2015). Interestingly, these responses to α-LCMs occurred by means of transcriptional effects on inducible NO synthase, cycloxygenase-2, and interleukin-1β. In vitro data also demonstrated the superiority of α-13′-COOH and δ-13′-COOH with respect to the corresponding TOH precursors as proapoptotic agents in HepG2 hepatocarcinoma cells (with EC50 values of 13.5 and 6.5 μM, respectively) (Birringer et al., 2010), and a role of these acid metabolites and GA in the modulation of cell cycle and programmed cell-death pathways was also demonstrated in C6 glioblastoma cells (Mazzini et al., 2009). Recently α-13′-COOH has been demonstrated to form in immune cells and inflammatory exudates of mice (Pein et al., 2018), and to selectively inhibit the biosynthesis of 5-LOX-derived lipid mediators, a property that was already described for the 13′-LCMs formed by the enzymatic metabolism of desmethyl tocochromanols (Jiang et al., 2011 and references therein). This activity was associated with efficient suppression of inflammation and bronchial hyperreactivity in mouse models of peritonitis and asthma (Pein et al., 2018), consistent with the hypothesis that immunoregulatory and antiinflammatory functions of α-TOH can depend on its endogenous metabolites formed at the inflammatory foci, potentially through immune cell 5-LOX inhibition. Biological activities of α-13′-COOH not shared with the parent compound α-TOH have also recently been reported in other contexts, such as in the activation response in LS 180 cellsof PXR nuclear receptor and P-glycoprotein protein expression and transport activity (Podszun et al., 2017). It is worth noting that neither α-TOH, nor α-T3, or γ-TOH and the corresponding SCMs α-CEHC and γ-CEHC, were found to affect PXR or P-glycoprotein expression and activity in these cells.

24.5 The metabolome of vitamin E: analytical aspects and study perspectives

The free radical-derived metabolites α-tocopheronic acid and α-tocopheronolactone, also known as Simon's metabolites, were the first to be identified in the urine of men given large oral doses of α-TOH (Eisengart et al., 1956), a discovery that dates back to the 1950s. Later, Pope et al. (2000) confirmed the presence of α-tocopheronolactone in urine as an endogenous product of vitamin E metabolism. To achieve a more reliable estimation of endogenous α-TOH oxidation by the reaction with lipid peroxyl radicals, it is preferable to investigate circulating metabolites, and especially α-tocopheryl quinone that is relatively more stable compared with Simon's metabolites. An example of the application of this analysis in the study of lipid peroxidation in fatty liver subjects and liver cells is reported in Torquato et al. (2018). By the way, being the metabolites lipid oxidation products, it is crucial that their measurements are performed by adopting validated methods and quality assurance procedures to avoid preanalytical and analytical artifacts (Mottier et al., 2002; Sharma et al., 2013; Torquato et al., 2019).

Among the subfamily of enzymatic metabolites, CEHCs have been the first to be identified and measured in biological samples under different experimental settings. In 1984, δ-CEHC was the first enzymatic metabolite identified in rat urine (Chiku et al., 1984). Then in the late 1990s the analogous forms deriving from α-TOH and γ-TOH metabolism were identified in human urine (Schultz et al., 1995; Wechter et al., 1996). In the early 2000s these pioneering findings paved the way to a series of studies that measured the SCMs in biological fluids other than urine, also assessing the in vivo metabolism of α-TOH and γ-TOH by the administration of deuterium-labeled vitamers (Galli et al., 2001, 2002, 2003). In the same years, Pope et al. (2000) reported the tentative identification of the MCMs α-CMBHC and γ-CMBHC which were further characterized by Birringer et al. (2001). On the other hand, Sontag and Parker (2002) were the first to identify the LCMs α-13′-OH, γ-13′-OH, α-13′-COOH, and γ-13′-COOH, in the lipid extract of human hepatocytes. A few years later Jiang and coworkers proved that, like SCMs, the LCMs γ-13′-COOH and γ-13′-OH are released in their conjugated forms in rat plasma and liver, mainly as sulfates (Jiang et al., 2007). More recently, the availability of liquid chromatography high-resolution mass spectrometry (LC-HRMS) platforms has allowed a more extensive characterization of the vitamin E metabolome and new types of urinary conjugated metabolites have been identified, such as γ-CEHC-glucoside, α-CEHC-glycine, α-CEHC-glycine-glucuronide, and α-CEHC-taurine (Cho et al., 2009; Johnson et al., 2012). On the other hand, we utilized LC coupled to tandem mass spectrometry (LC-MS/MS) to develop a quantitative method to simultaneously determine the entire set of vitamers and metabolites in the human metabolome of vitamin E (Giusepponi et al., 2017).

α-13′-COOH and α-13′-OH are the most active metabolites of α-TOH. These LCMs were identified for the first time in human serum in our laboratories (Ciffolilli et al., 2015; Wallert et al., 2014). Besides providing evidence for their systemic availability, we measured circulating levels of these LCMs that are present in the low nanomolar range. Interestingly, serum concentrations of α-13′-OH significantly increased in healthy adults after 1-week supplementation with a supranutritional dose (1000 IU/day) of RRR-α-TOH (from baseline levels lower than 10 to >30 nM) (Ciffolilli et al., 2015). Further analytical investigations carried out with the recently developed LC-MS/MS protocol and also applying a LC-HRMS (LC-Q-Orbitrap) platform have substantially confirmed these data, also detecting three unknown compounds (M1, M2 and M3) related to α-13′-OH and α-13′-COOH LCMs (Giusepponi et al., 2017). These new α-LCMs are present at higher concentrations in human plasma compared with α-13′-OH and α-13′-COOH isomers, and in total these metabolites (i.e., α-13′-OH + α-13′-COOH + M1 + M2 + M3) in healthy adults fed a diet close to vitamin E RDA (10 mg/day) reach fasting plasma concentrations between 30−90 nM. α-TOH supplementation (1000 IU α-TOH/day per 1 week) carried out with the same protocol described above and in (Ciffolilli et al., 2015) increased LCM levels by about one order of magnitude (290−350 nM). These levels are similar to those observed for the end product of this catabolism α-CEHC. It is worth noting that the concentrations of these plasma metabolites decrease by about one order of magnitude in chronic kidney disease patients compared with healthy controls (Giusepponi et al., 2017), compatible with a disease-specific defect of vitamin E metabolism in these patients combined with increased levels of α-CEHC by the reduced renal excretion of this hydrophilic SCM (Galli et al., 2004c; Himmelfarb et al., 2003).

24.6 Conclusion

This chapter summarizes the available knowledge on the molecular aspects of vitamin E metabolism and function. In the light of recent findings on the gene response to vitamin E molecules (and especially to LCMs), the concept of "essentiality" for this vitamin has now been critically reconsidered by several authors and the hypothesis that α-TOH, similarly to other fat-soluble vitamins, could represent a provitamin, is gaining credit (Galli et al., 2017; Schmolz et al., 2016; Taylor et al., 2018). Now advanced lipidomics and bioinformatics tools are available to shed light on the multifaceted biological roles that this vitamin and its metabolites produce on human cells and tissues. Of particular interest is the exploration of the lipid−lipid and lipid−protein interactions that embody the functional interactome of this vitamin. Some of these interactions and their explorative strategies are presented in this chapter along with the protocols recently developed to investigate the metabolome of vitamin E. Now these aspects represent one of the hot topics of lipidomics and human nutrition.

References

Abe, C., Uchida, T., Ohta, M., Ichikawa, T., Yamashita, K., Ikeda, S., 2007. Cytochrome P450-dependent metabolism of vitamin E isoforms is a critical determinant of their tissue concentrations in rats. Lipids 42, 637–645.

Abidi, P., Leers-Sucheta, S., Azhar, S., 2004. Suppression of steroidogenesis and activator protein-1 transcription factor activity in rat adrenals by vitamin E deficiency-induced chronic oxidative stress. J. Nutr. Biochem. 15, 210–219.

Arai, H., Nagao, A., Terao, J., Suzuki, T., Takama, K., 1995. Effect ofd-α-tocopherol analogues on lipoxygenase-dependent peroxidation of phospholipid-bile salt micelles. Lipids 30, 135–140.

Arita, M., Nomura, K., Arai, H., Inoue, K., 1997. alpha-tocopherol transfer protein stimulates the secretion of alpha-tocopherol from a cultured liver cell line through a brefeldin A-insensitive pathway. Proc Natl Acad Sci U S A 94, 12437–12441.

Azzi, A., 2018. Many tocopherols, one vitamin E. Mol. Asp. Med. 61, 92–103.

Bardowell, S.A., Duan, F., Manor, D., Swanson, J.E., Parker, R.S., 2012. Disruption of mouse cytochrome p450 4f14 (Cyp4f14 gene) causes severe perturbations in vitamin E metabolism. J Biol Chem 287, 26077–26086.

Bartolini, D., Torquato, P., Barola, C., Russo, A., Rychlicki, C., Giusepponi, D., et al., 2017. Nonalcoholic fatty liver disease impairs the cytochrome P-450-dependent metabolism of alpha-tocopherol (vitamin E). J Nutr Biochem 47, 120–131.

Behrens, W.A., Thompson, J.N., Madere, R., 1982. Distribution of alpha-tocopherol in human plasma lipoproteins. Am J Clin Nutr 35, 691–696.

Birringer, M., Drogan, D., Brigelius-Flohe, R., 2001. Tocopherols are metabolized in HepG2 cells by side chain omega-oxidation and consecutive beta-oxidation. Free Radic. Biol. Med. 31, 226–232.

Birringer, M., Lington, D., Vertuani, S., Manfredini, S., Scharlau, D., Glei, M., et al., 2010. Proapoptotic effects of long-chain vitamin E metabolites in HepG2 cells are mediated by oxidative stress. Free Radic. Biol. Med. 49, 1315–1322.

Birringer, M., Pfluger, P., Kluth, D., Landes, N., Brigelius-Flohe, R., 2002. Identities and differences in the metabolism of tocotrienols and tocopherols in HepG2 cells. J Nutr 132, 3113–3118.

Blaner, W.S., 2013. Vitamin E: the enigmatic one!. J. Lipid Res. 54, 2293–2294.

Boscoboinik, D., Szewczyk, A., Hensey, C., Azzi, A., 1991. Inhibition of cell proliferation by alpha-tocopherol. Role of protein kinase C. J. Biol. Chem. 266, 6188–6194.

Brigelius-Flohe, R., 2009. Vitamin E: the shrew waiting to be tamed. Free Radic. Biol. Med. 46, 543–554.

Brigelius-Flohe, R., Galli, F., 2010. Vitamin E: a vitamin still awaiting the detection of its biological function. Mol. Nutr. Food Res. 54, 583–587.

Brown, W.J., Chambers, K., Doody, A., 2003. Phospholipase A2 (PLA2) enzymes in membrane trafficking: mediators of membrane shape and function. Traffic 4, 214–221.

Burton, G.W., Traber, M.G., Acuff, R.V., Walters, D.N., Kayden, H., Hughes, L., et al., 1998. Human plasma and tissue alpha-tocopherol concentrations in response to supplementation with deuterated natural and synthetic vitamin E. Am J Clin Nutr 67, 669–684.

Cachia, O., Benna, J.E., Pedruzzi, E., Descomps, B., Gougerot-Pocidalo, M.A., Leger, C. L., 1998. Alpha-tocopherol inhibits the respiratory burst in human monocytes. Attenuation ofp47(phox) membrane translocation and phosphorylation. J. Biol. Chem. 273, 32801–32805.

Chandra, V., Jasti, J., Kaur, P., Betzel, C., Srinivasan, A., Singh, T.P., 2002. First structural evidence of a specific inhibition of phospholipase A2 by alpha-tocopherol (vitamin E) and its implications in inflammation: crystal structure of the complex formed between phospholipase A2 and alpha-tocopherol at 1.8 A resolution. J. Mol. Biol. 320, 215–222.

Chang, S.J., Lin, J.S., Chen, H.H., 2000. Alpha-tocopherol downregulates the expression of GPIIb promoter in HEL cells. Free Radic. Biol. Med. 28, 202–207.

Chiku, S., Hamamura, K., Nakamura, T., 1984. Novel urinary metabolite of d-delta-tocopherol in rats. J. Lipid Res. 25, 40–48.

Cho, J.Y., Kang, D.W., Ma, X., Ahn, S.H., Krausz, K.W., Luecke, H., et al., 2009. Metabolomics reveals a novel vitamin E metabolite and attenuated vitamin E metabolism upon PXR activation. J. Lipid Res. 50, 924–937.

Chung, S., Ghelfi, M., Atkinson, J., Parker, R., Qian, J., Carlin, C., et al., 2016. Vitamin E and phosphoinositides regulate the intracellular localization of the hepatic alpha-tocopherol transfer protein. J. Biol. Chem. 291, 17028–17039.

Ciffolilli, S., Wallert, M., Bartolini, D., Krauth, V., Werz, O., Piroddi, M., et al., 2015. Human serum determination and in vitro anti-inflammatory activity of the vitamin E metabolite alpha-(13′-hydroxy)-6-hydroxychroman. Free Radic. Biol. Med. 89, 952–962.

Clevidence, B.A., Lehmann, J., 1989. Alpha- and gamma-tocopherol levels in lipoproteins fractionated by affinity chromatography. Lipids 24, 137–140.

Cohn, W., Goss-Sampson, M.A., Grun, H., Muller, D.P., 1992. Plasma clearance and net uptake of alpha-tocopherol and low-density lipoprotein by tissues in WHHL and control rabbits. Biochem J 287 (Pt 1), 247–254.

Comitato, R., Leoni, G., Canali, R., Ambra, R., Nesaretnam, K., Virgili, F., 2010. Tocotrienols activity in MCF-7 breast cancer cells: involvement of ERbeta signal transduction. Mol. Nutr. Food Res. 54, 669–678.

De Pascale, M.C., Bassi, A.M., Patrone, V., Villacorta, L., Azzi, A., Zingg, J.M., 2006. Increased expression of transglutaminase-1 and PPARgamma after vitamin E treatment in human keratinocytes. Arch. Biochem. Biophys. 447, 97–106.

Douglas, C.E., Chan, A.C., Choy, P.C., 1986. Vitamin E inhibits platelet phospholipase A2. Biochim. Biophys. Acta 876, 639–645.

Drevon, C.A., 1991. Absorption, transport and metabolism of vitamin E. Free Radic Res Commun 14, 229–246.

Egger, T., Hammer, A., Wintersperger, A., Goti, D., Malle, E., Sattler, W., 2001. Modulation of microglial superoxide production by alpha-tocopherol in vitro: attenuation ofp67(phox) translocation by a protein phosphatase-dependent pathway. J. Neurochem. 79 (1169-1182).

Eisengart, A., Milhorat, A.T., Simon, E.J., Sundheim, L., 1956. The metabolism of vitamin E. II. Purification and characterization of urinary metabolites of alpha-tocopherol. J. Biol. Chem. 221, 807–817.

Flohe, L., Brigelius-Flohe, R., Saliou, C., Traber, M.G., Packer, L., 1997. Redox regulation of NF-kappa B activation. Free Radic. Biol. Med. 22, 1115–1126.

Freiser, H., Jiang, Q., 2009. Optimization of the enzymatic hydrolysis and analysis of plasma conjugated gamma-CEHC and sulfated long-chain carboxychromanols, metabolites of vitamin E. Anal Biochem 388, 260–265.

Galli, F., Lee, R., Dunster, C., Atkinson, J., Floridi, A., Kelly, F.J., 2001. Gamma-tocopherol metabolism and its relationship with alpha-tocopherol in humans: a stable isotope supplementation study. Biofactors 15, 65–69.

Galli, F., Lee, R., Dunster, C., Kelly, F.J., 2002. Gas chromatography mass spectrometry analysis of carboxyethyl-hydroxychroman metabolites of alpha- and gamma-tocopherol in human plasma. Free Radic. Biol. Med. 32, 333–340.

Galli, F., Lee, R., Atkinson, J., Floridi, A., Kelly, F.J., 2003. Gamma-tocopherol biokinetics and transformation in humans. Free Radic. Res. 37, 1225–1233.

Galli, F., Stabile, A.M., Betti, M., Conte, C., Pistilli, A., Rende, M., et al., 2004a. The effect of alpha- and gamma-tocopherol and their carboxyethyl hydroxychroman metabolites on prostate cancer cell proliferation. Arch. Biochem. Biophys. 423, 97–102.

Galli, F., Piroddi, M., Lannone, A., Pagliarani, S., Tomasi, A., Floridi, A., 2004b. A comparison between the antioxidant and peroxynitrite-scavenging functions of the vitamin E metabolites alpha- and gamma-carboxyethyl-6-hydroxychromans. Int. J. Vitam. Nutr Res. 74, 362–373.

Galli, F., Floridi, A.G., Floridi, A., Buoncristiani, U., 2004c. Accumulation of vitamin E metabolites in the blood of renal failure patients. Clin. Nutr. 23, 205–212.

Galli, F., Polidori, M.C., Stahl, W., Mecocci, P., Kelly, F.J., 2007. Vitamin E biotransformation in humans. Vitam. Horm. 76, 263–280.

Galli, F., Azzi, A., Birringer, M., Cook-Mills, J.M., Eggersdorfer, M., Frank, J., et al., 2017. Vitamin E: emerging aspects and new directions. Free Radic. Biol. Med. 102, 16–36.

Giusepponi, D., Torquato, P., Bartolini, D., Piroddi, M., Birringer, M., Lorkowski, S., et al., 2017. Determination of tocopherols and their metabolites by liquid-chromatography coupled with tandem mass spectrometry in human plasma and serum. Talanta 170, 552–561.

Grammas, P., Hamdheydari, L., Benaksas, E.J., Mou, S., Pye, Q.N., Wechter, W.J., et al., 2004. Anti-inflammatory effects of tocopherol metabolites. Biochem. Biophys. Res. Commun. 319, 1047–1052.

Grau, A., Ortiz, A., 1998. Dissimilar protection of tocopherol isomers against membrane hydrolysis by phospholipase A2. Chem. Phys. Lipids 91, 109–118.

Grebenstein, N., Schumacher, M., Graeve, L., Frank, J., 2014. alpha-Tocopherol transfer protein is not required for the discrimination against gamma-tocopherol in vivo but protects it from side-chain degradation in vitro. Mol Nutr Food Res 58, 1052–1060.

Hacquebard, M., Carpentier, Y.A., 2005. Vitamin E: absorption, plasma transport and cell uptake. Curr Opin Clin Nutr Metab Care 8, 133–138.

Hermann, P.M., Watson, S.N., Wildering, W.C., 2014. Phospholipase A2–nexus of aging, oxidative stress, neuronal excitability, and functional decline of the aging nervous system? Insights from a snail model system of neuronal aging and age-associated memory impairment. Front. Genet. 5, 419.

Himmelfarb, J., Kane, J., McMonagle, E., Zaltas, E., Bobzin, S., Boddupalli, S., et al., 2003. Alpha and gamma tocopherol metabolism in healthy subjects and patients with end-stage renal disease. Kidney Int 64, 978–991.

Horiguchi, M., Arita, M., Kaempf-Rotzoll, D.E., Tsujimoto, M., Inoue, K., Arai, H., 2003. pH-dependent translocation of alpha-tocopherol transfer protein (alpha-TTP) between hepatic cytosol and late endosomes. Genes Cells 8, 789–800.

Hosomi, A., Arita, M., Sato, Y., Kiyose, C., Ueda, T., Igarashi, O., et al., 1997. Affinity for α-tocopherol transfer protein as a determinant of the biological activities of vitamin E analogs. FEBS Letters 409, 105–108.

Jiang, Q., Elson-Schwab, I., Courtemanche, C., Ames, B.N., 2000. Gamma-tocopherol and its major metabolite, in contrast to alpha-tocopherol, inhibit cyclooxygenase activity in macrophages and epithelial cells. Proc. Natl. Acad. Sci. USA 97, 11494–11499.

Jiang, Q., Freiser, H., Wood, K.V., Yin, X., 2007. Identification and quantitation of novel vitamin E metabolites, sulfated long-chain carboxychromanols, in human A549 cells and in rats. J. Lipid Res. 48, 1221–1230.

Jiang, Q., Yin, X., Lill, M.A., Danielson, M.L., Freiser, H., Huang, J., 2008. Long-chain carboxychromanols, metabolites of vitamin E, are potent inhibitors of cyclooxygenases. Proc. Natl. Acad. Sci. USA 105, 20464–20469.

Jiang, Z., Yin, X., Jiang, Q., 2011. Natural forms of vitamin E and 13′-carboxychromanol, a long-chain vitamin E metabolite, inhibit leukotriene generation from stimulated neutrophils by blocking calcium influx and suppressing 5-lipoxygenase activity, respectively. J. Immunol. 186, 1173–1179.
Johnson, C.H., Slanar, O., Krausz, K.W., Kang, D.W., Patterson, A.D., Kim, J.H., et al., 2012. Novel metabolites and roles for alpha-tocopherol in humans and mice discovered by mass spectrometry-based metabolomics. Am. J. Clin. Nutr. 96, 818–830.
Kagan, V.E., Mao, G., Qu, F., Angeli, J.P., Doll, S., Croix, C.S., et al., 2017. Oxidized arachidonic and adrenic PEs navigate cells to ferroptosis. Nat. Chem. Biol. 13, 81–90.
Kamal-Eldin, A., Frank, J., Razdan, A., Tengblad, S., Basu, S., Vessby, B., 2000. Effects of dietary phenolic compounds on tocopherol, cholesterol, and fatty acids in rats. Lipids 35, 427–435.
Kantoci, D., Wechter, W.J., Murray Jr., E.D., Dewind, S.A., Borchardt, D., Khan, S.I., 1997. Endogenous natriuretic factors 6: the stereochemistry of a natriuretic gamma-tocopherol metabolite LLU-alpha. J. Pharmacol. Exp. Ther. 282, 648–656.
Kempna, P., Reiter, E., Arock, M., Azzi, A., Zingg, J.M., 2004. Inhibition of HMC-1 mast cell proliferation by vitamin E: involvement of the protein kinase B pathway. J. Biol. Chem. 279, 50700–50709.
Khanna, S., Roy, S., Ryu, H., Bahadduri, P., Swaan, P.W., Ratan, R.R., et al., 2003. Molecular basis of vitamin E action: tocotrienol modulates 12-lipoxygenase, a key mediator of glutamate-induced neurodegeneration. J. Biol. Chem. 278, 43508–43515.
Khanna, S., Parinandi, N.L., Kotha, S.R., Roy, S., Rink, C., Bibus, D., et al., 2010. Nanomolar vitamin E α-tocotrienol inhibits glutamate-induced activation of phospholipase A2 and causes neuroprotection. J. Neurochem. 112, 1249–1260.
Khor, H.T., Ng, T.T., 2000. Effects of administration of alpha-tocopherol and tocotrienols on serum lipids and liver HMG CoA reductase activity. Int. J. Food Sci. Nutr. 51 (Suppl), S3–11.
Kluth, D., Landes, N., Pfluger, P., Muller-Schmehl, K., Weiss, K., Bumke-Vogt, C., et al., 2005. Modulation of Cyp3a11 mRNA expression by alpha-tocopherol but not gamma-tocotrienol in mice. Free Radic. Biol. Med. 38, 507–514.
Kolleck, I., Schlame, M., Fechner, H., Looman, A.C., Wissel, H., Rustow, B., 1999. HDL is the major source of vitamin E for type II pneumocytes. Free Radic Biol Med 27, 882–890.
Kono, N., Ohto, U., Hiramatsu, T., Urabe, M., Uchida, Y., Satow, Y., et al., 2013. Impaired α-TTP-PIPs interaction underlies familial vitamin E deficiency. Science 340, 1106–1110.
Kostner, G.M., Oettl, K., Jauhiainen, M., Ehnholm, C., Esterbauer, H., Dieplinger, H., 1995. Human plasma phospholipid transfer protein accelerates exchange/transfer of alpha-tocopherol between lipoproteins and cells. Biochem J 305 (Pt 2), 659–667.
Landes, N., Pfluger, P., Kluth, D., Birringer, M., Ruhl, R., Bol, G.F., et al., 2003. Vitamin E activates gene expression via the pregnane X receptor. Biochem. Pharmacol. 65, 269–273.
Lemaire-Ewing, S., Desrumaux, C., Neel, D., Lagrost, L., 2010. Vitamin E transport, membrane incorporation and cell metabolism: Is alpha-tocopherol in lipid rafts an oar in the lifeboat? Mol Nutr Food Res 54, 631–640.
Mahoney, C.W., Azzi, A., 1988. Vitamin E inhibits protein kinase C activity. Biochem. Biophys. Res. Commun. 154, 694–697.
Mardones, P., Strobel, P., Miranda, S., Leighton, F., Quinones, V., Amigo, L., et al., 2002. Alpha-tocopherol metabolism is abnormal in scavenger receptor class B type I (SR-BI)-deficient mice. J Nutr 132, 443–449.

Mazzini, F., Betti, M., Netscher, T., Galli, F., Salvadori, P., 2009. Configuration of the vitamin E analogue garcinoic acid extracted from *Garcinia kola* seeds. Chirality 21, 519–524.

McNally, A.K., Anderson, J.M., 2003. Foreign body-type multinucleated giant cell formation is potently induced by alpha-tocopherol and prevented by the diacylglycerol kinase inhibitor R59022. Am. J. Pathol. 163, 1147–1156.

Mottier, P., Gremaud, E., Guy, P.A., Turesky, R.J., 2002. Comparison of gas chromatography-mass spectrometry and liquid chromatography-tandem mass spectrometry methods to quantify alpha-tocopherol and alpha-tocopherolquinone levels in human plasma. Anal. Biochem. 301, 128–135.

Murphy, R.C., Gijon, M.A., 2007. Biosynthesis and metabolism of leukotrienes. Biochem. J. 405, 379–395.

Murray Jr, E.D., Kantoci, D., DeWind, S.A., Bigornia, A.E., D'Amico, D.C., King Jr., J. G., et al., 1995. Endogenous natriuretic factors 3: isolation and characterization of human natriuretic factors LLU-alpha, LLU-beta 1, and LLU-gamma. Life Sci. 57, 2145–2161.

Mustacich, D.J., Leonard, S.W., Devereaux, M.W., Sokol, R.J., Traber, M.G., 2006. Alpha-tocopherol regulation of hepatic cytochrome P450s and ABC transporters in rats. Free Radic. Biol. Med. 41, 1069–1078.

Parker, R.S., Sontag, T.J., Swanson, J.E., 2000. Cytochrome P4503A-dependent metabolism of tocopherols and inhibition by sesamin. Biochem Biophys Res Commun 277, 531–534.

Pein, H., Ville, A., Pace, S., Temml, V., Garscha, U., Raasch, M., et al., 2018. Endogenous metabolites of vitamin E limit inflammation by targeting 5-lipoxygenase. Nat. Commun. 9, 3834.

Podszun, M.C., Jakobi, M., Birringer, M., Weiss, J., Frank, J., 2017. The long chain alpha-tocopherol metabolite alpha-13′-COOH and gamma-tocotrienol induce P-glycoprotein expression and activity by activation of the pregnane X receptor in the intestinal cell line LS 180. Mol. Nutr. Food Res. (3), 61. Available from: https://doi.org/10.1002/mnfr.201600605.

Pope, S.A., Clayton, P.T., Muller, D.P., 2000. A new method for the analysis of urinary vitamin E metabolites and the tentative identification of a novel group of compounds. Arch. Biochem. Biophys. 381, 8–15.

Poynter, M.E., Daynes, R.A., 1998. Peroxisome proliferator-activated receptor alpha activation modulates cellular redox status, represses nuclear factor-kappaB signaling, and reduces inflammatory cytokine production in aging. J. Biol. Chem. 273, 32833–32841.

Qian, J., Morley, S., Wilson, K., Nava, P., Atkinson, J., Manor, D., 2005. Intracellular trafficking of vitamin E in hepatocytes: the role of tocopherol transfer protein. J Lipid Res 46, 2072-20.

Ran, L., Liu, A.B., Lee, M.-J., Xie, P., Lin, Y., et al., 2019. Effects of antibiotics on degradation and bioavailability of different vitamin E forms in mice. Biofactors . Available from: https://doi.org/10.1002/biof.1492.

Ricciarelli, R., Tasinato, A., Clement, S., Ozer, N.K., Boscoboinik, D., Azzi, A., 1998. Alpha-tocopherol specifically inactivates cellular protein kinase C alpha by changing its phosphorylation state. Biochem. J. 334 (Pt 1), 243–249.

Roager, H.M., Sulek, K., Skov, K., Frandsen, H.L., Smedsgaard, J., Wilcks, A., et al., 2014. Lactobacillus acidophilus NCFM affects vitamin E acetate metabolism and intestinal bile acid signature in monocolonized mice. Gut Microbes 5, 296–303.

Rode, S., Rubic, T., Lorenz, R.L., 2008. Alpha-tocopherol disturbs macrophage LXRalpha regulation of ABCA1/G1 and cholesterol handling. Biochem. Biophys. Res. Commun. 369, 868–872.

Ross, A.B., Chen, Y., Frank, J., Swanson, J.E., Parker, R.S., Kozubek, A., et al., 2004. Cereal alkylresorcinols elevate gamma-tocopherol levels in rats and inhibit gamma-tocopherol metabolism in vitro. J Nutr 134, 506–510.
Russo, A., Bartolini, D., Torquato, P., Giusepponi, D., Barola, C., Galarini, R., et al., 2017. CYP4F2 repression and a modified alpha-tocopherol (vitamin E) metabolism are two independent consequences of ethanol toxicity in human hepatocytes. Toxicol. In Vitro 40, 124–133.
Schmolz, L., Wallert, M., Heise, J., Galli, F., Werz, O., Birringer, M., et al., 2014. Regulation of inflammatory pathways by an a-tocopherol long-chain metabolite and a d-tocotrienol-related natural compound. Free Radic. Biol. Med. 75 (Suppl 1), S48.
Schmolz, L., Birringer, M., Lorkowski, S., Wallert, M., 2016. Complexity of vitamin E metabolism. World J. Biol. Chem. 7, 14–43.
Schmolz, L., Wallert, M., Rozzino, N., Cignarella, A., Galli, F., Glei, M., et al., 2017. Structure-function relationship studies in vitro reveal distinct and specific effects of long-chain metabolites of vitamin E. Mol. Nutr. Food Res. Available from: https://doi.org/10.1002/mnfr.201700562.
Schmolz, L., Schubert, M., Kirschner, J., Kluge, S., Galli, F., Birringer, M., et al., 2018. Long-chain metabolites of vitamin E: interference with lipotoxicity via lipid droplet associated protein PLIN2. Biochim. Biophys. Acta Mol. Cell Biol. Lipids 1863, 919–927.
Schubert, M., Kluge, S., Schmolz, L., Wallert, M., Galli, F., Birringer, M., et al., 2018. Long-chain metabolites of vitamin E: metabolic activation as a general concept for lipid-soluble vitamins? Antioxidants (Basel) 7.
Schultz, M., Leist, M., Petrzika, M., Gassmann, B., Brigelius-Flohe, R., 1995. Novel urinary metabolite of alpha-tocopherol, 2,5,7,8-tetramethyl-2(2'-carboxyethyl)-6-hydroxychroman, as an indicator of an adequate vitamin E supply? Am. J. Clin. Nutr. 62, 1527S–1534S.
Sharma, G., Muller, D.P., O'Riordan, S.M., Bryan, S., Dattani, M.T., Hindmarsh, P.C., et al., 2013. Urinary conjugated alpha-tocopheronolactone–a biomarker of oxidative stress in children with type 1 diabetes. Free Radic Biol Med 55, 54–62.
Siragusa, L., Spyrakis, F., Goracci, L., Cross, S., Cruciani, G., 2014. BioGPS: the music for the chemo- and bioinformatics Walzer. Mol. Inform. 33, 446–453.
Sontag, T.J., Parker, R.S., 2002. Cytochrome P450 omega-hydroxylase pathway of tocopherol catabolism. Novel mechanism of regulation of vitamin E status. J. Biol. Chem. 277, 25290–25296.
Sontag, T.J., Parker, R.S., 2007. Influence of major structural features of tocopherols and tocotrienols on their omega-oxidation by tocopherol-omega-hydroxylase. J Lipid Res 48, 1090–1098.
Stahl, W., van den Berg, H., Arthur, J., Bast, A., Dainty, J., Faulks, R.M., et al., 2002. Bioavailability and metabolism. Mol Aspects Med 23, 39–100.
Suzuki, Y.J., Packer, L., 1993. Inhibition of NF-kappa B activation by vitamin E derivatives. Biochem. Biophys. Res. Commun. 193, 277–283.
Tanabe, M., Fukushima, T., Usui, N., Aoyama, N., Tsunoda, M., Imai, K., 2004. Intravenous administration of 2,7,8-trimethyl-2-(beta-carboxyethyl)-6-hydroxy chroman (gamma-CEHC) to rats and determination of its plasma concentration and urinary sodium excretion. Biomed Chromatogr 18, 727–734.
Takeda, A.A., dos Santos, J.I., Marcussi, S., Silveira, L.B., Soares, A.M., Fontes, M.R., 2004. Crystallization and preliminary X-ray diffraction analysis of an acidic phospholipase A(2) complexed with p-bromophenacyl bromide and alpha-tocopherol inhibitors at 1.9- and 1.45-A resolution. Biochim. Biophys. Acta 1699, 281–284.

Taylor, L., Krueger, N., Malysheva, O., Atkinson, J., Parker, R.S., 2018. ω-Hydroxylation of α-tocopheryl quinone reveals a dual function for cytochrome P450-4F2 in vitamin E metabolism. Bioorg. Med. Chem 26 (20), 5555–5565.

Terashima, K., Shimamura, T., Tanabayashi, M., Aqil, M., Niwa, A.J.A.M., 1997. Constituents of the seeds of *Garcinia kola*: two new antioxidants, garcinoic acid and garcinal. Heterocycles 45, 1559–1566.

Thillai, K., Lam, H., Sarker, D., Wells, C.M., 2017. Deciphering the link between PI3K and PAK: an opportunity to target key pathways in pancreatic cancer? Oncotarget 8, 14173–14191.

Torquato, P., Bartolini, D., Giusepponi, D., Saluti, G., Russo, A., Barola, C., et al., 2016. Alpha-13′-OH is the main product of a-tocopherol metabolism and influences CYP4F2 and PPAR gamma gene expression in HepG2 human hepatocarcinoma cells. Free Radic. Biol. Med. 96, S19–S20.

Torquato, P., Bartolini, D., Giusepponi, D., Piroddi, M., Sebastiani, B., Saluti, G., et al., 2018. Increased plasma levels of the lipoperoxyl radical-derived vitamin E metabolite alpha-tocopheryl quinone are an early indicator of lipotoxicity in fatty liver subjects. Free Radic. Biol. Med. 131, 115–125.

Torquato, P., Giusepponi, D., Galarini, R., Bartolini, D., Piroddi, M., Galli, F., 2019. Analysis of vitamin E metabolites. In: Niki, E. (Ed.), Vitamin E: Chemistry and Nutritional Benefits. The Royal Society of Chemistry.

Traber, M.G., 2004. Vitamin E, nuclear receptors and xenobiotic metabolism. Arch. Biochem. Biophys. 423, 6–11.

Traber, M.G., 2010. Regulation of xenobiotic metabolism, the only signaling function of alpha-tocopherol? Mol. Nutr. Food Res. 54, 661–668.

Traber, M.G., 2013. Mechanisms for the prevention of vitamin E excess. J. Lipid Res. 54, 2295–2306.

Tran, K., Proulx, P.R., Chan, A.C., 1994. Vitamin E suppresses diacylglycerol (DAG) level in thrombin-stimulated endothelial cells through an increase of DAG kinase activity. Biochim. Biophys. Acta 1212, 193–202.

Viola, V., Pilolli, F., Piroddi, M., Pierpaoli, E., Orlando, F., Provinciali, M., et al., 2012. Why tocotrienols work better: insights into the in vitro anti-cancer mechanism of vitamin E. Genes Nutr. 7, 29–41.

Viola, V., Ciffolilli, S., Legnaioli, S., Piroddi, M., Betti, M., Mazzini, F., et al., 2013. Mitochondrial-dependent anticancer activity of delta-tocotrienol and its synthetic derivatives in HER-2/neu overexpressing breast adenocarcinoma cells. Biofactors 39, 485–493.

Wallert, M., Mosig, S., Rennert, K., Funke, H., Ristow, M., Pellegrino, R.M., et al., 2014. Long-chain metabolites of alpha-tocopherol occur in human serum and inhibit macrophage foam cell formation in vitro. Free Radic. Biol. Med. 68, 43–51.

Wallert, M., Schmolz, L., Koeberle, A., Krauth, V., Glei, M., Galli, F., et al., 2015. Alpha-tocopherol long-chain metabolite alpha-13′-COOH affects the inflammatory response of lipopolysaccharide-activated murine RAW264.7 macrophages. Mol. Nutr. Food Res. 59, 1524–1534.

Wechter, W.J., Kantoci, D., Murray Jr., E.D., D'Amico, D.C., Jung, M.E., Wang, W.H., 1996. A new endogenous natriuretic factor: LLU-alpha. Proc. Natl. Acad. Sci. USA 93, 6002–6007.

Wu, D., Mura, C., Beharka, A.A., Han, S.N., Paulson, K.E., Hwang, D., et al., 1998. Age-associated increase in PGE2 synthesis and COX activity in murine macrophages is reversed by vitamin E. Am. J. Physiol. 275, C661–C668.

Wu, D., Liu, L., Meydani, M., Meydani, S.N., 2005. Vitamin E increases production of vasodilator prostanoids in human aortic endothelial cells through opposing effects on cyclooxygenase-2 and phospholipase A2. J. Nutr. 135, 1847–1853.

Yamauchi, J., Iwamoto, T., Kida, S., Masushige, S., Yamada, K., Esashi, T., 2001. Tocopherol-associated protein is a ligand-dependent transcriptional activator. Biochem. Biophys. Res. Commun. 285, 295–299.

Zhang, W.X., Thakur, V., Lomize, A., Pogozheva, I., Panagabko, C., Cecchini, M., et al., 2011. The contribution of surface residues to membrane binding and ligand transfer by the alpha-tocopherol transfer protein (alpha-TTP). J Mol Biol 405, 972–988.

Zhou, C., Tabb, M.M., Sadatrafiei, A., Grun, F., Blumberg, B., 2004. Tocotrienols activate the steroid and xenobiotic receptor, SXR, and selectively regulate expression of its target genes. Drug Metab. Dispos. 32, 1075–1082.

Zimmer, S., Stocker, A., Sarbolouki, M.N., Spycher, S.E., Sassoon, J., Azzi, A., 2000. A novel human tocopherol-associated protein: cloning, in vitro expression, and characterization. J. Biol. Chem. 275, 25672–25680.

Zingg, J.M., 2007. Modulation of signal transduction by vitamin E. Mol. Asp. Med. 28, 481–506.

Zingg, J.M., 2015. Vitamin E: a role in signal transduction. Annu. Rev. Nutr. 35, 135–173.

Zingg, J.M., Libinaki, R., Lai, C.Q., Meydani, M., Gianello, R., Ogru, E., et al., 2010. Modulation of gene expression by alpha-tocopherol and alpha-tocopheryl phosphate in THP-1 monocytes. Free Radic. Biol. Med. 49, 1989–2000.

CHAPTER 25

Linking vitamin E and nitric oxide in liver disease

Ghazaleh Hajiluian and Farzad Shidfar
Department of Nutrition, School of Public Health, Iran University of Medical Sciences, Tehran, Iran

Contents

Key facts

- The liver is an organ that is severely attacked by reactive oxygen species (ROS) and reactive nitrogen species (RNS) free radicals, especially nitric oxide (NO).
- NO can induce elevation or reduction of pathophysiologic responses in various types of liver diseases, which shows the dual manner of this small molecule in the body.

Molecular Nutrition
DOI: https://doi.org/10.1016/B978-0-12-811907-5.00016-6

- When free radical production increases in the liver, hemostasis may be disrupted and this can result in oxidative/nitrosative stress pathologic conditions.
- If liver function is lost, the patients enter a type of liver disease that may be acute or chronic and will quickly disrupt the normal functions of the liver or disruption may occur over several months to several years.
- More than 100 types of liver disease are known that are significantly related to morbidity and mortality worldwide.
- Because of oxidative/nitrosative stress pathogenesis in liver diseases, an antioxidant system is required for disease prevention and treatment.
- Indeed an antioxidant system can be an enzymatic and nonenzymatic system in harmony with each other, modulating the cellular balance against ROS and RNS.
- Several studies have been performed to assess the effects of antioxidants, especially vitamin E, in liver diseases and the appropriate therapeutic approaches for the prevention and treatment of liver diseases.

Summary points

- This chapter focuses on linking vitamin E and NO in liver disease.
- One of the most important factors in the pathogenesis of liver disease is oxidative/nitrosative stress.
- NO is one of the most important RNS free radicals and is involved in various types of liver disease.
- NO is a dual molecule that can increase or decrease pathophysiologic responses in liver disease.
- Antioxidative therapy has investigated whether vitamins, especially vitamin E, are the most effective diet supplements for patients with liver disease.
- The biological activity of vitamin E is not limited to its antioxidant properties, and it could be involved in the regulation of inflammatory response, gene expression, enzymes attached to membrane, and modulation of cell signaling and proliferation.
- Vitamin E can protect liver functions against NO attacks via various mechanisms.

Word definition

***Free radicals*:** Free radicals are highly unstable and reactive atoms or molecules that have uncoupled electrons. In the body of living organisms, these radicals are derived from reactive oxygen species and reactive nitrogen species (RNS).

***Oxidative/nitrosative stress*:** Imbalances in the production and removal of reactive oxygen species and RNS result in oxidative/nitrosative stress that can cause an impairment in antioxidant production and consequently disruption in the normal function of organs.

***Nitric oxide*:** Nitric oxide is a dual, small, and distributable molecule that plays a role in the regulation of physiologic and pathologic processes of organs and is an important cellular signaling molecule.

***Nitric oxide synthase*:** Nitric oxide synthase is a family of enzymes catalyzing the production of nitric oxide (NO) from L-arginine. There are three isoforms of nitric oxide synthase enzyme in the liver, endothelial nitric oxide synthase, neuronal nitric oxide synthase, and inducible nitric oxide synthase.

***Antioxidant*:** Antioxidants scavenge free radicals from the body's cells, and prevent or reduce the damage caused by oxidation.

***Vitamin E*:** Vitamin E is one of the most important fat-soluble antioxidants that is mainly found in the lipid bilayer membrane. This vitamin fights with oxidants and inhibits free radical production. So it protects lipids, proteins, carbohydrates, and nucleic acids against free radical attacks.

***Vitamin C*:** Vitamin C is a strong water-soluble antioxidant that plays a role as an electron donor and in reduction. This vitamin is known as scavenger of reactive oxygen species and RNS.

***Nonenzymatic antioxidants*:** Nonenzymatic antioxidants are categorized into metabolic antioxidants and dietary antioxidants, which can inhibit or reduce the accumulation of free radicals.

***Enzymatic antioxidants*:** Enzymatic antioxidants include catalase, superoxide dismutase, and glutathione peroxidase, which enable the consumption of different types of reactive oxygen species and RNS radicals via catalysis of chemical reactions, removal of free radical precursors, and chelation of minerals transportation catalyzers.

***Viral hepatitis*:** Viral hepatitis is liver inflammation due to a viral infection. It may present in an acute form as a recent infection with relatively rapid onset, or in a chronic form. There are five main hepatitis viruses, referred to as types A, B, C, D, and E.

***Liver cirrhosis*:** Cirrhosis is a late stage of scarring (fibrosis) of the liver caused by many forms of liver diseases and conditions, such as hepatitis and chronic alcoholism. Cirrhosis occurs in response to damage to the liver.

***Hepatocellular carcinoma*:** Hepatocellular carcinoma (HCC) is the most common type of primary liver cancer. HCC occurs most often in patients with chronic liver diseases, such as cirrhosis caused by hepatitis B or hepatitis C infection.

Abbreviations

BH3	tri hydro biopterin
BH4	tetra hydro biopterin
CAT	catalase
DNA	deoxyribonucleic acid

eNOS	endothelial nitric oxide synthase
FAD	flavin adenine dinucleotide
FMN	flavin mononucleotide
GCH	guanosine tri-phosphate cyclohydrolase
GF	growth factor
GR	glutathione reductase
GSH-Px	glutathione peroxidase
HSCs	hepatic stellate cells
IFN-γ	interferon-γ
IL-1	interlukin-1
IL-12	interlukin-12
iNOS	inducible nitric oxide synthase
JAK	janus kinase
LDL	low density lipoprotein
MAPK	mitogen activated protein kinase
MPO	myeloperoxidase
NADPH	nicotinamide adenine dinucleotide phosphate
NF-κB	nuclear factor-κB
nNOS	neuronal nitric oxide synthase
NO	nitric oxide
NOS	nitric oxide synthase
PI3K	phospho inositide-3-kinase
PKC	protein kinase C
PP2A	protein phosphatase 2A
PPAR	peroxisome proliferator-activated receptor
PTP	protein tyrosine phosphatase
PUFA	polyunsaturated fatty acid
RNS	reactive nitrogen species
ROS	reactive oxygen species
SECs	sinusoidal endothelial cells
SOD	super oxide dismutase
TGF-β	tumor growth factor-beta
TK	tyrosine kinase
TLRs	toll like receptors
TNF-α	tumor necrosis factor-α
VEGF	vascular endothelial growth factor
XO	xanthine oxidase

25.1 Introduction

More than 100 types of liver diseases are known that are significantly related to morbidity and mortality worldwide. Liver diseases are life-threatening conditions that need emergency medical care.

The liver is an organ that is severely attacked by free radicals, so there is an antioxidant system for redox hemostasis maintenance in the liver. When, reactive oxygen species (ROS) and reactive nitrogen species

(RNS) production increases in the liver, hemostasis may be disrupted and this can result in oxidative/nitrosative stress pathologic conditions. These stresses may result in liver disorders via irreversible alterations in lipids, proteins, carbohydrates, nucleic acid, and more importantly pathways that control normal biological functions. Thus one of the most important factors in the pathogeneses of different types of liver diseases is oxidative/nitrosative stress. In this case nitric oxide (NO) is one of the most important RNS free radicals that is involved in various types of liver diseases.

NO is a dual and small molecule that plays a role in the regulation of physiologic and pathologic processes of organs. Also NO acts as a cytoprotective factor in physiological conditions and as a cytotoxic factor in pathological conditions in liver disease. However, NO production can be induced by various factors. Because of oxidative/nitrosative stress pathogenesis in liver diseases, the existence of an antioxidant system at the appropriate time for their prevention and treatment is required. An antioxidant system can be an enzymatic and nonenzymatic system in harmony with each other, modulating the cellular balance against ROS and RNS.

Several studies have been performed to evaluate the effects in liver disease of the antioxidants that showed an appropriate therapeutic effect for the prevention and treatment of liver disease. Based on investigations into antioxidative therapy, vitamins, especially vitamin E, are the most effective diet supplements for patients with liver disease. Vitamins counteract oxidants and inhibit ROS and RNS production. Thus they protect lipids, proteins, carbohydrates, and DNA, against free radical attacks and can maintain liver functions against NO attacks via various mechanisms.

25.2 Liver

The liver is the biggest organ of the body that is composed of different cells with various functions which are described below.

Hepatocytes comprise more than 80% of total liver mass and have a vital role in the metabolism of amino acids, lipids, carbohydrates, vitamins, minerals, hormones, ammonia, and detoxification. Hepatic stellate cells (HSCs) are the main storage mechanism for fat-soluble vitamins that are important for hepatic damage and fibrosis. Sinusoidal endothelial cells (SECs) are one half of the nonparenchymal hepatic cells and play a role in the transportation of nutrients between the bloodstream and liver parenchyma, the expression of scavenger receptors, and antigen-presenting cells. Hepatic Kupffer cells are the biggest storage macrophages of the body and cope with the toxins in the portal circulation. These cells are the most essential sources for the production of cytokines that are effective with regards to nutritional status. Bile duct epithelial cells play a role not only in the expression of transporters but also in the transportation of water and bile.

In physiologic conditions all hepatic cells play their role in harmony with each other; however, liver disorders and their progression disrupt the functions of the liver and finally will affect the whole body.

25.3 Liver diseases

More than 100 types of liver diseases are known that are significantly related to morbidity and mortality worldwide. At first liver disease may not have any symptoms or only have mild symptoms such as nausea, decreased appetite, fatigue, and diarrhea, which progress to more serious symptoms such as icterus, lack of blood agglutination, swollen stomach, hepatic encephalopathy, drowsiness, coma, and finally death. Thus liver diseases are life-threatening conditions that need emergency medical care.

Liver diseases are either acute and chronic, which will either quickly disrupt the normal functions of the liver or disrupt the functions over several months to several years, respectively. Chronic liver diseases include hepatitis B and C, long-term use of alcohol, cirrhosis, hemochromatosis, and malnutrition, whereas acute liver diseases include hepatitis A, reaction to chemical and herbal medicines, toxic fungi usage, and acetaminophen overdose (Mahan and Raymond, 2016; Ross et al., 2014).

25.4 Pathogenesis of liver disease

Free radicals are highly unstable and reactive atoms or molecules that have uncoupled electrons. In the body of living organisms, these radicals are derived from ROS and RNS. ROS include peroxyl, hydroxyl, peroxides, and superoxide, and RNS include nitric oxide, nitrogen dioxide, and peroxynitrite (Zhu et al., 2012). Free radicals are produced by various sources, such as lipoxygenase (LOX), cytochrome P450 (CYP), myeloperoxidase (MPO), xanthine oxidase (XO), nicotinamide adenine dinucleotide phosphate (NADPH) oxidase, the electron transport chain, and nitric oxide synthase (NOS) (Li and Jackson, 2002).

In physiologic conditions (redox homeostasis), low amounts of ROS and RNS radicals are required for vital functions such as the expression of growth and apoptosis genes, the signal transduction pathway, and the elimination of pathogen microorganisms (Fig. 25.1A) (McCord, 2000). In contrast, an imbalance in the generation and elimination of ROS and RNS by various factors results in oxidative/nitrosative stress that can cause an impairment in antioxidant productions, and consequently disruption in the normal function of organs, leading to various diseases. Moreover, intracellular signal transduction and the expression of proinflammatory and antiinflammatory genes are affected and result in the onset of inflammatory reactions (Fig. 25.1B) (McCord, 2000).

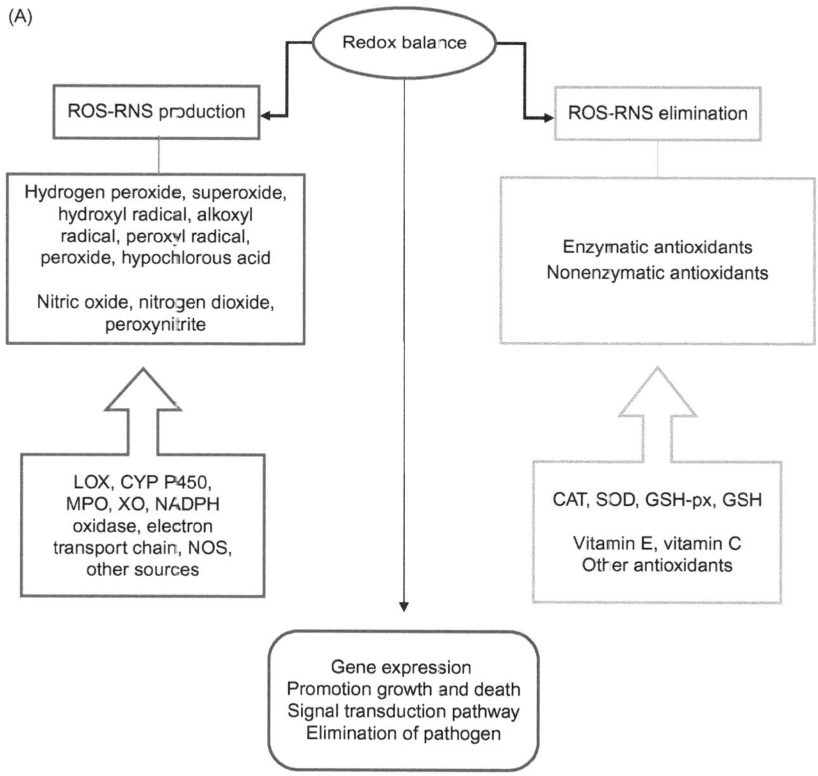

Figure 25.1 The redox physiologic (A) and pathological (B) conditions in the liver. (A) In physiologic conditions a redox balance status exists. Low levels of reactive oxygen species (ROS) and reactive nitrogen species (RNS) radicals are required for vital functions in the body. (B) In pathophysiologic conditions a redox imbalance status exists. The imbalance in the generation and elimination of ROS and RNS by various factors results in oxidative/nitrosative stress that can cause impaired function.

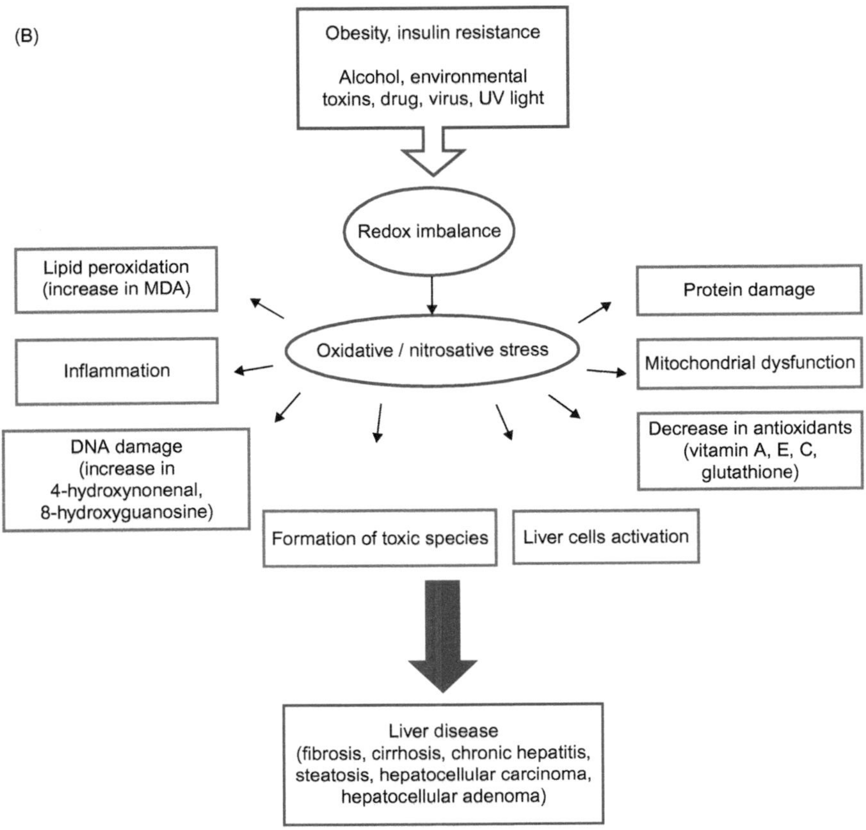

Figure 25.1 Continued.

The liver is an organ that is severely attacked by free radicals, so there is an antioxidant system for redox hemostasis maintenance in the liver. When ROS and RNS production increases in the liver, hemostasis may be disrupted and can result in oxidative/nitrosative stress pathologic conditions (Li et al., 2014). These stresses may result in liver disorders via irreversible alterations in lipids, proteins, carbohydrates, nucleic acid, and more importantly pathways that control normal biological functions (Singal et al., 2011). Thus one of the most important factors in the pathogenesis of different types of liver diseases is oxidative/nitrosative stress (Li et al., 2015). Nitric oxide is one of the most important RNS free radicals that is involved in various types of liver diseases (Iwakiri and Kim, 2015).

25.5 Liver and nitric oxide

Nitric oxide (NO) is a dual, small, and distributable molecule that plays a role in the regulation of physiologic and pathologic processes of organs (Table 25.1) (Moncada, 1991). NO quickly converts to nitrite and nitrate metabolites that can enter the bloodstream. NO has a very short biological half-life and direct measurement of NO is not easy (Schmidt et al., 1993; Moncada, 1991).

In the physiologic concentration NO results in the inhibition of proinflammatory platelet aggregation, proinflammatory-induced gene expression, integrin-mediated adhesion, and vascular inflammation (Moncada, 1991; Schmidt et al.,;1993; Hon et al., 2002).

NO is produced by L-arginine substrate, O_2, and NADPH cosubstrates, flavin adenine dinucleotide (FAD), flavin mononucleotide (FMN), and tetrahydrobiopterin (BH4) cofactors that using by NOS enzyme (Fig. 25.2) (Webb and Twedt, 2008).

There are three isoforms of NOS enzyme in the liver, including endothelial nitric oxide synthase (eNOS), neuronal nitric oxide synthase (nNOS), and inducible nitric oxide synthase (iNOS) that have different properties. eNOS and iNOS have the main role in liver biology, whereas

Table 25.1 The dual effects of nitric oxide.

Physiological effects
Inhibition of proinflammatory platelet aggregation
Inhibition of proinflammatory-induced gene expression
Inhibition of vascular inflammation
Antifibrosis
Vasodilation
Chain-breaking antioxidant (scavenges lipid peroxyl radicals)
Participates in liver regeneration
Antiapoptotic in liver inflammation
Inhibition of integrin-mediated adhesion
Pathological effects
Forms nitrogen mediators and cell dysfunction
Stimulates immune mechanisms
DNA degradation and depletion of cellular pyridine
Cytochrome oxidase inactivation and inhibits mitochondrial function
Cell cycle arrest and apoptosis
Liver disease

NO exerts dual functions in various circumstances. Which, translate either in to a protective or in to toxic actions.

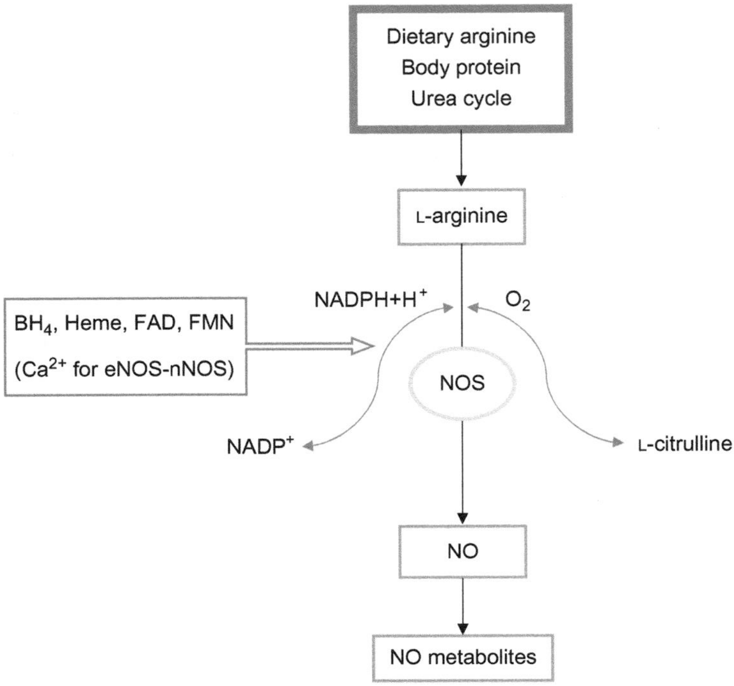

Figure 25.2 Enzymatic nitric oxide (NO) synthesis pathway. L-Arginine is transformed to NO and citrulline by NOS enzyme in the presence of nicotinamide adenine dinucleotide phosphate and O_2. This pathway depends on indispensable cofactors including tetra hydro biopterin, heme, flavin adenine dinucleotide, and flavin mononucleotide (Ca^{2+} for eNOS–nNOS) for their activity.

the role of nNOS is not completely known. NO derived from the eNOS isoforms has functions in physiologic homeostasis in the liver. By contrast, in the pathological liver conditions iNOS is expressed in all liver cells, such as hepatocytes, Kupffer cells, hepatic endothelial cells, and stellate cells. So it could be responsible for several liver diseases via NO production (Geller et al., 1993a, 1994; Harbrecht et al., 1995; Rockey and Chung, 1996). Moreover, inflammatory cells that are placed in the liver (such as neutrophils, eosinophils, and macrophages) can also produce low amounts of NO (Webb and Twedt, 2008).

NO has dual functions in the liver, acting as a cytoprotective factor in the physiologic condition and as a cytotoxic factor in the pathological condition (Zima and Kalousová, 2005). Several mechanisms may result in cellular toxicity via NO and are mentioned below:

NO can directly react with mitochondrial targets, resulting in cytochrome oxidase inactivation and disruption to the mitochondrial function.

It can result in DNA degradation, cell cycle arrest, and apoptosis via activation of the C-JUN N-terminal. Moreover, NO may result in liver disorders via the production of nitrogen mediators such as peroxynitrite and nitrogen oxide (Table 25.1) (Webb and Twedt, 2008; Geller et al., 1993b; Rockey and Shah, 2004).

Peroxynitrite is a strong oxidant molecule that can react with proteins, lipids, carbohydrates, and DNA. This results in irreversible inhibition of mitochondrial respiration and damage to the different components of mitochondria via oxidation reactions (Bartosz, 1996). Also this may result in the modification of some enzymes involved in the inflammatory processes and vascular functions, such as prostaglandin endoperoxidase, 5-lipooxygenase, synthase, and cytochrome p450. Peroxynitrite oxidize unsaturated fatty acids via a reaction with low-density lipoprotein (LDL), and the reaction of peroxynitrite with unsaturated fatty acids can also result in the onset of lipid peroxidation. Thus an increase in peroxide level is considered to be an important marker in liver diseases (Webb and Twedt, 2008; Hogg and Kalyanaraman, 1999).

Nitrogen oxide can also react with biomolecules, such as thiols, amines, and hydroxyls, resulting in conformation changes in protein structures via *S*-nitrosothiol production, for example, nitrosoglutathion products that cause a reduction in activity of glutathione peroxidase antioxidant enzymes, and the levels of some antioxidants such as thiol, ascorbic acid, and vitamin E. Moreover, it may result in the degradation of pyrimidine nucleotides, DNA breakage, and hepatic cellular necrosis via the production of reaction mediators (Webb and Twedt, 2008; Hogg and Kalyanaraman, 1999).

However, NO production in liver disease can be induced by various factors at different levels (Fig. 25.3):

First, iNOS activity is regulated and modified via cellular receptor molecules such as toll-like receptors (TLRs) and CD14. CD14 is a lipopolysaccharide receptor that plays an important role in proinflammatory responses in monocytes and macrophages via activation of the nuclear factor-κB (NF-κB) pathway.

Interferon γ (IFN-γ) can also induce iNOS via the JAK-STAT signaling pathway. Thus stimulation of the JAK-STAT signaling pathway can increase iNOS induction and consequently NO production (Aktan, 2004).

Moreover, it is reported that there is a complicated relationship between inflammatory status and the pathologic factors of nitrosative/oxidative stress. Proinflammatory cytokines, such as interlukin-1 (IL-1), tumor necrosis factor-α (TNF- α), and IL-6, in liver diseases may result

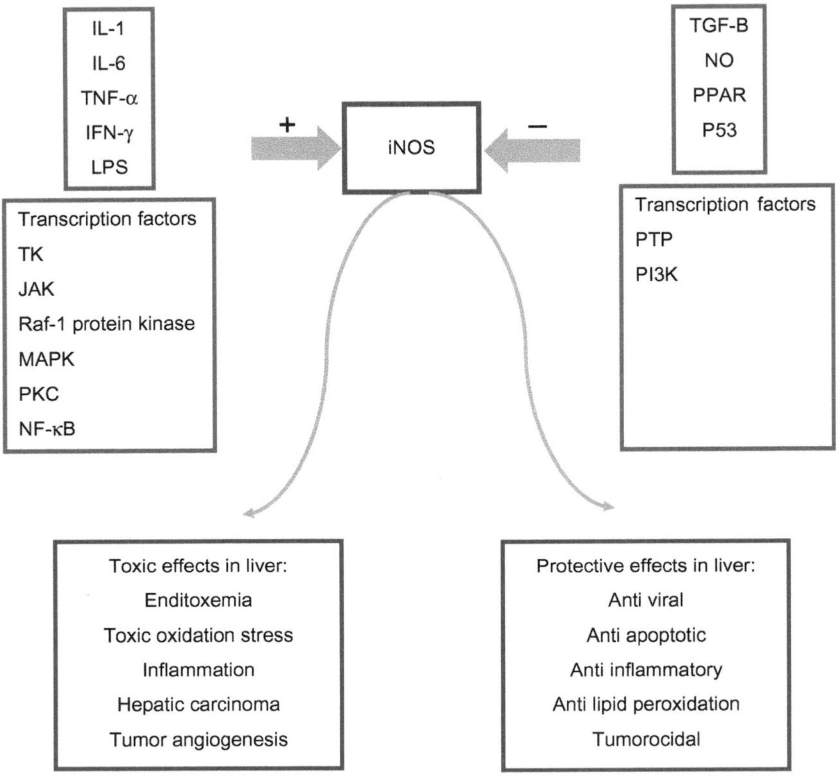

Figure 25.3 The inhibitor and activator factors of inducible nitric oxide synthase (iNOS) in the liver. iNOS is expressed in various liver cells including hepatocytes, Kupffer, vascular endothelial, and stellate cells. Although the amount of iNOS expression and activity are dependent on various factors, it can be either protective or toxic.

in hepatic iNOS stimulation, pathologic NO synthesis, peroxynitrite, nitrogen oxide production, and eventually oxidative/nitrosative stress. In contrast, oxidative/nitrosative stress itself can amplify inflammatory conditions, increase inflammatory cytokines production, attack the host, and lead to liver degradation (Diesen and Kuo, 2010).

The regulation of NO synthesis by NOS can be performed at transcriptional level. Molecular mechanisms involved in iNOS gene transcription can be related to the transcription of activation/ inhibition factors.

Transcription activator factors are those such as tyrosine kinase (TK), janus kinase (JAK), Raf-1 protein kinase, mitogen activated protein kinase (MAPK), and protein kinase C (PKC) that play important roles in iNOS mRNA maintenance (Aktan, 2004). Besides, NF-κB transcription factor can be effective for increasing the transcription and expression of NOS enzyme, and consequently NO production. NF-κB is found to occur as an IκB—NF-κB inactive complex in the cytosol. This complex is phosphorylated by IκB kinase via exogenous (such as LPS) and endogenous (such as proinflammatory cytokines) stimulators, resulting in the transportation of free NF-κB from the cytosol to the nucleus and the induction of iNOS gene expression (Mirzaei and Khazaei, 2017).

Transcription inhibitor factors that are involved in the degradation of mRNA iNOS include protein tyrosine phosphatase (PTP) and phosphoinositide-3-kinase (PI3K) (Aktan, 2004). Moreover, cell exposure with tumor growth factor-β (TGF-β) results in the inhibition of iNOS enzyme induction and NO production. TGF-β is a multifunction growth factor (GF) that regulates different cell functions including proliferation, differentiation, migration, and apoptosis and its signaling pathway inhibits the growth of tumor cells. iNOS expression is also related to the peroxisome proliferator-activated receptor (PPAR) that inhibits iNOS transcription activation factors.

Regulation of NO synthesis by iNOS could occur not only at transcriptional levels, but also at translational and posttranslational levels. NO synthesis could be regulated via BH4 cofactor that is required for NOS catalysis. Guanosine triphosphate cyclohydrolase (GCH) is a key enzyme in BH4 synthesis that can be induced or inhibited by specific cytokines. Also phosphorylation and dephosphorylation modification is another regulatory mechanism for NO synthesis. Posttranslational alterations are seen in the iNOS of macrophages via tyrosine kinase, which is required for iNOS function. Phosphorylation of proteins by tyrosine kinase at the tyrosine amino acid residue has an important role in the regulation of cell growth, cell proliferation, and cell signaling events in the immune system (Aktan, 2004).

25.6 Liver disease and nitric oxide

NO can elevate or reduce pathophysiologic responses in various types of liver disease, which shows the complicated manner of this small molecule in the body. Probable roles of NO in liver disease are mentioned below (Hon et al., 2002):

25.7 Liver damage during inflammation

In inflammatory conditions NO could have advantageous and disadvantageous effects. In inflammatory conditions cytokines such as TNF-α, IL-1, and IL-6 are produced in the liver and stimulate the iNOS enzyme and NO synthesis (Kaplowitz, 2000). iNOS inhibition in inflammatory conditions may increase liver damage showing the advantageous effect to the liver of NO during inflammation. Mechanisms of this process include the inhibition of proinflammatory cytokines synthesis and antiapoptotic function via caspase 3 inhibition. Moreover, increasing liver blood flow, reducing oxidative stress, scavenging lipid radicals, and the inhibition of lipid peroxidation could be effective for the maintenance of a healthy liver (Harbrecht et al., 1992, 1995; Zhu and Fung, 2000; Kim et al., 1997; Li and Billiar, 1999).

In contrast to NO's advantages, it has also disadvantageous effects. The reaction between NO and superoxide anion results in the production of hydroxyl and peroxynitrite radicals, which may play a role in the pathogenesis of liver damage due to inflammation (Bartosz, 1996; Sass et al., 2001).

The dual useful and harmful effects of NO could be due to varying redox status in the liver. At the onset of liver damage NO production level is low and the vasodilation, antioxidant, and antiapoptotic effects of NO may protect the liver, but as the damage progresses the oxidative/nitrosative stress and high level of NO production may result in the death of liver cells (Hon et al., 2002; Rockey and Shah, 2004).

25.8 Viral hepatitis infection

During viral hepatitis the elevation of NO synthesis can have two functions. First, NO may act as an antiviral agent. This helps the host via the inhibition of the transcription and expression of DNA–RNA viruses, the inhibition of viral growth, and apoptosis (Croen, 1993; Lowenstein et al., 1996). Second, because of the genotoxic properties of NO, its long-term elevation during chronic hepatitis can affect cellular DNA and result in the mutagenesis and production of *N*-nitroso hepatocarcinogenic components. So the known correlation between viral hepatitis infection and an increase in the risk of hepatic carcinoma could be due to the enhancement of NO production (Burney et al., 1999; Pan et al., 2001).

25.9 Liver cirrhosis

NO has disadvantageous effects in the pathogenesis of liver cirrhosis. In this disease NO elevation results in a vascular hyperdynamic occurrence that can increase endotoxemia. Endotoxemia itself causes excessive production of NO via an increase in number of cytokines. In conditions where NO enhancement results in a hyperdynamic status, NO reduction is advantageous (Rockey and Chung, 1998; Rees et al., 1990).

25.10 Hepatocellular carcinoma

The effects of NO on the different stages of hepatocellular carcinoma (HCC) are not same, and its effects could be different depending on the time, location, and levels of NO synthesis (Hon et al., 2002; Wink et al., 1998). NO is induced by hepatic tissue surrounding HCC via the mechanisms described below.

Tumor cells directly stimulate Kupffer cells and macrophages in the liver. HCC is the cause of the production of different cytokines that can play a role in the stimulation of hepatocytes. Moreover, shunting and portosystemic enhancement will occur and these are effective in increasing the production of NO. NO that is produced in the early stages of the disease will protect the liver because of its cytotoxic properties, via nitrosating important proteins in tumor cells. Moreover, other functional cells that surround a tumor could have tumoricidal, apoptotic, and antitumor properties due to NO production (Kurose et al., 1996; Saito et al., 1996).

In contrast, the most destructive effects of NO occur due to its reaction with superoxide anions and the synthesis of potential toxic mediators (such as peroxynitrite and hydroxyl), which result in DNA degradation (Burney et al., 1999; Hon et al., 2002). As the tumor progresses, NO released by tumor cells can increase angiogenesis, causing fast growth of the tumor, and facilitating the metastatic process via increasing expression of proangiogenic factors such as vascular endothelial growth factor (VEGF) and decreasing expression of antiangiogenesis factors (Suzuki et al., 1996). Also the genotoxic property of NO can be a cause of mutations in tumor suppressor genes, such as p53. Therefore NO has an important role in the progression of HCC (Li and Billiar, 1999; Wink et al., 1991).

25.11 Ischemia/reperfusion injury and shock

In this condition, NO can cause peroxynitrite synthesis or the induction of the expression of inflammatory factors (such as TNF-α and IL-1) via reaction with ROS, which consequently increases oxidative stress

(Hon et al., 2002; Sass et al., 2001). Therefore because of oxidative/nitrosative stress pathogenesis in liver diseases, the existence of an antioxidant system at the appropriate time for disease prevention and treatment is required.

Indeed, the antioxidant system can be an enzymatic and nonenzymatic system that are in harmony with each other and modulate the cellular balance against ROS and RNS (Webb and Twedt, 2008).

25.12 Enzymatic antioxidants

Enzymatic antioxidants, including catalase (CAT), superoxide dismutase (SOD), and glutathione peroxidase (GSH-PX), can result in the consumption of different types of ROS and RNS radicals via the catalysis of chemical reactions, removal of free radical precursors, and the chelation of mineral transportation catalyzers. The final product of the reaction is often a harmless component such as water and metabolites that are responsible for antioxidant reactions (Matés et al., 1999; McCall and Frei, 1999; Zhu et al., 2012; Webb and Twedt, 2008; Burton, 1994).

25.13 Nonenzymatic antioxidants

Nonenzymatic antioxidants are categorized into metabolic antioxidants and dietary antioxidants, which can inhibit or reduce the accumulation of free radicals (Webb and Twedt, 2008). Moreover, most of them have antiinflammatory properties. Metabolic antioxidants are related to endogenous antioxidants that are produced via the body's metabolism. These include coenzyme Q10, arginine, glutathione, lipoid acid, transferrin, bilirubin, uric acid, and melatonin.

In contrast, dietary antioxidants are exogenous and are not produced by the body, and most of them enter the body via food or supplements; such as carotenoids, flavonoids, omega-3, omega-6, vitamin C, and specially vitamin E (McCall and Frei, 1999; Matés et al., 1999; Zhu et al., 2012). Several studies have been performed to evaluate the effects of the antioxidants in liver diseases (Table 25.2).

25.14 Vitamin E

Vitamin E is one of the most important fat-soluble antioxidants that is mainly found in the lipid bilayer membrane (Ku, 1989). The role of

Table 25.2 The effects of some antioxidants on oxidative and nitrosative stress in liver damage.

Models	Antioxidants	Effects	References
Liver damage	Vitamin E and Se	Increase in *GSH-Px*, Se-*GSH-Px*	Ozkan et al. (2007)
Acute liver failure	Vitamin E	Increase in *SOD*, *GSH-Px*, *CAT*, *GST* Decrease in lipid peroxidation	Singh et al. (2014)
Liver injury	Vitamins E and C	Decrease in *ALT*, *AST*, *ALP*, *MDA*	Sutcu et al. (2006)
Hepatic damage	α-Tocopherol	Antioxidation	Zhang et al. (2013)
Liver damage	*Nigella sativa*	Increase in antioxidant enzyme Decrease in lipid peroxidation hepatoprotection	Kanter et al. (2005)
Ischemia/ reperfusion in fatty liver	Melatonin	Increase in antioxidant enzyme Decrease in *ALT*, *AST*, *MDA*, *NO* metabolites	Kireev et al. (2013)
Liver fibrosis	Garlic	Increase in *GSH*, decrease in *MDA*, *TNF-α*, *TGF-β*, *MMP-13*	Mahmoud et al. (2014)
Hepatotoxicity	coriander	Antioxidant; decrease in *ALT*, *AST*, *ALP*, *TBARS*, *MPO*, *NO*	Moustafa et al. (2014)
Hepatotoxicity	Allopurinol	Modulation of oxidative stress transcription factors, Modulation of *NF-κB* cytokine production	Demirel et al. (2012)

GSH-Px, Glutathione peroxidase; *Se-GSH-Px*, Selenium-dependent glutathione peroxidase; *SOD*, Superoxide dismutase; *CAT*, Catalase; *GST*, Glutathione S-transferase; *ALT*, Alanine transaminase; *AST*, Aspartate transaminase; *ALP*, Alkaline phosphatase; *MDA*, Malondialdehyde; *NO*, Nitric oxide; *TNF-α*, Tumor necrosis factor-α; *TGF-β*, Tumor growth factor-β; *TBARS*, Thiobarbituric acid reactive substances; *MPO*, Myeloperoxidase; *NF-κB*, Nuclear factor-κB.

vitamin E as an antioxidant was first discovered in 1937 by Olcott (Olcott and Emerson, 1937). Although tocopherols and tocotrienols are used instead of vitamin E, α-tocopherol has more vitamin E activity and consequently more antioxidant properties. α-Tocopherol is more common in plasma than γ-tocopherol (approximately five times higher). However, γ-tocopherol is more common in the diet and its metabolization is faster than α-tocopherol (Burton et al., 1983; Lehmann et al., 1986).

Based on investigations into antioxidative therapy, vitamins, especially vitamin E, are the most effective diet supplement for patients with liver diseases. This vitamin fights oxidants in the body and inhibits ROS and RNS production. Thus it protects lipids, proteins, carbohydrates, and DNA against free radical attacks (Wolf, 1997).

The ability for vitamin E to act as an antioxidant could be due to the following reasons:

Vitamin E has a hydroxyl group in its tocochromanols aromatic rings that gives hydrogen to a lipid peroxyl radical and converts it to a lipid hydroperoxide and a α-tocopheroxyl radical (Hadi et al., 2018). These products should be removed before being converted into free radical sources. The reaction of α-tocopherol with a peroxyl radical is faster than the reaction of peroxyl with a polyunsaturated fatty acid (PUFA) group. Thus low amounts of α-tocopherol could preserve high amounts of PUFA. The tocopheroxyl radical should also be inactive against oxygen or PUFA. Eventually the tocopheroxyl radical again reacts with another tocopheroxyl radical or a peroxyl radical to produce nonradical products, stop lipid peroxidation, and preserve the cellular membrane (Bowry et al., 1992; Burton, 1994; Bowry and Stocker, 1993; Ingold et al., 1987). This reaction also needs another antioxidant, such as vitamin C, to occur. In contrast, without other antioxidants, vitamin E performs its activity as a prooxidant to facilitate the entry of free radicals to LDL particles and lipid peroxidation (Bowry and Stocker, 1993; Burton, 1994). Therefore the presence of other antioxidants significantly alters the properties of vitamin E from a prooxidant to an antioxidant via a reaction with a tocopheroxyl radical, reproduction of vitamin E, and the transportation of free radicals from fat particles.

The biological activity of vitamin E is not limited to its antioxidant properties, and it could be involved in the regulation of inflammatory response, gene expression, enzymes attached to the membrane, and the modulation of cell signaling and proliferation. Thus vitamin E protects liver function against NO attacks via various mechanisms (Hadi et al., 2018).

α-Tocopherol reacts with nitrogen free radicals and oxidizes to form quinone-α tocopherol, while γ-tocopherol oxidizes to 5-nitro-γ-tocopherol and tocored. Thus vitamin E inhibits the reaction of NO with other active species and the synthesis of nitrogen mediators, such as nitrogen oxide and peroxynitrite, in order to protect the liver against damage from nitrogen mediators (Wolf, 1997). Moreover, vitamin E enables the trapping of membrane-soluble electrophilic nitrogen oxide, and produces stable and harmless products (Christen et al., 1997).

Vitamin E reduces the stimulation of TLR and CD14 receptors in response to pathogens. The stimulation of these receptors in the presence of pathogens starts a cascade of events, such as pathogen endocytosis into a phagosome, PKC activity, MAPK cascade, activity of the enzymatic NADPH oxidase complex, and the production of free radicals ROS and RNS that play an important role in the elimination of pathogens (Chapple et al., 2013).

Vitamin E can cause the reduction of IFN-γ endogenous signaling via decreasing the production of IL-12 by macrophages that consequently cause a lack of iNOS stimulation by IFN-γ (Tanaka et al., 2007). Moreover, vitamin E can have a direct effect on the reduction of iNOS enzyme expression and NO production in the liver (Calvisi et al., 2004).

The biological activity of vitamin E in association with NO function could be due to its inflammatory response modulation in liver diseases. Vitamin E plays a role in the elevation of antiinflammatory cytokine levels, such as IL-4 and IL-2, and the reduction of proinflammatory cytokines, such as IL-1, TNF-α, and IL-6, that consequently result in the inhibition of iNOS activity and NO production (Hadi et al., 2018). Moreover, vitamin E can reduce IL-1β mRNA and protein expression, and inhibit the stimulation and activity of iNOS (Wallert et al., 2014).

Vitamin E can also regulate NO synthesis at a transcriptional level that inhibits iNOS protein and mRNA expression in hepatic macrophages via the degradation of IκB kinase, leading to the lack of NF-κB-IκB phosphorylation and thus the inhibition of NF-κB transportation into the nucleus.

Vitamin E inhibits the induction of iNOS enzyme and NO production in various cells, such as hepatic monocytes, macrophages, and neutrophils, via the activation of protein phosphatase 2A (PP2A), PKC dephosphorylation, and consequently its inactivation (Hadi et al., 2018; Mirzaei and Khazaei, 2017).

Moreover, PKC inhibition via vitamin E results in NADPH oxidase inhibition in monocytes, and consequently causes the reduction of superoxide free radical production (Hadi et al., 2018). Besides, vitamin E can directly inhibit NADPH oxidase which leads to the inhibition of inflammatory factors including TNF-α and NF-κB, as well as NO production stimulation (Calvisi et al., 2004). On the other hand, vitamin E can inhibit the PPARs transcription factor that stimulates iNOS transcription and NO production.

Vitamin E can affect iNOS enzyme functions via the regulation of transcription activator/inhibitor factors such as MAPK and TGF-β (Hadi et al., 2018).

In contrast to other vitamins (such as vitamin C), vitamin E has no effect on the cofactors required for the iNOS enzyme such as BH4 at the translation and posttranslation regulatory levels (d'Uscio et al., 2003).

Moreover, vitamin E plays a role in the functions of tyrosine kinase and protein tyrosine phosphatase, one of the regulatory mechanisms of iNOS function and NO production at transcription and translation levels (Hadi et al., 2018).

Therefore as has been mentioned previously, the consequence of the elevation or reduction of NO in liver disease could be different depending on the type, duration, stages, oxidative status, and severity of disease, and thus antioxidative therapy using vitamin E can be an effective therapeutic approach in liver disease.

25.15 Comparing the activities of other vitamins

Vitamin C is a strong water-soluble antioxidant that plays a role as an electron donor and in reduction. This vitamin is known to be a scavenger of ROS and RNS free radicals (Webb and Twedt, 2008). It degenerates superoxide free radicals, and inhibits their reactions with NO and the production of peroxynitrite and hydroxyl radicals that are harmful for the liver. Moreover, vitamin C increases the activity of iNOS enzyme via increasing total biopeterin level, returning BH3 radicals to BH4, and consequently increases NO production that could be useful for liver diseases in some of the mentioned cases (d'Uscio et al., 2003). Other antioxidative effects of vitamin C occur alongside the vitamin E redox cycle that removes an electron from lipid hydroperoxyl and protects against lipid peroxidation (Kojo, 2004). In addition, vitamin C can increase the activity and levels of GSH-Px and glutathione reductase (GR) in the liver. So, it has a synergistic effect for the function of other antioxidants, such as vitamin E and GSH-Px, resulting in their storage and the maintenance of their levels.

Moreover, vitamin A can increase NO synthesis by stimulating macrophages, via an elevation in iNOS mRNA, and protein expression in some organs, such as liver, kidney, and spleen. In contrast, vitamin A can inhibit iNOS gene transcription and NO production in other cells. The opposed effects of vitamin A on iNOS can be attributed to various cell types and their actions.

1,25-Dihydroxyvitamin D-3 (the active form of vitamin D) increases iNOS expression and NO production in a human macrophage-like cell line. In contrast, the experimental studies show that vitamin D inhibits iNOS expression in inflammatory cells of the rat brain.

Other vitamins, including niacin and vitamin K_2, also inhibit iNOS expression and inducible NO (Wu and Meininger, 2002)

References

Aktan, F.J. (2004). iNOS-mediated nitric oxide production and its regulation. Life Sci. 75, 639-653.

Bartosz, G., 1996. Peroxynitrite: mediator of the toxic action of nitric oxide. Acta Biochim. Pol. Eng. Ed. 43, 645–660.

Bowry, V.W., Stocker, R., 1993. Tocopherol-mediated peroxidation. The prooxidant effect of vitamin E on the radical-initiated oxidation of human low-density lipoprotein. J. Am. Chem. Soc. 115, 6029–6044.

Bowry, V.W., Ingold, K.U., Stocker, R., 1992. Vitamin E in human low-density lipoprotein. When and how this antioxidant becomes a pro-oxidant. Biochem. J. 288, 341–344.

Burney, S., Caulfield, J.L., Niles, J.C., Wishnok, J.S., Tannenbaum, S.R., 1999. The chemistry of DNA damage from nitric oxide and peroxynitrite. Mutat. Res. Fundam. Mol. Mech. Mutagenesis 424, 37–49.

Burton, G.W., 1994 Vitamin E: molecular and biological function. Proc. Nutr. Soc. 53, 251–262.

Burton, G., Cheeseman, K., Doba, T., Ingold, K., Slater, T., 1983. Vitamin E as an antioxidant in vitro and in vivo. Biology of Vitamin E. Ciba Foundation Symposium, pp. 4–18.

Calvisi, D.F., Ladu, S., Hironaka, K., Factor, V.M., Thorgeirsson, S.S., 2004. Vitamin E down-modulates iNOS and NADPH oxidase in c-Myc/TGF-α transgenic mouse model of liver cancer. J. Hepatol. 41, 815–822.

Chapple, I.L., Matthews, J.B., Wright, H.J., Scott, A.E., Griffiths, H.R., Grant, M.M., 2013. Ascorbate and α-tocopherol differentially modulate reactive oxygen species generation by neutrophils in response to FcγR and TLR agonists. Innate Immun. 19, 152–159.

Christen, S., Woodall, A.A., Shigenaga, M.K., Southwell-Keely, P.T., Duncan, M.W., Ames, B.N., 1997. γ-Tocopherol traps mutagenic electrophiles such as NOx and complements α-tocopherol: physiological implications. Proc. Natl. Acad. Sci. U.S.A. 94, 3217–3222.

Croen, K.D., 1993. Evidence for antiviral effect of nitric oxide. inhibition of herpes simplex virus type 1 replication. J. Clin. Invest. 91, 2446–2452.

Demirel, U., Yalnız, M., Aygün, C., Orhan, C., Tuzcu, M., Sahin, K., et al., 2012. Allopurinol ameliorates thioacetamide-induced acute liver failure by regulating cellular redox-sensitive transcription factors in rats. Inflammation 35, 1549–1557.
Diesen, D.L., Kuo, P.C., 2010. Nitric oxide and redox regulation in the liver: Part I. General considerations and redox biology in hepatitis. J. Surg. Res. 162, 95–109.
d'Uscio, L.V., Milstien, S., Richardson, D., Smith, L., Katusic, Z.S., 2003. Long-term vitamin C treatment increases vascular tetrahydrobiopterin levels and nitric oxide synthase activity. Circ. Res. 92, 88–95.
Geller, D.A., Di Silvio, M., Nussler, A.K., Wang, S.C., Shapiro, R.A., Simmons, R.L., et al., 1993a. Nitric oxide synthase expression is induced in hepatocytes in vivo during hepatic inflammation. J. Surg. Res. 55, 427–432.
Geller, D.A., Nussler, A.K., Di Silvio, M., Lowenstein, C.J., Shapiro, R.A., Wang, S.C., et al., 1993b. Cytokines, endotoxin, and glucocorticoids regulate the expression of inducible nitric oxide synthase in hepatocytes. Proc. Natl. Acad. Sci. U.S.A. 90, 522–526.
Geller, D.A., Freeswick, P.D., Nguyen, D., Nussler, A.K., Di Silvio, M., Shapiro, R.A., et al., 1994. Differential induction of nitric oxide synthase in hepatocytes during endotoxemia and the acute-phase response. Arch. Surg. 129, 165–171.
Hadi, H.E., Vettor, R., Rossato, M., 2018. Vitamin E as a treatment for nonalcoholic fatty liver disease: reality or myth? Antioxidants (Basel) 7, 12.
Harbrecht, B., Billiar, T., Stadler, J., Demetris, A., Ochoa, J., Curran, R., et al., 1992. Inhibition of nitric oxide synthesis during endotoxemia promotes intrahepatic thrombosis and an oxygen radical-mediated hepatic injury. J. Leukoc. Biol. 52, 390–394.
Harbrecht, B.G., Mcclure, E.A., Simmons, R.L., Billiar, T.R., 1995. Prostanoids inhibit Kupffer cell nitric oxide synthesis. J. Surg. Res. 58, 625–629.
Hogg, N., Kalyanaraman, B., 1999. Nitric oxide and lipid peroxidation. Biochim. Biophys. Acta 1411, 378–384.
Hon, W.M., Lee, K.H., Khoo, H.E., 2002. Nitric oxide in liver diseases: friend, foe, or just passerby? Ann. N. Y. Acad. Sci. 962, 275–295.
Ingold, K., Burton, G., Foster, D., Hughes, L., Lindsay, D., Webb, A., 1987. Biokinetics of and discrimination between dietary RRR- and SRR-α-tocopherols in the male rat. Lipids 22, 163–172.
Iwakiri, Y., Kim, M.Y., 2015. Nitric oxide in liver diseases. Trends Pharmacol. Sci. 36, 524–536.
Kanter, M., Coskun, O., Budancamanak, M., 2005. Hepatoprotective effects of *Nigella sativa* L and *Urtica dioica* L on lipid peroxidation, antioxidant enzyme systems and liver enzymes in carbon tetrachloride-treated rats. World J. Gastroenterol. 11, 6684–6688.
Kaplowitz, N., 2000. Cell death at the millennium: implications for liver diseases. Clin. Liver. Dis. 4, 1–23.
Kim, Y.-M., De Vera, M.E., Watkins, S.C., Billiar, T.R., 1997. Nitric oxide protects cultured rat hepatocytes from tumor necrosis factor-α-induced apoptosis by inducing heat shock protein 70 expression. J. Biol. Chem. 272, 1402–1411.
Kireev, R., Bitoun, S., Cuesta, S., Tejerina, A., Ibarrola, C., Moreno, E., et al., 2013. Melatonin treatment protects liver of Zucker rats after ischemia/reperfusion by diminishing oxidative stress and apoptosis. Eur. J. Pharmacol. 701, 185–193.
Kojo, S., 2004. Vitamin C: basic metabolism and its function as an index of oxidative stress. Curr. Med. Chem. 11, 1041–1064.
Ku, I., 1989. Vitamin E as an in vitro and in vivo antioxydant. Ann. N.Y. Acad. Sci. 570, 7–22.
Kurose, I., Higuchi, H., Yonei, Y., Ebinuma, H., Watanabe, N., Hokari, R., et al., 1996. Rat kupffer cell-derived nitric oxide suppresses proliferation and induces apoptosis of syngeneic hepatoma cells. Gastroenterology 111, 1058–1070.

Lehmann, J., Martin, H., Lashley, E., Marshall, M., Judd, J., 1986. Vitamin E in foods from high and low linoleic acid diets. J. Am. Diet. Assoc. 86, 1208–1216.
Li, C., Jackson, R.M., 2002. Reactive species mechanisms of cellular hypoxia-reoxygenation injury. Am. J. Physiol. -Cell. Physiol. 282, C227–C241.
Li, J., Billiar, T.R., 1999. The anti-apoptotic actions of nitric oxide in hepatocytes. Cell Death Differ. 6, 952.
Li, A.-N., Li, S., Zhang, Y.-J., Xu, X.-R., Chen, Y.-M., Li, H.-B., 2014. Resources and biological activities of natural polyphenols. Nutrients 6, 6020–6047.
Li, S., Tan, H.-Y., Wang, N., Zhang, Z.-J., Lao, L., Wong, C.-W., et al., 2015. The role of oxidative stress and antioxidants in liver diseases. Int. J. Mol. Sci. 16, 26087–26124.
Lowenstein, C.J., Hill, S.L., Lafond-Walker, A., Wu, J., Allen, G., Landavere, M., et al., 1996. Nitric oxide inhibits viral replication in murine myocarditis. J. Clin. Invest. 97, 1837–1843.
Mahan, L.K., Raymond, J.L., 2016. Krause's Food and The Nutrition Care Process-e-Book. Elsevier Health Sciences.
Mahmoud, M.F., Zakaria, S., Fahmy, A., 2014. Aqueous garlic extract alleviates liver fibrosis and renal dysfunction in bile-duct-ligated rats. Z. Naturforsch. C. 69, 133–141.
Matés, J.M., Pérez-Gómez, C., De Castro, I.N., 1999. Antioxidant enzymes and human diseases. Clin. Biochem. 32, 595–603.
Mccall, M.R., Frei, B., 1999. Can antioxidant vitamins materially reduce oxidative damage in humans? Free Radic. Biol. Med. 26, 1034–1053.
McCord, J.M., 2000. The evolution of free radicals and oxidative stress. Am. J. Med. 108, 652–659.
Mirzaei, F., Khazaei M.J., 2017. Role of nitric oxide in biological systems: a systematic review. J. Mazandaran Univ. Med. Sci 27, 192–222.
Moncada, S., 1991. Nitric oxide: physiology, pathophysiology, and pharmacology. Pharmacol. Rev. 43, 109–142.
Moustafa, A.H., Ali, E.M., Moselhey, S.S., Tousson, E., El-Said, K.S., 2014. Effect of coriander on thioacetamide-induced hepatotoxicity in rats. Toxicol. Ind. Health 30, 621–629.
Olcott, H., Emerson, O., 1937. Antioxidants and the autoxidation of fats. IX. The antioxidant properties of the tocopherols. J. Am. Chem. Soc. 59, 1008–1009.
Ozkan, A., Fiskin, K., Ayhan, A.G.J.B., 2007. Effect of vitamin E and selenium on antioxidant enzymes in brain, kidney and liver of cigarette smoke-exposed mice. Biologia 62, 360–364.
Pan, J., Duan, L.-X., Sun, B.S., Feitelson, M.A., 2001. Hepatitis B virus X protein protects against anti-Fas-mediated apoptosis in human liver cells by inducing NF-κB. J. Gen. Virol. 82, 171–182.
Rees, D., Cellek, S., Palmer, R., Moncada, S., 1990. Dexamethasone prevents the induction by endotoxin of a nitric oxide synthase and the associated effects on vascular tone: an insight into endotoxin shock. Biochem. Biophys. Res. Commun. 173, 541–547.
Rockey, D., Chung, J.J., 1996. Regulation of inducible nitric oxide synthase in hepatic sinusoidal endothelial cells. Am. J. Physiol. -Gastrointest. Liver Physiol. 271, G260–G267.
Rockey, D.C., Chung, J.J., 1998. Reduced nitric oxide production by endothelial cells in cirrhotic rat liver: endothelial dysfunction in portal hypertension. Gastroenterol. 114, 344–351.
Rockey, D.C., Shah, V., 2004. Nitric oxide biology and the liver: report of an AASLD research workshop. Hepatology 39, 250–257.

Ross, A.C., Caballero, B., Cousins, R.J., Tucker, K.L., Ziegler, T.R., 2014. Modern Nutrition in Health and Disease. Lippincott Williams & Wilkins.

Saito, H., Kurose, I., Ebinuma, H., Fukumura, D., Higuchi, H., Atsukawa, K., et al., 1996. Kupffer cell-mediated cytotoxicity against hepatoma cells occurs through production of nitric oxide and adhesion via ICAM-1/CD18. Int. Immunol. 8, 1165–1172.

Sass, G., Koerber, K., Bang, R., Guehring, H., Tiegs, G., 2001. Inducible nitric oxide synthase is critical for immune-mediated liver injury in mice. J. Clin. Invest. 107, 439–447.

Schmidt, H.H., Lohmann, S.M., Walter, U., 1993. The nitric oxide and cGMP signal transduction system: regulation and mechanism of action. Biochim. Biophys. Acta (BBA) Mol. Cell. Res. 1178, 153–175.

Singal, A.K., Jampana, S.C., Weinman, S.A., 2011. Antioxidants as therapeutic agents for liver disease. Liver Int. 31, 1432–1448.

Singh, S., Mondal, P., Trigun, S.K., 2014. Acute liver failure in rats activates glutamine-glutamate cycle but declines antioxidant enzymes to induce oxidative stress in cerebral cortex and cerebellum. PLoS One 9, e95855.

Sutcu, R., Altuntas, I., Yildirim, B., Karahan, N., Demirin, H., Delibas, N., 2006. The effects of subchronic methidathion toxicity on rat liver: role of antioxidant vitamins C and E. Cell Biol. Toxicol. 22, 221–227.

Suzuki, K., Hayashi, N., Miyamoto, Y., Yamamoto, M., Ohkawa, K., Ito, Y., et al., 1996. Expression of vascular permeability factor/vascular endothelial growth factor in human hepatocellular carcinoma. Cancer Res. 56, 3004–3009.

Tanaka, Y., Wood, L.A., Cooney, R.V., 2007. Enhancement of intracellular γ-tocopherol levels in cytokine-stimulated C3H 10T1/2 fibroblasts: relation to NO synthesis, isoprostane formation, and tocopherol oxidation. BMC Chem. Biol. 7, 2.

Wallert, M., Schmölz, L., Galli, F., Birringer, M., Lorkowski, S., 2014. Regulatory metabolites of vitamin E and their putative relevance for atherogenesis. Redox Biol. 2, 495–503.

Webb, C., Twedt, D., 2008. Oxidative stress and liver disease. Vet. Clin. N. Am.: Small Anim. Pract. 38, 125–135.

Wink, D.A., Kasprzak, K.S., Maragos, C.M., Elespuru, R.K., Misra, M., Dunams, T.M., et al., 1991. DNA deaminating ability and genotoxicity of nitric oxide and its progenitors. Science 254, 1001–1003.

Wink, D.A., Vodovotz, Y., Laval, J., Laval, F., Dewhirst, M.W., Mitchell, J.B., 1998. The multifaceted roles of nitric oxide in cancer. Carcinog. 19, 711–721.

Wolf, G., 1997. σ-Tocopherol: an efficient protector of lipids against nitric oxide—initiated peroxidative damage. Nutr. Rev. 55, 376–378.

Wu, G., Meininger, C.J., 2002. Regulation of nitric oxide synthesis by dietary factors. Annu. Rev. Nutr. 22, 61–86.

Zhang, Y.-K.J., Wu, K.C., Klaassen, C.D., 2013. Genetic activation of Nrf2 protects against fasting-induced oxidative stress in livers of mice. PLoS One 8, e59122.

Zhu, W., Fung, P., 2000. The roles played by crucial free radicals like lipid free radicals, nitric oxide, and enzymes NOS and NADPH in CCl4-induced acute liver injury of mice. Free Rad. Bio. Med. 29, 870–880.

Zhu, R., Wang, Y., Zhang, L., Guo, Q., 2012. Oxidative stress and liver disease. Hepatol. Res. 42, 741–749.

Zima, T., Kalousová, M., 2005. Oxidative stress and signal transduction pathways in alcoholic liver disease. Alcohol. Clin. Exp. Res. 29, 110S–115S.

CHAPTER 26

Vitamin E and reproductive health

Siti Syairah Mohd Mutalip
Department of Pharmaceutical Life Sciences, Faculty of Pharmacy, Universiti Teknologi MARA (UiTM), Selangor, Malaysia

Contents

Key facts

- Vitamin E was first discovered in 1922 by Evans and Bishop through the finding of a particular "antisterility factor X" that was necessary for reproduction.
- Extensive research throughout the decades has introduced vitamin E as a powerful lipid-soluble antioxidant.
- In the earlier years, alpha-tocopherol was referred to as vitamin E.

Molecular Nutrition
DOI: https://doi.org/10.1016/B978-0-12-811907-5.00025-7

- Massive interest in tocotrienols only emerged in the 1980s following the discoveries of their potential in cholesterol-lowering and acting as anticancer agent.
- To date vitamin E has been widely reported to have beneficial effects against cancer cells, hypocholesterolemia, skin diseases, aging, cardiovascular diseases, nervous system disease, bone impairment, radioprotection, and many more.

Summary points

- This chapter focuses on vitamin E which is an antioxidant that is present naturally in a number of plants.
- Vitamin E comprises two major substances which are the tocopherols and tocotrienols.
- Vitamin E is a lipid-soluble antioxidant and is involved in numerous cellular regulations to maintain body health.
- Benefits of vitamin E in numerous health issues have been well-documented, especially for its effect as an antioxidant and anticancer agent.
- However, specific reports on its effects on reproductive-related health (other than reproductive cancers) are considerably lacking.
- Therefore this chapter intends to provide a summary of the available reports on the benefits of vitamin E on reproductive health (other than reproductive cancers) to help provide further guidelines for future vitamin E-based research.

Definitions of words and terms

Antioxidant: Antioxidants are natural substances that function to regulate the overproduction of reactive oxygen species (ROS). There are two types of antioxidants, the enzymatic and nonenzymatic antioxidants.

Fertilization: Fertilization is a process of the fusion of two gametes—the sperm and the ovum cell to produce a new individual.

Oxidative stress (*OS*): OS is a condition that occurs when there is an imbalance in the presence of antioxidants and prooxidants in the body.

Reactive oxygen species (ROS): ROS are generated to induce OS when there are excessive prooxidants present in the body. ROS are highly reactive and unstable. They acquire electrons from nucleic acids, lipids, proteins, carbohydrates, or any nearby molecule causing a string of chain reactions to become stable. These chain reactions result in cellular damage and diseases.

Vitamins: Vitamins are biogenic substances that play essential roles in human growth and nutrition through their biological functions, structures, and interactions with other molecules.

Abbreviations

OS oxidative stress
TOC tocopherol
TCT tocotrienol
TRF tocotrienol-rich fraction
ZP zona pellucida

26.1 Introduction

26.1.1 Vitamin E

Vitamin E was first discovered by Evans and Bishop in 1922 through the finding of a particular "antisterility factor X" that was necessary for reproduction (Evans and Bishop 1922). Following that, vitamin E has been extensively studied and eventually has become a well-recognized powerful lipid-soluble antioxidant (Tappel, 1962; Burton and Ingold 1986; Esterbauer et al., 1991). Ironically, although vitamin E is known as the vitamin for reproduction, it was widely recognized as a powerful lipid-soluble antioxidant and extensively studied for its role against oxidative stress. The great interest on its role as an antioxidant has left behind the research into its precious value as the "fertility booster." In reproduction-related studies, to date, reports on the role of vitamin E in infertility and sterility are far lacking, with most studies emphasizing the antioxidant activity of vitamin E.

26.2 Vitamin E

26.2.1 Sources of vitamin E

Vitamin E is available in a number of foods and plants, ranging from edible oils to nuts, including wheat, rice bran, barley, oat, coconut, palm, and annatto (Sheppard et al., 1993; Ramaswamy et al., 2012). Other sources of vitamin E include rye, amaranth, walnut, hazelnut, poppy, safflower, maize, and the seeds of grape and pumpkins. In addition, vitamin

E derivatives have also been detected in human milk (Kobayashi et al., 1975) and palm date (*Phoenix canariensis*) (Nehdi et al., 2010).

26.2.2 Structures of vitamin E homologs

Vitamin E comprises two substances, namely the tocopherols (TOCs) and tocotrienols (TCTs), that are synthesized by plants from homogentisic acid (Rimbach et al., 2010). These substances are present in eight different homologs, namely α-TOC, β-TOC, γ-TOC, δ-TOC, α-TOC, β-TOC, γ-TOC, and δ-TOC (IUPAC-IUB Joint Commission on Biochemical Nomenclature, 1982). The four TOC homologs (α-, β-, γ-, and δ-TOC) have a fully saturated 16-carbon isoprenoid side chain, whereas TCT homologs have a similar isoprenoid chain containing three double bonds (unsaturated side chain). Each of the homologs are named according to the position and number of the methyl groups on the phenol ring, with the α-, β-, γ-, and δ- homologs containing three, two, two, and one methyl groups, respectively (Fig. 26.1). These structural differences determine the biological activity of the homologs, with α-homologs being the most biologically active (Rimbach et al., 2002).

26.2.3 Vitamin E on general health

During the earlier period of vitamin E research, TCTs were not been studied as extensively as TOCs. However, there were a few reports that stated that α-TCT possesses better antioxidant properties than α-TOC (Serbinova et al., 1991; Serbinova and Packer 1994) due to the unsaturated side chain of TCTs that allows for better distribution through efficient penetration of tissue membranes with saturated fatty layers (Suzuki et al., 1993). The benefits of TCTs gained attention only during the late 1980s, when their cholesterol-lowering potential (Qureshi et al., 1986) and anticancer effects were published (Kato et al., 1985; Sundram et al., 1989). Since then the benefits of TCTs have been extensively studied, including their effects on hypocholesterolemia (Qureshi et al., 2002), skin protection (Traber et al., 1997, 1998; Weber et al., 1997), antiaging (Schaffer et al., 2005), cardiovascular diseases (Slyvester and Theriault, 2003; Thuhairah et al., 2016), nervous system disease (Sen et al., 2004), cancer (Conte et al., 2004; Nesaretnam et al., 2004), and bone health (Norazlina et al., 2002; Ima-Nirwana and Suhaniza, 2004; Nizar et al., 2012; Chin et al., 2016).

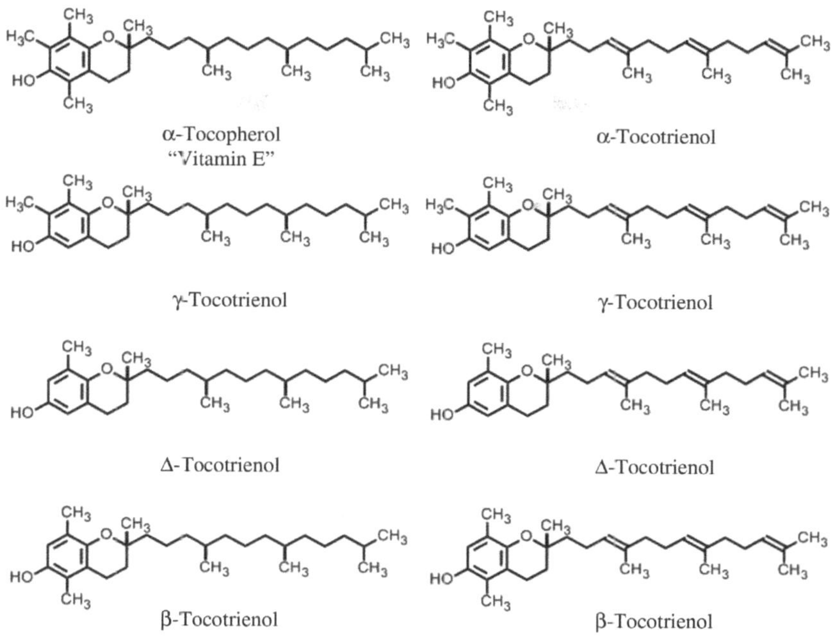

Figure 26.1 (A) Structure differences between tocopherols (TOCs) and tocotrienols (TCTs). (B) TOCs are present with saturated side chains while TCTs are present with unsaturated side chains, shown by the presence of double bond in TCTs. *Source: http://www.vita-dose.com/structure-of-vitamin-e.html.*

26.3 Reproduction

26.3.1 Fertilization

Fertilization is a process that involves the fusion of two haploid gametes, the sperm and the oocyte (egg) cell, to produce a new genetically distinct individual (Paul et al., 2001; Knobil and Neil, 2006). Fertilization normally occurs in the fallopian tubes and forms a "*zygote.*" The *zygote* will continue to grow along the way from the fallopian tubes to the uterus for implantation into the uterine wall.

26.3.2 Preimplantation embryonic growth

The preimplantation embryonic growth which begins from the 1-cell stage (*zygote*) is a critical and unique period that involves a number of developmental processes. The processes include the first mitotic divisions, the establishment of cellular contacts and the differentiation of the first cell lineages. At this time the embryos are free-floating, having no direct

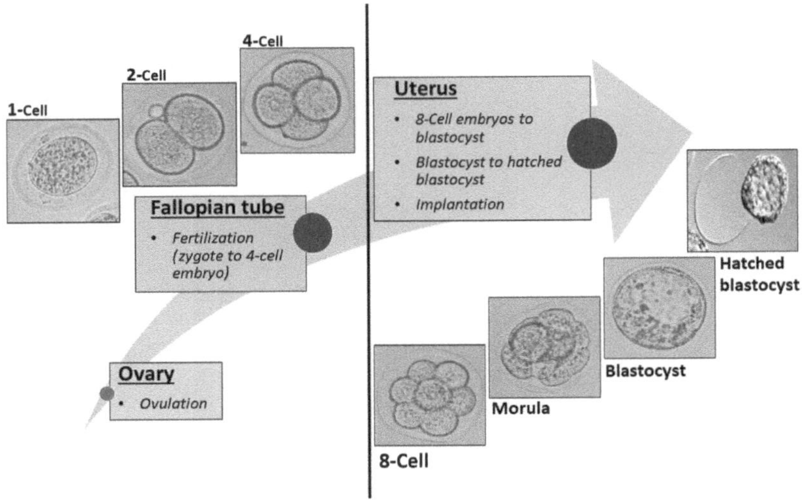

Figure 26.2 (A) Preimplantation stages during the embryonic growth. (B) The symmetrical cleavage of blastomeres until the 8-cell stage is followed by the asymmetrical cleavage of blastomeres in the morula and blastocyst stages.

cell to cell contact, lack a blood supply, are exposed to a dynamic fluid environment (Hardy and Spanos, 2002), and are dependent on autocrine and paracrine growth factors to support their growth and development.

The newly formed zygotes develop into the 2-cell, 4-cell, 8-cell, morula, and blastocyst stages prior to implantation into the uterine lining. The preimplantation embryonic developments are characterized by a relatively synchronous doubling of cell numbers until the 8-cell stage, followed by asynchronous cell divisions after compaction at the morula stage (Fig. 26.2) (Rebecca et al., 2011). The first events of cellular differentiation also occur during the morula stage. At the 8-cell to 16-cell stage (early morula stage), the embryos will enter into the uterine environment and continue developing into blastocysts (Fig. 26.3) (Wang and Dev, 2006). During the blastocyst stage, the embryos will hatch from the surrounding zona pellucida (ZP) and subsequently implant into the endometrium wall of the uterus (Wang and Dev, 2006). The embryonic growth will further be continued with postimplantation development.

The embryos at the blastocyst stage comprise the epithelial trophectoderm (TE), which is a layer of cells that surrounds the embryos and will develop into the extra embryonic tissues, and the inner cell mass (ICM), which consists of the pluripotent cells that will later differentiate into the fetus (Fig. 26.4). These embryonic components are vital for continuous

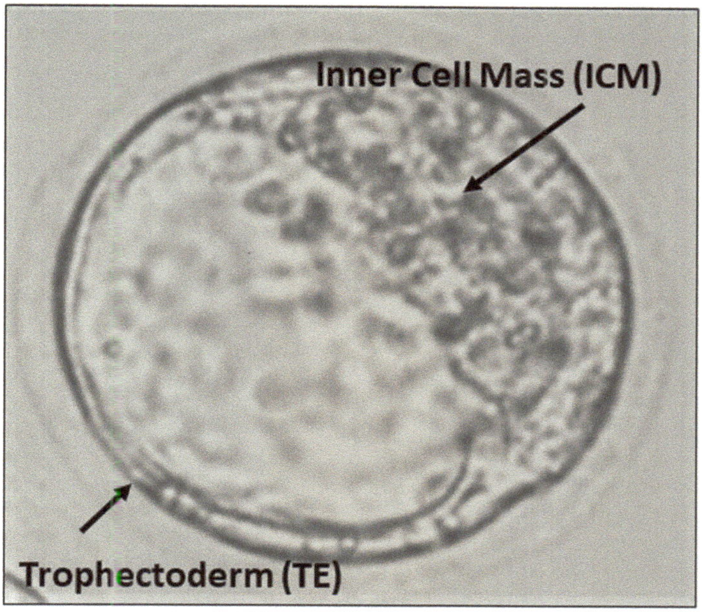

Figure 26.3 (A) The preimplantation embryonic development from ovary to uterus. (B) Embryos develop through the 2-cell, 4-cell, 8-cell, morula, and blastocyst stages. During the early morula stage, the embryos will enter into the uterine environment and continue developing into blastocysts prior to implantation.

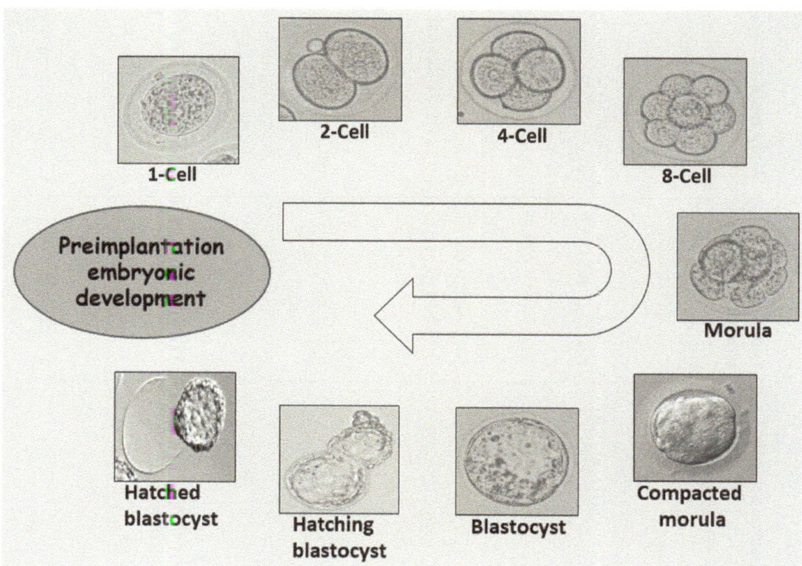

Figure 26.4 (A) A picture of embryo at the blastocyst stage. (B) Blastocysts comprise the epithelial trophectoderm (TE), the layer of cells surrounds the embryos and will develop into the extra embryonic tissues. The inner cell mass (ICM) consists of the pluripotent cells that will later differentiate into the fetus.

Table 26.1 Summary of the reported studies of vitamin E on male reproductive health in the years 2008–2018 (excluding reproductive cancers).

Experimental subjects	Types of vitamin E	Study result(s)	References
Human(clinical patients)	Vitamin E	Daily supplementation of selenium (200 μg) in combination with vitamin E (400 units) for 100 day resulted in 52.6% of total improvement in sperm motility, morphology, or both, and 10.8% of spontaneous pregnancy.	Moslemi and Tavanbakhsh (2011)
	Vitamin E	Daily cotreatment with 25 mg/day clomiphene citrate and 400 mg/day vitamin E for 6 months significantly improved the mean sperm concentration, and the total sperm motility was also improved.	ElSheikh et al. (2015)
	Meta-analysis study	Meta-analysis study revealed that the majority of reported studies showed that administration of supplements like L-carnitine, selenium, vitamin C, and vitamin E may lead to improved sperm concentration, motility, and morphology, and sometimes DNA integrity.	Ahmadi et al. (2016)
	Systematic review	Antioxidant types and doses in male infertility reported a significant positive effect on basic semen parameters, advanced sperm function, outcomes of assisted reproductive therapy, and live-birth rate, with vitamin E among one of the most commonly used antioxidants.	Reviewed in Ahmad and Ashok (2018)
In vitro studies/in vivo laboratory animal models	Vitamin E	• Coadministration of sodium arsenite and vitamin E significantly compensate for the harmful effects of sodium arsenite on sperm number, motility, viability, and morphology. • Rats treated with vitamin E alone significantly increased the sperm viability and motility.	Momeni and Eskandari (2012)
	Vitamin E	Coadministration of 400 mg/kg valproic acid (VPA) and 50 mg/kg vitamin E to male Wistar rats for 28 days restored the antioxidant potential and prevented oxidative damage on testes and epididymides; and restored sperm motility.	Giovana et al. (2016)

(Continued)

Table 26.1 (Continued)

Experimental subjects	Types of vitamin E	Study result(s)	References
Domestic animals	Vitamin E	Supplementation with 80 IU/goat/day and 320 IU/goat/day of vitamin E in diets significantly simulates the development of reproductive organs in Boer goats.	Hong et al. (2009)
	Vitamin E	• Supplementation with 70 IU of dietary vitamin E/kg diet to pigs resulted in the highest number of mounts, combats, head-kicks, and anogenital sniffs with the shortest reaction time. • Boar group supplemented with 70 IU of vitamin E produced semen with the highest semen volume, sperm cell motility, progressive movement, acrosomal normal apical ridge, percentage live sperm, sperm concentration per mL semen volume, and total number of sperm per ejaculate.	Umesiobi (2012)
	DL-α-Tocopherol acetate	Higher supplementation of dietary vitamin E helps to improve the semen characteristics of local *kampong* chicken after 4 weeks of supplementation.	Mohamad Asrol and Abdul Rashid (2017)

Table 26.2 Summary of the reported studies of vitamin E on female reproductive health in the years 2008–2018 (excluding reproductive cancers).

Experimental subjects	Types of vitamin E	Study result(s)	References
Human		Very low birth weight in Tunisian neonates resulted from vitamin A, D, and E deficiencies and were associated with preeclampsia.	Fares et al. (2014)
In vitro studies/in vivo laboratory animal models	Tocotrienol-rich fraction (TRF)	• Coadministration with 5 mg/kg/day of nicotine and 60 mg/kg/day of TRF increased pregnancy outcome to 83.3% in rats. • An estimate of 25.7% of the embryos developed into 2- and 4-cell stage in rats treated with both nicotine and TRF.	Mokhtar et al. (2008)
	Palm γ-TCT	The detrimental effects of nicotine on the ultrastructure of the oocytes were reduced.	Rajikin et al. (2009)
	Palm-TCT	Concurrent treatment with 90 mg/kg and 120 mg/kg of palm-TCT and 10 mg/kg corticosterone (CORT) reduced the numbers of abnormal embryos induced by CORT.	Nasibah et al. (2012a)
		Cotreatment with CORT and 120 mg/kg TCT significantly increased the number of implantation sites and reduced the resorption rate.	Nasibah et al. (2012b)
	Palm γ-TCT	Embryonic development in nicotine-induced mice were improved following treatment with palm γ-TCT.	Kamsani et al. (2013)
	γ-TCT	Coincubation in media supplemented with γ-TCT and hydrogen peroxide (H_2O_2) improved the development of porcine embryos through modulation of apoptotic *BCL-XL* and *BAX* genes.	Lee et al. (2014)
	Palm-TCT	• One-month supplementation with 150 mg/kg/day of palm-TCT significantly increased the percentage of normal embryos. • TCT is suggested to delay the effect of aging.	Saidatul et al. (2014)
	Annatto δ-TCT and Soy α-TOC	Intervention with annatto δ-TCT and soy α-TOC protected against the *Pik3ca* gene expression in preimplantation embryos of nicotine-treated mice.	Syairah et al. (2014)

(Continued)

Table 26.2 (Continued)

Experimental subjects	Types of vitamin E	Study result(s)	References
	Tocotrienol-rich fraction (TRF)	Concomitant supplementation of TRF with anticancer prodrug, cyclophosphamide (CPA) on ovarian cells protected against oxidative stress (OS)-induced apoptosis in ovaries.	Saleh et al. (2014, 2015)
	Annatto δ-TCT and Soy α-TOC	Supplementation with annatto δ-TCT(s) and soy α-TOC resulted in increased number of morula.	Syairah et al. (2015)
	Annatto δ-TCT and soy α-TOC	• Annatto δ-TCT reversed the body weight loss in nicotine-treated mice. • The development of 8-cell embryos was improved.	Rajikin et al. (2015)
	Annatto δ-TCT	• Annatto δ-TCT did not reversed the DNA damages induced by nicotine. • Treatment with annatto δ-TCT alone in normal mice did not affect the normal chromosomal arrangements.	Syairah et al. (2016)
	Tocotrienol-rich fraction (TRF)	• TRF supplementation significantly reduced the percentage of DNA damage in oocytes cells. • TRF supplementation upregulated the expression of antiaging gene, *SIRT1* and downregulated the expression of *CDKN2A* and *E2F1* genes.	Nuraliza et al. (2017)
	Tocotrienol-rich fraction (TRF)	• Concurrent treatment with 3 mg/kg bw/day of nicotine and 60 mg/kg bw/day of TRF resulted in the increased actin intensity in 2-cell and 8-cell embryos. • The same trend was seen in tubulin at 2-cell and 8-cell embryos. • Both actin and tubulin structures were enhanced in the groups treated with TRF alone.	Hamirah et al. (2017)
	Tocotrienol-rich fraction (TRF)	• The expression level of *CHEK1* gene (responsible for the detection of DNA damages) in group concurrently treated with CORT and TRF was found to be normal as the control value. • Intervention with TRF reduced the zona pellucida thickness of oocytes in mice exposed to exogenous CORT towards control.	Nuraliza et al. (2018)

(*Continued*)

Table 26.2 (Continued)

Experimental subjects	Types of vitamin E	Study result(s)	References
	Tocotrienol-rich fraction (TRF)	• Two-month supplementation with TRF at doses of 90, 120, and 150 mg/kg resulted in significantly higher percentages of normal oocytes and lower percentages of fragmented oocytes. • Significant changes were detected in metabolic pathways that include fatty acids, amino acids metabolism, and steroid hormone biosynthesis.	Norrabiatul et al. (2018)
	α-TOCPalm-TRF	• Palm-TRF produced significantly higher numbers of normal 2-cell embryos. • Alpha-tocopherol produced higher survival rate to the blastocyst stage. • TRF treatment produced more vacuolated mitochondria in 8-cell embryos.	Mimi et al. (2018)
	Soy α-TOC	• Intervention with α-TOC increased the average number of ovarian follicles compared to treatment with nicotine alone • Intervention with α-TOC showed increment in the measurement of thickness of the endometrium	Azmil et al. (2018)
	Annatto δ-TCT and soy α-TOC	• Supplementation with annatto δ-TCT(s) and soy α-TOC protected against embryonic malformations in nicotine-treated mice through alterations in PI3K/Akt-Cyclin D1 pathway. • Treatment in normal mice promoted the 2-cell murine preimplantation embryonic growth.	Syairah et al. (2019)

embryonic development and also in establishing an effective maternal–embryonic interface for the maintenance of pregnancy.

26.3.3 Vitamin E on reproductive health: the reported studies

Focused reports on the effects of vitamin E on reproductive-related health problems including fertility and preimplantation embryonic development are evidently lacking, despite numerous studies reporting on its benefits for health. Although vitamin E has been long known as the vitamin for reproduction, attempts to study this area have only been actively made in the last decade. The available research reports from the last 10 years (2008–2018) on vitamin E and male and female reproductive health (excluding reproductive cancers such as in breast, cervix, prostate, ovaries, etc.) are summarized in Tables 26.1 and 26.2, respectively.

26.4 Conclusion

Vitamin E has been acknowledged as one of the powerful lipid-soluble antioxidants long ago. Despite the large number of published reports on its health benefits, a lot of work on human and animal studies are still warranted in order to gain a comprehensive understanding of the effects of vitamin E, especially in regards to reproductive health. Future studies on the effects of vitamin E on clinical aspects should also be taken into account including the important factors such as the optimum dose intakes, synergistic effects of vitamin E with other compounds/drugs, severity of the patients, and other related factors.

References

Ahmad, M., Ashok, A., 2018. Systematic review of antioxidant types and doses in male infertility: benefits on semen parameters, advanced sperm function, assisted reproduction and live-birth rate. Arab J. Urol. 16 (1), 113–124.

Ahmadi, S., Bashiri, R., Ghadiri-Anari, A., Nadjarzadeh, A., 2016. Antioxidant supplements and semen parameters: an evidence based review. Int. J. Reprod. Biomed. (Yazd, Iran) 14 (12), 729–736.

Azmil, M.A., Shahrizal, M.S., Shahrul, M.N.M.I., Syairah, S.M.M., 2018. Histological analysis of murine ovaries and uteruses following supplementation with alpha-tocopherol in nicotine injected mice. IJET 7 (4.38), 1496–1498.

Burton, G.W., Ingold, K.U., 1986. Vitamin E application of the principles of physical organic chemistry to the exploration of its structure and function. Acc. Chem. Res. 19, 194–201.

Chin, K.-Y., Gengatharan, D., Mohd Nasru, F.S., Khairussam, R.A., Ern, S.L.H., Aminuddin, S.A.W., et al., 2016. The effects of annatto tocotrienol on bone biomechanical strength and bone calcium content in an animal model of osteoporosis due to testosterone deficiency. Nutrients 8, 808. Available from: https://doi.org/10.3390/nu8120808.

Conte, C., Floridi, A., Aisa, C., Piroddi, M., Floridi, A., Galli, F., 2004. Gamma-tocotrienol metabolism and antiproliferative effect in prostate cancer cells. Ann. N. Y. Acad. Sci. 1031, 391–394.

ElSheikh, M.G., Hosny, M.B., Elshenoufy, A., Elghamrawi, H., Fayad, A., Abdelrahman, S., 2015. Combination of vitamin E and clomiphene citrate in treating patients with idiopathic oligoasthenozoospermia: a prospective, randomized trial. Andrology 3, 864–867.

Esterbauer, H., Dieber-Rotheneder, M., Striegl, G., Waeg, G., 1991. Role of vitamin E in preventing the oxidation of low density lipoprotein. Am. J. Clin. Nutr. 53, 314S–321S.

Evans, H.M., Bishop, K.S., 1922. On the existence of a hitherto unrecognized dietary factor essential for reproduction. Science 56, 650–651.

Fares, S., Sethom, M.M., Khouaja-Mokrani, C., Jabnoun, S., Feki, M., Kaabachi, N., 2014. Vitamin A, E, and deficiencies in Tunisian very low birth weight neonates: prevalence and risk factors. Pediatr. Neonatol. 55, 196–201. Available from: https://doi.org/10.1016/j.pedneo.2013.09.006.

Ourique, G.M., Saccol, E.M., Pês, T.S., Glanzner, W.G., Schiefelbein, S.H., Woehl, V. M., et al., 2016. Protective effect of vitamin E on sperm motility and oxidative stress in valproic acid treated rats. Food Chem. Toxicol. 95, 159–167.

Hamirah, N.K., Kamsani, Y.S., Mohamed Nor Khan, N.A., Ab Rahim, S., Rajikin, M. H., 2017. Effects of nicotine and tocotrienol-rich fraction supplementation on cytoskeletal structures of murine pre-implantation embryos. Med. Sci. Monit. Basic Res. 23, 373–379.

Hardy, K., Spanos, S., 2002. Growth factor expression and function in the human and mouse preimplantation embryo. J. Endocrinol. 172 (2), 221–236.

Hong, Z., Hailing, L., Hui, M., Guijie, Z., 2009. Effect of vitamin E supplementation on development of reproductive organs in Boer goat. Anim. Reprod. Sci. 113 (1–4), 93–101. Available from: https://doi.org/10.1016/j.anireprosci.2008.05.076.

Ima-Nirwana, S., Suhaniza, S.J., 2004. Effects of tocopherols and tocotrienols on body composition and bone calcium content in adrenalectomized rats replaced with dexamethasone. J. Med. Food 7 (1), 45–51.

IUPAC-IUB Joint Commission on Biochemical Nomenclature, 1982. Nomenclature of tocopherols and related compounds. (Recommendations 1981). Eur. J. Biochem. 123, 473–475.

Kamsani, Y.S., Rajikin, M.H., Nor-Ashikin, M.N.K., Nuraliza, A.S., Chatterjee, A., 2013. Nicotine-induced cessation of embryonic development is reversed by γ-tocotrienol in mice. Med. Sci. Monit. Basic Res. 19, 87–92.

Kato, A., Yamaoka, M., Tanaka, A., Komiyama, K., Umezawa, I., 1985. Physiological effect of tocotrienol. J. Jpn. Oil Chem. Soc. 34 (5), 375–376. Available from: https://doi.org/10.5650/jos1956.34.375.

Knobil, E., Neill, J.D., 2006. Chapter 2: Fertilization in mammals. Physiology of Reproduction. Gulf Professional Publishing, Houston, TX, pp. 55–112.

Kobayashi, H., Kanno, C., Yamauchi, K., Tsugo, T., 1975. Identification of alpha-, beta-, gamma-, and delta-tocopherols and their contents in human milk. Biochim. Biophys. Acta 380 (2), 282–290.

Lee, E., Min, S.-H., Song, B.-S., Yeon, J.-Y., Kim, J.-W., Bae, J.-H., et al., 2014. Exogenous γ-tocotrienol promotes preimplantation development and improves the quality of porcine embryos. Reprod. Fertil. Dev. 27 (3), 481–490. Available from: https://doi.org/10.1071/RD13167.

Mimi, S.S., Zolkapli, E., Nor Shahida, N.A.R., Thalhah, A.A.A., Rajikin, M.H., Nooraain, H., et al., 2018. Palm tocotrienol-rich-fraction yields higher numbers of normal embryos whereas alpha-tocopherol produces higher preimplantation survival in murine embryos. Malays. J. Fundam. Appl. Sci. 14 (3), 407–410.

Mohamad Asrol, K., Abdul Rashid, B., 2017. Effect of vitamin E supplementation on semen quantity and quality of local Kampong roosters. Malays. J. Anim. Sci. 20 (1), 37–43.

Mokhtar, N., Rajikin, M.H., Zakaria, Z., 2008. Role of tocotrienol-rich palm vitamin E on pregnancy and preimplantation embryos in nicotine treated rats. Biomed. Res. 19, 181–184.

Momeni, H.R., Eskandari, N., 2012. Effect of vitamin E on sperm parameters and DNA integrity in sodium arsenite-treated rats. Iran. J. Reprod. Med. 10 (3), 249–256.

Moslemi, M.K., Tavanbakhsh, S., 2011. Selenium-vitamin E supplementation in infertile men: effects on semen parameters and pregnancy rate. Int. J Gen. Med. 4, 99–104. Available from: https://doi.org/10.2147/IJGM.S16275.

Nasibah, A., Rajikin, M.H., Nor-Ashikin, M.N.K., Nuraliza, A.S., 2012a. Tocotrienol improves the quality of impaired mouse embryos induced by corticosterone. In: Proceeding of the Symposium on Humanities, Science and Engineering Research (SHUSER2012), Kuala Lumpur, Malaysia, pp. 135–138.

Nasibah, A., Rajikin, M.H., Nor-Ashikin, M.N.K., Nuraliza, A.S., 2012b. Effects of tocotrienol supplementation on pregnancy outcome in mice subjected to maternal corticosterone administration. J. Oil Palm Res. 24, 1550–1558.

Nehdi, I., Omri, S., Khalil, M.I., Al-Resayes, S.I., 2010. Characteristics and chemical composition of date palm (*Phoenix canariensis*) seeds and seed oil. Ind. Crops Prod. 32, 360–365.

Nesaretnam, K., Ambra, R., Selvaduray, K.R., Radhakrishnan, A., Canali, R., Virgili, F., 2004. Tocotrienol-rich fraction from palm oil and gene expression in human breast cancer cells. Ann. N. Y. Acad. Sci. 1031, 143–157.

Nizar, A.M., Norazlina, M., Ahmad, N.S., 2012. Effects of low-dose versus high dose γ-tocotrienol on the bone cells exposed to the hydrogen peroxide-induced oxidative stress and apoptosis. Evid. Based Complem. Altern. Med. Available from: https://doi.org/10.1155/2012/680834.

Norazlina, M., Ima-Nirwana, S., Gapor, M.T.A., Kadir, K.B.A., 2002. Tocotrienols are needed for normal bone calcification in growing female rats. Asia Pac. J. Clin. Nutr. 11 (3), 194–199.

Norrabiatul, A.A., Fathimah, M., Nuraliza, A.S., 2018. Impact of tocotrienol-rich fraction supplementation on the ovarian metabolome and quality of oocytes in aging mice. In: Proceedings for International Conference on Antioxidants and Degenerative Diseases 2018 (ICADD2018), Kuala Lumpur, Malaysia, vol. 1, no. 1, p. 23.

Nuraliza, A.S., Saidatul, A.K., Norerlyda, H., Nasibah, A., Muhamad, M., 2017. Tocotrienol-rich fraction supplementation improves oocytes quality in aging mice and upregulates the expression of anti-aging genes in mouse ovary. Hum. Reprod. 32, i214–i215.

Nuraliza, A.S., Zaid, W.A.R., Norrabiatul, A.A., Nasibah, A., Mudiana, M., 2018. Effects of tocotrienol-rich fraction supplementation on the expression of DNA damage response genes in ovary and oocytes quality in mice exposed to corticosterone-induced oxidative damage. Hum. Reprod. 33, 234.

Paul, M.W., Luca, J., Eveline, S.L., 2001. A profile of fertilization in mammals. Nat. Cell Biol. 3, E59–E64. Available from: https://doi.org/10.1038/3505517.

Qureshi, A.A., Burger, W.C., Peterson, D.M., Elson, C.E., 1986. The structure of an inhibitor of cholesterol biosynthesis isolated from barley. The Journal of Biological Chemistry 261, 10544–10550.

Qureshi, A.A., Sami, S.A., Salser, W.A., Khan, F.A., 2002. Dose-dependent suppression of serum cholesterol by tocotrienol-rich fraction (TRF 25) of rice bran in hypercholesterolemic humans. Atherosclerosis 161, 199–207.

Rajikin, M.H., Latif, E.S., Mar, M.R., Mat Top, A.G., Mokhtar, N.M., 2009. Deleterious effects of nicotine on the ultrastructure of oocytes: role of gamma-tocotrienol. Med. Sci. Monit. 15 (12), BR378–BR383.

Rajikin, M.H., Syairah, S.M.M., Sharaniza, A.R., 2015. Effects of supplementation with annatto (*Bixa orellana*)-derived δ-tocotrienol on the nicotine induced reduction in body weight and 8-cell preimplantation embryonic development in mice. Int. J. Biol. Biomol., Agric., Food Biotechnol. Eng. 9 (7), 750–753.

Ramaswamy, K., Subash, C.G., Ji, H.K., Bharat, B.A., 2012. Tocotrienols fight cancer by targeting multiple cell signaling pathways. Genes Nutr. 7 (1), 43–52. Available from: https://doi.org/10.1007/s12263-011-0220-3.

Rebecca, J.C., John, C., James, H.S., Alan, H.D., Randall, D.A., 2011. Environmental and epigenetic effects upon preimplantation embryo metabolism and development. Tr. Endocr. Metab. 22 (10), 412–420. Available from: https://doi.org/10.1016/j.tem.2011.05.005.

Rimbach, G., Minihane, A.M., Majewicz, J., Fischer, A., Pallauf, J., Virgli, F., et al., 2002. Regulation of cell signalling by vitamin E. Proc. Nutr. Soc. 61, 415–425.

Rimbach, G., Jennifer, M., Patricia, H., John, K.L., 2010. Gene-regulatory activity of α-tocopherol. Molecules 15, 1746–1761. Available from: https://doi.org/10.3390/molecules15031746.

Saidatul, A.K., Nasibah, A., Esa, N.Y., Nuraliza, A.S., 2014. Time-dependant effect of tocotrienol supplementation on the quality of aging mouse embryo. Malays. J. Microsc. 10, 6–12.

Saleh, H., Omar, E., Froemming, G., Said, R., 2014. Tocotrienol rich fraction supplementation confers protection on the ovary from cyclophasphamide induced apoptosis. Asian Pac. J. Trop. Dis. 4 (3), 234. Available from: https://doi.org/10.1016/S2222-1808(14)60532-6.

Saleh, H., Omar, E., Froemming, G., Said, R., 2015. Tocotrienol preserves ovarian function in cyclophosphamide therapy. Hum. Exp. Toxicol. 34 (10), 946–952. Available from: https://doi.org/10.1177/0960327114564793.

Schaffer, S., Muller, W.E., Eckert, G.P., 2005. Tocotrienols: constitutional effects in aging and disease. J. Nutr. 135 (2), 151–154.

Sen, C.K., Khanna, S., Roy, S., 2004. Tocotrienol: the natural vitamin E to defend the nervous system? Ann. N. Y. Acad. Sci. 1031, 127–142.

Serbinova, E.A., Packer, L., 1994. Antioxidant properties of alpha-tocopherol and alpha-tocotrienol. Methods Enzymol. 234, 354–366.

Serbinova, E.A., Kagan, V., Han, D., Packer, L., 1991. Free radical recycling and intramembrane mobility in the antioxidant properties of alpha-tocopherol and alpha-tocotrienol. Free Radic. Biol. Med. 10 (5), 263–275.

Sheppard, A.J., Pennington, J.A.T., Weihrauch, J.L., 1993. Analysis and distribution of vitamin E in vegetable oils and foods. In: Packer, L., Fuchs, J. (Eds.), Vitamin E in Health and Disease. Marcel Dekker, New York, pp. 9–31.

Sundram, K., Khor, H.T., Ong, A.S., Pathmanathan, R., 1989. Effect of dietary palm oils on mammary carcinogenesis in female rats induced by 7, 12-dimethylbenz(a)anthracene. Cancer Res. 49 (6), 1447–1451.

Suzuki, Y.J., Tsuchiya, M., Wassall, S.R., Choo, Y.M., Govil, G., Kagan, V.E., et al., 1993. Structural and dynamic membrane properties of alpha-tocopherol and alpha-tocotrienol: implication to the molecular mechanism of their antioxidant potency. Biochemistry 32 (40), 10692–10699.

Syairah, S.M.M., Rajikin, M.H., Sharaniza, A.-R., Nor-Ashikin, M.N.K., Anne, T., Barrie, T., 2014. Annatto (*Bixa orellana*) derived δ-tocotrienol supplementation suppresses *PIK3CA* oncogene expression in 2- and 4-cell embryos of nicotine-induced mice. Anticancer Res. 34, 6064.

Syairah, S.M.M., Rajikin, M.H., Sharaniza, A.-R., 2015. Supplementation of annatto (*Bixa orellana*)-derived δ-tocotrienol produced high number of morula through increased expression of 3-phosphoinositide dependent protein kinase-1 (PDK1) in mice. Int. J. Biol. Biomol. Agric. Food Biotechnol. Eng. 9 (7), 741−745.

Syairah, S.M.M., Rajikin, M.H., Sharaniza, A.R., Nor-Ashikin, M.N.K., Kamsani, Y.S., 2016. Chromosomal status in murine preimplantation 2-cell embryos following annatto (*Bixa orellana*)-derived pure delta-tocotrienol supplementation in normal and nicotine-treated mice. World Appl. Sci. J. 34 (12), 1855−1859. Available from: https://doi.org/10.5829/idosi.wasj.1855.1859.

Syairah, S.M.M., Rajikin, M.H., Sharaniza, A.R., Nor-Ashikin, M.N.K., 2019. Annatto (*Bixa orellana*) δ-TCT supplementation protection against embryonic malformations through alterations in PI3K/Akt-Cyclin D1 pathway. Biomolecules 9 (1), 1−15. Available from: https://doi.org/10.3390/biom9010019.

Sylvester, P.W., Theriault, A., 2003. Role of tocotrienols in the prevention of cardiovascular disease and breast cancer. Curr. Top. Nutraceut. Res. 1 (2), 121−136.

Tappel, A.L., 1962. Vitamin E as the biological lipid antioxidant. Vitam. Horm. 20, 493−510.

The structure of vitamin E and related compounds, 2016. Available from: <http://www.vita-dose.com/structure-of-vitamin-e.html>, November 23.

Thuhairah, A.R., Noor, F.H., Nurmazni, Z., Suhaila, M., Kaslina, N.K., Hapizah, N., 2016. Atheroprotective effects of pure tocotrienol supplementation in the treatment of rabbits with experimentally induced early and established atherosclerosis. Food Nutr. Res. 60. Available from: https://doi.org/10.3402/fnr.v60.31525.

Traber, M.G., Podda, M., Weber, C., Thiele, J., Rallis, M., Packer, L., 1997. Diet derived topically applied tocotrienols accumulate in skin and protect the tissue against UV light-induced oxidative stress. Asia Pacific J. Clin. Nutr. 6, 63−67.

Traber, M.G., Rallis, M., Podda, M., Weber, C., Maibach, H.I., Packer, L., 1998. Penetration and distribution of alpha-tocopherol, alpha- or gamma-tocotrienols applied individually onto murine skin. Lipids 33 (1), 87−91.

Umesiobi, D.O., 2012. The effect of vitamin E supplementation on the libido and reproductive capacity of large white boars. S. Afr. J. Anim. Sci. 42 (5), 559−563.

Wang, H., Dev, S.K., 2006. Roadmap to embryo implantation: clues from mouse models. Nat. Rev. Genet. 7, 185−199. Available from: https://doi.org/10.1038/nrg1808.

Weber, C., Podda, M., Rallis, M., Thiele, J.J., Traber, M.G., Packer, L., 1997. Efficacy of topically applied tocopherols and tocotrienols in protection of murine skin from oxidative damage induced by UV-irradiation. Free Radic. Biol. Med. 22 (5), 761−769.

CHAPTER 27

Vitamins in chronic kidney disease

Magdalena Jankowska
Department of Nephrology, Transplantology and Internal Medicine, Medical University of Gdansk, Gdansk, Poland

Contents

Molecular Nutrition
DOI: https://doi.org/10.1016/B978-0-12-811907-5.00023-3

Abbreviations

AA	ascorbic acid
CKD	chronic kidney disease
DOPPS	Dialysis Outcomes and Practice Patterns Study
EGR	erythrocyte glutathione reductase
ESKD	end-stage kidney disease
HD	hemodialysis
HDF	hemodiafiltration
KDIGO	Kidney Disease: Improving Global Outcomes
MIA	malnutrition–inflammation–atherosclerosis syndrome
MGP	matrix γ-carboxyglutamic acid protein
PD	peritoneal dialysis
PEW	protein–energy wasting
PLP	pyridoxal phosphate
PTH	parathyroid hormone
RCT	randomized controlled trial
RRT	renal replacement therapy
RBP	retinol-binding protein
RTx	renal transplantation

27.1 Introduction

27.1.1 Chronic kidney disease

Chronic kidney disease (CKD) is defined as a decrease of the estimated glomerular filtration rate below 60 mL/min/m^2 or (and) increase of the urinary albumin/creatinine ratio above 30 mg/g, or any kind of structural kidney impairment that lasts for more than 3 months (Kidney Disease: Improving Global Outcomes (KDIGO) CKD Work Group 2013). The progressive character of the disease is reflected by its consecutive stages, which are described in detail in Table 27.1.

The prevalence of CKD affects 10%–15% of the population and is rising worldwide, especially in elderly individuals and in low-income countries (Levin et al., 2017). The most severe and devastating consequence of progressing CKD is end-stage kidney disease (ESKD). ESKD is kidney failure that is fatal unless treated with renal replacement therapy (RRT). There are three methods of RRT: hemodialysis (HD), peritoneal dialysis (PD), and renal transplantation (RTx) (Table 27.2).

Clinically, CKD can have a plethora of different presentations depending on the underlying kidney disease, comorbidities, the stage of CKD, and the method of treatment. Nevertheless, most clinical presentations of CKD are nonspecific and could be indistinguishable from other chronic conditions. Interestingly, the same symptomatology (Table 27.3) could be

Table 27.1 Stages of chronic kidney disease (CKD) according to Kidney Disease Improving Global Outcomes (KDIGO).

CKD stages	GFR category (G)Albuminuria category (A)	Description/definition
1	G1	Normal/highGFR >90 mL/min/1.73 m^2
2	G2	Mildly decreasedGFR = 60–89 mL/min/1.73 m^2
3	G3a	Mildly to moderately decreasedGFR = 45–59 mL/min/1.73 m^2
	G3b	Moderately to severely decreasedGFR = 30–44 mL/min/1.73 m^2
4	G4	Severely decreasedGFR = 15–29 mL/min/1.73 m^2
5	G5	Kidney failureGFR < 15 mL/min/1.73 m^2
	A1	Normal/mildly increased < 30 mg/g or <3 mg/mmol
	A2	Moderately increased30–300 mg/g or 3 to 300 mg/mmol
	A3	Severely increased > 300 mg/g or >30 mg/mmol

KDIGO established definitions that describe varying degrees of CKD and taking into account kidney function and persistent albuminuria. This terminology was accepted worldwide and is commonly used as a measure of the severity of the disease.

ascribed to both CKD and vitamin inadequacy. Hence, the suboptimal vitamin status can be easily misdiagnosed and overlooked.

27.1.2 Malnutrition and chronic kidney disease

Malnutrition is a common feature of the uremic phenotype and is a highly prevalent complication of CKD, especially in its advanced stages (CKD stage 4 and 5). In ESKD loss of protein and energy stores is commonly accompanied by inflammation and multiple metabolic derangements, including atherosclerosis, oxidative stress, endothelial dysfunction, and vascular calcification, that create a separate clinical entity, named malnutrition–inflammation–atherosclerosis syndrome (MIA) (Stenvinkel et al., 1999). The specific pathways by which the association between MIA and CKD might be mediated are still not well-known. Nonetheless, the overall effect is a persistence of the self-enhanced inflammatory cascade, that exacerbates the wasting and contributes to adverse outcomes. It is recommended to call the malnutrition component of this syndrome with a term of protein–energy wasting (PEW) (Fouque et al., 2008). PEW is diagnosed based on the presence of the biochemical (low

Table 27.2 Key facts of the renal replacement therapy (RRT).

• Patients in the most advanced stage of chronic kidney disease, called end-stage kidney disease, need a therapy substituting for kidney function to survive. There are several methods of such a treatment, and they are called RRT.
• RRT may take a form of dialysis or kidney transplantation.
• There are two modalities of dialysis: hemodialysis (HD) and peritoneal dialysis (PD).
• HD is a modality of treatment in which the patient's blood is purified extracorporeally with the use of a machine pumping the blood through a filter consisting of capillaries of a semipermeable membrane that are rinsed by disposable dialysis fluid. HD procedure is intermittent and is performed for a total of 12–15 h a week divided into three sessions.
• According to the type of the dialyzer membrane, filters are classified as low-flux (low water permeability) and high-flux (increased water permeability) and differ in the capability of removal of middle-sized uremic toxins.
• Hemodiafiltration (HDF) is a modality of treatment based on conventional HD with the addition of convection clearance, which is gained from the removal of a substantial amount of plasma water and substituting it with a solution free from toxins and waste products.
• PD is an intracorporeal modality of RRT in which a semipermeable membrane is the own peritoneal membrane of the patient. In this method, disposable dialysis fluid is placed inside a patient's peritoneal cavity and removed after some time of dwelling. This method is performed daily and in most cases continuously.
• Kidney transplantation is a surgical procedure in which a human kidney is placed in the body of a patient. The source of the organ can be from a living donor or a deceased donor. After the transplantation, the recipient needs to be treated with immunosuppressive agents in order to prevent organ rejection. Kidney transplantation is the best method of RRT.

albumin, prealbumin, or cholesterol), anthropometric, and dietary indices (Fouque et al., 2008).

27.1.3 Micronutrient malnutrition in chronic kidney disease

It should be noted that the term of PEW, albeit aptly describing the specificities of malnutrition in CKD, is not entirely satisfactory. It refers to depletion of protein and energy reserves, whereas CKD and ESKD predispose to also other nutritional derangements, including deficiencies of vitamins (Lodebo et al., 2018).

Although malnutrition is an acknowledged feature of CKD, alterations in micronutrients are much less recognized. Even if CKD distinctly predisposes to disorders of vitamins, the evidence for the prevalence and

Table 27.3 Symptoms of altered vitamin status in chronic kidney disease (CKD).

Premature aging
Increased mortality
Enhanced atherosclerosis
Inflammation
Impaired immune response
Oxidative stress
Bone and mineral disorder
Anemia
Polyneuropathy
Encephalopathy
Weakness and fragility
Muscle cramps
Insomnia
Depression

Symptoms and consequences of vitamin insufficiency are commonly similar to those of CKD and may be clinically indistinguishable. The clinical diagnosis of altered vitamin status is challenging.

consequences of suboptimal micronutrient levels remain scarce (Jankowska et al., 2017b). The same mechanisms are responsible for malnutrition and inadequate micronutrient status in CKD. A multitude of contributors to vitamin inadequacy in CKD are depicted in Fig. 27.1. Although altered vitamin status is mostly associated with deficiencies, it needs to be mentioned that in individuals with compromised renal function there is also a potential for an accumulation of micronutrients, and/or their metabolites (Jankowska et al., 2017c,d; Moradi and Said, 2016).

27.2 Contributors to altered vitamin status in chronic kidney disease

27.2.1 Dietary intake

Decreased dietary intake of nutrients is observed already in stage 3 of CKD (Kopple et al., 2000). The accumulation of nephrogenic toxins, endocrine disorders, and gastrointestinal complications that occur as a consequence of declining GFR, lead to anorexia, nausea, and impaired ingestion. Also well-intended dietary counseling and nutritional restrictions contribute to decreased dietary intake. Modification of diet is an important and widely recognized element of CKD management (Kalantar-Zadeh et al., 2015). However, dietary restrictions, especially of potassium, critically affect water-soluble vitamins intake, mostly folic acid and vitamin

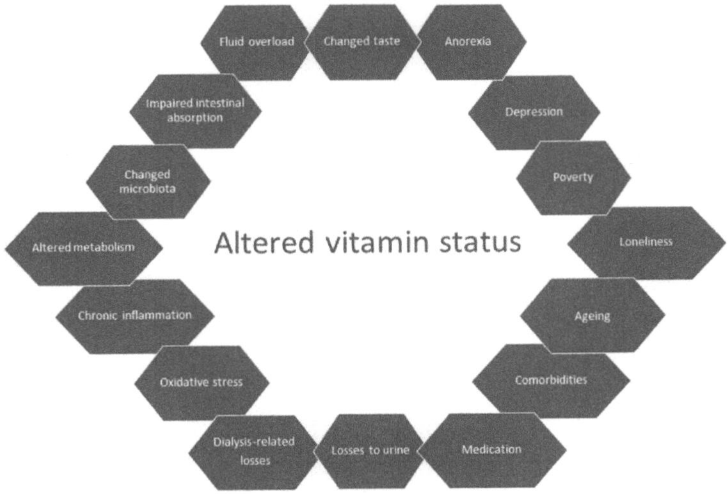

Figure 27.1 Contributors to altered vitamin status in chronic kidney disease. Causes of suboptimal vitamin status are multifactorial and frequently overlapping in chronic kidney disease. They include contributors to decreased dietary intake, specificities of renal replacement therapy, gastrointestinal complications, medication, comorbidities, and a range of psychosocial and demographic issues.

C (Jankowska et al., 2016; Kalantar-Zadeh et al., 2002). Vitamin intake is strongly associated with the energy content of the diet and most plausibly depends on the overall dietary pattern. This points to important psychosocial problems, such as impoverishment, solitude, depression, and physical inability to prepare or buy meals, that are typically found in CKD patients. Such contributors are potentially modifiable and overcoming them accompanied by meticulous and professional dietary counseling may play a pivotal role in the prevention of malnutrition CKD.

Low intake of vitamins is present in advanced CKD irrespective of the method of treatment. Even successful RTx does not warrant nutritional adequacy. However, the greatest risk of deficient vitamin intake is observed repeatedly in patients treated with HD (Bossola et al., 2014; Kalantar-Zadeh et al., 2002), while in general the diet of RTx individuals is the most satisfactory (Jankowska et al., 2016 Rho et al., 2013). Other factors that may influence vitamin intake in CKD include patients' nutritional and inflammatory status, dialysis adequacy, and the preservation of residual renal function (Martín-del-Campo et al., 2012; Wang et al., 2002).

27.2.2 Low sunlight exposure

All the above mentioned psychosocial concerns are also responsible for the decreased physical activity and time spent outdoors. CKD, and especially RTx, patients are advised to avoid sunlight to prevent skin cancer and drug photosensitization. As a consequence, the low sunlight exposure contributes additionally to low vitamin D supplies.

27.2.3 Impaired absorption

Several factors ascribed to CKD may importantly influence vitamin absorption. First, most water-soluble vitamins are absorbed from the intestine in a specific carrier-mediated process and CKD may influence the expression of vitamin-specific carriers (Bukhari et al., 2011). It has been shown that CKD is associated with the downregulation of folate and thiamin transporters in several tissues, including intestine (Bukhari et al., 2011). Also reduced intestinal uptake of biotin, riboflavin, and pyridoxine have been shown in an animal model of CKD (Barbari et al., 1989; Said et al., 1992; Vaziri et al., 1985).

Second, CKD profoundly alters intestinal microbial flora (Vaziri et al., 2016). The normal flora is a source of vitamin K, vitamin B12, and small amounts of other group B vitamins (such as biotin, folates, nicotinic acid, pantothenic acid, pyridoxine, riboflavin, and thiamine) (LeBlanc et al., 2013). It seems plausible that the synthesis of those vitamins is affected by the uremic milieu. What is more, there are grounds to hypothesize that an altered gut microbiome is capable of producing vitamin antimetabolites that are consecutively absorbed but are not effectively removed due to decreased kidney clearance. For example, such a compound is oxythiamine (4-hydroxythiamine), an antimetabolite of vitamin B1, leading to its functional deficiency (Moradi and Said, 2016).

Third, a fluid overload, frequently found in CKD patients, results in vascular congestion and increased permeability of gastrointestinal tract (Terpstra et al., 2016). Loss of absorptive surface, exudation from intestinal mucosa, and changes in gastrointestinal transit are mechanisms that may be at play in such a setting.

27.2.4 Urinary losses

Kidney pathology results in excessive urinary losses of water-soluble vitamins. Vitamins are freely filtered into the glomerular filtrate and may be lost in a case of tubular dysfunction or decreased activity of protein carriers (Handelman and Levin, 2011). The presence of proteinuria increases losses of fat-soluble vitamins, as they are transported in a protein-bound manner. Nephrotic range proteinuria may increase the urinary excretion of 25(OH)D by 10- to even 100-fold as compared to physiological urinary losses (Sato, 1982).

Further, administration of loop diuretics, widely used in CKD, is yet another enhancer of urinary vitamin losses. Thiamine, vitamin C, and vitamin B6 have been lost in this way, and the excretion of most vitamins depends on urinary flow rate (Mydlík et al., 1999; Suter and Vetter, 2000).

27.2.5 Medication

Several known drug–vitamin interactions may occur during treatment of renal diseases with commonly used drugs (e.g., trimethoprim or methotrexate). Still, CKD predisposes to several less obvious or subtle interferences. The most apparent example is the administration of erythropoiesis stimulating agents. Prolonged erythropoiesis stimulation may easily deplete stores of those vitamins that are used in a synthesis of heme, or iron metabolism (folate, vitamin B6, vitamin B12, and vitamin C). Another specific interaction is the potential of phosphate binders to limit the bioavailability of vitamin K (Neradova et al., 2017).

Immunosuppressive therapy, implemented after RTx, could in turn, influence the status of vitamin B6, involved in processes of immunological response and inflammation (Jankowska et al., 2013, 2014).

27.2.6 Dialysis-related losses

Molecular weight and protein binding determine dialysis-related losses of vitamins. Accordingly, vitamins that are not protein bound are most susceptible to an intradialytic removal.

The modality of treatment is yet another contributor to vitamin losses. In general, fat-soluble vitamins are not lost through the filter membrane in HD, whereas losses were reported in PD patients. HD patients may lose a substantial amount of water-soluble vitamins during a single dialysis session, while PD patients seem to have moderate losses unless peritonitis is present (Boeschoten et al., 1988; Jankowska et al., 2017a).

High-flux HD has little impact on clearances of small molecular weight vitamins, but may influence the middle molecules, that is, vitamin

B12 (Chandna et al., 1997; Heinz et al., 2008; Jankowska et al., 2017c). Middle molecules, that are not lost during conventional HD, can be lost during a procedure of hemodiafiltration (HDF) that is used as a modality of RRT. However, switching to HDF did not adversely affect vitamin B12 status in a single study with a 12-month follow-up period (Cross and Davenport, 2011).

27.2.7 Altered metabolism

Interestingly associations between measures of vitamin status and their most apparent contributors, intake or dialysis-related losses, are rather weak. It points to a role of other mechanisms of impaired vitamin status in CKD. One of them seems to be altered metabolism of vitamins in the uremic milieu. Indeed, the most obvious example is the metabolism of vitamin D. Kidneys play the central role in the activation of vitamin D, by its key and final step, 1-alpha-hydroxylation (Fraser and Kodicek, 1970). As a consequence, circulating levels of 1,25(OH)2D decline with the progression of CKD.

There is also some evidence that the accumulation of vitamin metabolites to potentially harmful concentrations may occur. For example, metabolites of nicotinamide, *N*-methyl-2-pyridone-5-carboxamide and *N*-methyl-4-pyridone-5-carboxamide, that are physiologically removed with urine, accumulate in CKD and constitute novel uremic toxins (Rutkowski et al., 2012). A metabolite of pyridoxine, 4-pyridoxic acid, increases with a decrease of GFR in a manner similar to the retention of other small molecular weight compounds and interferes with the synthesis of a biologically active form of vitamin B6 (Coburn et al., 2002). It is also conceivable, albeit not proven yet, that severe hyperphosphatemia, commonly found in CKD, may interfere with important steps in the transport and activation of numerous vitamins that are dependent on their phosphorylation and dephosphorylation.

Finally, functional vitamin deficiency is characteristically found in ESKD. Red blood cell transketolase activity is importantly decreased in ESKD patients, but is partially reversed after HD session or alleviated by an administration of high doses of thiamine (Zhang et al., 2016). This phenomenon has been recently explained by the GFR-dependent accumulation of a competitive inhibitor of transketolase, oxythiamine (Zhang et al., 2016). Similar functional abnormalities have also been known for other molecules, like vitamin E. As early as at CKD stage 3, the accumulation of the vitamin E metabolite, carboxyethyl hydroxychromans, is observed and may adversely influence vitamin E functional status (Galli et al., 2004). These observations allow for a hypothesis that functional vitamin deficiency is a characteristic feature of CKD.

27.3 Water-soluble vitamins

27.3.1 Vitamin B1 (thiamine)

Dietary intakes of vitamin B1 are low, especially in patients treated with HD. Thiamine has the shortest time for depletion of its body stores in humans, and several series of cases of Wernicke's encephalopathy, a vitamin B1 avitaminosis, were reported in dialysis patients. Wernicke's encephalopathy is a life-threatening and often misdiagnosed condition, but its occurrence seems generally rare. Thiamine plasma levels were mostly normal or increased in the CKD population. On the other hand, plasma concentration is not the best indicator of thiamine adequacy, and erythrocyte transketolase activity, a measure of thiamine functional status, was increased in CKD stage 4 and 5 (Frank et al., 2000).

Dialysis therapy has limited influence on thiamine status. Peritoneal losses are small and HD clearance ranges from 13 to 40 mL/min. A single HD procedure decreases levels of vitamin B1 in blood, but it does not affect overall thiamine status (Jankowska et al., 2017c).

27.3.2 Vitamin B2 (riboflavin)

A low protein diet, frequently prescribed in stages 3–5 of CKD, may impose a risk of riboflavin deficiency. Indeed, the percentage of individuals with increased α-erythrocyte glutathione reductase (EGR) index, which is a measure of functional deficiency of vitamin B2, rose with a reduction of dietary protein intake. HD losses are small, about 6%–7% per procedure, with a clearance of 27–52 mL/min. Although the peritoneal losses may be high compared to physiological urinary excretion (Boeschoten et al., 1988), most studies report the adequate status of this vitamin in ESKD. Supplementation with doubled RDA leads to a decreased EGR index suggesting an excessive intake (Mydlík et al., 1985). Due to the photosensitizing properties of riboflavin, high doses of this vitamin should be avoided.

27.3.3 Vitamin B3 (niacin, nicotinic acid)

There is no evidence that CKD patients are vitamin B3-deficient, although the dietary intake of this compound could be lower than recommended (Jankowska et al., 2016). Most probably, niacin is not lost during the dialysis procedure, even if small amounts of it are found in the peritoneal effluent. The niacin concentration in the whole blood and erythrocytes were within normal range in a group of HD patients followed for 12 months and not receiving supplementation (Ramirez et al., 1986). Interestingly, high doses of niacin were administered to ESKD patients to lower hyperphosphatemia and were effective and regarded safe (Berns, 2008; Musso et al., 2008; Young et al., 2009). Also there seems to be no need for a dose adjustment of an extended release formulation of nicotinic acid in CKD patients (Reiche et al., 2011).

27.3.4 Vitamin B5 (pantothenic acid)

The data on this vitamin are scarce, and there is no evidence of its deficiency in CKD. Pantothenic acid is lost with HD with a clearance of 30 mL/min, while peritoneal losses are unknown.

27.3.5 Vitamin B6 (pyridoxine)

There is no clear consensus regarding the status of vitamin B6 in CKD. The reports are conflicting, and their results range from severe deficiency to normal and even increased levels. This may result from different measures used to assess vitamin B6 status, from the multitude of biological forms of this vitamin present in human tissues and the functional deficiency of this vitamin typical for CKD. A biologically active form of the vitamin, pyridoxal phosphate (PLP), is albumin-bound and despite this, quite easily lost in HD with a clearance from 54 to 173 mL/min (Chazot et al., 2016). Plasma PLP drops after single HD of 29%–37% (Heinz et al., 2008), while peritoneal losses are low.

Plausibly the best measure of vitamin B6 functional status is EGTP index, which is increased compared to healthy individuals in virtually all CKD stages. Increased EGTP index is indicative of PLP deficiency and normalizes after administration of 10 mg of pyridoxine HCl daily.

27.3.6 Biotin (vitamin B7)

In a few studies measuring biotin in CKD patients no deficiency of this vitamin was found. On the contrary, levels of biotin were higher than in the general population or healthy individuals and increased with dialysis vintage and loss of residual renal function (Descombes et al., 1993; Livaniou et al., 1987; Oguma et al., 2012). The clinical consequences of these findings are unknown. Surprisingly, despite an apparent excess of this vitamin in ESKD, the supplementation with biotin had some beneficial effect on peripheral neuropathy and muscle cramps in HD patients (Oguma et al., 2012).

27.3.7 Folate (vitamin B9)

Dietary restrictions in rich potassium food, a molecular weight of 441 Da and a low ability for protein binding, make folate prone to be deficient in CKD patients. However, counterintuitively, both plasma and erythrocyte levels of this compound proved to be normal in CKD and even increased after initiation of RRT. Dialysis modality seems to influence folate status. Serum folate reduction after single HD treatment is above 30%, while RBC folate does not change (Heinz et al., 2008). PD losses are negligible. As a consequence, PD patients have better folate status and respond with very elevated folate values after supplementation. Folate administration in otherwise not deficient CKD individuals may have a homocysteine-lowering effect (De Vecchi et al., 2001), but disappointing results of the Homocysteine (HOST) study (Jamison et al., 2007) and Folic Acid for Vascular Outcome Reduction in Transplantation (FAVORIT) Trial (Bostom et al., 2011) discouraged the pursuit of this therapeutic approach.

27.3.8 Vitamin B12 (cobalamin)

Vitamin B12 has a unique characteristic as compared to other water-soluble vitamins. Due to its molecular weight of 1355 Da, it fulfills the definition of a middle molecule, and thus it is virtually not lost to the dialysate. Physiologically it is excreted through bile (Shinton, 1972). It explains the negligible impact of CKD on the incidence of B12 deficiency. High-flux HD, but astonishingly, not HDF, may remove vitamin B12 more effectively, with a clearance of 9 mL/min (Chandna et al., 1997).

27.3.9 Hyperhomocysteinemia

Hyperhomocysteinemia is commonly found in CKD patients and is responsible for increased oxidative stress and cardiovascular mortality in this population. Vitamins B6, B9, and B12 are involved in homocysteine metabolism. Homocysteine is metabolized through two pathways: remethylation to methionine, or transsulfuration to cystathionine and then to cysteine. Folate and vitamin B12 are involved in the first and the biologically active form of vitamin B6 in the second pathway. Numerous studies investigated associations between B vitamin status and homocysteine, as well as the influence of vitamin supplementation on homocysteine levels in CKD patients, giving conflicting results. However, two large RCTs showed that vitamin supplementation lowers homocysteine (Heinz et al., 2010; Jamison et al., 2007) but at the same time has no impact on important clinical outcomes, including mortality.

27.3.10 Vitamin C (ascorbic acid)

Vitamin C is a vitamin most efficiently cleared during the dialysis procedure. It is a consequence of its low molecular weight (176 DA) and not being protein bound. A median ascorbic acid (AA) dialyzer clearance is 212 mL/min (Wang et al., 1999), which may result in losses as high as 320 mg per procedure (Sirover et al., 2015). In PD the vitamin C level in dialysis effluent was estimated at 60% of the concentration in blood and average daily losses in nonsupplemented continuous PD patients were about 50 mg daily (Shah et al., 1991).

The common concern regarding vitamin C supplementation in ESKD patients is a risk of oxalosis. Oxalate is a metabolite of AA that used to be poorly removed by the dialysis procedure and thus accumulate. Therefore high doses of vitamin C supplements were not recommended. However, contemporary dialysis technique seems to be thoroughly efficient in clearing oxalate, and cases of oxalosis have not been reported recently. Also the relatively high intravenous doses of AA used in the treatment of anemia were well-tolerated in several reports.

Low vitamin C levels predict adverse cardiovascular outcomes in HD patients and this supports routine AA supplementation, especially when dietary intakes are low and dialysis-related loses are substantial.

27.4 Fat-soluble vitamins

27.4.1 Vitamin A

Plasma levels of vitamin A increase in CKD patients. This is related to the accumulation of retinol-binding protein 4 (RBP-4), a protein physiologically metabolized in kidney and regulating a release of retinol from liver stores. Interestingly, higher retinol and RBP plasma levels are associated with lower mortality in HD patients, while lower quartiles of, otherwise still high, concentrations are related to the increased risk of sudden death and overall mortality. This relation is believed to be a simple surrogate of a well-known association between mortality and nutritional status and not a direct biological function of retinol (Bataille et al., 2017). Accordingly, vitamin A supplements are not recommended in CKD patients.

27.4.2 Vitamin D

Low 1,25(OH)D is an expected finding, taking into account that 1-αhydroxylase activity is dependent on fibroblast growth factor that increases in CKD. However, other forms of vitamin D are also deficient in CKD, especially in its later stages and during RRT (Wolf et al., 2007). It points to yet another mechanism of decreased 1,25(OH)D, which is a reduced substrate for hydroxylation. 25(OH)D deficiency can be found in all stages of CKD, although it is most prevalent in dialysis patients. PD patients are at higher risk than those on HD, but the suboptimal status is universal.

Vitamin D is the most extensively studied micronutrient in CKD and there is mounting evidence on its influence on important outcomes, including cardiovascular disease and mortality. These effects are plausibly attained in several mechanisms including the downregulation of the renin–angiotensin–aldosterone system, modulation of the inflammatory response, anticoagulant activity, decreasing insulin resistance, and slowing down atherosclerosis and vascular calcification (Gluba-Brzózka et al., 2018). Numerous studies demonstrated the inverse association between 25 (OH)D levels and parathyroid hormone (PTH), as well as a decline of PTH as a result of supplementation of 25(OH)D, its analogs, or calcitriol.

The recent Kidney Disease Improving Global Outcomes (KDIGO) guidelines recommend screening for low serum 25(OH)D and supplementing it on an individualized basis. There is no consensus regarding the dose and form of the supplement. Supplements and analogs of vitamin D are regarded as safe. Nevertheless, caution is advocated while administering supraphysiological doses because of adverse effects including hypercalcemia and hyperphosphatemia.

27.4.3 Vitamin E

Studies assessing α-tocopherol in ESKD patients gave equivocal results, showing low, normal or even increased levels. It is possible that plasma levels of vitamin E do not reflect its functional status, especially that the accumulation of its competing metabolites is observed in parallel to the decrease of GFR. Theoretically, an increase of oxidative stress in CKD should increase the need for vitamin E, known for its antioxidant properties.

Although the dietary intakes of this agent were reduced (Galli et al., 2004), the supplementation of vitamin E in the Heart Outcomes Prevention Evaluation (HOPE) trial did not show any beneficial outcomes. Further, the extension of the trial under the acronym HOPE-TOO, raised important safety concerns, as an increased risk of heart failure was found in the arm receiving vitamin E supplementation. On the other hand, the SPACE study, a multicenter, randomized, prospective trial in HD patients with preexisting cardiovascular disease, reported that oral vitamin E supplementation (800 IU/day) significantly reduced the primary composite variable consisting of myocardial infarction (fatal and nonfatal), ischemic stroke, peripheral vascular disease (excluding the arteriovenous fistula), and unstable angina (Boaz et al., 2000). Notably, there was no difference in total and cardiovascular mortality between study arms.

A specific measure to overcome oxidative stress ensuing HD procedure is the use of dialyzers with vitamin E-coated membranes. Indeed, many in vivo and in vitro studies have shown antioxidative effects of such an approach, both in human and animal models. Also an increase in vitamin E levels in erythrocytes and the amelioration of anemia management were reported (Huang et al., 2015). Nevertheless, this way of treatment is not routinely recommended unless studies measuring mortality outcomes are conducted.

27.4.4 Vitamin K

There is mounting evidence that CKD patients suffer from vitamin K deficiency (Holden et al., 2010; Schurgers, 2013). The deficiency is present in CKD stages 3–5, is more pronounced in dialysis patients, and seems to be only partially reversed by kidney transplantation (Holden et al., 2010; Jansz et al., 2018). These facts may be of the utmost importance, as the main cause of death in CKD patients is cardiovascular disease strongly associated with vascular calcification. Vascular calcification, in turn, is actively inhibited by vitamin-K-dependent matrix γ-carboxyglutamic acid protein (MGP) and uremia impairs carboxylation of MGP. In such a setting, attempts at alleviating vascular calcification with the use of vitamin K supplementation should not come as a surprise. However, although some promising outcomes have been achieved in an animal model of CKD and non-CKD humans, there is still a lack of sound, confirming data from RCTs. Also, the dose of the supplement is highly debatable, as low doses of vitamin K had been shown to promote vascular calcification, while high doses had an opposite effect (McCabe et al., 2013). Several trials of the benefits of vitamin K supplementation are ongoing currently, and hopefully, they will provide some answers for the most important questions.

27.5 Recommendations on supplementation

There is little high-quality data from the research on vitamins in the CKD field (Table 27.4). That explains not only the scarcity and low grade of published recommendations on vitamin supplementation in CKD but also the fact that current recommendations have not been revised for at least 10 years (Cano et al., 2006; Fouque et al., 2007; Toigo et al., 2000). Obviously, the low level of evidence does not necessarily imply the weakness of the recommendation. Despite the unavailability of RCTs, there is a very clear clinical consensus that all water-soluble vitamins should be supplemented in doses at least equal to the recommended daily allowance. Interestingly, the clinical application of this recommendation is rather meager. The analysis of data from 308 representative dialysis facilities taking part in the Dialysis Outcomes and Practice Patterns Study (DOPPS I) showed that median administration of water-soluble supplements was 28.6% and varied substantially in different countries (Table 27.5) (Fissell et al., 2004). The study also reported a strong and significant association between lower mortality and regular use of water-soluble vitamins in HD patients (Fissell et al., 2004).

27.6 Conclusions

The status of most vitamins is suboptimal in the CKD population, and the vitamin inadequacy is further aggravated by the functional deficiency, typical for the uremic milieu. Although there is no sound evidence that vitamin supplements reduce mortality or major cardiovascular events in patients with CKD, it is possible that some health benefits, including improved cognition, alleviated sleep disorders, improved immunity, or reduced muscle cramps are present. Existing evidence suggests that vitamin supplements are overall safe in this group of patients. Although sufficiently powered RCTs are highly needed to assess the effects of vitamin therapy reliably and to expand our knowledge in this field, we should not

Table 27.4 Recommendations on daily dose of vitamin supplements in chronic kidney disease patients (compared to dietary reference intake, DRI, in general population).

Vitamin	DRI	CKD		HD		PD	
		EBPG-ERA/EDTA	ESPEN	EBPG-ERA/EDTA	ESPEN	EBPG-ERA/EDTA	ESPEN
A (μg retinol activity equivalents/24 h)	700–900	–	–	Not recommended	–	–	–
D (μg/24 h)	15	–	–	Individualized	–	–	–
E	15 mg	15 mg		400–800 IU	–	–	–
K (μg/24 h)	90–120[a]	–	–	Not recommended	–	–	–
B1 (mg/24 h)	1.1–1.2	–	–	1.1–1.2	–	1.1–1.2	–
B2 (mg/24 h)	1.1–1.3	–	–	1.1–1.3	–	1.1–1.3	–
B3 (mg/24 h)	14–16	–	–	14–16	–	16	–
B5 (mg/24 h)Pantothenic acid	5	–	–	5		5	–
B6 (mg/24 h)	1.3–1.7	–	5	10	10	10	10–20
B7 (μg/24 h)Biotin	30	–	–	30	–	30	–
B9 (μg/24 h)Folate	400	–	–	1000	1000	1000	1000
B12 (μg/24 h)	2.4	–	–	2.4	–	2.4	–
C (mg/24 h)	75–90	–	30–60	75–90	30–60	90	30–60

European Best Practice Guidelines of European Renal Association/European Dialysis and Transplantation Association (EBPG-ERA/EDTA) and European Society of Parenteral and Enteral Nutrition (ESPEN) approach in their documents on nutrition the issue of vitamin supplements. Due to the scarcity of evidence, the data are mostly based on expert opinions and have not been revised for several years.

[a]Adequate intake.

Table 27.5 Country variations in a number of patients supplemented with water-soluble vitamins according to DOPPS I (Fissell et al., 2004).

Country	Median percentage of patients administered water-soluble vitamins in a facility
Japan	0.0
Italy	1.9
United Kingdom	2.3
France	3.4
Germany	5.9
Spain	19.9
United States	65.5

The recommendation to supplement water-soluble vitamins in dialysis patients is generally widely accepted. However, countries and single dialysis facilities may vary substantially as regards the implementation of this recommendation, as showed in the analyzes of DOPPS I study. It is a consequence of variations in reimbursement policy, costs, adherence, and individual expert opinion because there is still no unequivocal evidence in favor of such an approach.

expect them in the near future. In this setting the most prudent approach is meticulous nutritional counseling and prescribing vitamin supplements according to existing guidelines.

References

Barbari, A., Vaziri, N.D., Benavides, I., Chen, Y.T., Said, H., Pahl, M.V., 1989. Intestinal transport of pyridoxine in experimental renal failure. Life Sci. 45, 663–669.

Bataille, S., Landrier, J.F., Astier, J., Cado, S., Sallette, J., Serveaux, M., et al., 2017. Plasma Retinol Concentration Is Mainly Driven by Transthyretin in Hemodialysis Patients. J Ren Nutr. 27, 395–401.

Berns, J.S., 2008. Niacin and related compounds for treating hyperphosphatemia in dialysis patients. Semin. Dial. 21, 203–205.

Boaz, M., Smetana, S., Weinstein, T., Matas, Z., Gafter, U., Iaina, A., et al., 2000. Secondary prevention with antioxidants of cardiovascular disease in endstage renal disease (SPACE): randomised placebo-controlled trial. Lancet 356, 1213–1218.

Boeschoten, E.W., Schrijver, J., Krediet, R.T., Schreurs, W.H., Arisz, L., 1988. Deficiencies of vitamins in CAPD patients: the effect of supplementation. Nephrol. Dial. Transpl. 3, 187–193.

Bossola, M., Di Stasio, E., Viola, A., Leo, A., Carlomagno, G., Monteburini, T., et al., 2014. Dietary intake of trace elements, minerals, and vitamins of patients on chronic hemodialysis. Int. Urol. Nephrol. 46, 809–815.

Bostom, A.G., Carpenter, M.A., Kusek, J.W., Levey, A.S., Hunsicker, L., Pfeffer, M.A., et al., 2011. Homocysteine-lowering and cardiovascular disease outcomes in kidney transplant recipients: primary results from the Folic Acid for Vascular Outcome Reduction in Transplantation trial. Circulation 123, 1763–1770.

Bukhari, F.J., Moradi, H., Gollapudi, P., Ju Kim, H., Vaziri, N.D., Said, H.M., 2011. Effect of chronic kidney disease on the expression of thiamin and folic acid transporters. Nephrol. Dial. Transpl. 26, 2137–2144.

Cano, N., Fiaccadori, E., Tesinsky, P., Toigo, G., Druml, W., Kuhlmann, M., et al., 2006. ESPEN Guidelines on Enteral Nutrition: adult renal failure. Clin. Nutr. 25, 295–310.

Chandna, S.M., Tattersall, J.E., Nevett, G., Tew, C.J., O'Sullivan, J., Greenwood, R.N., et al., 1997. Low serum vitamin B12 levels in chronic high-flux haemodialysis patients. Nephron 75, 259–263.

Chazot, C., Jean, G., Kopple, J.D., 2016. Can outcomes be improved in dialysis patients by optimizing trace mineral, micronutrient, and antioxidant status?: the impact of vitamins and their supplementation. Semin. Dial. 29, 39–48.

Coburn, S.P., Reynolds, R.D., Mahuren, J.D., Schaltenbrand, W.E., Wang, Y., Ericson, K.L., et al., 2002. Elevated plasma 4-pyridoxic acid in renal insufficiency. Am. J. Clin. Nutr. 75, 57–64.

Cross, J., Davenport, A., 2011. Does online hemodiafiltration lead to reduction in trace elements and vitamins? Hemodial. Int. 15, 509–514.

De Vecchi, A.F., Patrosso, C., Novembrino, C., Finazzi, S., Colucci, P., De Franceschi, M., et al., 2001. Folate supplementation in peritoneal dialysis patients with normal erythrocyte folate: effect on plasma homocysteine. Nephron 89, 297–302.

Descombes, E., Hanck, A.B., Fellay, G., 1993. Water soluble vitamins in chronic hemodialysis patients and need for supplementation. Kidney Int. 43, 1319–1328.

Fissell, R.B., Bragg-Gresham, J.L., Gillespie, B.W., Goodkin, D.A., Bommer, J., Saito, A., et al., 2004. International variation in vitamin prescription and association with mortality in the Dialysis Outcomes and Practice Patterns Study (DOPPS). Am. J. Kidney Dis. 44, 293–299.

Fouque, D., Vennegoor, M., ter Wee, P., Wanner, C., Basci, A., Canaud, B., et al., 2007. EBPG guideline on nutrition. Nephrol. Dial. Transpl. 22 (Suppl. 2), ii45–87.

Fouque, D., Kalantar-Zadeh, K., Kopple, J., Cano, N., Chauveau, P., Cuppari, L., et al., 2008. A proposed nomenclature and diagnostic criteria for protein-energy wasting in acute and chronic kidney disease. Kidney Int. 73, 391–398.

Frank, T., Czeche, K., Bitsch, R., Stein, G., 2000. Assessment of thiamin status in chronic renal failure patients, transplant recipients and hemodialysis patients receiving a multivitamin supplementation. Int. J. Vitam. Nutr. Res. 70, 159–166.

Fraser, D.R., Kodicek, E., 1970. Unique biosynthesis by kidney of a biological active vitamin D metabolite. Nature 228, 764–766.

Galli, F., Buoncristiani, U., Conte, C., Aisa, C., Floridi, A., 2004. Vitamin E in uremia and dialysis patients. Ann. N.Y. Acad. Sci. 1031, 348–351.

Gluba-Brzózka, A., Franczyk, B., Ciałkowska-Rysz, A., Olszewski, R., Rysz, J., 2018. Impact of vitamin D on the cardiovascular system in advanced chronic kidney disease (CKD) and dialysis patients. Nutrients 10, 709.

Handelman, G.J., Levin, N.W., 2011. Guidelines for vitamin supplements in chronic kidney disease patients: what is the evidence? J. Ren. Nutr. 21, 117–119.

Heinz, J., Domröse, U., Westphal, S., Luley, C., Neumann, K.H., Dierkes, J., 2008. Washout of water-soluble vitamins and of homocysteine during haemodialysis: effect of high-flux and low-flux dialyser membranes. Nephrology (Carlton) 13, 384–389.

Heinz, J., Kropf, S., Domröse, U., Westphal, S., Borucki, K., Luley, C., et al., 2010. B vitamins and the risk of total mortality and cardiovascular disease in end-stage renal disease: results of a randomized controlled trial. Circulation 121, 1432–1438.

Holden, R.M., Morton, A.R., Garland, J.S., Pavlov, A., Day, A.G., Booth, S.L., 2010. Vitamins K and D status in stages 3-5 chronic kidney disease. Clin. J. Am. Soc. Nephrol. 5, 590–597.

Huang, J., Yi, B., Li, A.M., Zhang, H., 2015. Effects of vitamin E-coated dialysis membranes on anemia, nutrition and dyslipidemia status in hemodialysis patients: a meta-analysis,. Ren. Fail. 37, 398–407.
Jamison, R.L., Hartigan, P., Kaufman, J.S., Goldfarb, D.S., Warren, S.R., Guarino, P.D., et al., 2007. Effect of homocysteine lowering on mortality and vascular disease in advanced chronic kidney disease and end-stage renal disease: a randomized controlled trial. JAMA 298, 1163–1170.
Jankowska, M., Marszałł, M., Dębska-Ślizień, A., Carrero, J.J., Lindholm, B., Czarnowski, W., et al., 2013. Vitamin B6 and the immunity in kidney transplant recipients. J. Ren. Nutr. 23, 57–64.
Jankowska, M., Trzonkowski, P., Dębska-Ślizień, A., Marszałł, M., Rutkowski, B., 2014. Vitamin B6 status, immune response and inflammation markers in kidney transplant recipients treated with polyclonal anti-thymocyte globulin. Transpl. Proc. 46, 2631–2635.
Jankowska, M., Szupryczyńska, N., Dębska-Ślizień, A., Borek, P., Kaczkan, M., Rutkowski, B., et al., 2016. Dietary intake of vitamins in different options of treatment in chronic kidney disease: is there a deficiency? Transpl. Proc. 48, 1427–1430.
Jankowska, M., Lichodziejewska-Niemierko, M., Małgorzewicz, S., Rutkowski, B., 2017a. Biologically active form of vitamin B1 in human peritoneal effluent. Adv. Clin. Exp. Med. 26, 1405–1410.
Jankowska, M., Lichodziejewska-Niemierko, M., Rutkowski, B., Dębska-Ślizień, A., Małgorzewicz, S., 2017b. Water soluble vitamins and peritoneal dialysis state of the art. Clin. Nutr. 36, 1483–1489.
Jankowska, M., Rudnicki-Velasquez, P., Storoniak, H., Rutkowski, P., Rutkowski, B., Krzymiński, K., et al., 2017c. Thiamine diphosphate status and dialysis-related losses in end-stage kidney disease patients treated with hemodialysis. Blood Purif. 44, 294–300.
Jankowska, M., Rutkowski, B., Dębska-Ślizień, A., 2017d. Vitamins and microelement bioavailability in different stages of chronic kidney disease. Nutrients 9, E 282.
Jansz, T.T., Neradova, A., van Ballegooijen, A.J., Verhaar, M.C., Vervloet, M.G., Schurgers, L.J., et al., 2018. The role of kidney transplantation and phosphate binder use in vitamin K status. PLoS One 13, e0203157.
Kalantar-Zadeh, K., Kopple, J.D., Deepak, S., Block, D., Block, G., 2002. Food intake characteristics of hemodialysis patients as obtained by food frequency questionnaire. J. Ren. Nutr. 12, 17–31.
Kalantar-Zadeh, K., Tortorici, A.R., Chen, J.L., Kamgar, M., Lau, W.L., Moradi, H., et al., 2015. Dietary restrictions in dialysis patients: is there anything left to eat? Semin. Dial. 28, 159–168.
Kidney Disease: Improving Global Outcomes (KDIGO) CKD Work Group, 2013. KDIGO clinical practice guideline for the evaluation and management of chronic kidney disease. Kidney Int. Suppl. 1–150.
Kopple, J.D., Greene, T., Chumlea, W.C., Hollinger, D., Maroni, B.J., Merrill, D., et al., 2000. Relationship between nutritional status and the glomerular filtration rate: results from the MDRD study. Kidney Int. 57, 1688–1703.
Levin, A., Tonelli, M., Bonventre, J., Coresh, J., Donner, J.A., Fogo, A.B., et al., 2017. Global kidney health 2017 and beyond: a roadmap for closing gaps in care, research, and policy. Lancet 390, 1888–1917.
LeBlanc, J.G., Milani, C., de Giori, G.S., Sesma, F., van Sinderen, D., Ventura, M., 2013. Bacteria as vitamin suppliers to their host: a gut microbiota perspective. Curr. Opin. Biotechnol. 24, 160–168.
Livaniou, E., Evangelatos, G.P., Ithakissios, D.S., Yatzidis, H., Koutsicos, D.C., 1987. Serum biotin levels in patients undergoing chronic hemodialysis. Nephron 46, 331–332.

Lodebo, B.T., Shah, A., Kopple, J.D., 2018. Is it important to prevent and treat protein-energy wasting in chronic kidney disease and chronic dialysis patients? J. Ren. Nutr. 8, 369–379.

Martín-del-Campo, F., Batis-Ruvalcaba, C., González-Espinoza, L., Rojas-Campos, E., Angel, J.R., Ruiz, N., et al., 2012. Dietary micronutrient intake in peritoneal dialysis patients: relationship with nutrition and inflammation status. Perit. Dial. Int. 32, 183–191.

McCabe, K.M., Booth, S.L., Fu, X., Shobeiri, N., Pang, J.J., Adams, M.A., et al., 2013. Dietary vitamin K and therapeutic warfarin alter the susceptibility to vascular calcification in experimental chronic kidney disease. Kidney Int. 83, 835–844.

Moradi, H., Said, H.M., 2016. Functional thiamine deficiency in end-stage renal disease: malnutrition despite ample nutrients. Kidney Int. 90, 252–254.

Musso, C.G., Reynaldi, M.J., Aparicio, C., Frydenlund, S., Imperiali, N., Algranati, L., 2008. Hyperphosphatemia and nicotinic acid in peritoneal dialysis patients. Int Urol Nephrol 40, 229–230.

Musso Mydlík, M., Derzsiová, K., Válek, A., Szabó, T., Dandár, V., Takác, M., 1985. Vitamins and continuous ambulatory peritoneal dialysis (CAPD). Int. Urol. Nephrol. 17, 281–286.

Mydlík, M., Derzsiová, K., Zemberová, E., 1999. Influence of water and sodium diuresis and furosemide on urinary excretion of vitamin B(6), oxalic acid and vitamin C in chronic renal failure. Miner Electrolyte Metab. 25, 352–356.

Neradova, A., Schumacher, S.P., Hubeek, I., Lux, P., Schurgers, L.J., Vervloet, M.G., 2017. Phosphate binders affect vitamin K concentration by undesired binding, an in vitro study. BMC Nephrol. 18, 149.

Oguma, S., Ando, I., Hirose, T., Totsune, K., Sekino, H., Sato, H., et al., 2012. Biotin ameliorates muscle cramps of hemodialysis patients: a prospective trial. Tohoku J. Exp. Med. 227, 217–223.

Ramirez, G., Chen, M., Boyce, H.W., Fuller, S.M., Butcher, D.E., Brueggemeyer, C.D., et al., 1986. The plasma and red cell vitamin B levels of chronic hemodialysis patients: a longitudinal study. Nephron 42, 41–46.

Reiche, I., Westphal, S., Martens-Lobenhoffer, J., Tröger, U., Luley, C., Bode-Böger, S. M., 2011. Pharmacokinetics and dose recommendations of Niaspan® in chronic kidney disease and dialysis patients. Nephrol. Dial. Transpl. 26, 276–282.

Rho, M.R., Lim, J.H., Park, J.H., Han, S.S., Kim, Y.S., Lee, Y.H., et al., 2013. Evaluation of nutrient intake in early post kidney transplant recipients. Clin. Nutr. Res. 2, 1–11.

Rutkowski, B., Rutkowski, P., Słomińska, E., Smolenski, R.T., Swierczyński, J., 2012. Cellular toxicity of nicotinamide metabolites. J. Ren. Nutr. 22, 95–97.

Sato, K.A.G., Lemann Jr, R.W.J., 1982. Urinary excretion of 25-hydroxyvitamin D in health and the nephrotic syndrome. J. Lab. Clin. Med. 325–330.

Said, H.M., Vaziri, N.D., Oveisi, F., Hussienzadha, S., 1992. Effect of chronic renal failure on intestinal transport of biotin in the rat. J. Lab. Clin. Med. 120, 471–475.

Schurgers, L.J., 2013. Vitamin K: key vitamin in controlling vascular calcification in chronic kidney disease. Kidney Int. 83, 782–784.

Shah, G.M., Ross, E.A., Sabo, A., Pichon, M., Bhagavan, H., Reynolds, R.D., 1991. Ascorbic acid supplements in patients receiving chronic peritoneal dialysis. Am. J. Kidney Dis. 18, 84–90.

Shinton, N.K., 1972 Vitamin B 12 and folate metabolism. Br. Med. J. 1, 556–559.

Sirover, W.D., Liu, Y., Logan, A., Hunter, K., Benz, R.L., Prasad, D., et al., 2015. Plasma ascorbic acid concentrations in prevalent patients with end-stage renal disease on hemodialysis. J. Ren. Nutr. 25, 292–300.

Stenvinkel, P., Heimbürger, O., Paultre, F., Diczfalusy, U., Wang, T., Berglund, L., et al., 1999. Strong association between malnutrition, inflammation, and atherosclerosis in chronic renal failure. Kidney Int. 55, 1899–1911.

Suter, P.M., Vetter, W., 2000. Diuretics and vitamin B1: are diuretics a risk factor for thiamin malnutrition? Nutr. Rev. 58, 319–323.

Terpstra, M.L., Singh, R., Geerlings, S.E., Bemelman, F.J., 2016. Measurement of the intestinal permeability in chronic kidney disease. World J. Nephrol. 5, 378–388.

Toigo, G., Aparicio, M., Attman, P.O., Cano, N., Cianciaruso, B., Engel, B., et al., 2000. Expert working group report on nutrition in adult patients with renal insufficiency (Part 2 of 2). Clin. Nutr. 19, 281–291.

Vaziri, N.D., Said, H.M., Hollander, D., Barbari, A., Patel, N., Dang, D., et al., 1985. Impaired intestinal absorption of riboflavin in experimental uremia. Nephron 41, 26–29.

Vaziri, N.D., Zhao, Y.Y., Pahl, M.V., 2016. Altered intestinal microbial flora and impaired epithelial barrier structure and function in CKD: the nature, mechanisms, consequences and potential treatment. Nephrol. Dial. Transpl. 31, 737–746.

Wang, S., Eide, T.C., Sogn, E.M., Berg, K.J., Sund, R.B., 1999. Plasma ascorbic acid in patients undergoing chronic haemodialysis. Eur. J. Clin. Pharmacol. 55, 527–532.

Wang, A.Y., Sea, M.M., Ip, R., Law, M.C., Chow, K.M., Lui, S.F., et al., 2002. Independent effects of residual renal function and dialysis adequacy on dietary micronutrient intakes in patients receiving continuous ambulatory peritoneal dialysis. Am. J. Clin. Nutr. 76, 569–576.

Wolf, M., Shah, A., Gutierrez, O., Ankers, E., Monroy, M., Tamez, H., et al., 2007. Vitamin D levels and early mortality among incident hemodialysis patients. Kidney Int. 72, 1004–1013.

Young, D.O., Cheng, S.C., Delmez, J.A., Coyne, D.W., 2009. The effect of oral niacinamide on plasma phosphorus levels in peritoneal dialysis patients. Perit. Dial. Int. 29, 562–567.

Zhang, F., Masania, J., Anwar, A., Xue, M., Zehnder, D., Kanji, H., et al., 2016. The uremic toxin oxythiamine causes functional thiamine deficiency in end-stage renal disease by inhibiting transketolase activity. Kidney Int. 90, 396–403.

CHAPTER 28

Inflammatory bowel disorders and fat-soluble vitamins

Mikołaj Świerczyński, Jakub Fichna and Agata Szymaszkiewicz
Department of Biochemistry, Faculty of Medicine, Medical University of Lodz, Lodz, Poland

Contents

Key facts of inflammatory bowel diseases

- The precise etiology of inflammatory bowel disease (IBD) remains unknown, however, the involvement of autoimmune, genetic, and environmental factors is suggested.

Molecular Nutrition
DOI: https://doi.org/10.1016/B978-0-12-811907-5.00024-5

- Although IBD affects mainly European and North American populations, the prevalence of this condition is still increasing in Eastern countries.
- The manifestations of IBD are both intestinal and extraintestinal.
- Ulcerative colitis (UC) affects distal part of the colon and leads to the manifestations like: blood in the stools, diarrhea, and pain in the left lower abdomen which deteriorates with the bowel movements.
- Crohn's disease can affect any segment of the gastrointestinal tract, therefore its manifestations are more diversified than those in UC.

Key facts of fat-soluble vitamins

- There are four fat-soluble vitamins: A, D, E, and K.
- The hallmark of the fat-soluble vitamins is their hydrophobicity, which results in their ability to be stored and the involvement of numerous factors in their absorption (such as the presence of fat in diet).
- In the course of IBD, the fat-soluble vitamin deficiency is related to malnutrition, malabsorption, reduced oral intake, and increased intestinal loss.
- Vitamin A has three active forms with similar molecular structures: retinal, retinol, and retinoic acid.
- Vitamin D appears in two different forms: D_2 and D_3, which undergo subsequent transformations resulting in active, double-hydroxylated forms.
- Vitamin E is a group of eight closely related compounds including four tocopherols and four tocotrienols.
- Vitamin K has two main forms: K1 (a single compound named phylloquinone) and K2 (a group of closely related structures, called menaquinones).

Summary points

- Inflammatory bowel disease (IBD) is a group of chronic, relapsing, and highly problematic conditions that affect the gastrointestinal system.
- The course of IBD poses a real danger to the patients' nutritional status (micro- and macronutrients deficiencies).
- Among patients with IBDs, lower levels of fat-soluble vitamins (A, D, E, and K) are observed more frequently than in healthy population.

- Vitamin A is involved in the process of inflammation which suggests its possible role in the pathogenesis of IBD.
- Vitamin E is an antioxidant with the ability to prevent inflammation, and this ability varies between different forms of vitamin E.
- Vitamin K is crucial for the synthesis of coagulation factors and the process of calcification.
- Vitamin D is the most important vitamin in the pathogenesis of IBD as it affects the immune system, intestinal microbiota, and mucosal integrity.
- According to the guidelines, vitamin D is the only fat-soluble vitamin which requires supplementation in patients with IBD.

Abbreviations

CD	Crohn's disease
GGCX	γ-carboxyglutamyl carboxylase
GI	gastrointestinal
Gla	γ-carboxyglutamate
IBD	inflammatory bowel disease
IOM	US Institutes of Medicine
MDP	muramyl dipeptide
Ω-3	omega-3
NOD2	nucleotide-binding oligomerization domain containing 2
PLTP	phospholipid transfer protein
PMBC	peripheral mononuclear blood cells
PUFA	polyunsaturated fatty acid
RA	retinoic acid
RAR	retinoic acid receptor
RXR	retinoid X receptor
Th	T helper
TLR	Toll-like receptors
Tregs	T regulatory cells
UC	ulcerative colitis
ucOC	uncarboxylated osteocalcin
VAD	vitamin A deficiency
VDR	vitamin D receptor
VKD proteins	vitamin K-dependent proteins

28.1 Inflammatory bowel disease

The term inflammatory bowel disease (IBD) encompasses a group of chronic, relapsing, and highly problematic conditions that affect the gastrointestinal (GI) system. Among IBD two main types can be distinguished: ulcerative colitis (UC) and Crohn's disease (CD) (Hendrickson et al., 2002).

Despite the fact that IBD affects over 1.5 million of people in North America and over 2 million in Europe and that the IBD prevalence is still increasing (Ananthakrishnan, 2015), the precise etiology remains unknown. Many studies emphasize the multifactorial nature of IBD and the involvement of autoimmune, genetic, and environmental factors.

UC is a condition with mucosal inflammation that affects the distal part of the colon. The onset of UC is limited to the rectum or distal colon and it spreads upwards to its right side. According to the extension of inflammation, UC can be defined as proctitis, left-sided colitis, or extensive colitis (Silverberg et al., 2005). UC is associated with blood appearing in the stools, diarrhea, and pain in the left lower part or even whole abdomen which deteriorates when the bowels move.

In contrast to UC, CD is a transmural inflammation of any segment of the GI tract, from the oral part of pharynx to the area around the anus (Hendrickson et al., 2002). However, the most characteristic site is the distal part of the ileum. In CD the healthy regions ("skip areas") can be found between affected parts of the GI system. The manifestations of CD are related to the location of inflammation and the onset of CD is not as typical as in the case of UC. Usually, CD is associated with postprandial pain that radiates to the navel. If the inflammation is located in the upper GI tract (esophagus, stomach, or duodenum), patients experience difficulties in swallowing (dysphagia), vomiting, and early satiety. In addition, because the whole thickness of intestinal wall is inflamed, there is a risk of the development of fistulas and abscesses (Hendrickson et al., 2002).

Even though IBD is thought to affect mainly the GI tract, about half of the patients experience extraintestinal symptoms (Hendrickson et al., 2002). The comparisons of intestinal and extraintestinal manifestations of IBD are summarized in Table 28.1.

28.2 Nutritional state and malnutrition in inflammatory bowel disease

The course of IBD poses a real danger to the patients' nutritional status by forcing them to limit oral intake and also increasing nutrient requirements, disrupting nutrients absorption, and causing intestinal loss (steatorrhea, diarrhea, and hemorrhage). It should be noticed that the

Table 28.1 Comparison of intestinal and extraintestinal IBD manifestations.

Intestinal manifestations				
Feature	**Ulcerative colitis**	**Crohn's disease**	**Comments**	**References**
Location	Distal colon and rectum	Any part of GI tract; most common in ileocecal area	–	Hendrickson et al. (2002)
Extension of changes within the intestinal wall	Limited to the mucosa	Transmural	Transmural inflammation in CD can result in formation of fistulas or abscesses	
The histology of changes	Crypt abscesses, loss of mucosal glands and goblet cells	Superficial ulcerations, focal chronic inflammation, sometimes noncaseating granuloma	Presence of cells typical of inflammatory reactions is observed, mainly polymorphonuclear leukocytes and mononuclear cells	
Abdominal pain	Left lower part of abdomen, diffuse pain in abdomen in pancolitis	Most often in right lower part of abdomen; generally diffuse pain	• Abdominal pain accompanies the onset or aggravation of IBD in 50%–70% of patients • 20%–50% of patients experience pain during clinical remission of the disease • The pathogenesis of pain involves peripheral (e.g., afferent hyperalgesia) and central nervous systems (e.g., impact of stress)	
Presence of blood in the stool	Characteristic	Only when colon is affected	Bloody diarrhea is helpful in diagnosis of UC	

(*Continued*)

Table 28.1 (Continued)

		Intestinal manifestations		
Feature	**Ulcerative colitis**	**Crohn's disease**	**Comments**	**References**
Extraintestinal manifestations				
Fever	Present in 40% of IBD patients		Usually prolonged and mild; High fever occurs during aggravation/exacerbation	Hendrickson et al. (2002)
Loss of weight	Present in both, but more common in CD		Observed more consistently in children	
Developmental delay in children	Present in 6%–12% of patients	Present in 60%–88% of patients	May be the first sign of IBD in children	
Oral lesions	Rarely seen	The disease affects buccal cavity in 9% of patients	Usually aphthous ulcers are found	
Ocular manifestations	• Present in 2%–5% of IBD patients • Ocular manifestations include: scleritis, episcleritis, uveitis, and conjunctivitis • Symptoms: blurred vision, burning or itchy eyes, ocular pain, photophobia, conjunctival or scleral hyperemia, loss of visual acuity			Petrelli et al. (1982)
Renal manifestations	Kidney stones built up of uric acid	Kidney stones built up of oxalate	Renal manifestations that are rife among IBD patients are: • Nephrolithiasis • Tubulointerstitial nephritis • Glomerulonephritis • Amyloidosis The nephrolithiasis is more common in CD than UC	Corica and Romano (2015)

Referred pain	Generally experienced on the skin, commonly in mid-lower back, abdomen, and lower limbs	Farrell et al. (2014)
Hepatobiliary manifestations	About 5% of adults with IBD also suffer from chronic liver disease. In these patients primary sclerosing cholangitis is predominantly detected, which in 70% is linked to UC	Fousekis et al. (2018)
Bones	Osteopenia (23%–67%) and osteoporosis (7%–35%) appears frequently among CD and UC patients	Mouli and Ananthakrishnan (2014)
Arthritis	Often in IBD patients, sometimes prior to the development of intestinal symptoms. Both peripheral and axial joints can be affected (e.g., ankylosing spondylitis)	Hendrickson et al. (2002)
Loss of hearing	Sensorineural hearing loss (SNHL) is more frequent in UC. SNHL is said to be symptomless or scanty in manifestations even in 40% of UC patients	Loos et al. (2018)

drug–nutrient interactions may be another possible factor predisposing to malnutrition (Hwang et al., 2012).

Several products such as spicy food, legumes, beans, corn, and peas are frequently eliminated by patients from their diet. For example, the main reason for the avoidance of spicy food in IBD is related to the action of capsaicin and its physiological outcomes, such as a burning sensation, which additionally aggravate IBD symptoms (Evangelista, 2014). Moreover, dietary fiber, fructans (in raw vegetables), and galactooligosaccharides may cause diarrhea (Gearry et al., 2009). Obviously, in an active phase of IBD food avoidance is much more common than in remission and pertains to a wider range of food items with restricted or eliminated consumption. Generally, the avoidance is much more noticeable in CD than in UC; however, the difference between CD and UC becomes even more significant during remission of the disease (Bergeron et al., 2016).

Malnutrition is the most common issue in the course of IBD. Statistically, the nutritional status (assessed on the basis of dietary intake, body composition, biochemical tests, and strength of muscles) of even 80% of patients in the active phase of CD and 40% in remission is unsatisfactory (Benjamin et al., 2008). Massironi et al. (2013) revealed that the problems with patients' nutritional status were much more prominent in CD (about 14%), because, in contrast to UC (about 5.8%), the disease can affect any part of digestive tract. However, in UC the patient can become malnourished much more rapidly than in CD. Therefore it was suggested that the malnutrition was associated with the activity or duration of the illness, respectively, rather than the type of the disease (Massironi et al., 2013).

Malnutrition in IBD can relate to both: macroelements (protein and energy supply) and microelements (minerals, trace elements, and vitamins). Patients that suffer from IBD in its active and severe form are at risk of developing so-called "protein–energy malnutrition." Moreover, IBD can also evoke micronutrient deficiencies, which can develop in mild to severe disease or even during remission.

The major micronutrient deficiencies (besides fat-soluble vitamins) are summarized in Table 28.2.

28.3 Fat-soluble vitamins: structures, roles, sources

The hallmark of the fat-soluble vitamins is their hydrophobicity. Their specific chemical structure implicates the ability of being stored, as well as

Table 28.2 Most common micronutrient deficiencies in inflammatory bowel disease (IBD) (fat-soluble vitamins not included).

Deficient micronutrient	Deficiency prevalence	Comments	References
Iron	36%–90% of IBD patients	The prevalence of anemia in IBD patients was reported to be in the range of 6%–74% with the average of 17%. Iron deficiency is responsible for majority of these cases	Gomollón and Gisbert (2009)
Calcium	Around 13% adult patients with CD and 10% with UC	Potential cause of osteoporosis	Bjarnason et al. (1997)
Magnesium	13%–88% of IBD patients	Risk factor of hypocalcemia	Hwang et al. (2012)
Zinc	Prevalence of deficiency is difficult to assess because of zinc body distribution with relatively low concentration in serum	An important cofactor of over 100 enzymes Zinc supports wound healing	
Folate (vitamin B9)	20%–60% of IBD patients	Potential cause and exacerbating factor of anemia	Massironi et al. (2013)
Vitamin B12	Prevalence of deficiency differs (20%–100%) depends on affected part of GI tract The highest prevalence (up to 100%) occurs in patients after extensive ileal resection	Deficiency leads to hyperhomocysteinemia	
Vitamin C	Deficiency is common in IBD patients, but does not correlate with activity of the disease	Participates in collagen synthesis and wound healing. Decreased consumption is more likely to be the cause of deficiency	Hwang et al. (2012)

the involvement of numerous factors in their absorption (such as the presence of fat in diet). The most important risk factors of developing fat-soluble vitamin deficiency in IBD are malnutrition, malabsorption, reduced oral intake, and increased intestinal loss (e.g., steatorrhea) (Hwang et al., 2012).

Four fat-soluble vitamins are distinguished: vitamins A, E, K, and D, which has the most vital role in IBD pathogenesis. The structural formulae of these vitamins are presented in Fig. 28.1.

28.4 Vitamin A

Vitamin A possesses three active forms with similar molecular structures: retinal, retinol, and retinoic acid (RA), which is the most active form of vitamin A (Hoag et al., 2002). Vitamin A is produced from carotenoids (among them β-carotene has the highest biological vitamin A-related activity). The active forms of vitamin A can be supplied with diet (food of animal origin) or dietary supplements, while fruits, vegetables (like carrot, pumpkin, spinach, or batata), fish, and dairy products contain carotenoids (Bai et al., 2010).

Because of its fat-soluble structure, the absorption of vitamin A requires salts of bile acids. Vitamin A passes through the enterocytes and gets to the bloodstream by being packed into chylomicrons. Subsequently, the majority of vitamin A (50%–80%) is stored in the liver and from there it is distributed to other tissues through the bloodstream as retinol. Due to its hydrophobic character, retinol requires a transporting agent to circulate in the bloodstream, namely retinol binding protein, which is synthesized in a zinc-dependent manner (Bai et al., 2010).

Vitamin A is involved in numerous processes and therefore belongs to the group of indispensable compounds for humans. Among the active forms of vitamin A, RA plays a pivotal role by engaging in processes including embryonic development, epithelial cells growth (as it acts like a growth factor), wound healing (through increasing the number of macrophages and monocytes), and promoting collagen synthesis by fibroblasts. It can interact with cells by means of two types of receptors: the retinoic acid receptor (RAR) and the retinoid X receptor (RXR) which both act as transcription factors (Bai et al., 2010).

Vitamin A has an impact on the immune system, especially adaptive immunity cells. Iwata et al. (2003) found that RA acted directly by RAR receptor (but not RXR) on naive T cells and supported their differentiation into Th2 cells, while suppressing Th1 cell development. Interestingly, RA added at the initiation of naive T cells stimulation gave the contradictory effect by blocking their transformation to Th2 cells (Iwata et al., 2003). However, there is an alternative and indirect way

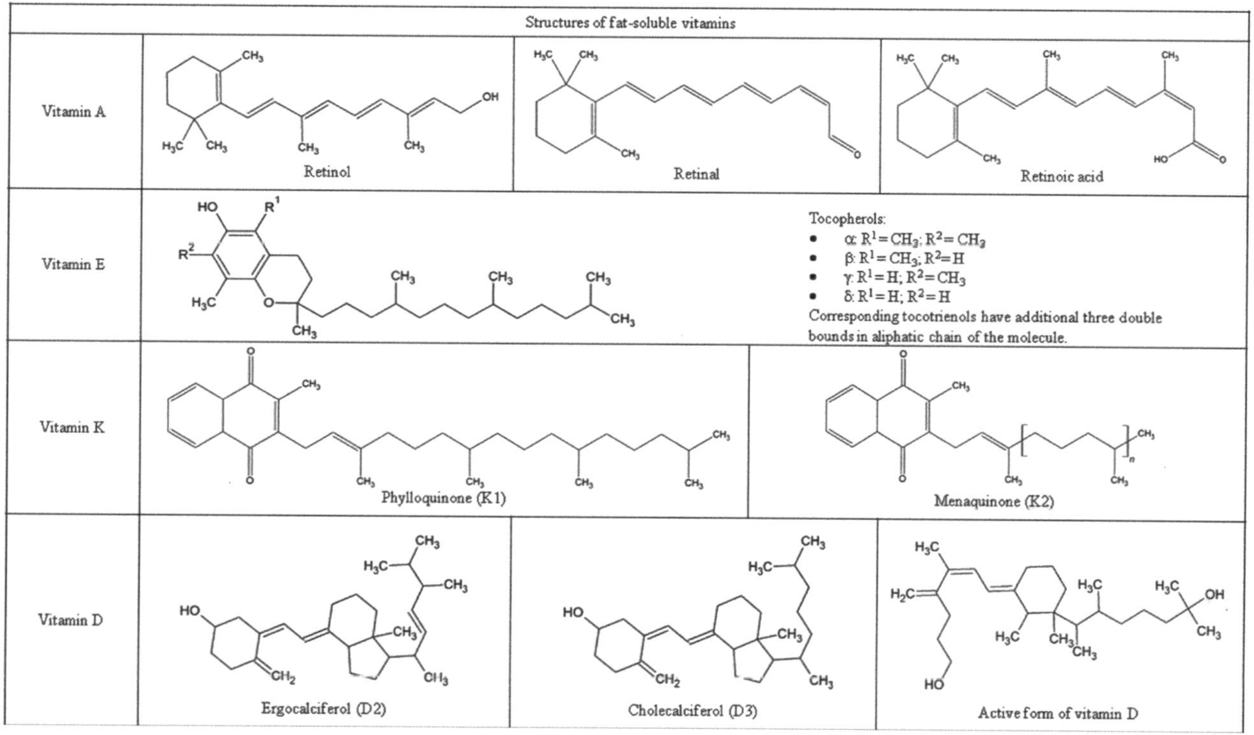

Figure 28.1 The structures of various forms of fat-soluble vitamins. Retinol, retinal, and retinoic acid are major forms of vitamin A. Vitamin E is considered as group of four tocopherols and four tocotrienols (α, β, γ, δ). Vitamin K can be found in form of phylloquinones (K1) and menaquinones (K2). Finally, vitamin D appears in two possible forms (D_2 and D_3) which then are activated in two subsequent hydroxylation processes.

leading to similar effects by influencing antigen-presenting cells (APCs) (Hoag et al., 2002).

There is yet another way in which vitamin A limits the progression of inflammation. A special group of T lymphocytes, so-called T regulatory cells (Tregs), are responsible for the inhibition of inflammation and other immune responses, protecting against uncontrolled immune activation in autoimmunity (Vignali et al., 2009). Tregs' activation by TGF-β is enhanced by RA. Therefore RA supports the activity of Tregs which in turn limits proinflammatory Th17 cells (Mucida et al., 2007).

Finally, vitamin A is crucial for immune responses that involve immunoglobulin A (IgA) (Tokuyama and Tokuyama, 1999). It was discovered that RA intensified the production of IgA by splenic B lymphocytes previously stimulated by lipopolysaccharide. However, RA alone was not able to influence the IgA production; such effects were observed in the presence of IL-5 or IL-6 which exhibit supportive properties for this process (Mora et al., 2006; Sato et al., 2003).

28.5 Vitamin A and inflammatory bowel disease

In both groups of patients suffering from either CD or UC, lower concentrations of retinol in serum were reported. This tendency did not relate to the presence of inflammation in any concrete part of the GI tract (Janczewska et al., 1991). It is worth mentioning that the serum retinol level may not be as reliable parameter of vitamin A deficiency (VAD) as hepatic retinol, because the vast majority of vitamin A is stored in the liver (Soares-Mota et al., 2015). A decrease of vitamin A level in the course of IBD was observed in correlation with their duration: the longer the disease, the lower the concentrations of vitamin A (Fabisiak et al., 2017).

Importantly, VAD is associated with the development of inflammation and fibrosis. Reifen (2002) suggested that VAD induced inflammation in the colon in rats as it increased the activity of NF-κB, potentiated oxidative stress, and promoted collagen deposition. Moreover, in rats with VAD, several histological alterations in the colon were observed: villi shortage, or inflammatory cell infiltration, and hyperplasia. Furthermore, it was reported that VAD deteriorated colitis, while it was ameliorated with vitamin A supplementation (Reifen, 2002). Additionally, VAD was linked to decreased food intake, reduced weight gain (Uni et al., 1998) and changes in taste preference (increased threshold for sweet) (Reifen et al., 1998).

The activity of vitamin A seems to have unique value in the case of IBD, where large amounts of Th1 cells accumulate in lamina propria and produce cytokines that harm colonic tissue (Monteleone et al., 1997). Because vitamin A has the ability to increase the number of Th2 at the expense of Th1 cells, it can reinstate the equilibrium between them and therefore RA is believed to present therapeutic properties in IBD (Bai et al., 2010).

A more recent hypothesis about the involvement of vitamin A and mitochondria in inflammation has been tested. A report by Tirosh et al. (2007) showed that necrosis of tissues, which occurred during inflammation, was associated with a decrease in oxygen consumption rate. Another study carried out on rats revealed that in rat model of colitis reduction of mitochondrial respiration, decreased amounts of mitochondrial DNA and expression of mitochondrial proteins were observed. In this experiment vitamin A counteracted these changes (Reifen et al., 2015).

Supplementation of vitamin A alleviated colitis in rats through limitation of the NF-κB level and oxidative stress reduction (Reifen et al., 2002). However, the supplementation is not recommended in IBD patients because of the possible toxic influence of excessive amounts of vitamin A (bone fractures, liver damage). Therefore prolonged vitamin A intake with doses exceeding daily recommended intake values (males, 900 μg/d; females, 700 μg/d) should be carefully considered before implementation (Hwang et al., 2012).

28.6 Vitamin E

Vitamin E is defined as a group of eight closely related compounds including four tocopherols and four tocotrienols (Fig. 28.1). The main structural difference is the presence of three unsaturated double bounds in the aliphatic chain of tocotrienols, while such chains in tocopherols are saturated. Each of this group consists of structures (α, β, γ, δ) varying in quantity and localization of the methyl substituents attached to the aromatic ring [Institute of Medicine (US) Panel on Dietary Antioxidants and Related, 2000].

Vitamin E is absorbed with fatty meals in the small intestine; its absorption requires pancreatic esterases and bile acids; the micellization was recognized to be the most important part of this process. Similarly to vitamin A, vitamin E gets to the bloodstream by being transported within chylomicrons. In their interaction with endothelial lipoprotein lipase, chylomicron remnants are created and subsequently taken up by the liver. In contrast to vitamin A and vitamin D, the secretion of vitamin E from the liver to other tissues involves very-low-density lipoproteins without any specific transporters (Borel and Desmarchelier, 2018).

Vitamin E in the blood is spread between all types of lipoproteins by phospholipid transfer protein (PLTP) (Kostner et al., 1995). Interestingly, recent studies revealed that PLTP can modulate immunity on different levels, from inflammation and phagocytosis to even adaptive immune cells, by changing the Th1/Th2 balance in favor of proinflammatory Th1 cells. Moreover, it was shown that the deficiency of PLTP in mice correlated with the reduced production of proinflammatory IL-18 and increased the level of α-tocopherol. In addition, α-tocopherol positively influenced T cells activity. Therefore it has been recently suggested that vitamin E favored antiinflammatory Th2 lymphocyte development, but further research is necessary (Desrumaux and Lagrost, 2018).

Most importantly vitamin E is an antioxidant that stops the cascade of lipid peroxidation. It reacts with peroxyl radicals instead of polyunsaturated fatty acids (PUFA), because the reactivity of the peroxyl radical with vitamin E is about 1000 times higher than with PUFA (Burton et al., 1985). Even though α-tocopherol has been attracting the greatest interest among researchers so far, the specific activity of other forms of vitamin E may play key roles in human health. For example, γ-tocopherol was discovered to be a better inhibitor of cyclooxygenase than α-tocopherol, which made it more efficient in inflammation prevention (with a similar mechanism as typical nonsteroidal antiinflammatory drugs) (Jiang, 2003).

28.7 Vitamin E and inflammatory bowel disease

In IBD patients the level of vitamin E was lowered in comparison to healthy controls (Fabisiak et al., 2017). However, the deficiencies are not very common, since vitamin E can be found in a variety of food sources like margarine, corn, sunflowers, and also safflower and soybean oils (Hwang et al., 2012). In fact Alkhouri et al. (2013) reported that vitamin E deficiency was more frequent in the control group (8%) than among IBD patients (5%). Another study showed that cholesterol levels in CD patients were lowered proportionally to vitamin E, which elicited a hypothesis about decreased cholesterol concentration as the cause of vitamin E deficiency (Geerling et al., 1998). In contrast to vitamin A and K, the serum concentrations of vitamin E did not correlate with the duration of IBD (Fabisiak et al., 2017).

28.8 Vitamin K

Similarly to other fat-soluble vitamins, vitamin K is not just one well-defined compound. The naturally occurring organic structures of vitamin K can be divided into two main groups: vitamin K1 and vitamin K2. Vitamin K1 is a single compound named phylloquinone that can be supplied with a diet enriched with leafy vegetables. Whereas, vitamin K2 is a group of closely related structures, called menaquinones. As vitamin K synthesis is performed by lactic acid bacteria, it is produced locally in the intestines. The source of vitamin K2 are fermented dairy products (Shearer and Okano, 2018).

The majority of vitamin K is absorbed in the proximal part of the small intestine. In further steps, vitamins K1 and K2 are distributed to different destinations:

- Vitamin K1: to the liver where it participates in the synthesis of coagulation factors: II, VII, IX, and X (examples of vitamin K-dependent (VKD) proteins).
- Vitamin K2: to the bones or vascular walls where it participates in the regulation of the activity of proteins containing γ-carboxyglutamate (Gla), such as osteocalcin.

Vitamin K is a cofactor of the microsomal enzyme called γ-carboxyglutamyl carboxylase (GGCX) which participates in the post-translational modification of proteins that involves the transformation of glutamate (Glu) into Gla by the addition of a carboxyl group (Shearer and Okano, 2018).

The presence of Gla in the structure of VKD proteins is crucial for their functions. Taking into consideration the place of origin, hepatic and extrahepatic VKD proteins can be distinguished. For example, the coagulation factor proteins have modules containing Gla, which are responsible for binding Ca^{2+} ions due to the presence of a negatively charged carboxyl group. The two main representatives of extrahepatic VKD proteins are osteocalcin and matrix Gla protein. Both are specifically engaged in physiological and pathological calcification (Willems et al., 2014).

Moreover, a synergistic influence of vitamin K and vitamin D on bones and the cardiovascular system was revealed. The key to the explanation of this relationship seems to be the ability of vitamin D to increase the amount of VKD proteins and also the impact of vitamin K on vitamin D receptors (VDRs) that can undergo γ-carboxylation (Van Ballegooijen et al., 2017).

Because of the activity of GGCX, the concentration of uncarboxylated osteocalcin (ucOC) increases in conditions of vitamin K insufficiency. Therefore the measurement of ucOC is used in the assessment of vitamin K intake—the higher concentration of ucOC, the more significant the vitamin K insufficiency (Fabisiak et al., 2017).

28.9 Vitamin K and inflammatory bowel disease

In IBD patients the deficiency of vitamin K appeared more frequently than in healthy controls (Fabisiak et al., 2017); in CD patients, lower levels of vitamin K correlated with the activity of inflammation. Additionally, the ucOC concentration in CD was significantly higher than in UC, which implicated that CD patients were more predisposed to vitamin K deficiency (Nakajima et al., 2011).

It was suggested that vitamin K deficiency, together with vitamin D, may participate in pathogenesis of osteoporosis in IBD patients. In fact about 10%–12% of CD patients suffer from osteoporosis and even 30% from osteomalacia. This activity stems (at least partially) from the ability of vitamin K to reduce the production of prostaglandin E2 in osteoclasts, which induces bone resorption (Bjarnason et al., 1997).

However, the findings mentioned above do not seem to be convincing enough to use vitamin K supplementation routinely in IBD.

28.10 Vitamin D

There are two forms of vitamin D in humans: vitamin D_2 (ergocalciferol) and vitamin D_3 (cholecalciferol) (Fig. 28.1). Both are synthesized under the influence of ultraviolet B radiation and can be supplied with meals. Each form of vitamin D has a different origin: vitamin D_2 is produced by mushrooms, while vitamin D_3 can be found in fish like salmon, mackerel, or herring. The majority of vitamin D is synthesized in the skin as D_3 (Jeon and Shin, 2018).

Vitamin D acts through VDR which are nuclear receptors with transcription factor activity. These receptors are abundantly expressed in adaptive and innate immune cells. Additionally, VDR are expressed in the

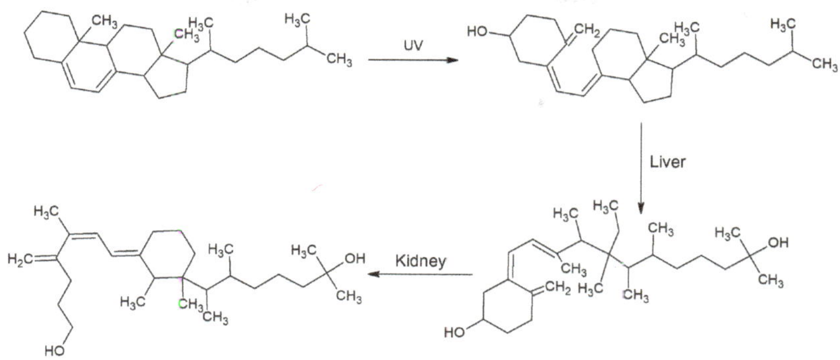

Figure 28.2 The scheme of $1,25(OH)_2D_3$ synthesis, which is an active form of vitamin D. Three steps of this process take place in the skin, liver, and finally in the kidney.

central nervous system, renal tubules, intestine, pancreas, heart, skin, reproductive system, and also placenta (Lee et al., 2018).

Both vitamins, vitamins D_2 and D_3, are inactive at the moment of supply to the human body or, in case of D_3, genesis in the skin. Their activation is achieved in two consecutive hydroxylations: first in the liver (in position 25 in the structure of vitamin D) and then in the kidneys (hydroxylation in position 1). The first step results in 25(OH)D which is used in analyses as a marker of vitamin D status. The whole process ends with the formation of double-hydroxylated structures ($1,25(OH)_2D_2$ and $1,25(OH)_2D_3$) of a fully active vitamin, so-called calcitriol (Jeon and Shin, 2018). The scheme of synthesis of $1,25(OH)_2D_3$ is shown in Fig. 28.2.

The activation of vitamins D_2 and D_3 includes the same steps, however, there are some significant differences in their activity in the organism. It was shown that supplementation of vitamin D_3 was much more efficient in increasing the concentration of 25(OH)D and duration of this increase than in groups where vitamin D_2 was administered (Tripkovic et al., 2012).

Vitamin D is considered as an important regulator of immune response. The VDR are expressed on leukocytes, peripheral mononuclear blood cells (PMBCs), APCs, T lymphocytes, $CD4^+$, and $CD8^+$ (Veldman et al., 2000).

28.11 Vitamin D and inflammatory bowel disease

For several years it has been suggested that vitamin D_3 deficiency is an important factor that contributes to the IBD pathogenesis (Lim et al., 2005).

Additionally, epidemiological studies revealed higher prevalence of IBD in the northern countries of Europe (the UK, Scandinavia) and North America (Canada) (Ananthakrishnan, 2015); in these regions patients were more susceptible to vitamin D deficiency through limited sun exposure. Moreover, the seasonal variability in the onset and exacerbation of IBD was reported: the highest rate of new, symptomatic cases of UC was observed in December (Moum et al., 1996), while for CD, the greater proportion of disease aggravation was noted in autumn and winter (Zeng & Anderson, 1996). Decreased vitamin D levels were observed in patients newly diagnosed with IBD with significantly lower vitamin D serum concentrations in comparison to healthy controls during winter (Schoon et al., 2000). Interestingly, among patients newly diagnosed with IBD, those with CD had significantly lower vitamin D level in comparison to UC patients (Lee et al., 2000).

The main causes of vitamin D deficiency in IBD patients are listed in Table 28.3.

The importance of vitamin D in IBD pathogenesis was confirmed in research on gene polymorphism; it was observed that VDR genes alterations correlated with patients' susceptibility to CD and UC (Simmons et al., 2000). Furthermore, the important role of vitamin D in IBD was confirmed in numerous animal studies. For example, Kong et al. (2008) discovered that in VDR-knockout mice colitis developed much quicker and with more severity than in controls. Similar results were reported by Froicu et al. They also proved that the aggravated IBD course in mice was a result of immune system alterations, and not disturbed calcium homeostasis (Froicu et al., 2003). Moreover, it was reported that supplementation of vitamin D_3 ameliorated IBD-related symptoms (diarrhea, waste, mortality) in IL-10 knockout mice, an animal model of IBD (Cantorna et al., 2000).

Hereafter we present possible linkages between the pathogenesis of IBD and vitamin D.

28.11.1 The mucosal barrier

The mucosal barrier comprises mucous stratum, glycocalyx, and epithelial cells; the latter are connected via desmosomes, adherens junctions, and tight junctions. The barrier consists of components like E-cadherin, claudin-1, ZO-1, and occludin proteins (Merga et al., 2014). One of the causes of IBD is defective mucosal barrier leading to chronic stimulation

Table 28.3 Main causes of vitamin D deficiency.

Cause of vitamin D deficiency	Comments	References
Insufficient exposure to sunlight	• In Ireland, CD patients in remission have the highest level of vitamin D in late summer which is similar to the lowest level of vitamin D in healthy controls in late winter	Mouli and Ananthakrishnan (2014), Rosen (2011)
Insufficient supply of vitamin D with diet	• 36% of IBD patients supply too low quantity of vitamin D with a diet	
Disturbed activation of vitamin D	• Liver or kidney failure • Inhibitory activity of fibroblast growth factor 23 (FGF-23) produced by osteocytes	
Protein losing enteropathy	• Decrease in the level of vitamin D binding protein DBP, a specialized transporter of vitamin D	
Increased excretion	• Nephrotic syndrome results in the loss of vitamin D with the urine	
Defective absorption	• May be deteriorated by resection of intestine or presence of inflammation in proximal part of the small intestine (the major location of vitamin D absorption) • Most often affects CD patients with involvement of proximal part of the small intestine • Seems not to be crucial since no significant difference in vitamin D status was found in comparison between CD and UC	
Impaired bile acids absorption	• Decreased absorption of bile acids in terminal ileum (often affected in CD) may result in impaired absorption of fat and fat-soluble substances, i.e., vitamin D	

of the local immune system (Hanauer, 2006). In patients with IBD the proteins involved in junctions between epithelial cells were lower in number and the scale of these changes correlated with inflammation activity (Gassler et al., 2001). Other research reported alterations in the location of these proteins (Oshitani et al., 2005). In consequence, bacteria commonly found in the lumen of GI tract seem to have the ability to aggravate the already pathologically increased permeability, cross the barrier, and eventually stimulate the immune system (Farrell and LaMont, 2002).

Vitamin D was reported to significantly influence the mucosal barrier's homeostasis. In mice with absent VDR, lower levels of E-cadherin, claudin-1, ZO-1, and occludin proteins were observed when compared to wild-type animals (Kong et al., 2008). It was discovered that vitamin D directly increased the number of junction proteins (but not occludin) and healing potential of mucosa. Moreover, vitamin D induced migration of epithelial cells that seemed helpful in the restoration of injured mucosa, since such a process was crucial in the creation of new crypts (Kong et al., 2008).

28.11.2 Toll-like receptors

The activity of Toll-like receptors (TLRs) is linked to innate immunity. These receptors are reactive to patterns of microbes and as a result they stimulate NF-κB and activator protein 1 production, which leads to the increase of proinflammatory cytokine levels and recruitment of adaptive immune cells (Akira et al., 2001). It was reported that the stimulation of TLRs by *Mycobacterium tuberculosis* resulted in increased expression of VDR and Cyp27B1 an enzyme converting 25(OH)D to the calcitriol (1,25(OH)2D). Immune cells, in the presence of 25(OH)D, upregulated the antimicrobial peptides and cathelicidin (which destroys bacteria) (Liu et al., 2006). Moreover, vitamin D supported autophagy by causing colocalization of autophagosomes and phagosomes containing pathogens (with the important role of cathelicidin) (Yuk et al., 2009).

TLRs are also present in the GI tract, on intestinal epithelial cells, but the pattern of TLRs on these cells partly differs from that on immune cells—on epithelial cells TLR3 and TLR5 are normally present, while the number of TLR2 and TLR4 is significantly lower (Fukata and Abreu, 2008). In the course of IBD, there are additional differences—immunohistochemical staining revealed that the expression of TLR2 and TLR4 in IBD is higher than in healthy controls (Hausmann et al., 2002). Because of the association between TLRs and proinflammatory NF-κB, the abnormally high activity of TLRs may lead to overstimulation of these receptors by commensal microbes and finally induce the inflammation in the intestines (Fukata and Abreu, 2008). Dionne et al. (2014) studied the role of 1,25D supplementation on TLR2-, TLR4-, and TLR7/8-induced cytokines released in PMBCs from patients with CD; the production of cytokines (TNF-α, IL-10, IL-23, IL-12p40) was lower after 1,25D pretreatment.

28.11.3 NOD2 receptor

NOD2 is an intracellular receptor that is crucial in host defense against pathogen invasion. The main effect of NOD2 stimulation is the activation of NF-κB (a major transcription factor responsible for proinflammatory effect) and induction of HBD2 transcription, a gene encoding defensin β2, which is a host defense peptide. By acting with the ingredient of peptidoglycan, so-called muramyl dipeptide (MDP), commonly found in bacteria, NOD2 can lead to autophagy and to the development of Th17 lymphocytes (Yuk et al., 2009).

The alterations in NOD2 gene expression are linked to CD, but not UC, and they are responsible for about 1/5 or even 1/4 of CD cases. People who are homozygous with a pair of defective genes are at approximately 20–40 times greater risk of developing CD than healthy controls (Hugot et al., 2001). Surprisingly, the defective NOD2 genes cause impairment of MDP-induced responses and the decrease of NF-κB activity in macrophages in healthy (non-IBD patients). It suggests that the response of the immune system should be inhibited, while in the IBD intestines are excessively inflamed (Abreu, 2002).

It was discovered that vitamin D increases the expression of NOD2 in epithelial and monocytic origin cells (Wang et al., 2010). However, in CD patients with an inactivating mutation of NOD2, vitamin D_3 treatment led to activation of genes encoding defensin β2 and cathelicidin (antimicrobial peptides) in response to bacterial MDP. This stimulatory effect was diminished in healthy patients. Notably, the supportive effect of vitamin D on defensin production was not observed in CD patients with inactivating polymorphism of NOD2 gene, supplying additional evidence of a significant connection between vitamin D and IBD (Wang et al., 2010).

In PBMC from CD patients the production of NOD2-stimulated cytokines (IL-23, IL-10, TNFα, but not IL-12) was significantly increased after vitamin D_3 pretreatment. In the control group (without vitamin D_3 supplementation) the cytokine levels remained low. In further experiments the secretion of cytokines upon simultaneous NOD2- and TLR stimulation and vitamin D_3 pretreatment was assessed. Vitamin D_3 induced the increase of TNFα and IL-23, while IL-12 secretion was

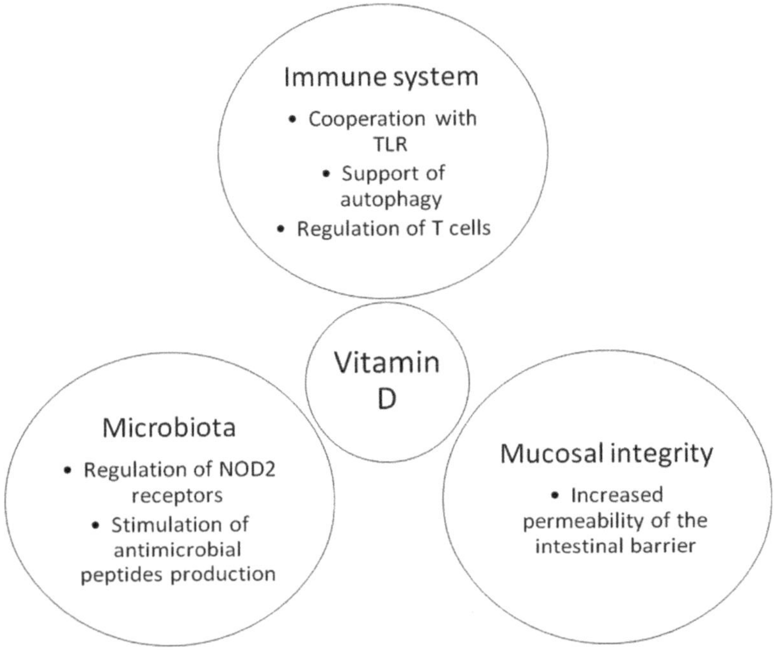

Figure 28.3 The summary of the comprehensive impact of vitamin D on IBD.

inhibited; the level of IL-10 remained unchanged. Moreover, it was evaluated whether the immunomodulatory effect of vitamin D_3 observed in CD was also present in UC and healthy controls; after NOD2- and TLR4 stimulation, the effect of vitamin D_3 treatment was similar between these three groups. However, the result of simultaneous stimulation of NOD2, TLR4, and TLR7/8 on cytokine production was consistent in CD and UC, but not healthy controls. These results indicate a significant role of vitamin D on immune response in IBD; nevertheless, the interactions between NOD2 and TLRs are complex and they are dependent on the type of TLR activated (Dionne et al., 2014).

The summary of the impact of vitamin D on IBD is included in Fig. 28.3.

28.12 Vitamin D supplementation

The gold standard for vitamin D serum concentration is about 40 ng/mL (Pludowski et al., 2018). It is important to emphasize that guidelines for vitamin D supplementation may be different according to the selected criteria. For example, the guidelines from US Institutes of Medicine (IOM) are based mainly on bone health and suggest a dosage of 400 IU/day for infants, 600 IU for children, adolescents, adults, and 800 IU for adults over 70 years of age; however it should not be used in IBD therapy, since those guidelines are created only for North Americans and based on "classical" vitamin D activity on bones. For this purposes, the Central European guidelines seem to be much more adequate and aim for a vitamin D concentration between 30 and 50 ng/mL (Pludowski et al., 2018).

Another aspect that should be taken into consideration is the possible impact of long-term supplementation of vitamin D. For the reasons mentioned above, the supplementation of vitamin D could pose a risk for the calcification of soft tissues by leading to relative deficiency of vitamin K and inadequate action of the VKD proteins (Peacock, 2010).

Vitamin D supplementation is an important factor for the effectiveness of antiTNF therapy in IBD. A prospective study performed by Santos-Antunes et al. (2016) showed that vitamin D deficiency correlates with a higher probability of failure of antiTNF treatment in IBD patients, which also had higher autoimmune potential. Therefore vitamin D should be measured and supplemented in the patients who are planned to receive the antiTNFαs.

According to the guidelines, vitamin D is the only fat-soluble vitamin that should be supplemented in IBD to prevent osteoporosis which is inseparably associated with corticosteroid therapy commonly seen in patients with IBD (Mouli and Ananthakrishnan, 2014).

28.13 Diet in inflammatory bowel disease

For many years the high prevalence of IBD was associated with regions representing the Western lifestyle (including contemporary alterations in common diet, like increased intake of sugar) such as North America, Europe, and Oceania. Now the incidence rate in these parts of the globe has been stable since 1990s, while the problem seems to be expanding with an increasing number of IBD cases reported in Japan, Hong Kong, and Korea, suggesting the correlation with the "Westernization" of lifestyle in those Eastern countries (Ananthakrishnan, 2015).

Some studies indicate that fruits and vegetables are indicated in the prevention of IBD (Owczarek et al., 2016). It was also reported that breastfeeding lowers the risk of IBD in later life (Owczarek et al., 2016).

Moreover, pediatric patients suffering from IBD have an increased concentration of antibodies against cow's milk proteins (like bovine serum albumin and β-lactoglobulins A and B). Taken together, this suggests the correlation between intolerance to cow's milk and IBD and promotes suckling for IBD prevention (Lerner et al., 1989).

The diet recommended for most IBD patients should be healthy and varied, without other more sophisticated indications. There is no doubt that for patients experiencing exacerbation of the disease, a low-fiber diet should be applied (Owczarek et al., 2016). However, there are no clear dietary recommendations for patients in remission. The fear of IBD symptom exacerbations contributes to diet restrictions and affects patients' social lives. Nevertheless, a modified carbohydrate diet with a limited amount of refined sugars and complex carbohydrates, semivegetarian diet, and use of prebiotics like geminated barley foodstuff gave promising results by maintaining remission in IBD patients, even when compared to pharmacotherapy (Owczarek et al., 2016).

Although there are no precise guidelines for IBD patients, some nutrients were reported to have positive impacts on the course of the disease, for example, omega-3 (Ω-3) PUFAs or fermentable fiber. The former, which are naturally found mainly in fish oils, are especially profitable dietary agents in the alleviation of prolonged inflammation. The antiinflammatory action of Ω-3 PUFAs results principally from the presence of their metabolic pathways' end products like prostaglandins, thromboxanes (both 3-series), and leukotrienes (5-series) (Massironi et al., 2013). The opposite effect was reported for omega-6 PUFAs, which are proinflammatory (Owczarek et al., 2016).

Fermentable fiber is much more beneficial for health than insoluble fiber. It is because of the process of fermentation conducted by colonic bacteria which ends with the formulation of short-chain fatty acids, including the most well-known, butyrate (Massironi et al., 2013). Butyrate is not only the fundamental substrate for epithelial cells in the colon but also probably decreases the endogenous synthesis of proinflammatory cytokines, helps in reactive oxygen species management, and stimulates the NF-κB pathway (Massironi et al., 2013).

In conclusion, as shown above, proper nutrition and diet have a great potential for IBD treatment. Since there are no standardized guidelines, further research is crucial for the development of efficient dietary interventions in IBD.

Acknowledgments

Supported by the grant from the Medical University of Lodz (#503/1-156-04/503-11-001 to JF) and National Science Center (#UMO-2017/25/B/NZ5/02848). AS is the recipient of the Polish L'Oréal UNESCO Awards for Women in Science.

References

Abreu, M.T., 2002. The pathogenesis of inflammatory bowel disease: translational implications for clinicians. Curr. Gastroenterol. Rep. 4 (6), 481–489.

Akira, S., Takeda, K., Kaisho, T., 2001. Toll-like receptors: critical proteins linking innate and acquired immunity. Nat. Immunol. 2 (8), 675–680.

Alkhouri, R.H., Hashmi, H., Baker, R.D., Gelfond, D., Baker, S.S., 2013. Vitamin and mineral status in patients with inflammatory bowel disease. J. Pediatr. Gastroenterol. Nutr. 56 (1), 89–92.

Ananthakrishnan, A.N., 2015. Epidemiology and risk factors for IBD. Nat. Rev. Gastroenterol. Hepatol. 12 (4), 205–217.

Bai, A., Lu, N., Zeng, H., Li, Z., Zhou, X., Chen, J., et al., 2010. All-trans retinoic acid ameliorates trinitrobenzene sulfonic acid-induced colitis by shifting Th1 to Th2 profile. J. Interf. Cytokine Res. 30 (6), 399–406.

Benjamin, J., Makharia, G., Kalaivani, M., Joshi, Y., 2008. Nutritional status of patients with Crohn's disease. Indian J. Gastroenterol. 27 (5), 195–200.

Bergeron, F., Bouin, M., D'Aoust, L., Lemoyne, M., Presse, N., 2016. Food avoidance in patients with inflammatory bowel disease: what, when and who? Clin. Nutr. 37 (3), 884–889.

Bjarnason, I., Macpherson, A., Mackintosh, C., Buxton-Thomas, M., Forgacs, I., Moniz, C., 1997. Reduced bone density in patients with inflammatory bowel disease. Gut 40 (2), 228–233.

Borel, P., Desmarchelier, C., 2018. Bioavailability of fat-soluble vitamins and phytochemicals in humans: effects of genetic variation. Annu. Rev. Nutr. 38 (1), 69–96.

Burton, G.W., Doba, T., Gabe, E.J., Hughes, L., Lee, F.L., Prasad, L., et al., 1985. Autoxidation of biological molecules. 4. Maximizing the antioxidant activity of phenols. J. Am. Chem. Soc. 107 (24), 7053–7065.

Cantorna, M.T., Munsick, C., Bemiss, C., Mahon, B.D., 2000. 1,25-Dihydroxycholecalciferol prevents and ameliorates symptoms of experimental murine inflammatory bowel disease. J. Nutr. 130 (11), 2648–2652.

Corica, D., Romano, C., 2015. Renal involvement in inflammatory bowel diseases. J. Crohn's Colitis 10 (2), 1–10.

Desrumaux, C., Lagrost, L., 2018. Plasma phospholipid transfer protein (PLTP) as an emerging determinant of the adaptive immune response. Cell. Mol. Immunol. 4, 12–14.

Dionne, S., Calderon, M.R., White, J.H., Memari, B., Elimrani, I., Adelson, B., et al., 2014. Differential effect of vitamin D on NOD2- and TLR-induced cytokines in Crohn's disease. Mucosal Immunol. 7 (6), 1405–1415.

Evangelista, S., 2014. Capsaicin receptor as target of calcitonin gene-related peptide in the gut. Prog. Drug. Res. 68, 259–276.

Fabisiak, N., Fabisiak, A., Watala, C., Fichna, J., 2017. Fat-soluble vitamin deficiencies and inflammatory bowel disease: systematic review and meta-analysis. J. Clin. Gastroenterol. 51 (10), 878–889.

Farrell, R.J., LaMont, J.T., 2002. Microbial factors in inflammatory bowel disease. Gastroenterol. Clin. North Am. 31 (1), 41–62.

Farrell, K.E., Callister, R.J., Keely, S., 2014. Understanding and targeting centrally mediated visceral pain in inflammatory bowel disease. Front. Pharmacol. 5, 1–4.

Fousekis, F.S., Theopistos, V.I., Katsanos, K.H., 2018. Hepatobiliary manifestations and complications in inflammatory bowel disease: a review. Gastroenterol. Res. 11 (2), 83–94.

Froicu, M., Weaver, V., Wynn, T.A., McDowell, M.A., Welsh, J.E., Cantorna, M.T., 2003. A crucial role for the vitamin D receptor in experimental inflammatory bowel diseases. Molec. Endocrinol. (Baltimore, MD.) 17 (12), 2386–2392.

Fukata, M., Abreu, M.T., 2008. What are toll-like receptors and what role may they have in IBD? Inflamm. Bowel Dis. 14, S90–S92.

Gassler, N., Rohr, C., Schneider, A., Kartenbeck, J., Bach, A., Obermüller, N., et al., 2001. Inflammatory bowel disease is associated with changes of enterocytic junctions. Am. J. Physiol. Gastrointest. Liver Physiol. 281, G216–G228.

Gearry, R.B., Irving, P.M., Barrett, J.S., Nathan, D.M., Shepherd, S.J., Gibson, P.R., 2009. Reduction of dietary poorly absorbed short-chain carbohydrates (FODMAPs) improves abdominal symptoms in patients with inflammatory bowel disease-a pilot study. J. Crohn's Colitis 3 (1), 8–14.

Geerling, B.J., Badart-Smook, A., Stockbrügger, R.W., Brummer, R.J.M., 1998. Comprehensive nutritional status in patients with long-standing Crohn disease currently in remission. Am. J. Clin. Nutr. 67, 919–926.

Gomollón, F., Gisbert, J.P., 2009. Anemia and inflammatory bowel diseases. World J. Gastroenterol. 15 (37), 4659–4665.

Hanauer, S.B., 2006. Inflammatory bowel disease: epidemiology, pathogenesis, and therapeutic opportunities. Inflamm. Bowel Dis. 12, S3–S9.

Hausmann, M., Kiessling, S., Mestermann, S., Webb, G., Spöttl, T., Andus, T., et al., 2002. Toll-like receptors 2 and 4 are up-regulated during intestinal inflammation. Gastroenterology 122 (7), 1987–2000.

Hendrickson, B.A., Gokhale, R., Cho, J.H., 2002. Clinical aspects and pathophysiology of inflammatory bowel disease. Clin. Microbiol. Rev. 15 (1), 79–94.

Hoag, K.A., Nashold, F.E., Goverman, J., Hayes, C.E., 2002. Retinoic acid enhances the T helper 2 cell development that is essential for robust antibody responses through its action on antigen-presenting cells. J. Nutr. 132 (12), 3736–3739.

Hugot, J.P., Chamaillard, M., Zouali, H., Lesage, S., Cézard, J.P., Belaiche, J., et al., 2001. Association of NOD2 leucine-rich repeat variants with susceptibility to Crohn's disease. Nature 411 (6837), 599–603.

Hwang, C., Ross, V., Mahadevan, U., 2012. Micronutrient deficiencies in inflammatory bowel disease: from A to zinc. Inflamm. Bowel Dis. 18 (10), 1961–1981.

Institute of Medicine (US) Panel on Dietary Antioxidants and Related, 2000. Dietary Reference Intakes for Vitamin C, Vitamin E, Selenium, and Carotenoids. *National Academy Press.*

Iwata, M., Eshima, Y., Kagechika, H., 2003. Retinoic acids exert direct effects on T cells to suppress Th1 development and enhance Th2 development via retinoic acid receptors. Int. Immunol. 15 (8), 1017–1025.

Janczewska, I., Bartnik, W., Butruk, E., Tomecki, R., Kazik, E., Ostrowski, J., 1991. Metabolism of vitamin A in inflammatory bowel disease. Hepato-Gastroenterology 38 (5), 391–395.

Jeon, S., Shin, E., 2018. Exploring vitamin D metabolism and function in cancer. Exp. Mol. Med. 50, 20.

Jiang, Q., 2003. γ-Tocopherol, but not α-tocopherol, decreases proinflammatory eicosanoids and inflammation damage in rats. FASEB J. 17 (8), 816–822.

Kong, J., Zhang, Z., Musch, M.W., Ning, G., Sun, J., Hart, J., et al., 2008. Novel role of the vitamin D receptor in maintaining the integrity of the intestinal mucosal barrier. Am. J. Physiol. Gastrointest. Liver Physiol. 294, G208–G216.

Kostner, G.M., Oettl, K., Jauhiainen, M., Ehnholm, C., Esterbauer, H., Dieplinger, H., 1995. Human plasma phospholipid transfer protein accelerates exchange/transfer of alpha-tocopherol between lipoproteins and cells. Biochem. J. 305 (Pt 2), 659–667.

Lee, S.H., Kim, H.J., Yang, S.K., Kim, W.H., Joo, Y.S., Dong, S.H., et al., 2000. Decreased trabecular bone mineral density in newly diagnosed inflammatory bowel disease patients in Korea. J. Gastroenterol. Hepatol. 15 (5), 512–518.

Lee, S.M., Meyer, M.B., Benkusky, N.A., O'Brien, C.A., Pike, J.W., 2018. The impact of VDR expression and regulation in vivo. J. Steroid Biochem. Molec. Biol. 177, 36–45.

Lerner, A., Rossi, T.M., Park, B., Albini, B., Lebenthal, E., 1989. Serum antibodies to cow's milk proteins in pediatric inflammatory bowel disease: Crohn's disease vs. ulcerative colitis. Acta Paediatr. Scand. 78 (1), 81–86.

Lim, W.C., Hanauer, S.B., Li, Y.C., 2005. Mechanisms of disease: vitamin D and inflammatory bowel disease. Nat. Clin. Pract. Gastroenterol. Hepatol. 2, 308–315.

Liu, P.T., Stenger, S., Li, H., Wenzel, L., Tan, B.H., Krutzik, S.R., et al., 2006. Toll-like receptor triggering of a vitamin D–mediated human antimicrobial response. Science 311 (March), 1770–1773.

Loos, E., Lemkens, P., Poorten, V.V., Humblet, E., Laureyns, G., 2018. Laryngeal manifestations of inflammatory bowel disease. J. Voice 33, 1–6.

Massironi, S., Rossi, R.E., Cavalcoli, F.A., Della Valle, S., Fraquelli, M., Conte, D., 2013. Nutritional deficiencies in inflammatory bowel disease: therapeutic approaches. Clin. Nutr. 32 (6), 904–910.

Merga, Y., Campbell, B.J., Rhodes, J.M., 2014. Mucosal barrier, bacteria and inflammatory bowel disease: possibilities for therapy. Dig. Dis. 32 (4), 475–483.

Monteleone, G., Biancone, L., Marasco, R., Morrone, G., Marasco, O., Luzza, F., et al., 1997. Interleukin 12 is expressed and actively released by Crohn's disease intestinal lamina propria mononuclear cells. Gastroenterology 112 (4), 1169–1178.

Mora, J.R., Iwata, M., Eksteen, B., Song, S.Y., Junt, T., Senman, B., et al., 2006. Generation of gut-homing IgA-secreting B cells by intestinal dendritic cells. Science 314 (5802), 1157–1160.

Mouli, V.P., Ananthakrishnan, A.N., 2014. Review article: vitamin D and inflammatory bowel diseases. Aliment. Pharmacol. Ther. 39 (2), 1–19.

Moum, B., Aadland, E., Ekbom, A., Vatn, M.H., 1996. Seasonal variations in the onset of ulcerative colitis. Gut 38 (3), 376–378.

Mucida, D., Park, Y., Kim, G., Turovskaya, O., Scott, I., Kronenberg, M., et al., 2007. Reciprocal TH17 and regulatory T cell differentiation mediated by retinoic acid. Science 317 (5835), 256–260.

Nakajima, S., Iijima, H., Egawa, S., Shinzaki, S., Kondo, J., Inoue, T., et al., 2011. Association of vitamin K deficiency with bone metabolism and clinical disease activity in inflammatory bowel disease. Nutrition 27 (10), 1023–1028.

Oshitani, N., Watanabe, K., Nakamura, S., Fujiwara, Y., Higuchi, K., Arakawa, T., 2005. Dislocation of tight junction proteins without F-actin disruption in inactive Crohn's disease. Int. J. Mol. Med. 15 (3), 407–410.

Owczarek, D., Rodacki, T., Domagała-Rodacka, R., Cibor, D., Mach, T., 2016. Diet and nutritional factors in inflammatory bowel diseases. World J. Gastroenterol. 22 (3), 895–905.

Peacock, M., 2010. Calcium metabolism in health and disease. Clin. J. Am. Soc. Nephrol. 5 (1), S23–30.

Petrelli, E.A., McKinley, M., Troncale, F.J., 1982. Ocular manifestations of inflammatory bowel disease. Ann. Ophthalmol. 14 (4), 356–360.

Pludowski, P., Holick, M.F., Grant, W.B., Konstantynowicz, J., Mascarenhas, M.R., Haq, A., et al., 2018. Vitamin D supplementation guidelines. J. Steroid Biochem. Molec. Biol. 175, 125–135.

Reifen, R., 2002. Vitamin A as an anti-inflammatory agent. Proc. Nutr. Soc. 61 (03), 397–400.

Reifen, R., Agami, O., Weiser, H., Biesalski, H., Naim, M., 1998. Impaired responses to sweet taste in vitamin A-deficient rats. Metabolism 47 (1), 1–2.

Reifen, R., Nur, T., Ghebermeskel, K., Zaiger, G., Urizky, R., Pines, M., 2002. Vitamin A deficiency exacerbates inflammation in a rat model of colitis through activation of nuclear factor-kappaB and collagen formation. J. Nutr. 132 (9), 2743–2747.

Reifen, R., Levy, E., Berkovich, Z., Tirosh, O., 2015. Vitamin A exerts its antiinflammatory activities in colitis through preservation of mitochondrial activity. Nutrition 31 (11–12), 1402–1407.

Rosen, C.J., 2011. Clinical practice. Vitamin D insufficiency. N. Engl. J. Med. 364, 248–254.

Santos-Antunes, J., Nunes, A.C.R., Lopes, S., Macedo, G., 2016. The relevance of vitamin D and antinuclear antibodies in patients with inflammatory bowel disease under anti-TNF treatment. Inflamm. Bowel Dis. 22 (5), 1101–1106.

Sato, A., Hashiguchi, M., Toda, E., Iwasaki, A., Hachimura, S., Kaminogawa, S., 2003. CD11b + Peyer's patch dendritic cells secrete IL-6 and induce IgA secretion from naive B cells. J. Immunol. 171 (7), 3684–3690.

Schoon, E.J., Blok, B.M., Geerling, B.J., Russel, M.G., Stockbrugger, R.W., Brummer, R.J., 2000. Bone mineral density in patients with recently diagnosed inflammatory bowel disease. Gastroenterology 119 (5), 1203–1208.

Shearer, M.J., Okano, T., 2018. Key pathways and regulators of vitamin K function and intermediary metabolism. Annu. Rev. Nutr. *4*(May), 1–25.

Silverberg, M.S., Satsangi, J., Ahmad, T., Arnott, I.D., Bernstein, C.N., Brant, S.R., et al., 2005. Toward an integrated clinical, molecular and serological classification of inflammatory bowel disease: report of a working party of the 2005 montreal world congress of gastroenterology. Can. J. Gastroenterol. 19 (Suppl. A), 5A–36A.

Simmons, J.D., Mullighan, C., Welsh, K.I., Jewell, D.P., 2000. Vitamin D receptor gene polymorphism: association with Crohn's disease susceptibility. Gut 47 (2), 211–214.

Soares-Mota, M., Silva, T.A., Gomes, L.M., Pinto, M.A.S., Mendonça, L.M.C., Farias, M.L.F., et al., 2015. High prevalence of vitamin A deficiency in Crohn's disease patients according to serum retinol levels and the relative dose-response test. World J. Gastroenterol. 21 (5), 1614–1620.

Tirosh, O., Levy, E., Reifen, R., 2007. High selenium diet protects against TNBS-induced acute inflammation, mitochondrial dysfunction, and secondary necrosis in rat colon. Nutrition 23 (11–12), 878–886.

Tokuyama, H., Tokuyama, Y., 1999. The regulatory effects of all-trans-retinoic acid on isotype switching: retinoic acid induces IgA switch rearrangement in cooperation with IL-5 and inhibits IgG1 switching. Cell. Immunol. 192 (1), 41–47.

Tripkovic, L., Lambert, H., Hart, K., Smith, C.P., Bucca, G., Penson, S., et al., 2012. Comparison of vitamin D2 and vitamin D3 supplementation in raising serum 25-hydroxyvitamin D status : a systematic review. Am. J. Clin. Nutr. 95, 1357–1364.

Uni, Z., Zaiger, G., Reifen, R., 1998. Vitamin A deficiency induces morphometric changes and decreased functionality in chicken small intestine. Br. J. Nutr. 80 (4), 401–407.

Van Ballegooijen, A.J., Pilz, S., Tomaschitz, A., Grübler, M.R., Verheyen, N., 2017. The synergistic interplay between vitamins D and K for bone and cardiovascular health: a narrative review. Int. J. Endocrinol. 2017, 1–12.

Veldman, C.M., Cantorna, M.T., DeLuca, H.F., 2000. Expression of 1,25-dihydroxyvitamin D(3) receptor in the immune system. Arch. Biochem. Biophys. 374 (2), 334–338.

Vignali, D.A., Collison, L.W., Workman, C.J., 2009. How regulatory T cells work. Nat. Rev.: Immunol. 8 (7), 523–532.
Wang, T.T., Dabbas, B., Laperriere, D., Bitton, A.J., Soualhine, H., Tavera-Mendoza, L. E., et al., 2010. Direct and indirect induction by 1,25-dihydroxyvitamin D3 of the NOD2/CARD15-defensin β2 innate immune pathway defective in crohn disease. J. Biol. Chem. 285 (4), 2227–2231.
Willems, B.A.G., Vermeer, C., Reutelingsperger, C.P.M., Schurgers, L.J., 2014. The realm of vitamin K dependent proteins: shifting from coagulation toward calcification. Molec. Nutr. Food Res. 58 (8), 1620–1635.
Yuk, J.M., Shin, D.M., Lee, H.M., Yang, C.S., Jin, H.S., Kim, K.K., et al., 2009. Vitamin D3 induces autophagy in human monocytes/macrophages via cathelicidin. Cell Host Microbe 6 (3), 231–243.
Zeng, L., Anderson, F.H., 1996. Seasonal change in the exacerbations of Crohn's disease. Scand. J. Gastroenterol. 31 (1), 79–82.

CHAPTER 29

Prostate cancer and applications of vitamin K

Smita Vinjamuri[1], Venkata Satish Dontaraju[2] and Gnanasekar Munirathinam[1]
[1]Department of Biomedical Sciences, University of Illinois-College of Medicine, Rockford, IL, United States
[2]Internal Medicine, Rockford Memorial Hospital, Rockford, IL, United States

Contents

Key facts

- Vitamin K is a fat-soluble vitamin that plays a vital role in the blood clotting process.
- Vitamin K1 is naturally present in green leafy vegetables while vitamin K2 is derived from bacteria or dairy and meat products.
- Vitamin K intake, especially vitamin K2, is inversely correlated with advanced prostate cancer (PCa).

Molecular Nutrition
DOI: https://doi.org/10.1016/B978-0-12-811907-5.00027-0

- Vitamin K2 inhibits both hormone-dependent and hormone-independent PCa in experimental studies.
- Vitamin K3 (synthetic vitamin K) in combination with ascorbic acid induces autoschizis type of cell death in PCa cells while vitamin K2 mainly induces apoptotic cell death.
- Vitamin K3-based therapy (Apatone) has shown promise in an open label, Phase I/IIa study of PCa patients by delaying biochemical progression.

Summary points

- The focus of this chapter is on the applications of vitamin K in prostate cancer (PCa).
- Vitamin K exists naturally in two forms, namely vitamin K1 (phylloquinone) and vitamin K2 (menaquinone).
- Vitamin K administration improves bone health, reduce fractures, and prevents calcium buildup in the arteries.
- Recent studies suggest that vitamin K2 may reduce fatal PCa incidence.
- Vitamin K and its derivatives can target multiple stages of PCa development by acting on various cellular mechanisms.
- However, before clinical use of vitamin K for PCa patients, rigorous clinical trials need to be undertaken.

Abbreviations

PCa prostate cancer
ADT androgen deprivation therapy
ROS reactive oxygen species
PSA prostate-specific antigen
K2 vitamin K2
K3 vitamin K3
K4 vitamin K4
MGP matrix-Gla protein

29.1 Introduction

29.1.1 Prostate cancer

Prostate cancer (PCa) is one of the leading causes of cancer-related death among men in the United States and the second leading cause of cancer worldwide (Stan and Singh, 2009). The American Cancer Society has estimated that in 2017 there will be approximately 161,360 new cases of PCa and 26,730 deaths from PCa. Some cases of PCa show clinical relevance from the beginning, whereas others acquire the clinical relevance as the cancer progresses (Geisler et al., 2015). In spite of the various methods of diagnosis available and the evolution of targeted therapies, this cancer proves to be devastating. The current treatment options available for PCa include surgery, radiation therapy, chemotherapy, and hormonal therapy (Geisler et al., 2015). Surgery, which is also called prostatectomy, is preferred only if the tumor is localized inside the prostate gland. But approximately one in three PCa patients tend to develop biochemical relapse after prostatectomy. These patients who develop biochemical relapse will eventually develop clinical relapse causing metastasis and leading to death. Radiation therapy is used to either treat the primary tumor within the prostate or serve as a curative treatment to prevent the recurrence of the cancer after prostatectomy (Antonarakis et al., 2015). Unfortunately, recurrence of cancer occurs in 30%–40% of the patients undergoing radiation therapy. Studies reveal that radiotherapy resistance is due to radiation-resistant PCa cells, the presence of cancer stem cells and the complexity of the tumor microenvironment (Antonarakis et al., 2015). Chemotherapy is the most conventional treatment for any cancer. Hormonal therapy, also called androgen deprivation therapy, is the most successful treatment for the initial stages of PCa, which is accomplished by lowering the level of hormones such as androgens, testosterone, and dihydrotestosterone in the patient's body. However, after 18–24 months of any kind of therapy the patients develop resistance known as castration-resistant prostate cancer (CRPC) (Antonarakis and Armstrong, 2011). This type of PCa is often highly aggressive, metastatic, and resistant to conventional treatments. Currently, there are six therapies available for treating CRPC in men, which have all shown prolonged survival in CRPC patients. These treatments include taxol-based chemotherapeutics (cabazitaxel and docetaxel), androgen receptor targeted therapies (enzalutamide and abiraterone), cell-based immunotherapy (Sipuleucel-T), and therapy for bone metastases using radioisotope (radium-223) (Antonarakis et al., 2015). Although these treatments are available for treating PCa patients, development of therapy resistance leads to poor survival rate.

There is no clear study that points exactly in the direction of why PCa occur in some people and not in others. However, scientists have identified many factors that raise a man's risk of disease, such as age, race, family history, and lifestyle. In patients with PCa an improvement in survival increases with the early detection and treatment. For people with localized PCa whether early detection and treatment can improve the chances of survival is under research. In the last two decades natural compounds have been attracting increased attention for the discovery of small molecules as effective anticancer chemotherapeutic agents. Studies show that more than 60% of the anticancer agents used for treating various cancers are from natural sources such as plants, microorganisms, and marine organisms (Bailon-Moscoso et al., 2017). There are currently more than 200 compounds from natural sources that are in preclinical/clinical trials or in clinical use (Bailon-Moscoso et al., 2017). Natural compounds are reported to have much less cytotoxic effects on patients than other chemically synthesized small molecules (Bailon-Moscoso et al., 2017). Epidemiological and preclinical studies show that intake of vitamin K, especially vitamin K2, is inversely associated with advanced PCa (Nimptsch et al., 2008, 2010). The use of vitamin K and its substituents in treating PCa is currently under intense research. In fact many clinical studies have proved that vitamin K is a potential anticancer agent for various types of cancers (Dasari et al., 2017).

29.1.2 What is vitamin K

The letter K is derived from the German term "Koagulation Vitamin", and this vitamin plays an important role in coagulation as well as being beneficial in managing various diseases such as osteoporosis, cardiovascular diseases, and cancer. Recent studies have revealed the potential anticancer role played by vitamin K and its derivatives as a promising treatment for PCa (Dasari et al., 2017, 2018; Schwalfenberg, 2017). Vitamin K is a fat-soluble vitamin, important for the function of numerous proteins within the body, such as the coagulation factors (II, VII, IX, X, and proteins C and S), osteocalcin (a bone-forming protein), and matrix-Gla protein (MGP) (an anticalcification protein), to name a few (Booth, 2009; Booth and Suttie, 1998; Krueger et al., 2009).

Vitamin K is a group of structurally related molecules that have a 2-methyl-1,4-naphthoquinone ring and a variable aliphatic chain. The variable aliphatic chain differentiates vitamin K into two naturally occurring forms: vitamin K1 (phylloquinone) and vitamin K2 (menaquinone). The synthetic form of vitamin K without the aliphatic chain is referred to as vitamin K3 or menadione which is used as a provitamin (Lamson and Plaza, 2003).

Vitamin K1 is found in green leafy vegetables such as broccoli, lettuce, spinach, fermented soy (natto), spring onions, and cabbage. The various forms of vitamin K2 (MK-4, MK-7, and MK-10) are mainly synthesized by bacteria, especially in nutrient products such as natto and yogurt (Knapen et al., 2015). Vitamin K2 (MK-4) is also found in meat, eggs, curd, and cheese products (Booth and Suttie, 1998).

Postintestinal absorption, vitamins K1 and K2 are carried to the liver by triglyceride-rich lipoprotein (Shearer et al., 1996; Schurgers and Vermeer, 2002). Vitamin K2 is transported from the low-density lipoproteins to extraliver tissues while vitamin K1 is excreted by the human body. High levels of vitamin K2 are accumulated in peripheral tissues and are detected in the brain, aorta, and pancreas, and low levels are present in the liver (Shearer et al., 1996; Schurgers and Vermeer, 2002).

29.1.3 Sources of vitamin K

As we have earlier stated, vitamin K exists as two major types, namely K1 and K2. Various forms of vitamin K are naturally present in different sources such as green leafy vegetables, fruits, meats, and dairy products (Booth and Suttie, 1998). Table 29.1 illustrates the various sources of vitamin K.

29.1.4 Deficiency of vitamin K

Most of the blood tests that are used to measure and treat the deficiency of vitamin K are not conclusive of the deficiency as the concentrations of vitamin K (plasma phylloquinone) fluctuate based on the dietary intake (DiNicolantonio et al., 2015). The poor status of vitamin K can be reflected based on the presence of a high percentage of undercarboxylated osteocalcin, but this is also not accurate as it varies when a recent intake of vitamin K is found in the test (Booth and Suttie, 1998; Booth and

Table 29.1 Various food sources of vitamin K.

Type of vitamin K	Food source
Vitamin K1	Vegetables such as spinach, broccoli, cabbage, and kale (Booth and Suttie, 1998)
Vitamin K2	Gut bacteria, meats, and dairy products (Booth and Suttie, 1998)

Al Rajabi, 2008). However, the presence of adequate levels of carboxylated MGP protein in the serum does not conclude that the status of vitamin K is normal as it can be suboptimal (abnormal) in the arteries to prevent vascular calcification (DiNicolantonio et al., 2015). Risk factors for vitamin K deficiency include lipid malabsorption, and patients undergoing anticoagulant therapy and antibiotic treatment. Hence, vitamin K deficiency could be counteracted with adequate vitamin K supplementation.

29.1.5 Osteoporosis and vitamin K

More than 200 million people are suffering from osteoporosis and it has been identified as a leading contributor to bone fractures (Sozen et al., 2017). It is estimated that by 2050, hip fractures will increase by 310% in men and 240% in women and this will cause an economic stress. Currently vitamin D is widely administered for managing osteoporosis but there is no epidemiological evidence that advocates that vitamin D intake has reduced fractures. Studies indicate that the intake of vitamin K can reduce hip fractures that are caused due to osteoporosis (Hamidi et al., 2013; Zittermann, 2001). Various health-promoting effects of vitamin K are summarized in Table 29.2.

29.1.6 Vitamin K and vascular calcification

Studies have shown that as and when kidney function declines, coronary artery calcium (CAC) has increased in patients (Krueger et al., 2009). It was observed that diets not sufficient with vitamin K can accentuate the development of vitamin K deficiency in as little as 7 days (Israels et al., 1997). With a higher intake of vitamin K2 (menaquinone) the risk of coronary heart disease and severe aortic calcifications were significantly lower when compared to other patients (Beulens et al., 2013; Geleijnse et al., 2004). It has been found that vitamin K1 is less effective compared

Table 29.2 Health-promoting effects of vitamin K.

Target pathology	Metabolic role
Hemorrhage	Promotes coagulation (Booth, 2009)
Osteoporosis	Improves bone health and prevents fracture (Hamidi et al., 2013; Zittermann, 2001)
Atherosclerosis	Inhibits vascular calcification (Shea et al., 2009)

to vitamin K2 for reversing arterial calcifications. Based on undercarboxylated osteocalcin and MGP many healthy patients were subclinically deficient in vitamin K content in the body (Cranenburg et al., 2007). In a clinical study done over 3 years with a double-blind, randomized controlled trial of 452 patients (229 patients on vitamin K1 and 223 patients in the control group) it was found that patients on vitamin K had a significantly lower rate of development of CAC (Shea et al., 2009).

29.1.7 Vitamin K and warfarin

It has been observed that there could be an increased arterial calcification in patients given warfarin as it directly leads to the inhibition of vitamin K. Many preclinical studies have proved that increased calcifications were observed upon warfarin treatment (Schurgers et al., 2007). Vitamin K deficiency can be exacerbated further when warfarin is initiated (Schurgers et al., 2007). The negative impact that warfarin can have on the body has long been recognized (Hall et al., 1980). It was observed that the arterial distensibility was restored when a high-dose administration of vitamin K1 or vitamin K2 levels brought back to the same levels seen in control rats (Schurgers et al., 2007). Experimental data indicate that vitamin K (K1 or K2) may be able to reverse arterial calcifications and at the same time improve arterial compliance. A vitamin K antagonist, warfarin has been shown to prevent the conversion of vitamin K1 to vitamin K2 (Nakamura et al., 1994).

29.1.8 Vitamin K and insulin sensitivity

A randomized, double-blind, controlled trial of an ancillary study has shown that vitamin k administration (500 μg/day for 3 years) increased insulin sensitivity in older men compared to older women based on homeostasis model assessment of insulin resistance (Yoshida et al., 2008a). Vitamin k effects on insulin resistance in older women appear to be inversely correlated with BMI. However, increased vitamin k consumption in observational study has shown to increase insulin sensitivity in both men and women (Yoshida et al., 2008b).

29.1.9 Vitamin K and cancer

Anticancer effects of vitamin K have been widely reported in various studies. For instance, vitamin K2 has been shown to successfully treat myelodysplastic syndrome and to induce differentiation in a myeloid leukemia cell line (Takami et al., 1999; Sakai et al., 1994). In two recent studies, vitamin K2 with a dosage of 45 mg/day showed a reduction in development of hepatocellular carcinoma (HCC) in patients with liver cirrhosis. The intake of vitamin K2 also reduced the recurrence of HCC after the curative treatment of HCC with a corresponding reduction in mortality (Kakizaki et al., 2007; Mizuta et al., 2006). Several anticancer mechanisms of vitamin K have been reported by various studies, which include arylation pathways (Carr et al., 2002), activation of growth arrest genes such as GAS6 (Vermeer, 2012), and increased c-Jun and c-Myc mRNA expression in hepatoma cells (Bouzahzah et al., 1995).

Many studies have shown that cancer cells have higher levels of reactive oxygen species (ROS) and thus are more vulnerable to cell death due to oxidative stress (Schumacker, 2006; Fang et al., 2009). This mechanism can be used to develop therapeutic approaches to treat various types of cancer. Chemotherapeutic compounds, such as cisplatin, buthionine sulfoximine, and imexon, increase ROS production by targeting scavenging systems, causing cell death by the accumulation of ROS in cancer cells (Bailon-Moscoso et al., 2017; Schumacker, 2006; Fang et al., 2009). Notably, redox cycling of menadione (vitamin K3) in cancer cells leads to increased synthesis of ROS, which surpasses the oxidative capacity of the cancer cells resulting in cell death. Cycling of quinones, as in the case of menadione, can produce either semiquinone radicals with one-electron reduction or hydroquinones with two-electron reduction (Nishikawa et al., 1995). By directly arylating nucleophiles such as glutathione and initiating one- or two-electron redox cycling, menadione was more cytotoxic at higher doses when compared to other forms of vitamin K, as phylloquinone and menaquinone undergo a lower rate of cycling with an increased proportion of two-electron transfer. Vitamin K3 involves the direct arylation of thiols within the cell by menadione, thereby causing a decrease of glutathione and/or sulfhydryl-containing proteins (Scott et al., 2005). There were other experimental studies that also investigated and supported the theory that vitamin K3-induced arylation can be an effective anticancer mechanism (Gant et al., 1988; Ross et al., 1985; Wilson et al., 1987; Morrison et al., 1984). Vitamin K analogs, such as 2-(2-mercaptoethanol)-3-methyl-1,4-naphthoquinone, were studied in Hep3B cells and showed cell growth inhibition that was antagonized by thiols, but not by nonthiol antioxidants, which further supports the mechanism of growth inhibition being sulfhydryl arylation (Nishikawa et al., 1995).

It was suggested that vitamin K3 acts by two different mechanisms on rat pancreatic cancer cells: at higher levels by initiating an oxidative action and necrosis or autoschizis, or at lower levels by a nonoxidative mechanism inducing apoptosis (Sata et al., 1997). Another mechanism that implicates the anticancer effect of vitamin K3 via induction of oxidative stress was proved using catalase as a counteracting agent (Sun et al., 2000). This was observed as catalase acts as a radical scavenger by neutralizing superoxide radical anions and hydrogen peroxide. When cancer cells were treated with small concentrations of menadione (20 μM), the apoptosis frequency was three per high power field. On the other hand, when higher concentrations of vitamin K3 in the range of 60–150 μM were added, they caused necrosis, but vitamin K2 with a concentration of 150 μM resulted in an apoptosis frequency of 1.5 with no necrosis (Sata et al., 1997).

The anticancer efficiency of vitamin K1 and vitamin K2 was based on anticancer mechanisms via the targeting of transcription factors, whereas vitamin K3's efficiency is via reducing oxidative stress and arylation (Lamson and Plaza, 2003). The nonoxidative effect of vitamin K which include orchestration of transcription factors that regulate apoptosis and cell cycle arrest (Lamson and Plaza, 2003). Transcription factors can be modulated by ROS, protein tyrosine kinases, and protein tyrosine phosphatases which controls the fate of cell growth. In response to cellular activation, protein kinases phosphorylate their target proteins. On the other hand, protein phosphatases antagonize the function of protein kinases by dephosphorylating the various enzymes and proteins (Lamson and Plaza, 2003).

VK3 can alter the expression of c-myc and c-fos proto-oncogenes which in turn effect apoptosis, differentiation, and cell cycle arrest (Wu et al., 1993). The oncogenic transcription factor c-Myc encoded from proto-oncogene c-myc can form heterodimeric complex with Max protein to activate other target genes (Bouchard et al., 1998). In association with Max transcription complex, c-Myc can promote cellular alterations such as differentiation and immortalization transformation, immortalization, cell differentiation, and induction of apoptosis (Cole and McMahon, 1999).

As a modulator of cellular function, c-myc proto-oncogene is one of the best studied gene markers for apoptosis and proliferation depending on its expression status (Hoffman and Liebermann, 1998; Evan et al., 1992). In particular, c-myc oncogene can enhance oncogenic transformation and promote cell growth. When vitamin K and its analogs (K1, K2, and K3) were added to cancer cells, the expression levels of proto-oncogenes c-Myc, c-Jun, and c-Fos were found to be altered (Wu et al., 1993).

In a study conducted by Wu et al. (1993) it was found that K3 transiently induced c-fos proto-oncogene expression in vitro in 1 hour, while c-myc proto-oncogene expression was increased 1−9 hours after treatment with a concomitant increase in c-Fos and c-myc transcription factors and the changes were correlated with cell cycle arrest and delay in apoptosis. This study and other reports suggest that K3 is the most potent stimulator, followed by K2 then K1 (Wu et al., 1993; Wang et al., 1995).

29.1.10 Beneficial effects of vitamin K in prostate cancer

A study conducted in the year 2003 by Nelson et al. (2003) suggested that the mortality rates due to higher PCa prevalence are higher in Western and European countries when compared to Asian countries because of diet and other lifestyle-related reasons. Based on the data available, it is estimated that less than 5% of all PCa is hereditary. However, a population-based case control study showed that PCa risk is increased in individuals with a family history of PCa (Hayes et al., 1995).

It is believed that PCa occurs after a sequence of at least eight genetic mutational events. The first event appears to be the loss of tumor suppressor genes, such as p53 which is mutated in up to 64% of tumors and p21 in up to 55%. It was also identified that p73 tumor suppressor gene has significant homology to p53 and also appears to be mutated in PCa. In PCa, MMAC1/p10 is the most mutated suppressor gene that contributes to the acquisition of the metastatic phenotype (Burton et al., 2000). The overexpression of mutant p53 and the bcl-2 family of proteins and amplification of the AR which appears to be related to hormone refractory phenotype (Apakama et al., 1996). Epidemiological studies conducted by Nimptsch et al. (2008) suggested that dietary intake of menaquinones are especially beneficial in preventing fatal PCa in patients. These studies are further supported by an open label, Phase I/IIa study using a vitamin K3-based therapy (Apatone) in which patients showed delayed biochemical progression (Tareen et al., 2008), suggesting that vitamin K-based treatments hold promise for end stage PCa patients. Different forms of vitamin K are reported to target various types of PCa cell lines (Table 29.3). For instance, vitamin K2 is shown to prevent malignant transformation of normal prostate epithelial cells (RWPE-1) by targeting

Table 29.3 Prostate cancer (PCa) cell lines sensitive to vitamin K.

Type of vitamin K	PCa cell line
Vitamin K2	LNCaP, DU 145, 22Rv1 (Samykutty et al., 2013), and VCaP (Dasari et al., 2018)
Vitamin K3	DU 145 (Taper et al., 2001), TRAMP (Gilloteaux et al., 2005)
Vitamin K4	PC-3 (Jiang et al., 2013)

hepatoma-derived growth factor (HDGF) expression and by modulating the apoptosis signaling pathway (Shetty et al., 2016). Experimental studies have also proved that vitamin K2 is effective against both androgen-dependent and -independent PCa types (Samykutty et al., 2013). Furthermore, vitamin K2 is shown to preferentially target the growth of castration-resistant VCaP cells that have wild-type AR, while no toxic effects were found when benign prostate cells (RWPE cells) were treated with vitamin K2 at the same doses as the treatment of the VCaP CRPC cells (Dasari et al., 2018). The results of this study also indicated that vitamin K2 can be a very potent inhibitor of invasion, growth, and metastasis of castration-resistant PCa cells. Taken together, these studies support the use of vitamin K2 as both a preventive and therapeutic agent for PCa (Fig. 29.1).

In clinical settings prostate-specific antigen (PSA) is considered to be a gold standard marker that is used in the diagnosis and monitoring of various treatment outcomes. The fact that vitamin K2 has the ability to suppress PSA expression in both androgen-dependent and castration-resistant PCa cells (Samykutty et al., 2013; Dasari et al., 2018) suggests that vitamin K2 could be a potential therapy targeting the AR signaling pathway. More importantly vitamin K2 was shown to potently inhibit the tumor growth of hormone-dependent and hormone-independent tumor growth in a mice model (Samykutty et al., 2013). Based on various experimental approaches, vitamin K2 was found to effectively prevent the malignant properties of VCaP CRPC cells by specifically targeting ROS-mediated apoptosis and cell cycle progression (Dasari et al., 2018). This study also suggested that vitamin K2 prevented metastasis by inhibiting key signaling molecules. Similarly, another study showed vitamin K4, an analog of menadione is effective against PC-3 bone metastatic PCa cells via the targeting of Bcl-2 antiapoptotic protein (Jiang et al., 2013). To ascertain

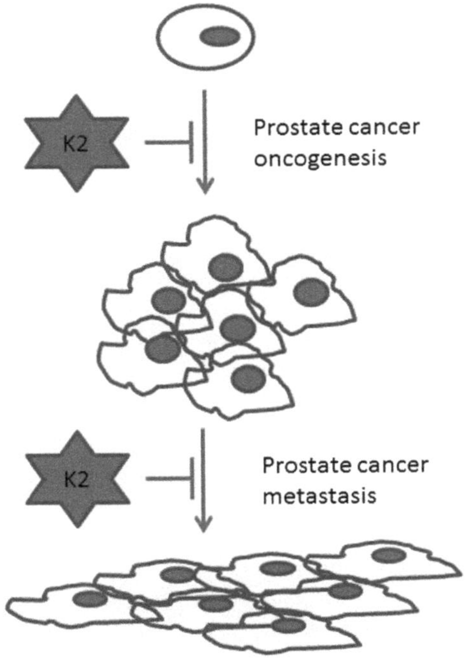

Figure 29.1 Schematic picture showing vitamin K2 inhibiting both prostate carcinogenesis and metastasis.

the results of these in vitro findings, more in vivo studies are certainly warranted to investigate the therapeutic effects of treating CRPC cells with vitamin K2.

Mechanistically, vitamin K2 was shown to target inflammation-related genes, such as HMGB1, RAGE, IL-6, and IL-8, in PCa cells in addition to inhibiting VEGF-A and AR expressions (Samykutty et al., 2013). Follow-up research to this study showed that vitamin K2 can indeed inhibit key antiapoptotic and stem cell markers (Bcl-2, Survivin, Mcl-1, Akt, c-Myc, Oct 3/4, Vimentin, HMGB1, and HMGB2) in VCaP PCa cells (Dasari et al., 2018). The key genes that are targeted by various forms of vitamin K are summarized in Table 29.4. A previous in vivo study conducted by Taper et al. (2001) advocated the use of a combination of K3 and vitamin C treatment for PCa. Their study was designed to assess the combination effect of vitamin C and vitamin K3 on the life span of nude mice bearing DU 145-derived prostate tumor growth. In this study, nude mice implanted with DU 145 cells when treated with the combination of

Table 29.4 Target genes of vitamin K in prostate cancer (PCa) cells.

Vitamin K form	Target genes
Vitamin K2	Hepatoma-derived growth factor (HDGF) (Shetty et al., 2016), androgen receptor (AR), Akt, NF-kB (Samykutty et al., 2013), and Survivin (Dasari et al., 2018)
Vitamin K3	Not known
Vitamin K4	Bcl-2 (Jiang et al., 2013)

Table 29.5 Type of cell death induced by vitamin K in prostate cancer (PCa) cells.

Vitamin K form	PCa cell death type
Vitamin K2	Apoptosis (Dasari et al., 2017; Samykutty et al., 2013)
Vitamin K3	Autoschizis (Taper et al., 2001; Gilloteaux et al., 2005)
Vitamin K4	Apoptosis (Jiang et al., 2013)

vitamin C and K3 lived significantly longer than those control mice bearing the DU 145 tumor which did not receive the treatment. This combination therapy appears to be a safe treatment as mice receiving vitamin C and K3 treatment did not exhibit any significant toxicity concerns. The underlying anticancer mechanism of this combination treatment is reported to be via autoschizis (Taper et al., 2001) which is further supported by other in vitro studies (Gilloteaux et al., 2005, 2014a,b). The types of cell death induced by different forms of vitamin K are presented in Table 29.5.

29.2 Conclusion

Given the nontoxic effects of vitamin K that have been reported in various clinical studies, the abundant availability of this vitamin in various food sources and the reported health benefits, especially in osteoporosis and cardiovascular disease, indicate that the clinical use of vitamin K for various types of cancers appears feasible. Based on the various epidemiological and experimental evidence, the use of vitamin K for managing PCa is particularly encouraging. However, before the clinical use of vitamin K for PCa patients, thorough preclinical and clinical trials need to be undertaken.

References

Antonarakis, E.S., Armstrong, A.J., 2011. Evolving standards in the treatment of docetaxel-refractory castration-resistant prostate cancer. Prostate Cancer Prostatic Dis. 14, 192–205.

Antonarakis, E.S., Lu, C., Luber, B., Wang, H., Chen, Y., Nakazawa, M., et al., 2015. Androgen receptor splice variant 7 and efficacy of taxane chemotherapy in patients with metastatic castration-resistant prostate cancer. JAMA Oncol. 1, 582–591.

Apakama, I., Robinson, M.C., Walter, N.M., Charlton, R.G., Royds, J.A., Fuller, C.E., et al., 1996. Bcl-2 overexpression combined with p53 protein accumulation correlates with hormone-refractory prostate cancer. Br. J. Cancer 74, 1258–1262.

Bailon-Moscoso, N., Cevallos-Solorzano, G., Romero-Benavides, J.C., Orellana, M.I., 2017. Natural compounds as modulators of cell cycle arrest: application for anticancer chemotherapies. Curr. Genomics 18, 106–131.

Beulens, J.W., Booth, S.L., van den Heuvel, E.G., Stoecklin, E., Baka, A., Vermeer, C., 2013. The role of menaquinones (vitamin K(2)) in human health. Br. J. Nutr. 110, 1357–1368.

Booth, S.L., 2009. Roles for vitamin K beyond coagulation. Annu. Rev. Nutr. 29, 89–110.

Booth, S.L., Suttie, J.W., 1998. Dietary intake and adequacy of vitamin K. J. Nutr. 128, 785–788.

Booth, S.L., Al Rajabi, A., 2008. Determinants of vitamin K status in humans. Vitam. Horm. 78, 1–22.

Booth, S.L., O'Brien-Morse, M.E., Dallal, G.E., Davidson, K.W., Gundberg, C.M., 1999. Response of vitamin K status to different intakes and sources of phylloquinone-rich foods: comparison of younger and older adults. Am. J. Clin. Nutr. 70, 368–377.

Bouchard, C., Staller, P., Eilers, M., 1998. Control of cell proliferation by Myc. Trends Cell Biol. 8, 202–206.

Bouzahzah, B., Nishikawa, Y., Simon, D., Carr, B.I., 1995. Growth control and gene expression in a new hepatocellular carcinoma cell line, Hep40: inhibitory actions of vitamin K. J. Cell Physiol. 165, 459–467.

Burton, J.L., Oakley, N., Anderson, J.B., 2000. Recent advances in the histopathology and molecular biology of prostate cancer. BJU Int. 85, 87–94.

Carr, B.I., Wang, Z., Kar, S., 2002. K vitamins, PTP antagonism, and cell growth arrest. J. Cell. Physiol. 193, 263–274.

Cole, M.D., McMahon, S.B., 1999. The Myc oncoprotein: a critical evaluation of transactivation and target gene regulation. Oncogene 18, 2916–2924.

Cranenburg, E.C., Schurgers, L.J., Vermeer, C., 2007. Vitamin K: the coagulation vitamin that became omnipotent. Thromb. Haemost. 98, 120–125.

Dasari, S., Ali, S.M., Zheng, G., Chen, A., Dontaraju, V.S., Bosland, M.C., et al., 2017. Vitamin K and its analogs: potential avenues for prostate cancer management. Oncotarget 8, 57782–57799.

Dasari, S., Samy, A., Kajdacsy-Balla, A., Bosland, M.C., Munirathinam, G., 2018. Vitamin K2, a menaquinone present in dairy products targets castration-resistant prostate cancer cell-line by activating apoptosis signaling. Food Chem. Toxicol. 115, 218–227.

DiNicolantonio, J.J., Bhutani, J., O'Keefe, J.H., 2015. The health benefits of vitamin K. Open Heart 2, e000300.

Evan, G.I., Wyllie, A.H., Gilbert, C.S., Littlewood, T.D., Land, H., Brooks, M., et al., 1992. Induction of apoptosis in fibroblasts by c-myc protein. Cell 69, 119–128.

Fang, J., Seki, T., Maeda, H., 2009. Therapeutic strategies by modulating oxygen stress in cancer and inflammation. Adv. Drug Deliv. Rev. 61, 290–302.

Gant, T.W., Rao, D.N., Mason, R.P., Cohen, G.M., 1988. Redox cycling and sulphydryl arylation; their relative importance in the mechanism of quinone cytotoxicity to isolated hepatocytes. Chem. Biol. Interact. 65, 157–173.

Geisler, C., Gaisa, N.T., Pfister, D., Fuessel, S., Kristiansen, G., Braunschweig, T., et al., 2015. Identification and validation of potential new biomarkers for prostate cancer diagnosis and prognosis using 2D-DIGE and MS. Biomed. Res. Int. 2015, 454256.

Geleijnse, J.M., Vermeer, C., Grobbee, D.E., Schurgers, L.J., Knapen, M.H., van der Meer, I.M., et al., 2004. Dietary intake of menaquinone is associated with a reduced risk of coronary heart disease: the Rotterdam study. J. Nutr. 134, 3100–3105.

Gilloteaux, J., Jamison, J.M., Neal, D.R., Summers, J.L., 2005. Cell death by autoschizis in TRAMP prostate carcinoma cells as a result of treatment by ascorbate: menadione combination. Ultrastruct. Pathol. 29, 221–235.

Gilloteaux, J., Jamison, J.M., Summers, J.L., 2014a. Pro-oxidant treatment of human prostate carcinoma (DU145) induces autoschizis cell death: autophagosomes build up out of injured endomembranes and mitochondria. Ultrastruct. Pathol. 38, 315–328.

Gilloteaux, J., Jamison, J.M., Neal, D., Summers, J.L., 2014b. Synergistic antitumor cytotoxic actions of ascorbate and menadione on human prostate (DU145) cancer cells in vitro: nucleus and other injuries preceding cell death by autoschizis. Ultrastruct. Pathol. 38, 116–140.

Hall, J.G., Pauli, R.M., Wilson, K.M., 1980. Maternal and fetal sequelae of anticoagulation during pregnancy. Am. J. Med. 68, 122–140.

Hamidi, M.S., Gajic-Veljanoski, O., Cheung, A.M., 2013. Vitamin K and bone health. J. Clin. Densitom. 16, 409–413.

Hayes, R.B., Liff, J.M., Pottern, L.M., Greenberg, R.S., Schoenberg, J.B., Schwartz, A. G., et al., 1995. Prostate cancer risk in U.S. blacks and whites with a family history of cancer. Int. J. Cancer 60, 361–364.

Hoffman, B., Liebermann, D.A., 1998. The proto-oncogene c-myc and apoptosis. Oncogene 17, 3351–3357.

Israels, L.G., Israels, E.D., Saxena, S.P., 1997. The riddle of vitamin K1 deficit in the newborn. Semin. Perinatol. 21, 90–96.

Jiang, Y., Yang, J., Yang, C., Meng, F., Zhou, Y., Yu, B., et al., 2013. Vitamin K4 induces tumor cytotoxicity in human prostate carcinoma PC-3 cells via the mitochondria-related apoptotic pathway. Pharmazie 68, 442–448.

Kakizaki, S., Sohara, N., Sato, K., Suzuki, H., Yanagisawa, M., Nakajima, H., et al., 2007. Preventive effects of vitamin K on recurrent disease in patients with hepatocellular carcinoma arising from hepatitis C viral infection. J. Gastroenterol. Hepatol. 22, 518–522.

Knapen, M.H., Braam, L.A., Teunissen, K.J., Zwijsen, R.M., Theuwissen, E., Vermeer, C., 2015. Yogurt drink fortified with menaquinone-7 improves vitamin K status in a healthy population. J. Nutr. Sci. 4, e35.

Krueger, T., Westenfeld, R., Schurgers, L., Brandenburg, V., 2009. Coagulation meets calcification: the vitamin K system. Int. J. Artif. Organs 32, 67–74.

Lamson, D.W., Plaza, S.M., 2003. The anticancer effects of vitamin K. Alternat. Med. Rev. 8, 303–318.

Mizuta, T., Ozaki, I., Eguchi, Y., Yasutake, T., Kawazoe, S., Fujimoto, K., et al., 2006. The effect of menatetrenone, a vitamin K2 analog, on disease recurrence and survival in patients with hepatocellular carcinoma after curative treatment: a pilot study. Cancer 106, 867–872.

Morrison, H., Jernstrom, B., Nordenskjold, M., Thor, H., Orrenius, S., 1984. Induction of DNA damage by menadione (2-methyl-1,4-naphthoquinone) in primary cultures of rat hepatocytes. Biochem. Pharmacol. 33, 1763–1769.

Nakamura, K., Toyohira, H., Kariyazono, H., Ishibashi, M., Saigenji, H., Shimokawa, S., et al., 1994. Anticoagulant effects of warfarin and kinetics of K vitamins in blood and feces. Artery 21, 148–160.
Nelson, W.G., De Marzo, A.M., Isaacs, W.B., 2003. Prostate cancer. N. Engl. J. Med. 349, 366–381.
Nimptsch, K., Rohrmann, S., Linseisen, J., 2008. Dietary intake of vitamin K and risk of prostate cancer in the Heidelberg Cohort of the European Prospective Investigation into Cancer and Nutrition (EPIC-Heidelberg). Am. J. Clin. Nutr. 87, 985–992.
Nimptsch, K., Rohrmann, S., Kaaks, R., Linseisen, J., 2010. Dietary vitamin K intake in relation to cancer incidence and mortality: results from the Heidelberg Cohort of the European Prospective Investigation into Cancer and Nutrition (EPIC-Heidelberg). Am. J. Clin. Nutr. 91, 1348–1358.
Nishikawa, Y., Carr, B.I., Wang, M., Kar, S., Finn, F., Dowd, P., et al., 1995. Growth inhibition of hepatoma cells induced by vitamin K and its analogs. J. Biol. Chem. 270, 28304–28310.
Ross, D., Thor, H., Orrenius, S., Moldeus, P., 1985. Interaction of menadione (2-methyl-1,4-naphthoquinone) with glutathione. Chem. Biol. Interact. 55, 177–184.
Sakai, I., Hashimoto, S., Yoda, M., Hida, T., Ohsawa, S., Nakajo, S., et al., 1994. Novel role of vitamin K2: a potent inducer of differentiation of various human myeloid leukemia cell lines. Biochem. Biophys. Res. Commun. 205, 1305–1310.
Samykutty, A., Shetty, A.V., Dakshinamoorthy, G., Kalyanasundaram, R., Zheng, G., Chen, A., et al., 2013. Vitamin k2, a naturally occurring menaquinone, exerts therapeutic effects on both hormone-dependent and hormone-independent prostate cancer cells. Evid. Based Complem. Alternat. Med. 2013, 287358.
Sata, N., Klonowski-Stumpe, H., Han, B., Haussinger, D., Niederau, C., 1997. Menadione induces both necrosis and apoptosis in rat pancreatic acinar AR4-2J cells. Free Radic. Biol. Med. 23, 844–850.
Schumacker, P.T., 2006. Reactive oxygen species in cancer cells: live by the sword, die by the sword. Cancer Cell 10, 175–176.
Schurgers, L.J., Vermeer, C., 2002. Differential lipoprotein transport pathways of K-vitamins in healthy subjects. Biochim. Biophys. Acta 1570, 27–32.
Schurgers, L.J., Spronk, H.M., Soute, B.A., Schiffers, P.M., DeMey, J.G., Vermeer, C., 2007. Regression of warfarin-induced medial elastocalcinosis by high intake of vitamin K in rats. Blood 109, 2823–2831.
Schwalfenberg, G.K., 2017. Vitamins K1 and K2: the emerging group of vitamins required for human health. J. Nutr. Metab. 2017, 6254836.
Scott, G.K., Atsriku, C., Kaminker, P., Held, J., Gibson, B., Baldwin, M.A., et al., 2005. Vitamin K3 (menadione)-induced oncosis associated with keratin 8 phosphorylation and histone H3 arylation. Mol. Pharmacol. 68, 606–615.
Shea, M.K., O'Donnell, C.J., Hoffmann, U., Dallal, G.E., Dawson-Hughes, B., Ordovas, J.M., et al., 2009. Vitamin K supplementation and progression of coronary artery calcium in older men and women. Am. J. Clin. Nutr. 89, 1799–1807.
Shearer, M.J., Bach, A., Kohlmeier, M., 1996. Chemistry, nutritional sources, tissue distribution and metabolism of vitamin K with special reference to bone health. J. Nutr. 126, 1181S–1186S.
Shetty, A., Dasari, S., Banerjee, S., Gheewala, T., Zheng, G., Chen, A., et al., 2016. Hepatoma-derived growth factor: a survival-related protein in prostate oncogenesis and a potential target for vitamin K2. Urol. Oncol. 34, 483 e481–483 e488.
Sozen, T., Ozisik, L., Basaran, N.C., 2017. An overview and management of osteoporosis. Eur. J. Rheumatol. 4, 46–56.

Stan, S.D., Singh, S.V., 2009. Transcriptional repression and inhibition of nuclear translocation of androgen receptor by diallyl trisulfide in human prostate cancer cells. Clin. Cancer Res. 15, 4895–4903.

Sun, L.K., Yoshii, Y., Miyagi, K., 2000. Cytotoxic effect through fas/APO-1 expression due to vitamin K in human glioma cells. J. Neurooncol. 47, 31–38.

Takami, A., Nakao, S., Ontachi, Y., Yamauchi, H., Matsuda, T., 1999. Successful therapy of myelodysplastic syndrome with menatetrenone, a vitamin K2 analog. Int. J. Hematol. 69, 24–26.

Taper, H.S., Jamison, J.M., Gilloteaux, J., Gwin, C.A., Gordon, T., Summers, J.L., 2001. In vivo reactivation of DNases in implanted human prostate tumors after administration of a vitamin C/K(3) combination. J. Histochem. Cytochem. 49, 109–120.

Tareen, B., Summers, J.L., Jamison, J.M., Neal, D.R., McGuire, K., Gerson, L., et al., 2008. A 12 week, open label, phase I/IIa study using apatone for the treatment of prostate cancer patients who have failed standard therapy. Int. J. Med. Sci. 5, 62–67.

Vermeer, C., 2012. Vitamin K: the effect on health beyond coagulation—an overview. Food Nutr. Res. 56.

Wang, Z., Wang, M., Finn, F., Carr, B.I., 1995. The growth inhibitory effects of vitamins K and their actions on gene expression. Hepatology 22, 876–882.

Wilson, I., Wardman, P., Lin, T.S., Sartorelli, A.C., 1987. Reactivity of thiols towards derivatives of 2- and 6-methyl-1,4-naphthoquinone bioreductive alkylating agents. Chem. Biol. Interact. 61, 229–240.

Wu, F.Y., Chang, N.T., Chen, W.J., Juan, C.C., 1993. Vitamin K3-induced cell cycle arrest and apoptotic cell death are accompanied by altered expression of c-Fos and c-Myc in nasopharyngeal carcinoma cells. Oncogene 8, 2237–2244.

Yoshida, M., Jacques, P.F., Meigs, J.B., Saltzman, E., Shea, M.K., Gundberg, C., et al., 2008a. Effect of vitamin K supplementation on insulin resistance in older men and women. Diabetes Care 31, 2092–2096.

Yoshida, M., Booth, S.L., Meigs, J.B., Saltzman, E., Jacques, P.F., 2008b. Phylloquinone intake, insulin sensitivity, and glycemic status in men and women. Am. J. Clin. Nutr. 88, 210–215.

Zittermann, A., 2001. Effects of vitamin K on calcium and bone metabolism. Curr. Opin. Clin. Nutr. Metab. Care 4, 483–487.

PART III

Genetic Machinery and its Function

CHAPTER 30

Vitamins and epigenetics

Simonetta Friso[1], Domenica De Santis[1], Francesca Pizzolo[1] and Silvia Udali[1]

[1]Department of Medicine, School of Medicine, University of Verona, Verona, Italy

Contents

Key facts of vitamins and epigenetics

- The regulation of gene expression is not only determined by the decoding of the DNA sequence but also by the interplay of other mechanisms that are superimposed on the DNA structure, which are called epigenetic phenomena.
- Epigenetics relates precisely to those features of DNA that regulate gene expression by conditioning the accessibility of proteins regulating gene expression to determine whether they should be active or silent despite their DNA sequence.
- Among the major epigenetic phenomena there are DNA methylation, consisting of the modification of the DNA base called cytosine by the addition of a methyl group, and other features, called modifications of histone proteins, that are mostly linked to the way in which the chromatin structure is modified into proteins in the functioning of the genome transcriptional machinery. Other epigenetic mechanisms relate to small RNA with a noncoding function.

Molecular Nutrition
DOI: https://doi.org/10.1016/B978-0-12-811907-5.00033-6

- Differently from genetic characteristics of DNA, the epigenetic characteristics are potentially modifiable by nutritional factors, among which folate-linked vitamins are recognized as the main players due to their role in the provision of methyl groups for the methylation of DNA—the most studied epigenetic phenomenon in mammalian cells, including human cells, and the most clearly linked to disease risk, especially cancer.
- Modulating gene expression through nutritional approaches is indeed a challenging but promising approach for disease prevention and therapy.

Summary points

- This chapter focuses on the role of vitamins with a recognized function in modulating epigenetic mechanisms.
- Epigenetics refers to the complex of somatically heritable states that regulate gene expression resulting from modifications in DNA and chromatin structure that occur without alterations in the DNA sequence.
- Epigenetic phenomena include DNA methylation, posttranslational histone modifications, chromatin remodeling mechanisms, and the role of small noncoding RNA.
- Folate, namely vitamin B9, is a major player in the link between vitamins and epigenetics because it is responsible for the transport of methyl groups for the methylation of DNA, one of the most significant epigenetic phenomena.
- While pathologic conditions are associated with severe vitamin deficiency, it is now known that even mild vitamin deficiencies, especially of the hydrosoluble B group, are related to the impairment of epigenetic features of DNA.
- Vitamin A status is also associated with the modification of DNA methylation and other epigenetic phenomena at histone tails sites.
- Altered epigenetic mechanisms are associated with major chronic diseases, with the relationship mostly defined for chronic diseases such as cancer.

Definitions of words and terms

BHMT betaine-homocysteine *S*-methyltransferase
DHF dihydrofolate
DHFR dihydrofolate reductase

DNMTs	DNA methyltransferases
dTMP	deoxythymidine monophosphate
dUMP	deoxyuridine monophosphate
GNMT	glycine *N*-methyltransferase
5hmC	5-hydroxymethylcytosine
MS	methionine synthase
MTHFR	methylenetetrahydrofolate
RA	retinoic acid
SAdoHcy	*S*-adenosylhomocysteine
SAdoMet	*S*-adenosylmethionine
SHMT	serine hydroxymethyltransferase
TET	ten-eleven translocation proteins
THF	tetrahydrofolate

30.1 Introduction

Nutrients have been clearly recognized to influence epigenetic phenomena, such as DNA methylation, histone modifications, noncoding RNAs expression, and chromatin remodeling mechanisms (Choi et al., 2013; Udali et al., 2013). They all significantly impact the transcriptional regulatory pathways and the phenotypic expression but, differently from genetic phenomena, the epigenetic gene regulation occurs without changing the DNA sequence (Bird, 2007; Mizzen and Allis, 1998; Robertson and Wolffe, 2000).

The most studied epigenetic feature of eukaryote cells is DNA methylation (Bird, 2002). Biological methylation, including that of DNA, is based upon the provision of methyl groups by the function of methyl donors and acceptors that takes place within one-carbon metabolism with a special task, in this context, for the B vitamins including folate and vitamin B12 (Friso and Choi, 2002).

The scope of the present review is to focus on the link between nutritional factors such as vitamins and gene expression regulation through epigenetics. Attention will be dedicated toward evidence based mainly on the role of one-carbon nutrients but also on other vitamins known to affect the main epigenetic features of DNA.

Vitamins are essential nutritional factors that need to be included in diet.

The charm of studying the link between vitamins and epigenetics is, therefore, due to the fact that gene expression regulation by epigenetic phenomena is, differently to genetics, potentially modifiable, and therefore it is likely that a deeper understanding in this field will open up novel ways for disease prevention and therapy (Berdasco and Esteller, 2019; Burton and Lillycrop, 2019).

30.1.1 Epigenetic mechanisms

Epigenetic mechanisms refer to the complex of heritable phenomena that regulate gene expression without modifying the DNA structural sequence (Bird, 2007; Mizzen and Allis, 1998; Robertson and Wolffe, 2000; Wolffe and Matzke, 1999). They are modalities of gene expression control and eventually of protein synthesis, hence they have been shown to be influenced by nutrients throughout life from early development toward aging (Bacalini et al., 2014; Kim et al., 2009; Lillycrop and Burdge, 2012; Park et al., 2012) and it is thus feasible that they are related to the risk, the onset, and the progression of several human diseases including cancer and cardiovascular illnesses (Friso et al., 2012; Heyn and Esteller, 2012; Udali et al., 2013) (Fig. 30.1).

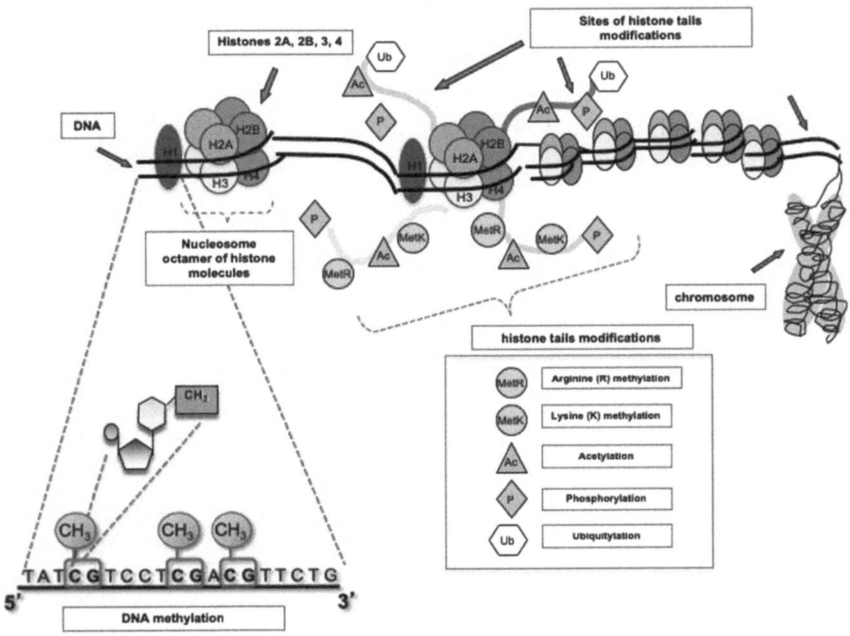

Figure 30.1 ***Schematic representation of the main epigenetic mechanisms.*** Histone modifications, such as arginine and lysine methylation, acetylation, phosphorylation, and ubiquitination, that occur on histone tails, and DNA methylation, the covalent addition of a methyl group to the 5′-carbon position of a cytosine placed inside a CpG dinucleotide sequence.

30.1.1.1 DNA methylation

Methylation of DNA refers to the transfer of a methyl group (one-carbon, $-CH_3$ group) to the 5′ position of a cytosine within the DNA sequence and this reaction is catalyzed by a number of DNA methyltransferases that regulate the transfer of methyl groups from *S*-adenosylmethionine (SAdoMet) (Costello and Plass, 2001). The provision of SAdoMet is regulated by one-carbon metabolism as shown in the scheme at Fig. 30.2. The 5′-methylcytosine in mammalian DNA is present in 5′-CpG-3′ dinucleotide sequences and exerts a number of functions in gene regulatory elements, such as promoters, enhancers, insulators, and repressors, where it generally suppresses the function of the gene (Friso and Choi, 2002; Robertson and Jones, 2000). But among the many functions of DNA methylation, so far the most clear seems to be gene silencing when the methylation occurs at a promoter site (Stein et al., 1982).

Another epigenetic phenomena that was initially considered to be only an intermediate product of the DNA methylation process

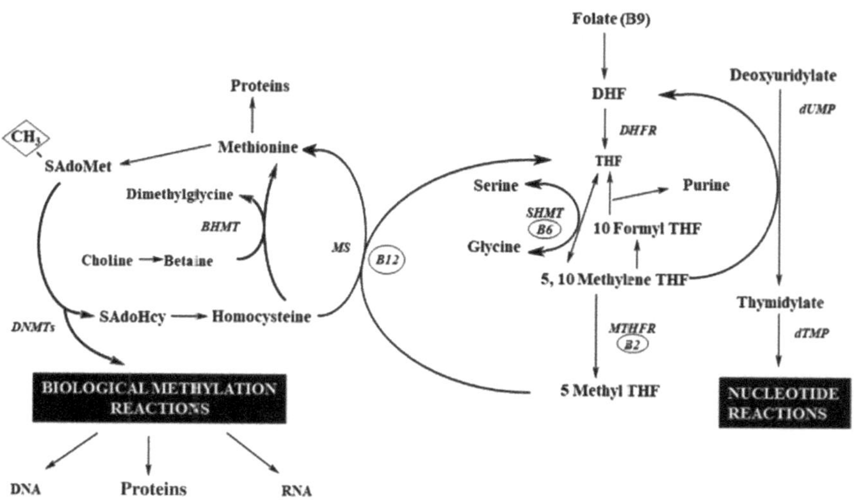

Figure 30.2 ***Overview of the nutrients, enzymes, and vitamins (cofactors) involved in folate-mediated/related one-carbon metabolism, connected to methylation and nucleotide reactions.*** *THF*, Tetrahydrofolate; *DHF*, dihydrofolate; *SAdoMet*, *S*-adenosylmethionine; *SAdoHcy*, *S*-adenosylhomocysteine; *dUMP*, deoxyuridine monophosphate; *dTMP*, deoxythymidine monophosphate; *DHFR*, dihydrofolate reductase; *MTHFR*, 5,10-methylenetetrahydrofolate reductase; *MS*, methionine synthase; *DNMTs*, DNA methyltransferases; *BHMT*, betaine-homocysteine S-methyltransferase; *SHMT*, serine hydroxymethyltransferase.

(Fu and He, 2012) but has been, most recently, gaining higher attention is DNA hydroxymethylation, namely the synthesis of 5-hydroxymethylcytosine (5hmC). The formation of 5hmC is mediated by methylcytosine oxygenase, namely by one of the ten-eleven translocation (TET) protein family, i.e., TET1 (Shukla et al., 2015; Tahiliani et al., 2009), and is mainly described in aging and cancer (Tammen et al., 2014).

30.1.1.2 Histone modifications

Short segments of 146 bp sequence of DNA are wrapped around blocks of histone proteins forming octamers of paired histones H2A, H2B, H3, and H4 called nucleosomes with another histone, called H1 that serves to anchor the DNA to each histone octamer, thereby stabilizing the nucleosome unit (Jenuwein and Allis, 2001) (Fig. 30.1). Attached to the histone proteins, sequences of amino acids called histone tails are the sites of the posttranslational histone changes, including methylation, acetylation, phosphorylation, biotinylation, ubiquitination, sumoylation, ADP-ribosylation, and other mechanisms, with the function of controlling the modulation of the chromatin structure to control gene expression (Gardner et al., 2011; Ruthenburg et al., 2007) (Fig. 30.1). Histone modifications of nucleosomes define the euchromatin from heterochromatin, namely the open versus the close chromatin status that regulates the accessibility to transcriptional factors as mainly studied in cancer diseases (Sabari et al., 2017). Histone modifications have been related to cancer and described in association with methyl groups-deficient diet in an animal model (Pogribny et al., 2006).

30.1.1.3 microRNAs

The role of small noncoding RNA molecules in gene expression regulation has recently gained importance because those RNA fragments are capable of modulating the expression of genes with a function in the cell transcriptional regulatory processes and disease development including cancer (Moutinho and Esteller, 2017). In fact, small noncoding RNA-mediated gene silencing was shown to be related to changes in histone modifications and consequently in chromatin structure at the targeted promoter conditioning the active or inactive state of a gene (Carthew and Sontheimer, 2009). The regulatory functions of microRNAs occur through the RNA-induced silencing complex to target specific microRNAs (Kunej et al., 2011; Masi et al., 2016; Esteller, 2011; Harries, 2012).

30.2 Vitamins and epigenetic mechanisms

Many nutrients are known to modulate DNA methylation, and an imbalance of nutritional components, including vitamins, in the diet can alter epigenetic mechanisms. Among the vitamins with a prominent role for the link with epigenetics, a special place is given to B vitamins since they act as coenzymes of one-carbon metabolism and regulate the provision of methyl groups for DNA and histone methylation. Vitamin A has been also described recently to have a role in epigenetics due to its active form, retinoic acid (RA).

30.2.1 Hydrosoluble B vitamins

30.2.1.1 Folate metabolism and epigenetics

Vitamin B9, most commonly known as folate, is the most extensively studied vitamin with regards to epigenetics because multiple forms of folate are involved in the supply of one-carbon units (MacKenzie, 1984; Shane, 1989) by acting as acceptors or donors of methyl groups for biological methylation reactions catalyzed by methyltransferases including those of DNA and histone proteins (Friso et al., 2002) (Fig. 30.2). Furthermore, the final product of the methyltransferases is *S*-adenosylhomocysteine (SAdoHcy), which is also a strong inhibitor of the methyltransferase-driven reactions (Friso and Choi, 2002).

Serine hydroxymethyltransferase (SHMT), a pyridoxal-5'-phosphate (vitamin B6)-containing enzyme, catalyzes the reversible transfer of a methyl group from serine to tetrahydrofolate (THF) to generate glycine and 5,10-methylene-THF. Then methylenetetrahydrofolate reductase (MTHFR), a flavin adenine dinucleotide (vitamin B2)-containing enzyme, irreversibly catalyzes the conversion of 5,10-methylene-THF to 5-methyl-THF, the primary methyl donor for the remethylation of homocysteine to methionine by methionine synthase (Fig. 30.2). The methionine synthase, an enzyme containing a cobalamin (vitamin B12) cofactor, drives the conversion of homocysteine to serve as a transporter of methyl groups from the serine compound. Methionine, which is either restored from homocysteine or, being an essential amino acid, is obtained directly from the diet, is converted into SAdoMet, the key player for the donation of 5-methyl-THF for biological methylation of DNA, RNA, proteins, phospholipids, and small molecules (Friso and Choi, 2002). Through a transsulfuration reaction, homocysteine condenses with serine to form cystathionine in an irreversible reaction catalyzed by the pyridoxal-5'-phosphate (vitamin B-6)-containing enzyme, cystathionine-β-synthase (Martinez et al., 2000). Cystathionine is subsequently hydrolyzed to form cysteine by cystathionase, another pyridoxal-5'-phosphate (vitamin B6)-containing enzyme (Fig. 30.2).

Because of this fundamental role in the provision of methyl groups, it is indeed well-known that an folate-deficient diet alters the epigenetic DNA methylation phenomenon, as demonstrated in human and in animal studies (Choi et al., 2005; Jacob et al., 1998; Rampersaud et al., 2000).

An impairment in folate status has been described to be associated with abnormal patterns of DNA methylation in several conditions, from early development processes to chronic diseases and aging (Bacalini et al., 2014). Maternal folate deficiency has long been known to cause neural tube defects in humans with a prevalence that differs worldwide (Zaganjor et al., 2016). An aberrant DNA methylation due to folate deficiency is claimed as one of the possible mechanisms underlying the link between folate deficiency and neural tube defects, because the low methyl availability is thought to induce an abnormal DNA methylation reprogramming during the critical stage of the embryonic development phase (Chang et al., 2011; Chang et al., 2013). The periconceptional maternal folic acid supplementation was associated, in a transgenerational study, with changes in methylation at a Differentially Methylated Region (DMR) of *IGF2* in the children from those supplemented mothers (Chang et al., 2011; Chang et al., 2013). Furthermore, it is known that the *IGF2* is a gene regulated by imprinting, in which the methylated allele at the DMR imprinted allele is repressed, and children of folic acid-supplemented mothers had a higher methylation at the *IGF2* DMR compared to controls (Steegers-Theunissen et al., 2009). Other authors demonstrated that methyl-deficient diet rats showed liver genomic DNA hypomethylation as compared to pair-fed control animals (Balaghi et al., 1993) a methyl-deficient diet was able to induce liver carcinogenesis in an animal model (Poirier and Beland, 1994; Powell et al., 2005). Other authors demonstrated, in a mouse model, that both genomic and *p16* promoter methylations of colonic DNA are modulated by dietary folate in old mice but not in young mice (Keyes et al., 2007). Jacob et al. (Jacob et al., 1998) observed the induction of genomic hypomethylation in human lymphocytic DNA in healthy human volunteers when placed on a long-term folate-deficient diet (56 μg folate/day) in a metabolic unit (Rampersaud et al., 2000). Interestingly, those effects were reversible when the deficiency was corrected (Rampersaud et al., 2000). In women affected by cervical intraepithelial neoplasia, researchers reported that serum folate levels and folate concentrations measured in the uterine cervix were significantly correlated with genomic DNA methylation (Fowler et al., 1998).

An interesting gene–nutrient interaction taking place within one-carbon metabolism has been also demonstrated to relate to a decreased genomic DNA methylation when subjects carrying the homozygote variant of the *MTHFR 677C > T* polymorphism, known to impair the enzyme function (Frosst et al., 1995), are under a low folate status, but not if folate concentrations are adequate. This therefore highlights the possibility of modulating the effect of an impaired enzyme function due to a genetic defect by correcting the vitamin B9 status (Friso et al., 2002). Moreover, the *MTHFR 677C > T* genotype and folate concentration in humans interact to determine the status of DNA methylation, so that *MTHFR 677TT* carriers with low folate have the lowest DNA methylation, and the impaired DNA methylation status relates to a higher prevalence of cancer history and risk of cancer development (Friso et al., 2013). This study, in fact, highlighted the possibility of using genomic methylation from peripheral blood mononuclear cells DNA, as a marker for cancer disease (Friso et al., 2013). A threshold for genomic DNA methylation defined according to MTHFR 677C > T genotype and folate status, allows to clearly cluster cancer-affected from cancer-free subjects and to identify those at-risk for cancer (Friso et al., 2013). Further and larger studies are certainly needed in this regard for possible uses of such epigenetic markers in disease prevention and possibly treatment.

Folate deficiency was also associated with a reduced histone methylation, mainly H3K4 methylation, and determined changes in gene expression (Sadhu et al., 2013). Deficiency of the major dietary sources of methyl groups, including methionine and folate, induced modifications in histone patterns associated with liver carcinogenesis in rodents and, more specifically, a progressive decrease of H3K9 and H4K20 trimethylation that were related to an increased genomic instability (Pogribny et al., 2007). Dobosy and colleagues analyzed the impact of a methyl-deficient diet in a similar rodent model on prostate tissue and observed an increased gene expression of the epigenetically regulated Igf2-H19 locus induced by histone modification with a decrease of the inhibitory dimethyl modification H3K9, and a concurrent increase of the activating histone dimethyl-H3K4 modification (Dobosy et al., 2008). Besides the function as a carrier of one-carbon units, folate has been proposed to participate in the enzymatic demethylation of histones by modulating lysine demethylase 1, an enzyme that catalyzes the removal of a methyl group from histone 3 lysine 4, defined also as a folate-binding protein, where the THF moiety serves as an acceptor of the formaldehyde that is produced from the removal of the methyl group (Garcia et al., 2016; Luka et al., 2011).

Some studies showed also a relationship between vitamin B9 and microRNA regulation. A rat model fed a methyl-deficient diet for 36 weeks demonstrated the downregulation of specific microRNAs, such as miR-122, and this change appeared tumor-specific since it did not occur in rats that were switched to a normal diet after the methyl-deficient diet period (Kutay et al., 2006). These rats, moreover, did not develop hepatocarcinoma (Kutay et al., 2006). In the livers of a rodent model in which methyl-deficiency induces hepatocarcinogenesis (Pogribny et al., 2008), the inhibition of tumor suppressors by miRNAs, in particular by the miR34a and the miR127, and the concurrent increase of specific target proteins suggest a causative role of the downregulation of these miRNAs in hepatocarcinogenesis (Pogribny et al., 2008). In a mouse model of non-alcoholic fatty liver disease, a choline- and folate-deficient diet induced a specific microRNAs profile modification leading to the progression of the hepatic disease toward the trigger of carcinogenetic processes by the methyl-deficient diet (Tryndyak et al., 2016).

30.2.1.2 Vitamin B12 and epigenetics

Vitamin B12 is involved in epigenetic phenomena by being a coenzyme for the function of methionine synthase within one-carbon metabolism (Fig. 30.2). By catalyzing the remethylation of homocysteine to methionine, vitamin B12 is, therefore, a potential limiting factor for the provision of methyl groups for methylation reactions. Piyathilake and colleagues evaluated, in a small study in humans, the tissue concentrations of vitamin B12 together with genomic DNA methylation status in tissue samples of squamous cell lung cancer paired with surrounding normal appearing bronchial mucosa, and both vitamin B12 concentrations and genomic DNA methylation were significantly lower in cancer tissue compared to the normal tissue samples (Piyathilake et al., 2000). The authors observed also a significant correlation between vitamin B12 and genomic DNA methylation indicating that vitamin B12 insufficiency is associated with genomic DNA hypomethylation (Piyathilake et al., 2000). In a rat model of vitamin B12 deficiency induced by gastrectomy and consequent deficiency of intrinsic factor, the specific transporter of vitamin B12 through the gastric cells, an altered DNA methylation was observed (Brunaud et al., 2003).

A deficient status of vitamin B12 in a rat model that was specifically designed to induce the sole deficiency of this water-soluble B vitamin by adding to the diet pectin, a heteropolysaccharide that inhibits vitamin B12 absorption, has been also shown to generate DNA hypomethylation in the rat colonic mucosa DNA (Choi et al., 2004). The vitamin B12-deficient diet was of inadequate severity to cause either anemia or any other overt severe illnesses but was, instead, sufficient to induce molecular aberrations in methylation patterns so to cause a significant global hypomethylation of the murine colonic epithelial DNA (Choi et al., 2004).

30.2.1.3 Lipophilic vitamin A

30.2.1.3.1 Retinoic acid and epigenetics

The active form of vitamin A is the RA metabolite that has been described to increase the activity of glycine *N*-methyltransferase (GNMT) that regulates the methyl group supply for the SAdoMet-dependent transmethylation reactions (Fig. 30.3), thereby leading to the reduction of methyl groups in a rat model (Ozias and Schalinske, 2003). Different epigenetic effects have been observed by RA (Table 30.1), such as a gene-specific DNA hypermethylation leading toward stem cell differentiation in a human cell culture model (Cheong et al., 2010) and a modulation of tumor suppressor genes mediated by methylation in human breast cancer cell models (Stefanska et al., 2010, 2012). RA was also observed to decrease the H3K27 trimethylation and induce the H3K4/9 acetylation, and then promote transcriptional activation in a human stem cells model (Kashyap and Gudas, 2010; Urvalek and Gudas, 2014). Vitamin A active metabolite induces also histone acetylation and phosphorylation modifications both in human and murine cell models (Angrisano et al., 2011;

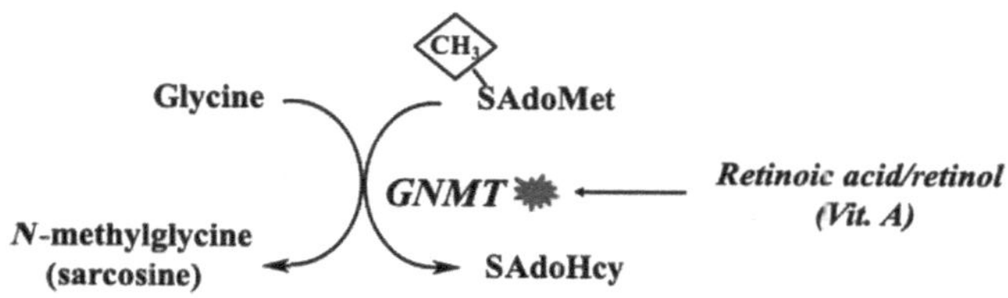

Figure 30.3 ***Vitamin A interaction with methyl group metabolism.*** Vitamin A promotes enzymatic activation of GNMT. *GNMT*, Glycine *N*-methyltransferase; *SAdoHcy*, *S*-adenosylhomocysteine; *SAdoMet*, *S*-adenosylmethionine.

Table 30.1 Main role in modulating the major epigenetic mechanisms of vitamin B9, vitamin B12, and vitamin A.

Vitamins	Epigenetic mechanisms	Study model	Main effects on epigenetics	References
Vitamin B9 (folate)	DNA methylation	Mouse and rodent models	Folate depletion decreases and folate supplementation increases global DNA methylation	Choi et al. (2005), Keyes et al. (2007)
		Human study	Subjects with low serum folate levels and MTHFR 677TT genotype present genomic hypomethylation	Friso et al. (2002)
		Human and animal studies	Maternal folate deficiency is associated with abnormal DNA methylation patterns leading to neural tube defects	Steegers-Theunissen et al. (2009), Chang et al. (2011, 2013)
	Histone modifications	In vitro study on yeast and human cells	Folate and methionine deficiency is associated with a decrease of histone methylation marks	Sadhu et al. (2013)
		In vitro studies	Folate binds to a specific Lysine demethylase (LSD1) and participates in the enzymatic demethylation of histones	Luka et al. (2011), Garcia et al. (2016)
	MicroRNAs	Rodent model	Folate and methyl-deficient diet induces changes of microRNAs expression profiles in the liver associated to hepatocarcinogenesis	Kutay et al. (2006), Pogribny et al. (2008), Tryndyak et al. (2016)
Vitamin B12	DNA methylation	Rodent model	Low vitamin B12 levels are associated with genomic DNA hypomethylation in gastrectomized rats	Brunaud et al. (2003)
			Vitamin B12 deficiency induces genomic DNA hypomethylation in the colonic mucosa	Choi et al. (2004)
	Histone modifications	Rodent model	Vitamin B12 and methyl-deficient diet induce histone modifications associated to genomic instability and carcinogenesis	Pogribny et al. (2008)
	MicroRNAs		Inhibition of tumor suppressors by miRNAs, in particular the miR34a and miR127, and concurrent increase of specific target proteins	Pogribny et al. (2008)

Vitamin A (retinoic acid, RA)	DNA methylation	In vitro studies on human embryonic stem cells	RA induces gene-specific DNA hypermethylation associated to stem cells differentiation	Cheong et al. (2010)
		In vitro study on human breast cancer cells	RA induces promoter demethylation of specific tumor suppressor genes	Stefanska et al. (2010, 2012)
	Histone modifications	In vitro studies on human stem cells	RA decreases the repressive marks H3K27me3 and induces the activation marks H3K4/9ac allowing the transcriptional activation of genes that regulate stem cell differentiation	Kashyap and Gudas (2010), Urvalek and Gudas (2014)
		In vitro studies on human and murine cancer cells	RA decreases H3K4me3 and increases histone H3 acetylation and phosphorylation	Angrisano et al. (2011), Lefebvre et al. (2002)
		In vitro studies on human T cells	RA induces histone acetylation and methylation promoting T cells differentiation	Lu et al. (2011), Kang et al. (2007)
	MicroRNAs		Role for RA and microRNAs regulation as an increases miR-3666 expression in surgical specimens of colorectal cancer in humans	Liu et al. (2018), Nervi and Grignani (2014)

Lefebvre et al., 2002) with a role in T cell differentiation processes (Kang et al., 2007; Lu et al., 2011). Some authors report a role for RA in microRNA regulation (Nervi and Grignani, 2014). In a study evaluating colon cancer specimens in humans a protective role of RA has been shown through an increase in microRNA3666 (Liu et al., 2018).

30.3 Conclusions

Epigenetic modifications are phenomena that, differently from the genetic ones, are involved in gene expression regulation without base pair changes in the DNA sequence. Epigenetic features of DNA are influenced by dietary factors such as vitamins and they are potentially modifiable by dietary approaches. Due to these characteristics, epigenetic phenomena, that include DNA methylation, histone modifications, chromatin remodeling, and miRNAs regulation, are among the most rapidly growing fields in molecular science. Indeed, epigenetics has revealed new mechanisms responsible for embryonic development and aging processes with clear involvement also in the onset of several major diseases including cancer. One of the most extensively studied epigenetic features in the eukaryote cell is DNA methylation, which regulates gene expression and preserves genome integrity by its strict link with other epigenetic features of DNA, such as histone modifications. Because DNA- and histone protein methylation are directly associated with SAdoMet, a unique methyl donor, and SAdoHcy, an inhibitor of methyltransferases, both of which are one-carbon metabolites, vitamins B9 and B12 are the most clearly associated with the modulation of epigenetics from cell culture, animal, and human studies. The active form of vitamin A, RA, has been also shown to be associated with modifications of epigenetic mechanisms, mostly in cell culture studies.

Due to their reversibility, epigenetic modifications are very attractive for possible nutritional intervention strategies in cancer and other major chronic diseases. Epigenetics may provide additional insights to genetics with regards to transcriptional regulation in many physiologic and pathologic processes.

This chapter discussed the effect of vitamins on DNA methylation and other main epigenetic features of DNA based on the current knowledge. Evidence is, however, still limited, especially regarding the combined effects of nutrients with other factors, including gene polymorphisms on the modification of epigenetic features, therefore more studies are needed to open up new perspectives for possible preventive or therapeutic intervention modalities in humans.

References

Angrisano, T., Sacchetti, S., Natale, F., Cerrato, A., Pero, R., Keller, S., et al., 2011. Chromatin and DNA methylation dynamics during retinoic acid-induced RET gene transcriptional activation in neuroblastoma cells. Nucleic Acids Res. 39, 1993–2006.

Bacalini, M.G., Friso, S., Olivieri, F., Pirazzini, C., Giuliani, C., Capri, M., et al., 2014. Present and future of anti-ageing epigenetic diets. Mech. Ageing Dev. 136-137, 101–115.

Balaghi, M., Horne, D.W., Wagner, C., 1993. Hepatic one-carbon metabolism in early folate deficiency in rats. Biochem. J. 291 (Pt 1), 145–149.

Berdasco, M., Esteller, M., 2019. Clinical epigenetics: seizing opportunities for translation. Nat. Rev. Genet. 20, 109–127.

Bird, A., 2002. DNA methylation patterns and epigenetic memory. Genes Dev. 16, 6–21.

Bird, A., 2007. Perceptions of epigenetics. Nature 447, 396–398.

Brunaud, L., Alberto, J.M., Ayav, A., Gerard, P., Namour, F., Antunes, L., et al., 2003. Vitamin B12 is a strong determinant of low methionine synthase activity and DNA hypomethylation in gastrectomized rats. Digestion 68, 133–140.

Burton, M.A., Lillycrop, K.A., 2019. Nutritional modulation of the epigenome and its implication for future health. Proc. Nutr. Soc. 1–8.

Carthew, R.W., Sontheimer, E.J., 2009. Origins and Mechanisms of miRNAs and siRNAs. Cell 136, 642–655.

Chang, H., Zhang, T., Zhang, Z., Bao, R., Fu, C., Wang, Z., et al., 2011. Tissue-specific distribution of aberrant DNA methylation associated with maternal low-folate status in human neural tube defects. J. Nutr. Biochem. 22, 1172–1177.

Chang, S., Wang, L., Guan, Y., Shangguan, S., Du, Q., Wang, Y., et al., 2013. Long interspersed nucleotide element-1 hypomethylation in folate-deficient mouse embryonic stem cells. J. Cell. Biochem. 114, 1549–1558.

Cheong, H.S., Lee, H.C., Park, B.L., Kim, H., Jang, M.J., Han, Y.M., et al., 2010. Epigenetic modification of retinoic acid-treated human embryonic stem cells. BMB Rep. 43, 830–835.

Choi, S.W., Friso, S., Ghandour, H., Bagley, P.J., Selhub, J., Mason, J.B., 2004. Vitamin B-12 deficiency induces anomalies of base substitution and methylation in the DNA of rat colonic epithelium. J. Nutr. 134, 750–755.

Choi, S.W., Friso, S., Keyes, M.K., Mason, J.B., 2005. Folate supplementation increases genomic DNA methylation in the liver of elder rats. Br. J. Nutr. 93, 31–35.

Choi, S.W., Claycombe, K.J., Martinez, J.A., Friso, S., Schalinske, K.L., 2013. Nutritional epigenomics: a portal to disease prevention. Adv. Nutr. 4, 530–532.

Costello, J.F., Plass, C., 2001. Methylation matters. J. Med. Genet. 38, 285–303.

Dobosy, J.R., Fu, V.X., Desotelle, J.A., Srinivasan, R., Kenowski, M.L., Almassi, N., et al., 2008. A methyl-deficient diet modifies histone methylation and alters Igf2 and H19 repression in the prostate. Prostate 68, 1187–1195.

Esteller, M., 2011. Non-coding RNAs in human disease. Nat. Rev. Genet. 12, 861–874.

Fowler, B.M., Giuliano, A.R., Piyathilake, C., Nour, M., Hatch, K., 1998. Hypomethylation in cervical tissue: is there a correlation with folate status? Cancer Epidemiol. Biomarkers Prev. 7, 901–906.

Friso, S., Choi, S.W., 2002. Gene–nutrient interactions and DNA methylation. J. Nutr. 132, 2382S–2387S.

Friso, S., Choi, S.W., Girelli, D., Mason, J.B., Dolnikowski, G.G., Bagley, P.J., et al., 2002. A common mutation in the 5,10-methylenetetrahydrofolate reductase gene affects genomic DNA methylation through an interaction with folate status. Proc. Natl. Acad. Sci. U.S.A. 99, 5606–5611.

Friso, S., Lotto, V., Choi, S.W., Girelli, D., Pinotti, M., Guarini, P., et al., 2012. Promoter methylation in coagulation F7 gene influences plasma FVII concentrations and relates to coronary artery disease. J. Med. Genet. 49, 192–199.

Friso, S., Udali, S., Guarini, P., Pellegrini, C., Pattini, P., Moruzzi, S., et al., 2013. Global DNA hypomethylation in peripheral blood mononuclear cells as a biomarker of cancer risk. Cancer Epidemiol. Biomarkers Prev. 22, 348–355.

Frosst, P., Blom, H.J., Milos, R., Goyette, P., Sheppard, C.A., Matthews, R.G., et al., 1995. A candidate genetic risk factor for vascular disease: a common mutation in methylenetetrahydrofolate reductase. Nat. Genet. 10, 111–113.

Fu, Y., He, C., 2012. Nucleic acid modifications with epigenetic significance. Curr. Opin. Chem. Biol. 16, 516–524.

Garcia, B.A., Luka, Z., Loukachevitch, L.V., Bhanu, N.V., Wagner, C., 2016. Folate deficiency affects histone methylation. Med. Hypotheses 88, 63–67.

Gardner, K.E., Allis, C.D., Strahl, B.D., 2011. Operating on chromatin, a colorful language where context matters. J. Mol. Biol. 409, 36–46.

Harries, L.W., 2012. Long non-coding RNAs and human disease. Biochem. Soc. Trans. 40, 902–906.

Heyn, H., Esteller, M., 2012. DNA methylation profiling in the clinic: applications and challenges. Nat. Rev. Genet. 13, 679–692.

Jacob, R.A., Gretz, D.M., Taylor, P.C., James, S.J., Pogribny, I.P., Miller, B.J., et al., 1998. Moderate folate depletion increases plasma homocysteine and decreases lymphocyte DNA methylation in postmenopausal women. J. Nutr. 128, 1204–1212.

Jenuwein, T., Allis, C.D., 2001. Translating the histone code. Science 293, 1074–1080.

Kang, S.G., Lim, H.W., Andrisani, O.M., Broxmeyer, H.E., Kim, C.H., 2007. Vitamin A metabolites induce gut-homing FoxP3+ regulatory T cells. J. Immunol. 179, 3724–3733.

Kashyap, V., Gudas, L.J., 2010. Epigenetic regulatory mechanisms distinguish retinoic acid-mediated transcriptional responses in stem cells and fibroblasts. J. Biol. Chem. 285, 14534–14548.

Keyes, M.K., Jang, H., Mason, J.B., Liu, Z., Crott, J.W., Smith, D.E., et al., 2007. Older age and dietary folate are determinants of genomic and p16-specific DNA methylation in mouse colon. J. Nutr. 137, 1713–1717.

Kim, K.C., Friso, S., Choi, S.W., 2009. DNA methylation, an epigenetic mechanism connecting folate to healthy embryonic development and aging. J. Nutr. Biochem. 20, 917–926.

Kunej, T., Godnic, I., Ferdin, J., Horvat, S., Dovc, P., Calin, G.A., 2011. Epigenetic regulation of microRNAs in cancer: an integrated review of literature. Mutat. Res. 717, 77–84.

Kutay, H., Bai, S., Datta, J., Motiwala, T., Pogribny, I., Frankel, W., et al., 2006. Downregulation of miR-122 in the rodent and human hepatocellular carcinomas. J. Cell. Biochem. 99, 671–678.

Lefebvre, B., Ozato, K., Lefebvre, P., 2002. Phosphorylation of histone H3 is functionally linked to retinoic acid receptor beta promoter activation. EMBO Rep. 3, 335–340.

Lillycrop, K.A., Burdge, G.C., 2012. Epigenetic mechanisms linking early nutrition to long term health. Best. Pract. Res. Clin. Endocrinol. Metab. 26, 667–676.

Liu, W., Song, Y., Zhang, C., Gao, P., Huang, B., Yang, J., 2018. The protective role of all-transretinoic acid (ATRA) against colorectal cancer development is achieved via

increasing miR-3666 expression and decreasing E2F7 expression. Biomed. Pharmacother. 104, 94–101.
Lu, L., Ma, J., Li, Z., Lan, Q., Chen, M., Liu, Y., et al., 2011. All-trans retinoic acid promotes TGF-beta-induced Tregs via histone modification but not DNA demethylation on Foxp3 gene locus. PLoS One 6, e24590.
Luka, Z., Moss, F., Loukachevitch, L.V., Bornhop, D.J., Wagner, C., 2011. Histone demethylase LSD1 is a folate-binding protein. Biochemistry 50, 4750–4756.
MacKenzie, R., 1984. Biogenesis and Interconversion of Substituted Tetrahydrofolates. Wiley, New York.
Martinez, M., Cuskelly, G.J., Williamson, J., Toth, J.P., Gregory 3rd, J.F., 2000. Vitamin B-6 deficiency in rats reduces hepatic serine hydroxymethyltransferase and cystathionine beta-synthase activities and rates of in vivo protein turnover, homocysteine remethylation and transsulfuration. J. Nutr. 130, 1115–1123.
Masi, L.N., Serdan, T.D., Levada-Pires, A.C., Hatanaka, E., Silveira, L.D., Cury-Boaventura, M.F., et al., 2016. Regulation of gene expression by exercise-related micrornas. Cell. Physiol. Biochem. 39, 2381–2397.
Mizzen, C.A., Allis, C.D., 1998. Linking histone acetylation to transcriptional regulation. Cell. Mol. Life Sci. 54, 6–20.
Moutinho, C., Esteller, M., 2017. MicroRNAs and Epigenetics. Adv. Cancer Res. 135, 189–220.
Nervi, C., Grignani, F., 2014. RARs and microRNAs. Subcell. Biochem. 70, 151–179.
Ozias, M.K., Schalinske, K.L., 2003. All-trans-retinoic acid rapidly induces glycine N-methyltransferase in a dose-dependent manner and reduces circulating methionine and homocysteine levels in rats. J. Nutr. 133, 4090–4094.
Park, L.K., Friso, S., Choi, S.W., 2012. Nutritional influences on epigenetics and age-related disease. Proc. Nutr. Soc. 71, 75–83.
Piyathilake, C.J., Johanning, G.L., Macaluso, M., Whiteside, M., Oelschlager, D.K., Heimburger, D.C., et al., 2000. Localized folate and vitamin B-12 deficiency in squamous cell lung cancer is associated with global DNA hypomethylation. Nutr. Cancer 37, 99–107.
Pogribny, I.P., Ross, S.A., Tryndyak, V.P., Pogribna, M., Poirier, L.A., Karpinets, T.V., 2006. Histone H3 lysine 9 and H4 lysine 20 trimethylation and the expression of Suv4-20h2 and Suv-39h1 histone methyltransferases in hepatocarcinogenesis induced by methyl deficiency in rats. Carcinogenesis 27, 1180–1186.
Pogribny, I.P., Tryndyak, V.P., Muskhelishvili, L., Rusyn, I., Ross, S.A., 2007. Methyl deficiency, alterations in global histone modifications, and carcinogenesis. J. Nutr. 137, 216S–222S.
Pogribny, I.P., Tryndyak, V.P., Ross, S.A., Beland, F.A., 2008. Differential expression of microRNAs during hepatocarcinogenesis induced by methyl deficiency in rats. Nutr. Rev. 66 (Suppl 1), S33–35.
Poirier, M.C., Beland, F.A., 1994. DNA adduct measurements and tumor incidence during chronic carcinogen exposure in rodents. Environ. Health Perspect. 102 (Suppl 6), 161–165.
Powell, C.L., Kosyk, O., Bradford, B.U., Parker, J.S., Lobenhofer, E.K., Denda, A., et al., 2005. Temporal correlation of pathology and DNA damage with gene expression in a choline-deficient model of rat liver injury. Hepatology 42, 1137–1147.
Rampersaud, G.C., Kauwell, G.P., Hutson, A.D., Cerda, J.J., Bailey, L.B., 2000. Genomic DNA methylation decreases in response to moderate folate depletion in elderly women. Am. J. Clin. Nutr. 72, 998–1003.
Robertson, K.D., Jones, P.A., 2000. DNA methylation: past, present and future directions. Carcinogenesis 21, 461–467.

Robertson, K.D., Wolffe, A.P., 2000. DNA methylation in health and disease. Nat. Rev. Genet. 1, 11–19.

Ruthenburg, A.J., Li, H., Patel, D.J., Allis, C.D., 2007. Multivalent engagement of chromatin modifications by linked binding modules. Nat. Rev. Mol. Cell Biol. 8, 983–994.

Sabari, B.R., Zhang, D., Allis, C.D., Zhao, Y.M., 2017. Metabolic regulation of gene expression through histone acylations. Nat. Rev. Mol. Cell Biol. 18, 90–101.

Sadhu, M.J., Guan, Q., Li, F., Sales-Lee, J., Iavarone, A.T., Hammond, M.C., et al., 2013. Nutritional control of epigenetic processes in yeast and human cells. Genetics 195, 831–844.

Shane, B., 1989. Folylpolyglutamate synthesis and role in the regulation of one-carbon metabolism. Vitam. Horm. 45, 263–335.

Shukla, A., Sehgal, M., Singh, T.R., 2015. Hydroxymethylation and its potential implication in DNA repair system: a review and future perspectives. Gene 564, 109–118.

Steegers-Theunissen, R.P., Obermann-Borst, S.A., Kremer, D., Lindemans, J., Siebel, C., Steegers, E.A., et al., 2009. Periconceptional maternal folic acid use of 400 microg per day is related to increased methylation of the IGF2 gene in the very young child. PLoS One 4, e7845.

Stefanska, B., Rudnicka, K., Bednarek, A., Fabianowska-Majewska, K., 2010. Hypomethylation and induction of retinoic acid receptor beta 2 by concurrent action of adenosine analogues and natural compounds in breast cancer cells. Eur. J. Pharmacol. 638, 47–53.

Stefanska, B., Salame, P., Bednarek, A., Fabianowska-Majewska, K., 2012. Comparative effects of retinoic acid, vitamin D and resveratrol alone and in combination with adenosine analogues on methylation and expression of phosphatase and tensin homologue tumour suppressor gene in breast cancer cells. Br. J. Nutr. 107, 781–790.

Stein, R., Razin, A., Cedar, H., 1982. In vitro methylation of the hamster adenine phosphoribosyltransferase gene inhibits its expression in mouse L cells. Proc. Natl. Acad. Sci. U.S.A. 79, 3418–3422.

Tahiliani, M., Koh, K.P., Shen, Y., Pastor, W.A., Bandukwala, H., Brudno, Y., et al., 2009. Conversion of 5-methylcytosine to 5-hydroxymethylcytosine in mammalian DNA by MLL partner TET1. Science 324, 930–935.

Tammen, S.A., Dolnikowski, G.G., Ausman, L.M., Liu, Z., Kim, K.C., Friso, S., et al., 2014. Aging alters hepatic DNA hydroxymethylation, as measured by liquid chromatography/mass spectrometry. J. Cancer Prev. 19, 301–308.

Tryndyak, V.P., Marrone, A.K., Latendresse, J.R., Muskhelishvili, L., Beland, F.A., Pogribny, I.P., 2016. MicroRNA changes, activation of progenitor cells and severity of liver injury in mice induced by choline and folate deficiency. J. Nutr. Biochem. 28, 83–90.

Udali, S., Guarini, P., Moruzzi, S., Choi, S.W., Friso, S., 2013. Cardiovascular epigenetics: from DNA methylation to microRNAs. Mol. Asp. Med. 34, 883–901.

Urvalek, A.M., Gudas, L.J., 2014. Retinoic acid and histone deacetylases regulate epigenetic changes in embryonic stem cells. J. Biol. Chem. 289, 19519–19530.

Wolffe, A.P., Matzke, M.A., 1999. Epigenetics: regulation through repression. Science 286, 481–486.

Zaganjor, I., Sekkarie, A., Tsang, B.L., Williams, J., Razzaghi, H., Mulinare, J., et al., 2016. Describing the prevalence of neural tube defects worldwide: a systematic literature review. PLoS One 11, e0151586.

CHAPTER 31

Transcriptional control of cells by vitamin D and its role in liver health and disease

Daniel Jahn[1] and Andreas Geier[2]
[1]Hepatology Research Laboratory, Division of Hepatology, Department of Internal Medicine II, University Hospital Würzburg, Würzburg, Germany
[2]Division of Hepatology, Department of Internal Medicine II, University Hospital Würzburg, Würzburg, Germany

Contents

Summary points

- Vitamin D needs to be taken up via the diet or can be synthesized endogenously via sunlight exposure of the skin.
- Vitamin D has pleiotropic functions in human health such as the regulation of calcium homeostasis and immune responses.

Molecular Nutrition
DOI: https://doi.org/10.1016/B978-0-12-811907-5.00030-0

- The metabolism of vitamin D includes various activation steps and catabolic reactions that are performed by different cytochrome P450 mixed-function oxidases expressed in different tissues.
- The nuclear vitamin D receptor (VDR) is the major molecular mediator of vitamin D's biological functions.
- VDR is a ligand-activated transcription factor belonging to the superfamily of nuclear hormone receptors.
- Vitamin D deficiency and impaired VDR function are associated with several human disorders including chronic liver diseases.
- Vitamin D and the activation of VDR seem to have beneficial therapeutic effects in nonalcoholic fatty liver disease.

Definition of words and term

Nonalcoholic fatty liver disease (NAFLD) A highly prevalent metabolic liver disease that is closely linked to obesity and type 2 diabetes. It comprises a spectrum of pathological changes in the liver that start with a bland (i.e., noninflammatory) accumulation of fat (i.e., steatosis) in parenchymal liver cells (i.e., hepatocytes). May progress to advanced disease stages (i.e., nonalcoholic steatohepatitis, NASH) in a subset of patients.

Nonalcoholic steatohepatitis (NASH) The progressive form of NAFLD which, in addition to liver steatosis, includes lobular liver inflammation (i.e., the infiltration of activated immune cells) as well as ballooning of hepatocytes (considered as a form of programmed cell death). The presence of these three criteria (steatosis, lobular inflammation, and hepatocyte ballooning) are essential for the diagnosis of bona fide NASH. This diagnosis can only be made on the histological level and therefore requires the examination of a liver biopsy by a trained pathologist. NASH can result in severe liver damage and is therefore a major risk factor for the development of end-stage liver disease including cirrhosis and cancer.

Vitamin D deficiency Commonly defined as circulating 25-OH vitamin D (25-OH VD) levels of 30 ng/mL or less.

Vitamin D receptor (VDR) Transcription factor that binds to and is activated by its primary ligand, 1,25(OH)2 vitamin D. Mediates most of the biological effects of vitamin D by activating (or repressing) gene expression on the level of RNA transcription.

Vitamin D response element (VDRE) Nucleotide sequence of the DNA that can be recognized and bound by VDR.

List of abbreviations

CYP	cytochrome P450 mixed-function oxidase
FGF23	fibroblast growth factor 23
LCA	lithocholic acid
NAFLD	nonalcoholic fatty liver disease

NASH	nonalcoholic steatohepatitis
RXR	retinoid X receptor
UV	ultraviolet
VDBP	vitamin D-binding protein
VDR	vitamin D receptor
VDRE	vitamin D response element

31.1 Vitamin D metabolism

31.1.1 Dietary uptake and endogenous synthesis of vitamin D

In contrast to other vitamins, the supply of vitamin D is not solely dependent on its dietary uptake because the human organism is able to produce it endogenously in the skin. In fact only a few foods (e.g., fatty fish) contain high levels of vitamin D. Therefore its intake from unfortified foods accounts only for a relatively small proportion that is usually not sufficient to ensure an adequate overall supply. Vitamin D exists in two different forms, namely cholecalciferol (vitamin D3), which is present in foods from animal origin, and ergocalciferol (vitamin D2), which is present in plants and fungi. In principle, both cholecalciferol and ergocalciferol can be converted into biologically active vitamin D metabolites (i.e., 1,25(OH)2 vitamin D3 and 1,25(OH)2 vitamin D2, respectively; see below). However, both forms have slightly different metabolic fates, resulting in slower metabolic turnover and greater biological activity of cholecalciferol over ergocalciferol (Hollis, 1984; Horst et al., 1986; Houghton and Vieth, 2006). As consequence the intake of cholecalciferol seems to be more efficient than that of ergocalciferol with regard to ensuring an adequate vitamin D status (Tripkovic et al., 2012).

Endogenous synthesis of cholecalciferol (vitamin D3) in the skin is a nonenzymatic two-step process that requires ultraviolet (UV) radiation from sunlight (Deluca, 2014) (Fig. 31.1). The substrate for the first step of this reaction is 7-dehydrocholesterol, an intermediate of the cholesterol synthesis pathway. In the skin, UV light breaks up the so-called B-ring of 7-dehydrocholesterol leading to the formation of previtamin D3. In the second step of the reaction, which is thermosensitive but also nonenzymatic, the previtamin D3 then isomerizes to vitamin D3.

Endogenous synthesis of vitamin D3 is dependent on various factors such as skin pigmentation, season, latitude, and altitude (Holick, 1987). Importantly, vitamin D3 synthesis is dependent of UV light with a specific wavelength of 280–315 nm, termed UV-B radiation. In contrast, UV-A light (315–380 nm) is much less efficient. The ratio between UV-A and

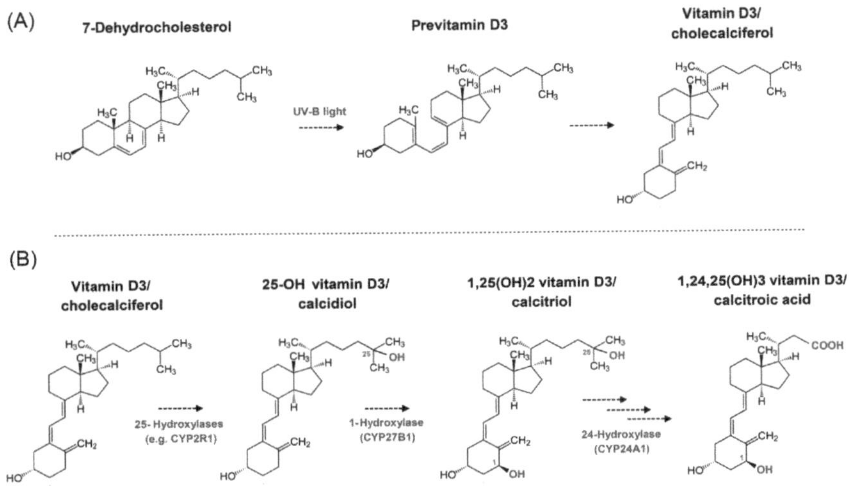

Figure 31.1 ***Synthesis, activation, and catabolism of vitamin D3 metabolites.*** (A) Endogenous synthesis of vitamin D3 is a nonenzymatic reaction that requires a 7-dehydrocholesterol substrate and UV-B light with a wavelength between 280 and 315 nm. The B-ring of the 7-dehydrocholesterol precursor is broken by UV-B light resulting in the formation of previtamin D3, which then isomerizes spontaneously to vitamin D3. (B) Vitamin D3 is actively hydroxylated at various positions by different cytochrome P450 mixed-function oxidases (CYPs). Hydroxylation at C25 is mediated by CYP2R1 (and others) resulting in the formation of 25-OH vitamin D3 as the major circulating form of vitamin D. Concomitantly, 1α-hydroxylation results in the formation of 1,25(OH)2 vitamin D3, which is regarded as the physiologically most active vitamin D metabolite. The 1α-hydroxylation is carried out by one single known enzyme termed CYP27B1. Finally, CYP24A1 is the most important catabolic enzyme which deactivates vitamin D by a series of reactions resulting in the formation of 1,24,25(OH)3 vitamin D3.

UV-B radiation reaching the surface of the earth is strongly dependent on the incidence angle of the sunlight. The efficient synthesis of vitamin D3 in the skin is therefore not possible in winter months in areas of the world exceeding a certain latitude, even when the weather is sunny (Engelsen et al., 2005). Hence the further people live from the equator, the less time of the year they can rely on solar exposure to ensure sufficient dermal production of vitamin D3. In addition to this, many aspects of modern lifestyle (e.g., indoor work, long clothing, and sunblocker) may hamper the sufficient production of vitamin D3 even in areas with favorable solar exposure. Due to these circumstances, vitamin D deficiency is a phenomenon frequently observed in the general population of many countries (Holick, 2007).

31.1.2 Vitamin D metabolites

After being synthesized in the skin or taken up from the diet, vitamin D is transported through the blood circulation and can thus be metabolized in other organs and cell types (Fig. 31.2). Only a very small fraction of all vitamin D metabolites (~1%) are transported as free molecules in the blood while the vast majority are bound to a carrier protein termed the

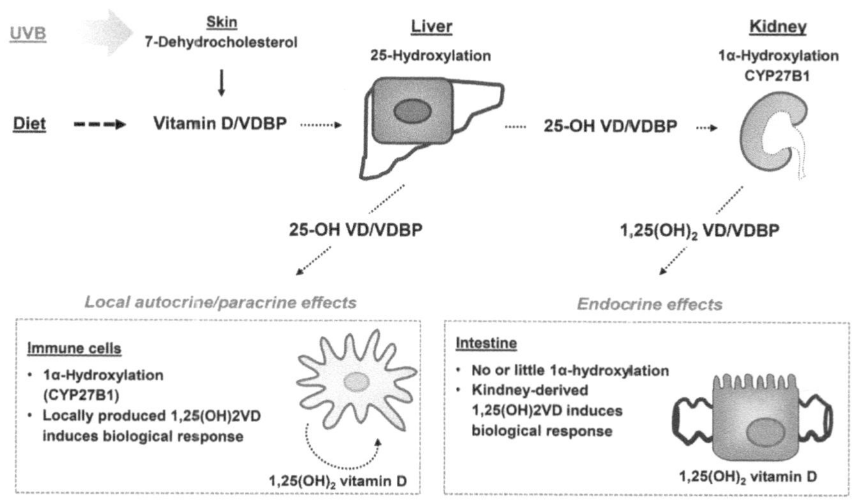

Figure 31.2 ***Various organs and cell types contribute to vitamin D metabolism.*** After its synthesis in the skin or its uptake from the diet, vitamin D is transported to the liver via the bloodstream. The liver is the major organ for the 25-hydroxylation of vitamin D resulting in the formation of 25-OH vitamin D (25-OH VD), which is the main vitamin D metabolite present in the circulation. In the kidney, 25-OH is converted into 1,25(OH)2 vitamin D (1,25(OH)2 VD) as the biologically active form of vitamin D. Kidney-derived 1,25(OH)2 vitamin D is released into the bloodstream and can act as an endocrine signaling molecule in vitamin D—responsive tissues expressing the vitamin D receptor (VDR). These tissues include, for example, the intestine. Here, active 1,25(OH)2 vitamin D is important for calcium homeostasis by regulating the expression of calcium transporters in enterocytes. Besides this endocrine function, vitamin D can also act as a signaling molecule in a locally more restricted manner. This is for example the case for various immune cell types, which express CYP27B1 and are therefore able to locally activate the 25-OH vitamin D present in the circulation. Most immune cells also express VDR and are therefore able to respond to 1,25(OH)2 vitamin D. With few exceptions, vitamin D—responsive cells are able to catabolize 1,25(OH)2 vitamin D via the action of CYP24A1 thus avoiding the accumulation of toxic levels. In general, the vast majority (~99%) of all vitamin D metabolites present in the circulation is bound to serum proteins such as albumin or the vitamin D-binding protein (VDBP).

vitamin D-binding protein (VDBP) (White and Cooke, 2000). The three major steps in the metabolism of vitamin D (either in the form of cholecalciferol or ergocalciferol) are 25-hydroxylation, 1α-hydroxylation, and 24-hydroxylation (Fig. 31.1). These reactions are performed by a group of different enzymes which are located in the mitochondria or the endoplasmic reticulum and belong to the protein family of cytochrome P450 mixed-function oxidases (CYPs) (Bikle, 2014).

The initial step of vitamin D metabolism is its 25-hydroxylation giving rise to either 25-OH vitamin D3/calcidiol or 25-OH vitamin D2 depending on which precursor is used as substrate. The liver is the major organ for the production of 25-OH vitamin D (25-OH VD), and studies in humans and mice demonstrated that this enzymatic reaction can be carried out by the microsomal protein CYP2R1. Moreover, these experiments suggested that CYP2R1 is probably the most important, although not the sole, 25-hydroxylase in both species (Cheng et al., 2003, 2004; Zhu et al., 2013). In addition, various other members of the CYP family may contribute to the overall vitamin D 25-hydroxylation activity of the liver (Bikle, 2014). Irrespective of the contributing enzymes, the 25-hydroxylation of vitamin D appears not to be a major target of regulation. Thus the 25-OH VD blood level is a valid indicator for the long-term overall supply with vitamin D that is routinely measured in clinical practice.

The second step in vitamin D metabolism is the 1α-hydroxylation of 25-OH vitamin D3 or 25-OH vitamin D2 to either 1,25(OH2) vitamin D3/calcitriol or 1,25(OH)2 vitamin D2, respectively. In contrast to 25-hydroxylation, 1α-hydroxylation is performed by one single enzyme in a physiologically tightly regulated process. The protein responsible for the generation of 1,25(OH)2 vitamin D is CYP27B1 which is highly expressed in the kidney (Fu et al., 1997; Shinki et al., 1997; St-Arnaud et al., 1997; Takeyama et al., 1997), but is also present in some other cell types including certain immune cells. The kidney is considered as the major source of 1,25(OH)2 vitamin D present in the circulation. Regulation of renal CYP27B1 expression and activity is complex and requires the integration of various endocrine signals including parathyroid hormone, fibroblast growth factor 23 (FGF23), and 1,25(OH)2 vitamin D itself (Bikle, 2014). In contrast, the regulation of extrarenal CYP27B1 differs and extrarenal CYP27B1 activity seems to be more important to produce 1,25(OH)2 vitamin D in a locally restricted manner (e.g., as a regulator of immune cell function; (Mora et al., 2008)). Independent of the tissue or cell type, 1α-hydroxylation can be regarded as the key activation step to produce 1,25(OH)2 vitamin D, which is the most potent natural ligand of the nuclear vitamin D receptor (VDR) and is therefore the biologically most active form of vitamin D.

The 24-hydroxylation is the third important step of vitamin D metabolism and is carried out by only one single known enzyme, namely CYP24A1. This reaction produces 1,24,25(OH)3 vitamin D3/calcitroic acid from 1,25(OH)2 vitamin D3 or 1,24,25(OH)3 vitamin D2 from 1,25 (OH)2 vitamin D2. Although 1,24,25(OH)3 vitamin D is biologically not completely inactive and can promote VDR-mediated gene expression, it is less potent than 1,25(OH)2 vitamin D (Teske et al., 2016; Yu and Arnold, 2016). In addition, the 1,24,25(OH)3 vitamin D metabolite is a substrate for further chemical modifications and subsequent urinary excretion. Thus 24-hydroxylation can be regarded as an initial catabolic reaction limiting the biological response to active vitamin D metabolites and avoiding their accumulation to toxic levels. Consistent with this notion, the deletion of *Cyp24a1* in mice or inactivating mutations of *CYP24A1* in humans cause several disease phenotypes including elevated 1,25(OH)2 vitamin D levels and severe hypercalcemia (Schlingmann et al., 2011; St-Arnaud et al., 2000). CYP24A1 can also hydroxylate 25-OH vitamin D to 24,25(OH)2 vitamin D and several lines of evidence suggest that the latter metabolite may also have some biological activity (Bikle, 2014).

31.2 The nuclear vitamin D receptor

31.2.1 Ligands of vitamin D receptor

Although vitamin D has some nongenomic actions (e.g., reviewed in Hii and Ferrante, 2016), most of its biological effects are directly mediated on the transcriptional level. Virtually all of these direct transcriptional effects of vitamin D require the nuclear VDR (Bouillon et al., 2008; Haussler et al., 1998). VDR is a ligand-activated transcription factor and a member of the superfamily of nuclear steroid hormone receptors. On the structural level, the VDR protein shares the general domain organization of nuclear receptors, which generally comprise three major parts: The N-terminal DNA-binding domain, the C-terminal ligand binding domain, and a flexible hinge domain in the middle part of the polypeptide (Fig. 31.3).

The ligand binding domain of VDR consists of 12 helices and, as the name suggests, mediates binding of VDR ligands to the protein. As already indicated above, 1,25(OH)2 vitamin D is generally regarded as the most potent natural ligand of VDR stimulating VDR's transcriptional

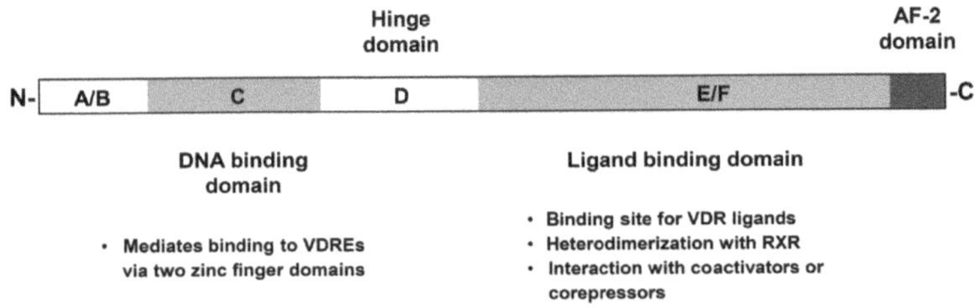

Figure 31.3 ***Protein domains of the vitamin D receptor (VDR).*** Human VDR exists in two isoforms: a shorter isoform of 427 amino acids and a longer variant of 477 amino acids with an N-terminal extension of the A/B domain. VDR is a member of the superfamily of nuclear hormone receptors. These share a common domain structure that comprises an N-terminal DNA-binding domain (C domain), a structurally flexible hinge domain in the middle (D domain), and a C-terminal ligand binding domain (E/F domain). In the case of VDR, the DNA-binding domain mediates binding to VDR response elements (VDREs) on the DNA via two zinc fingers. The ligand binding domain binds VDR ligands including 1,25(OH)2 vitamin D and lithocholic acid (LCA). Moreover, this domain is required for the interaction with retinoid X receptor (RXR) and other coactivator or corepressor proteins regulating VDR-mediated transcription. The AF-2 domain at the very C-terminus of the protein is thought to contribute to cofactor recruitment and is essential for VDR's ability to induce transcription of its target genes. The hinge domain in the middle part of the protein is important for structural flexibility and allows VDR to bind to different VDREs and different chromatin structures.

activity within the low nanomolar (nM) range. In contrast, other endogenous vitamin D metabolites including cholecalciferol, 25-OH VD, or 1,24,25(OH)3 vitamin D have much less or almost no activity on VDR. Another potent natural ligand of VDR is lithocholic acid (LCA), which activates human VDR at the low micromolar (μM) level (Makishima et al., 2002) (Fig. 31.4). In contrast to 1,25(OH)2 vitamin D, LCA is not a vitamin D metabolite, but is a secondary bile acid that is produced by intestinal bacteria from the primary bile acid chenodeoxycholic acid. LCA is a very hydrophobic molecule and is toxic to cells including hepatocytes and enterocytes at high concentrations. Activation of intestinal VDR by LCA leads to the induction of enzymes of the CYP family (CYP3A), thus promoting its detoxification and protecting cells from the toxic and potentially carcinogenic effects of LCA (Makishima et al., 2002).

Next to these natural VDR ligands, a number of synthetic VDR agonists have been developed and are either approved or currently being tested in clinical trials for the treatment of various human diseases including osteoporosis, psoriasis, cancer, and others (Bikle, 2014; Plum and DeLuca, 2010).

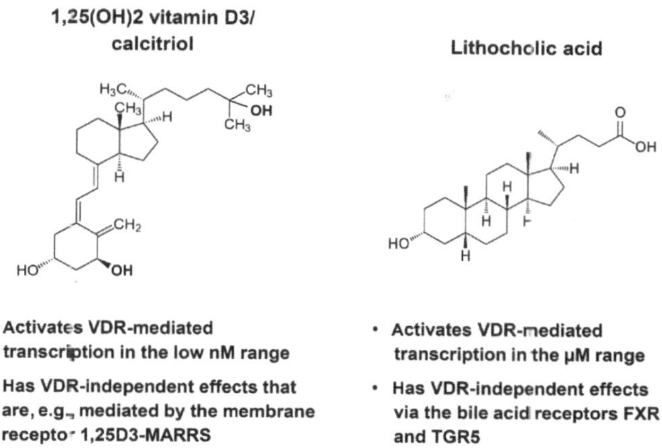

Figure 31.4 ***Chemical structures and biological properties of the two endogenous vitamin D receptor (VDR) ligands 1,25(OH)2 vitamin D and lithocholic acid (LCA).*** 1,25(OH)2 vitamin D is the most potent endogenous vitamin D metabolite activating VDR at the low nanomolar (nM) range. Besides VDR, some biological actions of 1,25 (OH)2 vitamin D are mediated via the membrane-associated rapid response steroid (MARRS) binding protein. In contrast to 1,25(OH)2 vitamin D, LCA is not a vitamin D metabolite but a secondary bile acid that is produced by intestinal bacteria from the primary bile acid chenodeoxycholic acid. LCA activates VDR in the micromolar (μM) range. Besides VDR, LCA also activates the bile acid receptors farnesoid X receptor (FXR) and Takeda G-protein receptor 5 (TGR5).

31.2.2 DNA binding of vitamin D receptor at vitamin D response elements

The DNA-binding domain of VDR mediates its binding to the DNA. This DNA–protein interaction is facilitated by two zinc finger domains within the VDR DNA-binding domain and is known to occur at discrete chromatin sites, so-called vitamin D response elements (VDREs). There is a substantial variability with regard to the nucleotide sequence of the DNA at these VDREs. However, most VDREs with high affinity for VDR are direct repeats of six nucleotides (i.e., on half-site) with a spacing of three nucleotides between the two half-sites. This sequence is therefore called a DR-3 motif (for "direct repeat 3"). Functional VDREs can be found at the proximal promoter regions of VDR target genes in close vicinity to their transcriptional start sites. However, VDR binding can also occur at regulatory elements in intronic or intergenic regions which are often located several kilobases away from the transcriptional start sites of their respective target genes (Pike and Meyer, 2014).

VDR and VDREs seem to regulate the expression of a substantial proportion of the genome in a very complex and highly cell type-specific manner. Various studies analyzed VDR-dependent gene regulation on a genome-wide scale using modern techniques such as chromatin immunoprecipitation coupled to next-generation sequencing. These studies suggest that the presence of 1,25(OH)2 vitamin D generally increases VDR binding to VDREs in the genome with several hundred sites being occupied under basal conditions (i.e., absence of 1,25(OH)2 vitamin D) and up to several thousand being occupied after 1,25(OH)2 vitamin D treatment. Importantly, collective analysis of the available datasets from different cells (e.g., osteoblasts, B cells, monocytes, colorectal cancer cells, and hepatic stellate cells) suggests that, although a certain degree of overlap exists, the usage of genomic VDREs differs considerably between distinct cell types (Ding et al., 2013; Heikkinen et al., 2011; Meyer et al., 2010, 2012; Pike and Meyer, 2014; Ramagopalan et al., 2010; Satoh and Tabunoki, 2013). These genome-wide data on VDR binding sites (i.e., the so-called VDR cistrome) are consistent with observations on the transcriptome level, indicating that 1,25(OH)2 vitamin D in fact regulates mRNA expression of distinct subsets of genes in a highly cell type- and tissue-specific manner (summarized in Haussler et al., 2010; Plum and DeLuca, 2010).

31.2.3 Interaction partners of vitamin D receptor

VDR interacts with many different proteins in multimeric complexes to regulate gene expression. These protein interactions are primarily mediated by the C-terminal ligand binding domain of VDR and, in addition to that, by a short additional domain at the very C-terminus, called the AF-2 domain. VDR's ability to transactivate or repress gene expression requires its interaction with many cofactors such as DNA modifying enzymes or proteins of the basal transcriptional machinery which are present in virtually all cells. In addition to that, VDR is thought to interact with various cofactors in a cell type- or tissue-specific manner (Campbell, 2014).

A major interaction partner of VDR, independent of the cell type, is the retinoid X receptor (RXR), which is a universal heterodimerization partner of many nuclear receptors. Heterodimerization of VDR with RXR seems to be an essential prerequisite for VDR-mediated transcriptional activation of most of its target genes (Kraichely and MacDonald, 1998). Consistent with this notion, a large proportion of VDR binding sites in the genome showed a significant overlap with RXR binding irrespective of the analyzed cell type (Pike and Meyer, 2014).

Similarly, it has been established as a general principle in many different cell types that activation of VDR leads to a more relaxed, "open," chromatin structure. This facilitates the recruitment of additional coactivators and, subsequently, the assembly of the basal transcriptional machinery including RNA polymerase. This relaxation of the chromatin structure is generally performed by histone acetyl transferases such as members of the CBP/p300 family. Vice versa gene repression by nonligand bound VDR is frequently associated with the recruitment of histone deacetylases or various corepressors such as hair growth associated or the nuclear corepressors NCOR1 and NCOR2 (reviewed in Campbell, 2014).

31.3 The role of vitamin D and vitamin D receptor in liver health and disease

31.3.1 The epidemiology and pathophysiology of nonalcoholic fatty liver disease as a prototypical chronic liver disease

From a clinical perspective, vitamin D deficiency is widely recognized in the general population and low vitamin D levels are thought to increase the risk for several human disorders including osteoporosis, autoimmune diseases, metabolic disorders, and cancer (Holick, 2007). Interestingly, reductions of circulating 25-OH VD levels are particularly pronounced in chronic liver diseases and are generally associated with increased fibrosis stage in both viral and nonviral etiologies (Baur et al., 2012; Geier, 2011; Petta et al., 2010; Stokes et al., 2013; Targher et al., 2007). A clear causal relationship between low vitamin D status and advanced liver damage can of course not be established from observational clinical studies. However, as pointed out above, the liver is the major organ responsible for the 25-hydroxylation of vitamin D. Moreover, the liver produces bile acids which are required for the intestinal absorption of lipid-soluble molecules including vitamins. One could therefore hypothesize that increased tissue damage in advanced liver disease may, at least in part, mechanistically contribute to the reduced levels of 25-OH VD present in the circulation.

The last part of this chapter will therefore provide a short overview on some clinical aspects of vitamin D metabolism and its molecular modes of action in the context of liver health and disease. This will be focused on the role of vitamin D in nonalcoholic fatty liver disease (NAFLD) as the prototypical chronic liver disease of our time. NAFLD represents an increasingly recognized disease entity with rising prevalence of about one-fourth of the global population. NAFLD is closely linked to obesity, insulin resistance, and type 2 diabetes mellitus. In these patient populations its prevalence increases to up to 70%–90% (Portillo-Sanchez et al., 2015; Younossi et al., 2016). In the early stage, NAFLD is characterized by a noninflammatory accumulation of lipid droplets (steatosis) in parenchymal liver cells (hepatocytes). As the major problem of the disease, it can progress to nonalcoholic steatohepatitis (NASH) which involves the activation of various nonparenchymal cell types such as Kupffer cells (i.e., liver-resident macrophages), infiltrating T cells, or hepatic stellate cells (Arab et al., 2018; Jahn et al., 2016). These processes can then lead to chronic liver inflammation and result in severe tissue damage and fibrosis in a subset of patients. In some affected individuals, NASH can eventually progress to liver cirrhosis and cancer (Fig. 31.5). Due to its high prevalence and its potential progression to end-stage liver disease, NASH is currently among the three most common causes of liver transplantation in the United States and is projected to become an even larger problem in the future (Charlton et al., 2011).

31.3.2 Observational and interventional clinical studies on vitamin D in nonalcoholic fatty liver disease

Vitamin D deficiency is commonly defined as circulating 25-OH VD levels of 30 ng/mL or less. A large body of observational clinical studies suggests a close association of vitamin D deficiency with obesity and metabolic disorders as well as with the incidence and progression of NAFLD. For example, low serum 25-OH VD levels are predictive of future hyperglycemia and insulin resistance in nondiabetic subjects (Forouhi et al., 2008) and are inversely associated with metabolic syndrome (Hypponen et al., 2008). Moreover, low vitamin D levels have been associated with a higher body fat mass and several markers of insulin resistance such as plasma glucose, insulin, HOMA-IR, and adiponectin (Dasarathy et al., 2014; Gannage-Yared et al., 2009; Liu et al., 2009). Decreased 25-OH vitamin D is furthermore closely associated with the histological severity of hepatic steatosis, necroinflammation, and fibrosis in NAFLD (Targher et al., 2007). In addition to that, vitamin D deficiency increases the likelihood of definitive NASH in patients with NAFLD (Nelson et al., 2016).

In addition to this, recent interventional clinical proof-of-concept studies suggest beneficial effects of vitamin D treatment on NAFLD and the metabolic syndrome (Amin et al., 2016; Beilfuss et al., 2012; Geier

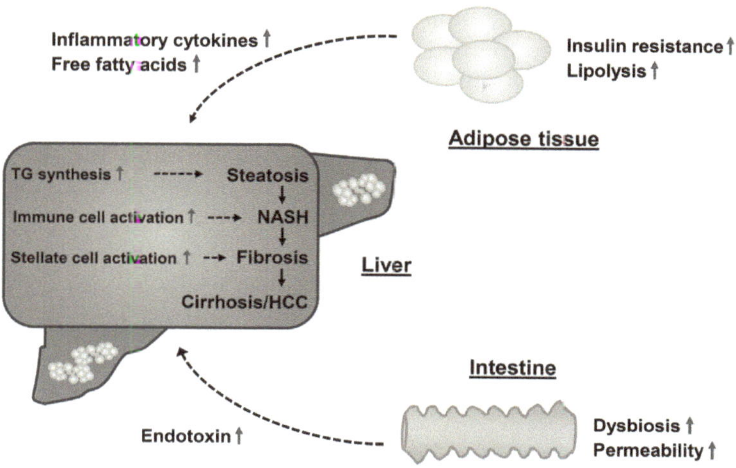

Figure 31.5 ***The pathophysiology of nonalcoholic fatty liver disease (NAFLD) as a prototypic chronic liver disease.*** NAFLD is a complex multiorgan disease involving metabolic and inflammatory changes in liver, adipose tissue, and intestine. Increased release of fatty acids from the insulin-resistant adipose tissue or increased de novo lipogenesis in the liver result in increased triglyceride (TG) accumulation in hepatocytes (liver steatosis). This can induce various metabolic stresses including mitochondrial dysfunction and the generation of reactive oxygen species that trigger the activation of immune cells. This results in disease progression from bland steatosis to nonalcoholic steatohepatitis (NASH). NASH can also be triggered or aggravated by proinflammatory signals coming from the inflamed adipose tissue (e.g., adipocytokines) or by bacterial metabolites such as endotoxin coming from the leaky gut. The metabolic and inflammatory changes present in NASH can lead to hepatocyte apoptosis/necrosis, tissue damage, and, subsequently, scar tissue formation (i.e., liver fibrosis) through the activity of hepatic stellate cells. In a subset of individuals, NASH can eventually progress to liver cirrhosis and/or hepatocellular carcinoma (HCC).

et al., 2018; Papapostoli et al., 2016; Sharifi et al., 2014). In general, these studies observed reductions in liver injury markers (e.g., measured as serum alanine aminotransferase and serum cytokeratin-18 fragments) and noninvasive measures of hepatic steatosis (e.g., ultrasound). Moreover, vitamin D supplementation was found to improve insulin resistance (e.g., measured by homeostatic model assessment; HOMA) as well as markers of systemic low grade inflammation and oxidative stress. As a major fact limiting our current knowledge about the efficacy of vitamin D treatment in progressed stages of NAFLD (i.e., NASH), the definitive diagnosis of NASH can only be made on the histological level and thus requires a liver biopsy. However, with a few exceptions (Geier et al., 2018), the currently available clinical studies have not addressed the effects of vitamin D on liver health in patients with biopsy-proven NASH. Thus further investigation of this aspect is warranted in further clinical trials in patients with histologically-defined NASH.

31.3.3 Vitamin D and vitamin D receptor directly target various pathophysiological processes in nonalcoholic fatty liver disease—insights from preclinical models

31.3.3.1 Effects on adipose tissue

In addition to the clinical data outlined above, there is substantial evidence to suggest direct beneficial effects of vitamin D and VDR on various pathophysiological aspects of NAFLD on the molecular level. The transition from bland liver steatosis to the inflammatory and fibrotic changes seen in NASH can be triggered and promoted by various pathophysiological events in various tissues and organs. These events include the obesity-associated inflammation of the adipose tissue. Adipose tissue inflammation in NAFLD causes two main problems for the liver: first, inflammation promotes adipose tissue insulin resistance leading to uncontrolled lipolysis and increased release of free fatty acids (FFAs) into the circulation. These FFAs are cleared by the liver and promote hepatic steatosis. Second, adipose tissue inflammation leads to an increased release of proinflammatory adipocytokines which act as endocrine signaling molecules and can promote the transition to NASH (Arab et al., 2018).

Macrophage infiltration and a shift from antiinflammatory M2 macrophages to proinflammatory M1 macrophages are thought to play a vital role in the process of adipose tissue inflammation (Boutens and Stienstra, 2016). Both adipocytes and macrophages express VDR and, interestingly, vitamin D has been reported to modulate the macrophage balance favoring M2 polarization in various disease models (Gunasekar et al., 2018; Wasnik et al., 2018; Zhang et al., 2014). The molecular mechanisms underlying these effects are not yet entirely clear. However, these observations suggest that a direct effect of vitamin D on adipocytes and adipose tissue macrophages could also contribute to the metabolic improvements of vitamin D treatment seen in NAFLD.

31.3.3.2 Intestinal effects

Besides adipose tissue, changes in the gut microbiota (i.e., "dysbiosis") and the intestinal immune system play a major role in the pathogenesis of NAFLD (Arab et al., 2018). Obesity-associated intestinal dysbiosis and inflammation can lead to impaired intestinal barrier function by downregulation of tight junction proteins (Al-Sadi and Ma, 2007; Luck et al., 2015;

Winer et al., 2016). Intestinal permeability (also termed "leaky gut") can, in turn, lead to the translocation of bacterial metabolites such as endotoxin or bacterial DNA into the portal and systemic circulation. Increased bacterial metabolites and subsequent activation of Toll-like receptor signaling contribute to metabolic complications in obesity and, in particular, to hepatic inflammation and fibrogenesis in NAFLD (Cani et al., 2008; Gabele et al., 2011; Harte et al., 2010; Rivera et al., 2007). Interestingly, VDR is strongly expressed in enterocytes and has been shown to directly contribute to multiple aspects of intestinal homeostasis. First, VDR regulates the expression of antimicrobial peptides directly on the transcriptional level and loss of VDR expression in $Vdr^{-/-}$ mice has a profound effect on the general composition of the gut microbiota (Campbell et al., 2012; Jin et al., 2015). Second, VDR has been shown to regulate the physiology of intestinal Paneth cells by transcriptional regulation of the autophagy-related *Atg16l1* gene (Wu et al., 2015). Third, vitamin D inhibits proinflammatory nuclear factor kappa B (NF-κB) signaling in intestinal cells via VDR and, fourth, upregulates the tight junction protein claudin-2 as a direct target gene of VDR (Liu et al., 2013; Zhang et al., 2015). These mechanistic studies suggest that vitamin D protects intestinal homeostasis at multiple levels via direct transcription effects on various VDR target genes.

31.3.3.3 Effects on hepatic immune cells and stellate cells

Finally, vitamin D and VDR are thought to exert protective functions directly in the liver tissue, which seem to be mostly mediated by nonparenchymal cells. Amongst other immune cell types, T cells play a major role in the pathogenesis of NAFLD. The progression to NASH is marked by an increased ratio of Th17/resting regulatory T cells in peripheral blood as well as an increased frequency of Th17 in the liver (Rau et al., 2016). Amongst other cytokines, Th17 cells produce IL-17 which promotes the development of NASH and eventually liver cancer in experimental mouse models (Gomes et al., 2016). Importantly, vitamin D has been found to downregulate IL-17 expression in human T cells and in a mouse model of autoimmune encephalomyelitis by a direct transcriptional mechanism involving VDR (Joshi et al., 2011). This suggests that the repression of Th17 cells and IL-17 production by VDR could, at least in part, mechanistically contribute to the beneficial effects of vitamin D supplementation in NAFLD. However, this hypothesis needs further experimental validation.

Liver fibrosis is a strong predictor for long-term mortality in NAFLD patients (Angulo et al., 2015). Consequently, efficient antifibrotic strategies seem to hold promising therapeutic potential for NASH and for the prevention of its progression to end-stage liver disease. Fibrotic changes in NASH are mainly driven by hepatic stellate cells which produce extracellular matrix proteins in response to liver injury, thus leading to scar tissue formation. Interestingly, active vitamin D inhibits the proliferation and profibrotic activity of murine and human hepatic stellate cells via VDR-dependent and independent effects in vitro (Beilfuss et al., 2015; Reiter et al., 2015). The hepatic fibrotic response is primarily governed by transforming growth factor beta (TGFβ) signaling which activates mothers against decapentaplegic homolog (SMAD) transcription factors to drive the expression of profibrotic genes. Detailed mechanistic in vivo studies in $Vdr^{-/-}$ mice have shown that ligand-activated VDR antagonizes SMAD chromatin binding in the context of profibrotic TGFβ signaling and thus protects from liver fibrosis (Ding et al., 2013).

In summary, several observational and interventional clinical studies suggest that vitamin D has multiple liver protective effects in human patients with NAFLD. Various lines of clinical and preclinical evidence suggest that these benefits are mostly mediated via direct transcriptional effects of VDR that occur in different tissues, including adipose tissue, the intestine, and the liver (Geier, 2011) (Table 31.1).

Table 31.1 Potential molecular mechanisms contributing to the therapeutic effects of vitamin D in nonalcoholic fatty liver disease.

Adipose tissue
• Amelioration of adipose tissue inflammation via regulation of M1/M2 macrophage balance.
Intestine
• Regulation of gut microbiota via protection of Paneth cells and production of antimicrobial peptides. • Promotion of intestinal barrier function via upregulation of tight function proteins. • Inhibition of proinflammatory nuclear factor kappa B (NF-κB) signaling.
Liver/systemic inflammation
• Reduction of proinflammatory IL-17 production from Th17 cells. • Antifibrotic effects in hepatic stellate cells by inhibition of TGFβ/SMAD signaling.

References

Al-Sadi, R.M., Ma, T.Y., 2007. IL-1 beta causes an increase in intestinal epithelial tight junction permeability. J. Immunol. 178, 4641–4649.

Amin, H.L., Agah, S., Mousavi, S.N., Hosseini, A.F., Shidfar, F., 2016. Regression of non-alcoholic fatty liver by vitamin D supplement: a double-blind randomized controlled clinical trial. Arch. Iran. Med. 19, 631–638.

Angulo, P., Kleiner, D.E., Dam-Larsen, S., Adams, L.A., Bjornsson, E.S., Charatcharoenwitthaya, P., et al., 2015. Liver fibrosis, but no other histologic features, is associated with long-term outcomes of patients with nonalcoholic fatty liver disease. Gastroenterology 149, 389-397 e310.

Arab, J.P., Arrese, M., Trauner, M., 2018. Recent insights into the pathogenesis of nonalcoholic fatty liver disease. Ann. Rev. Pathol. Mech. Disease 13, 321–350.

Baur, K., Mertens, J.C., Schmitt, J., Iwata, R., Stieger, B., Eloranta, J.J., et al., 2012. Combined effect of 25-OH vitamin D plasma levels and genetic vitamin D receptor (NR 1I1) variants on fibrosis progression rate in HCV patients. Liver Int. 32, 635–643.

Beilfuss, J., Berg, V., Sneve, M., Jorde, R., Kamycheva, E., 2012. Effects of a 1-year supplementation with cholecalciferol on interleukin-6, tumor necrosis factor-alpha and insulin resistance in overweight and obese subjects. Cytokine 60, 870–874.

Beilfuss, A., Sowa, J.P., Sydor, S., Beste, M., Bechmann, L.P., Schlattjan, M., et al., 2015. Vitamin D counteracts fibrogenic TGF-beta signalling in human hepatic stellate cells both receptor-dependently and independently. Gut 64, 791–799.

Bikle, D.D., 2014. Vitamin D metabolism, mechanism of action, and clinical applications. Chem. Biol. 21, 319–329.

Bouillon, R., Carmeliet, G., Verlinden, L., van Etten, E., Verstuyf, A., Luderer, H.F., et al., 2008. Vitamin D and human health: lessons from vitamin D receptor null mice. Endocr. Rev. 29, 726–776.

Boutens, L., Stienstra, R., 2016. Adipose tissue macrophages: going off track during obesity. Diabetologia 59, 879–894.

Campbell, M.J., 2014. Vitamin D and the RNA transcriptome: more than mRNA regulation. Front. Physiol. 5, 181.

Campbell, Y., Fantacone, M.L., Gombart, A.F., 2012. Regulation of antimicrobial peptide gene expression by nutrients and by-products of microbial metabolism. Eur. J. Nutr. 51, 899–907.

Cani, P.D., Bibiloni, R., Knauf, C., Neyrinck, A.M., Neyrinck, A.M., Delzenne, N.M., et al., 2008. Changes in gut microbiota control metabolic endotoxemia-induced inflammation in high-fat diet-induced obesity and diabetes in mice. Diabetes 57, 1470–1481.

Charlton, M.R., Burns, J.M., Pedersen, R.A., Watt, K.D., Heimbach, J.K., Dierkhising, R.A., 2011. Frequency and outcomes of liver transplantation for nonalcoholic steatohepatitis in the United States. Gastroenterology 141, 1249–1253.

Cheng, J.B., Motola D.L., Mangelsdorf, D.J., Russell, D.W., 2003. De-orphanization of cytochrome P450 2R1—a microsomal vitamin D 25-hydroxylase. J. Biol. Chem. 278, 38084–38093.

Cheng, J.B., Levine, M.A., Bell, N.H., Mangelsdorf, D.J., Russell, D.W., 2004. Genetic evidence that the human CYP2R1 enzyme is a key vitamin D 25-hydroxylase. Proc. Natl Acad. Sci. USA 101, 7711–7715.

Dasarathy, J., Periyalwar, P., Allampati, S., Bhinder, V., Hawkins, C., Brandt, P., et al., 2014. Hypovitaminosis D is associated with increased whole body fat mass and greater severity of non-alcoholic fatty liver disease. Liver Int. 34, e118–e127.

Deluca, H.F., 2014. History of the discovery of vitamin D and its active metabolites. Bonekey Rep. 3, 479.
Ding, N., Yu, R.T., Subramaniam, N., Sherman, M.H., Wilson, C., Rao, R., et al., 2013. A vitamin D receptor/SMAD genomic circuit gates hepatic fibrotic response. Cell 153, 601–613.
Engelsen, O., Brustad, M., Aksnes, L., Lund, E., 2005. Daily duration of vitamin D synthesis in human skin with relation to latitude, total ozone, altitude, ground cover, aerosols and cloud thickness. Photochem. Photobiol. 81, 1287–1290.
Forouhi, N.G., Luan, J., Cooper, A., Boucher, B.J., Wareham, N.J., 2008. Baseline serum 25-hydroxy vitamin D is predictive of future glycemic status and insulin resistance: the Medical Research Council Ely Prospective Study 1990–2000. Diabetes 57, 2619–2625.
Fu, G.K., Lin, D., Zhang, M.Y.H., Bikle, D.D., Shackleton, C.H.L., Miller, W.L., et al., 1997. Cloning of human 25-hydroxyvitamin D-1 alpha-hydroxylase and mutations causing vitamin D-dependent rickets type 1. Mol. Endocrinol. 11, 1961–1970.
Gabele, E., Dostert, K., Hofmann, C., Wiest, R., Scholmerich, J., Hellerbrand, C., et al., 2011. DSS induced colitis increases portal LPS levels and enhances hepatic inflammation and fibrogenesis in experimental NASH. J. Hepatol. 55, 1391–1399.
Gannage-Yared, M.H., Chedid, R., Khalife, S., Azzi, E., Zoghbi, F., Halaby, G., 2009. Vitamin D in relation to metabolic risk factors, insulin sensitivity and adiponectin in a young Middle-Eastern population. Eur. J. Endocrinol. 160, 965–971.
Geier, A., 2011. Shedding new light on vitamin D and fatty liver disease. J. Hepatol. 55, 273–275.
Geier, A., Eichinger, M., Stirnimann, G., Semela, D., Tay, F., Seifert, B., et al., 2018. Treatment of non-alcoholic steatohepatitis patients with vitamin D: a double-blinded, randomized, placebo-controlled pilot study. Scand. J. Gastroenterol. 53, 1114–1120.
Gomes, A.L., Teijeiro, A., Buren, S., Tummala, K.S., Yilmaz, M., Waisman, A., et al., 2016. Metabolic inflammation-associated IL-17A causes non-alcoholic steatohepatitis and hepatocellular carcinoma. Cancer Cell. 30, 161–175.
Gunasekar, P., Swier, V.J., Fleegel, J.P., Boosani, C.S., Radwan, M.M., Agrawal, D.K., 2018. Vitamin D and macrophage polarization in epicardial adipose tissue of atherosclerotic swine. PLoS One. 13 (10), e0199411.
Harte, A.L., da Silva, N.F., Creely, S.J., McGee, K.C., Billyard, T., Youssef-Elabd, E.M., et al., 2010. Elevated endotoxin levels in non-alcoholic fatty liver disease. J. Inflamm. (Lond.). 7, 15.
Haussler, M.R., Whitfield, G.K., Haussler, C.A., Hsieh, J.C., Thompson, P.D., Selznick, S.H., et al., 1998. The nuclear vitamin D receptor: biological and molecular regulatory properties revealed. J. Bone Miner. Res. 13, 325–349.
Haussler, M.R., Haussler, C.A., Whitfield, G.K., Hsieh, J.C., Thompson, P.D., Barthel, T.K., et al., 2010. The nuclear vitamin D receptor controls the expression of genes encoding factors which feed the "Fountain of Youth" to mediate healthful aging. J. Steroid Biochem. Mol. Biol. 121, 88–97.
Heikkinen, S., Vaisanen, S., Pehkonen, P., Seuter, S., Benes, V., Carlberg, C., 2011. Nuclear hormone 1 alpha,25-dihydroxyvitamin D-3 elicits a genome-wide shift in the locations of VDR chromatin occupancy. Nucleic Acids Res. 39, 9181–9193.
Hii, C.S., Ferrante, A., 2016. The non-genomic actions of vitamin D. Nutrients 8 (3), 135.
Holick, M.F., 1987. Photosynthesis of vitamin D in the skin: effect of environmental and life-style variables. Fed. Proc. 46, 1876–1882.
Holick, M.F., 2007. Vitamin D deficiency. N.Engl. J. Med. 357, 266–281.
Hollis, B.W., 1984. Comparison of equilibrium and disequilibrium assay conditions for ergocalciferol, cholecalciferol and their major metabolites. J. Steroid Biochem. Mol. Biol. 21, 81–86.

Horst, R.L., Reinhardt, T.A., Ramberg, C.F., Koszewski, N.J., Napoli, J.L., 1986. 24-Hydroxylation of 1,25-dihydroxyergocalciferol—an unambiguous deactivation process. J. Biol. Chem. 261, 9250−9256.

Houghton, L.A., Vieth, R., 2006. The case against ergocalciferol (vitamin D2) as a vitamin supplement. Am. J. Clin. Nutr. 84, 694−697.

Hypponen, E., Boucher, B.J., Berry, D.J., Power, C., 2008. 25-hydroxyvitamin D, IGF-1, and metabolic syndrome at 45 years of age: a cross-sectional study in the 1958 British Birth Cohort. Diabetes 57, 298−305.

Jahn, D., Rau, M., Wohlfahrt, J., Hermanns, H.M., Geier, A., 2016. Non-alcoholic steatohepatitis: from pathophysiology to novel therapies. Dig. Dis. 34, 356−363.

Jin, D.P., Wu, S.P., Zhang, Y.G., Lu, R., Xia, Y.L., Dong, H., et al., 2015. Lack of vitamin D receptor causes dysbiosis and changes the functions of the murine intestinal microbiome. Clin. Ther. 37, 996−1009.

Joshi, S., Pantalena, L.C., Liu, X.K., Gaffen, S.L., Liu, H., Rohowsky-Kochan, C., et al., 2011. 1,25-Dihydroxyvitamin D-3 ameliorates Th17 autoimmunity via transcriptional modulation of interleukin-17A. Mol. Cell. Biol. 31, 3653−3669.

Kraichely, D.M., MacDonald, P.N., 1998. Transcriptional activation through the vitamin D receptor in osteoblasts. Front. Biosci. 3, d821−d833.

Liu, E., Meigs, J.B., Pittas, A.G., McKeown, N.M., Economos, C.D., Booth, S.L., et al., 2009. Plasma 25-hydroxyvitamin d is associated with markers of the insulin resistant phenotype in nondiabetic adults. J. Nutr. 139, 329−334.

Liu, W.C., Chen, Y.Z., Golan, M.A., Annunziata, M.L., Du, J., Dougherty, U., et al., 2013. Intestinal epithelial vitamin D receptor signaling inhibits experimental colitis. J. Clin. Invest. 123, 3983−3996.

Luck, H., Tsai, S., Chung, J., Clemente-Casares, X., Ghazarian, M., Revelo, X.S., et al., 2015. Regulation of obesity-related insulin resistance with gut anti-inflammatory agents. Cell. Metab. 21, 527−542.

Makishima, M., Lu, T.T., Xie, W., Whitfield, G.K., Domoto, H., Evans, R.M., et al., 2002. Vitamin D receptor as an intestinal bile acid sensor. Science 296, 1313−1316.

Meyer, M.B., Goetsch, P.D., Pike, J.W., 2010. Genome-wide analysis of the VDR/RXR cistrome in osteoblast cells provides new mechanistic insight into the actions of the vitamin D hormone. J. Steroid Biochem. Mol. Biol. 121, 136−141.

Meyer, M.B., Goetsch, P.D., Pike, J.W., 2012. VDR-RXR and TCF4/beta-catenin cistromes in colonic cells of colorectal tumor origin: impact on c-FOS and c-MYC gene expression. Mol. Endocrinol. 26, 37−51.

Mora, J.R., Iwata, M., von Andrian, U.H., 2008. Vitamin effects on the immune system: vitamins A and D take centre stage. Nat. Rev. Immunol. 8, 685−698.

Nelson, J.E., Roth, C.L., Wilson, L.A., Yates, K.P., Aouizerat, B., Morgan-Stevenson, V., et al., 2016. Vitamin D deficiency is associated with increased risk of non-alcoholic steatohepatitis in adults with non-alcoholic fatty liver disease: possible role for MAPK and NF-kappaB? Am. J. Gastroenterol. 111, 852−863.

Papapostoli, I., Lammert, F., Stokes, C.S., 2016. Effect of short-term vitamin D correction on hepatic steatosis as quantified by controlled attenuation parameter (CAP). J. Gastrointest. Liver Dis. 25, 175−181.

Petta, S., Camma, C., Scazzone, C., Tripodo, C., Di Marco, V., Bono, A., et al., 2010. Low vitamin d serum level is related to severe fibrosis and low responsiveness to interferon-based therapy in genotype 1 chronic hepatitis C. Hepatology 51, 1158−1167.

Pike, J.W., Meyer, M.B., 2014. Fundamentals of vitamin D hormone-regulated gene expression. J. Steroid Biochem. Mol. Biol. 144, 5−11.

Plum, L.A., DeLuca H.F., 2010. Vitamin D, disease and therapeutic opportunities. Nat. Rev. Drug Discov. 9, 941−955.

Portillo-Sanchez, P., Bril, F., Maximos, M., Lomonaco, R., Biernacki, D., Orsak, B., et al., 2015. High prevalence of nonalcoholic fatty liver disease in patients with type 2 diabetes mellitus and normal plasma aminotransferase levels. J. Clin. Endocrinol. Metab. 100, 2231–2238.

Ramagopalan, S.V., Heger, A., Berlanga, A.J., Maugeri, N.J., Lincoln, M.R., Burrell, A., et al., 2010. A ChIP-seq defined genome-wide map of vitamin D receptor binding: Associations with disease and evolution. Genome Res. 20, 1352–1360.

Rau, M., Schilling, A.K., Meertens, J., Hering, I., Weiss, J., Jurowich, C., et al., 2016. Progression from nonalcoholic fatty liver to nonalcoholic steatohepatitis is marked by a higher frequency of Th17 cells in the liver and an increased Th17/resting regulatory T cell ratio in peripheral blood and in the liver. J. Immunol. 196, 97–105.

Reiter, F.P., Hohenester, S., Nagel, J.M., Wimmer, R., Artmann, R., Wottke, L., et al., 2015. 1,25-(OH)(2)-vitamin D-3 prevents activation of hepatic stellate cells in vitro and ameliorates inflammatory liver damage but not fibrosis in the Abcb4(−/−) model. Biochem. Biophys. Res. Commun. 459, 227–233.

Rivera, C.A., Adegboyega, P., van Rooijen, N., Tagalicud, A., Allman, M., Wallace, M., 2007. Toll-like receptor-4 signaling and Kupffer cells play pivotal roles in the pathogenesis of non-alcoholic steatohepatitis. J. Hepatol. 47, 571–579.

Satoh, J., Tabunoki, H., 2013. Molecular network of chromatin immunoprecipitation followed by deep sequencing-based vitamin D receptor target genes. Mult. Scler. J. 19, 1035–1045.

Schlingmann, K.P., Kaufmann, M., Weber, S., Irwin, A., Goos, C., John, U., et al., 2011. Mutations in CYP24A1 and idiopathic infantile hypercalcemia. N. Engl. J. Med. 365, 410–421.

Sharifi, N., Amani, R., Hajiani, E., Cheraghian, B., 2014. Does vitamin D improve liver enzymes, oxidative stress, and inflammatory biomarkers in adults with non-alcoholic fatty liver disease? A randomized clinical trial. Endocrine 47, 70–80.

Shinki, T., Shimada, H., Wakino, S., Anazawa, H., Hayashi, M., Saruta, T., et al., 1997. Cloning and expression of rat 25-hydroxyvitamin D3-1alpha-hydroxylase cDNA. Proc. Natl. Acad. Sci. USA 94, 12920–12925.

St-Arnaud, R., Messerlian, S., Moir, J.M., Omdahl, J.L., Glorieux, F.H., 1997. The 25-hydroxyvitamin D 1-alpha-hydroxylase gene maps to the pseudovitamin D deficiency rickets (PDDR) disease locus. J. Bone Miner. Res. 12, 1552–1559.

St-Arnaud, R., Arabian, A., Travers, R., Barletta, F., Raval-Pandya, M., Chapin, K., et al., 2000. Deficient mineralization of intramembranous bone in vitamin D-24-hydroxylase-ablated mice is due to elevated 1,25-dihydroxyvitamin D and not to the absence of 24,25-dihydroxyvitamin D. Endocrinology 141, 2658–2666.

Stokes, C.S., Volmer, D.A., Grunhage, F., Lammert, F., 2013. Vitamin D in chronic liver disease. Liver Int. 33, 338–352.

Takeyama, K., Kitanaka, S., Sato, T., Kobori, M., Yanagisawa, J., Kato, S., 1997. 25-Hydroxyvitamin D3 1alpha-hydroxylase and vitamin D synthesis. Science 277, 1827–1830.

Targher, G., Bertolini, L., Scala, L., Cigolini, M., Zenari, L., Falezza, G., et al., 2007. Associations between serum 25-hydroxyvitamin D3 concentrations and liver histology in patients with non-alcoholic fatty liver disease. Nutr. Metab. Cardiovasc. Dis. 17, 517–524.

Teske, K.A., Bogart, J.W., Sanchez, L.M., Yu, O.B., Preston, J.V., Cook, J.M., et al., 2016. Synthesis and evaluation of vitamin D receptor-mediated activities of cholesterol and vitamin D metabolites. Eur. J. Med. Chem. 109, 238–246.

Tripkovic, L., Lambert, H., Hart, K., Smith, C.P., Bucca, G., Penson, S., et al., 2012. Comparison of vitamin D2 and vitamin D3 supplementation in raising serum

25-hydroxyvitamin D status: a systematic review and meta-analysis. Am. J. Clin. Nutr. 95, 1357–1364.
Wasnik, S., Rundle, C.H., Baylink, D.J., Yazdi, M.S., Carreon, E.E., Xu, Y., et al., 2018. 1,25-Dihydroxyvitamin D suppresses M1 macrophages and promotes M2 differentiation at bone injury sites. JCI Insight 3, 98773.
White, P., Cooke, N., 2000. The multifunctional properties and characteristics of vitamin D-binding protein. Trends Endocrinol. Metab. 11, 320–327.
Winer, D.A., Luck, H., Tsai, S., Winer, S., 2016. The intestinal immune system in obesity and insulin resistance. Cell Metab. 23, 413–426.
Wu, S.P., Zhang, Y.G., Lu, R., Xia, Y.L., Zhou, D., Petrof, E.O., et al., 2015. Intestinal epithelial vitamin D receptor deletion leads to defective autophagy in colitis. Gut 64, 1082–1094.
Younossi, Z.M., Koenig, A.B., Abdelatif, D., Fazel, Y., Henry, L., Wymer, M., 2016. Global epidemiology of nonalcoholic fatty liver disease-meta-analytic assessment of prevalence, incidence, and outcomes. Hepatology 64, 73–84.
Yu, O.B., Arnold, L.A., 2016. Calcitroic acid—a review. ACS Chem. Biol. 11, 2665–2672.
Zhang, X.L., Guo, Y.F., Song, Z.X., Zhou, M., 2014. Vitamin D prevents podocyte injury via regulation of macrophage M1/M2 phenotype in diabetic nephropathy rats. Endocrinology 155, 4939–4950.
Zhang, Y.G., Wu, S.P., Lu, R., Zhou, D., Zhou, J.S., Carmeliet, G., et al., 2015. Tight junction CLDN2 gene is a direct target of the vitamin D receptor. Sci. Rep. 5, 10642.
Zhu, J.G., Ochalek, J.T., Kaufmann, M., Jones, G., DeLuca, H.F., 2013. CYP2R1 is a major, but not exclusive, contributor to 25-hydroxyvitamin D production in vivo. Proc. Natl Acad. Sci. USA 110, 15650–15655.

CHAPTER 32

Vitamin B3: niacin and transcriptome analysis in relation to the GPR109A receptor

Allison Bridges, Pragya Rajpurohit, Puttur D. Prasad and Muthusamy Thangaraju
Department of Biochemistry and Molecular Biology, Augusta University, Augusta, GA, United States

Contents

Key facts of GPR109A and tumor suppression

- Nicotinic acid-induced GPR109A activation potentiates antitumor immunity, antiinflammatory, and antitumor signaling in a number of cell types and tissues.
- Antiinflammatory effects of GPR109A on immune signaling have been demonstrated in retinal pigment epithelium and neurons, to protect against retinal degradation during diabetes and Parkinson's disease, respectively.

Molecular Nutrition
DOI: https://doi.org/10.1016/B978-0-12-811907-5.00031-2

- Butyrate-mediated activation of GPR109A has been demonstrated to improve inflammation in the colon through regulation of immune regulations and proliferation.
- This mediation of inflammation has been demonstrated to also decrease the incidence of colorectal cancer, presenting GPR109A as a potential tumor suppressor.
- The tumor suppressive effects of butyrate/GPR109A have been demonstrated in breast tissue as well, for the breast produces butyrate in significant quantities for activation during lactation.
- NA deficiency is associated with increased tumor incidence and NA supplementation, along with vitamin C, increases the overall survival from 10 to 122 months (~12 times more overall survival)

Summary points

- This chapter focuses on GPR109A, a Gαi protein-coupled receptor for vitamin B_3 or niacin.
- Niacin or nicotinic acid (NA) is an essential dietary supplement, which has been utilized as an antidyslipidemic drug for more than 50 years without its mechanism being fully understood.
- Although niacin is a ligand for GPR109A, the normal circulating level of NA (~0.2 μM) is not sufficient to activate GPR109A because the EC_{50} for NA to activate GPR10A is ~1.0 μM.
- The ketone body β-hydroxybutyrate and short-chain fatty acid butyrate are physiological endogenous ligands for GPR109A.
- Endogenous ligands have been demonstrated in a variety of studies to have tissue-specific effects in lipid regulation, cellular metabolism, and inflammation.
- Research in colon and breast cancer suggests that GPR109A is also a tumor suppressor and can be a valid target for further cancer therapeutic studies.

Abbreviations

AC	adenylate cyclase
cAMP	cyclic adenosine monophosphate
DNMT	DNA methyltransferases
FFAs	free fatty acids
HDAC	histone deacetylase
NA	nicotinic acid
NAD	nicotinamide adenine dinucleotide

NAM	niacinamide or nicotinamide
PD	parkinson's disease
RPE	retinal pigment epithelium
TAG	triacylglycerol
Trp	tryptophan
SMCT1 or SLC5A8	sodium-coupled monocarboxylate transporter

32.1 Introduction

GPR109A is a G protein-coupled receptor that belongs to a G_i ($G_{inhibitory}$) subfamily of receptors that includes GPR109B and GPR81 (Offermanns, 2006). While it is not utilized as a vitamin, GPR109A is the only known receptor for vitamin B_3, also known as niacin or nicotinic acid (NA). Deficiency in niacin was once quite common, a condition that would eventually lead to death. However, once the relevance of niacin's physiological importance was grasped, fortifying food types, particularly grain products, all but eliminated such a deficiency as a cause for malady. NA has also been utilized as an antidyslipidemic drug for several years, but only recently has its mechanism of action through GPR109A been understood. GPR109A is able to limit the release of free fatty acids, thereby lowering the levels of harmful lipids in the plasma that increase the risk factors associated with cardiovascular disease and elevating cardioprotective lipids. However, the effects of NA are not merely isolated to adipocyte regulation of fat storage. Following the discovery of GPR109A, its expression was found in significant levels in the spleen, immune cells, colon, retinal pigment epithelial cells, and breast tissue. While NA is the pharmacological agent primarily used to activate GPR109A, two endogenous ligands of GPR109A have been identified, the ketone body β-hydroxybuturate and short-chain fatty acid butyrate. These endogenous ligands have tissue-specific effects that play a role in cellular metabolism and, surprisingly, inflammation. GPR109A has been shown in several studies to have a role in regulating antiinflammatory and proinflammatory molecules in various tissues. Studies in breast and colon cancer have also suggested that GPR109A activation may also function as a tumor suppressor. GPR109A is therefore a unique receptor that has pleiotropic potential as a target for future therapeutics.

32.2 GPR109A: a receptor for niacin

32.2.1 Niacin: the antidyslipidemic vitamin

Niacin (NA), vitamin B3, is one of the most essential human nutrients with the molecular formula $C_6H_5NO_2$. NA is a colorless water-soluble

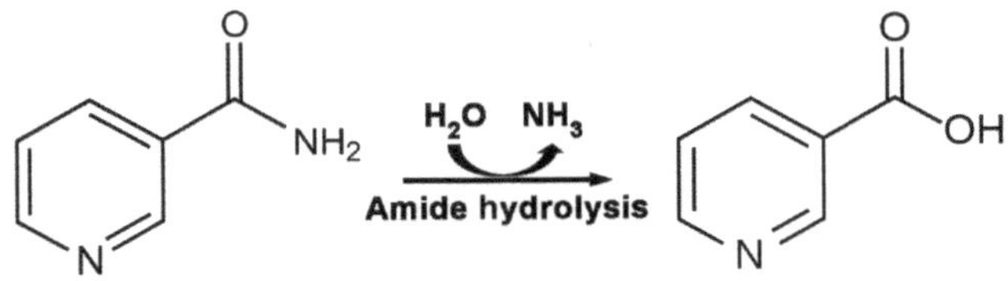

Figure 32.1 Conversion of nicotinamide nicotinamide (NAM) into niacin (NA): hydrolysis of NAM will release ammonia (NH_3) and produce NA.

vitamin and is a derivative of pyridine with a carboxyl group (COOH) at the 3-position (Fig. 32.1). NA and niacinamide or nicotinamide (NAM) are both often utilized as supplements, their names being used interchangeably in reference to their physiological effects. Both NA and NAM are the dietary precursors for the coenzyme nicotinamide adenine dinucleotide (NAD), the metabolic cofactor that is necessary for basic cellular metabolism, energy production, and certain enzymatic reactions that consume NAD to generate by-products (Srivastava, 2016). NAD is most often designated as NAD^+ to highlight its oxidized form and its potential to be reduced to NADH. NAD^+/NADH interconvert between their oxidized and reduced states to facilitate enzymatic reactions, redox reactions, and the generation of new components in different aspects of cellular metabolism (Fig. 32.2). From progression through glycolysis and the TCA cycle to providing the reduction reaction necessary at complex I of the electron transport chain to eventually generate adenosine triphosphate (ATP), the NAD^+/NADH ratio is essential for cell function, with changes in the ratio altering metabolism and changing energy production based upon the available resources. The largest source of NAD comes from the consumption of dietary NA, the recommended daily intake being 14–16 mg for adult men and women, respectively (Bogan and Brenner, 2008). NA or any of its various derivatives can then be converted into NAD^+ via the salvage pathway. NAD^+ can also be generated through de novo synthesis from tryptophan (Trp) but to a lesser extent. A deficiency in NA or Trp results in a disease known as pellagra, a reversible condition characterized by diarrhea, dermatitis, and dementia. Efforts made to eradicate this condition, which was once very common among the poor, even in the rural United States in the early 20th century, led to the discovery and subsequent understanding of NAD^+. Therefore today, due to the enrichment of many affordable foods with NA, cases of

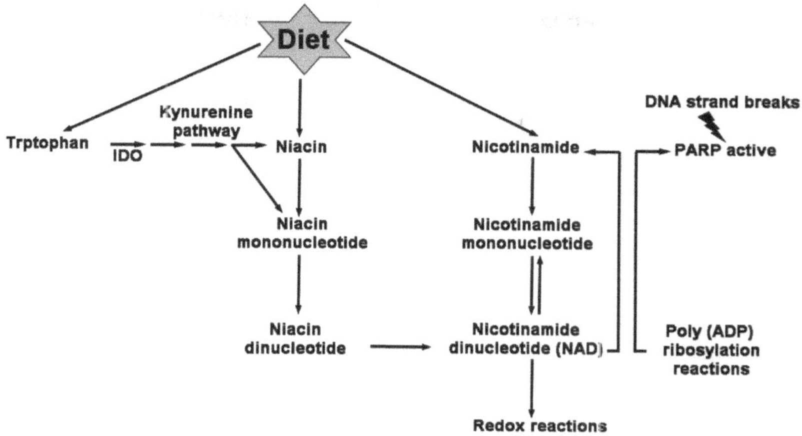

Figure 32.2 Synthesis of niacin from the amino acid tryptophan (Trp). Niacin can be also synthesized from the diet via the amino acid Trp through the kynurenine pathway. The first step is catalyzed by the extrahepatic enzyme indoleamine 2,3-dioxygenase (IDO), which is responsible for the oxidative cleavage of tryptophan, and leads to the synthesis of niacin (NA) nicotinamide (NAM) and nicotinamide adenine dinucleotide (NAD) In healthy individuals, less than 2% of dietary Trp is converted to NAD by this Trp oxidation pathway. On average 1 mg of NA can be synthesized from 60 mg of Trp.

pellagra are rare. However, these early studies with NA did more than just eliminate pellagra, demonstrating NA's greater importance to maintaining health as a whole.

In the 1950s NA was discovered to have properties for use as an antidyslipidemic drug (Altschul et al., 1955). Some of the first studies examined adipose tissue, where it was discovered NA was able to reduce the levels of free fatty acids (FFAs) that circulated in the plasma (Carlson and Oro, 1962). This altered the lipid profile, reducing triacylglycerol (TAG), very-low-density lipoprotein (VLDL), and low-density lipoprotein levels in the plasma, which was accompanied by an increase in high-density lipoprotein (HDL) levels and a decrease in Lp(a), a risk factor for coronary heart disease, suggesting that NA has both cardioprotective and antidyslipidemic effects (Carlson, 1963; Carlson et al., 1989; Shepherd et al., 1979). Further studies have confirmed its clinical usefulness. NA was marketed as the first antidyslipidemic drug rather than a cardioprotective agent, mainly due to the fact that high dosing of NA often results in the unexpected side effect of flushing (Carlson, 2005). Interestingly, NAM does not cause the flushing that is commonly associated with NA.

Therefore further studies sought to alleviate this side effect of NA and understand its mechanism of action.

It was demonstrated early on that NA had an effect on the accumulation of cyclic adenosine monophosphate (cAMP) in the isolated fat cells (Butcher et al., 1968). It was later reconfirmed and demonstrated that NA decreases the activity of adenylate cyclase (AC), the enzyme responsible for converting ATP to cAMP (Aktories et al., 1980). ACs are regulated by G protein-coupled receptors, meaning that NA has an indirect effect on AC through a specific G protein-coupled receptor (Sadana and Dessauer, 2009). This proposed mechanism of action helped to explain the immediate effects of NA on FFA levels, the production which is directly under cAMP control, and the delayed response on the rest of the lipoproteins altered. Therefore the search for the G protein-coupled receptor responsible began.

32.2.2 GPR109A receptor discovery and its agonists

Wise et al. (2003) discovered that there were two receptors for NA, following a screening of orphan G protein-coupled receptors that are highly expressed in adipose tissue and spleen. Low-affinity receptor HM74 and high-affinity receptor HM74A were their original designations; HM74A is a paralogue of HM74. PUMA-G was also discovered to be the mouse variant of HM74A. But Tunaru et al. (2003) in the same year took this study a step further and described a proposed mechanism for how NA works through its receptor. HM74A and PUMA-G were found to be highly expressed on white and brown adipose tissues of human and mouse, respectively, where NA bound with high affinity to both receptors, triggering the release of Ca^{2+} to inhibit AC activity and decrease FFA release from adipocytes. A parallel study conducted by Soga et al. (2003) further analyzed the binding of NA and found that NA bound with high affinity to human HM74A and mouse PUMA-G but with a much lower affinity to HM74, suggesting that NA effects are primarily mediated through HM74A/PUMA-G. Subsequently, PUMA-G-deficient mice were shown to have reduced NA binding affinity at adipocytes plasma membranes. NA also failed to decrease FFA release from adipocytes following starvation or to decrease TAG levels in PUMA-G-deficient mice placed on a high-fat diet. Nevertheless, PUMA-G and HM74A may mediate the effects of NA following treatment, but NA is not the physiological ligand of these receptors. NA plasma and serum concentrations are low under normal physiological conditions (100–400 nM), significantly lower than the given dosage in these experiments, suggesting another endogenous ligand for PUMA-G and HM74A must exist.

In 2005 Taggart et al. identified that the fatty acid-derived ketone body D-β-hydroxybuturate is the endogenous ligand for PUMA-G and HM74A (Taggart et al., 2005). Starvation requires the body to utilize its own resources to continue to generate ATP in the absence of dietary glucose (Puchalska and Crawford, 2017). Fat stores will be the first to be employed, producing acetyl CoA from β-oxidation of FFAs to generate ATP. This can also increase the accumulation of ketone bodies in the liver to ensure the maximum utilization of resources for energy production once released into the blood. In this study, it was demonstrated that both forms of the ketone body D-β-hydroxybuturate and L-β-hydroxybuturate could bind to HM74A and PUMA-G but not HM74 and increased the release of Ca^{2+} to limit FFA release (Taggart et al., 2005). PUMA-G-deficient mice also demonstrated no reduction in FFAs release from adipocytes despite increased levels of D-β-hydroxybuturate. It is believed that D-β-hydroxybuturate may serve as part of a homeostatic negative feedback mechanism by which this ketone body limits its own production rate by inhibiting lipolysis, thus attempting to conserve fat stores during extended periods of starvation. Some other small-chain fatty acids such as butyrate could activate HM74A and PUMA-G, but these small-chain fatty acids do not reach sufficient concentrations in the blood to be physiologically relevant for these receptors on adipose tissue.

While these groups published utilizing the HM74A/PUMA-G and HM74 designations for this G protein-coupled receptor, they have come to be known in the literature as GPR109A and GPR109B, respectively. Even though GPR109A and GPR109B are more than likely the result of gene duplication (Zellner et al., 2005), GPR109A binds NA with high affinity and mediates its antidyslipidemic effects, thus being the key receptor in the rest of our discussion.

32.3 The role of GPR109A in tissue

32.3.1 Adipocytes

It was also determined that GPR109A is the receptor through which NA-induced flushing is caused (Offermanns, 2006). Flushing is a harmless condition, but it can occur at even small doses of NA, usually on the upper body and face, accompanied by an intense burning sensation. Therefore many patients choose not to continue with NA treatment despite its perceived benefits. Interestingly, the flushing response to NA usually disappears within a week of continued NA use, while the antidyslipidemic effects have been reported to be maintained over long periods of time.

A study conducted by Benyo et al. (2005) demonstrated that GPR109A is the receptor that mediates the flushing response. PUMA-G-deficient mice did not exhibit flushing following NA treatment. However, transplantation of wild-type bone marrow into these mice restored NA-induced flushing, suggesting that bone marrow-derived cells are responsible. Further examination demonstrated that NA binding and activation of GPR109A led to an increased production of prostaglandin E_2 and prostaglandin D_2 through a COX-1-dependent mechanism in bone marrow-derived cells, namely macrophages. Prostaglandins are potent vasodilators, thereby easily inducing a flushing response (Eklund et al., 1979). Mice lacking COX-1 or any of the receptors necessary for prostaglandin activity demonstrated no NA-induced flushing. Langerhans cells, macrophages only found in the skin, have also been found to release prostaglandin D_2 in response to IFNγ (Maciejewski-Lenoir et al., 2006). These early studies point toward a distinct antiinflammatory role for GPR109A activity.

32.3.2 Immune cells

Other studies have demonstrated these antiinflammatory effects of GPR109A are not limited to one particular cell type and are certainly not limited to prostaglandin pathways. GPR109A was identified as a potential receptor for NA on the membranes of cells from adipocytes and spleen cells (Soga et al., 2003). Initial studies confirming the efficacy of NA effects through GPR109A also reported that PUMA-G expression is upregulated in macrophages by IFNγ (Tunaru et al., 2003; Wise et al., 2003). GPR109A expression has been determined to be the highest in immune cells, which include macrophages, monocytes, neutrophils, and dendritic cells. In particular, GPR109A stimulation on human monocytes resulted in decreased expression of TNF-α-mediated proinflammatory molecules IL-6 and MCP-1 following lipopolysaccharide (LPS) and heat killed listeria monocytogenes (HKLM) challenge, respectively (Digby et al., 2012). This was accomplished by the inhibition of its transcription factor NF-κB by NA. Prostaglandin or COX inhibition did not alter the effects of NA and GPR109A activity, demonstrating NA could work through GPR109A by a prostaglandin-independent mechanism in monocytes to protect against inflammation and potentially effect atherosclerosis.

These antiinflammatory effects are not solely mediated through traditional immune signaling molecules. In adipose tissue, short-term treatment with extended release of NA was found to increase the expression of adiponectin, an antiinflammatory protein expressed in adipose tissue that has been found to be cardioprotective and is inversely correlated with several risk factors with cardiovascular disease (Westphal et al., 2007). However, the dosing and time span of treatment in this set of experiments was not enough to observe the effects of the protein. Further study confirmed the ability of NA to increase both adiponectin and adipokine while decreasing the proinflammatory chemokines fractalkine (CX3CL1), MCP-1, and RANTES, all of which play important roles in the early stages of atherosclerosis (Digby et al., 2010). These data contributed to the determination that GPR109A has pleiotropic potential to combat both atherosclerosis and dyslipidemia.

32.3.3 Retinal pigment epithelium

GPR109A has been demonstrated to be expressed in the retinal pigment epithelium (RPE), specifically on its basement membrane (Gambhir et al., 2012). The RPE is known to secrete proinflammatory cytokines and antiinflammatory molecules to help to maintain the overall health of the retina. GPR109A was specifically shown to be regulated in diabetic retina, from not of mouse models of both type I and type II diabetes. Activation of GPR109A via NA and β-hydroxybuturate in cultured RPE suppressed proinflammatory cytokines IL-6 and CCL2 (MCP-1), even following stimulation of these cytokines by TNF-α. Inhibition of GPR109A antagonized the effects of NA and β-hydroxybuturate on IL-6 and CCL2 expression, solidifying the role of GPR109A in inflammatory regulation in the retina.

32.3.4 Neurons and Parkinson's disease

Many studies have also examined the potential of GPR109A antiinflammatory effects in the nervous system, particularly pertaining to Parkinson's disease (PD). Two case studies suggest that individuals who consume niacin-rich diets have a decreased risk of developing PD (Fall et al., 1999;

Hellenbrand et al., 1996). Another case study also suggested that niacin was able to decrease rigidity and bradykinesia in a PD patient with increasing dosage (Alisky, 2005). However, this increased dosage also appeared to increase the patient's sensitivity to severe nightmares and skin rash, necessitating the need for further study to be conducted.

Mouse studies have also confirmed the potential of niacin to be neuroprotective. Fluid percussion injury in mice mimics traumatic brain injury, and it has been reported that NAM treatment improved sensorimotor, working memory, and behavior impairments in such mice (Hoane et al., 2006). Similar neuroprotective effects of NAM were observed in two mouse models of PD, preventing against neuron cell death and striatal dopamine depletion (Anderson et al., 2008).

Niacin is unsurprisingly important for overall neural health, due to the role it plays in dopamine synthesis (Wakade and Chong, 2014). NAD and NADH and NADPH are required for the production of the coenzymes that are necessary to form dopamine from L-tyrosine. However, interferences with Trp metabolism can reduce niacin levels in PD patients. Trp metabolism itself may be impaired in individuals who have been diagnosed but not yet treated for PD (Ogawa et al., 1992). It has also been reported that Levodopa medicine given to PD patients disrupts Trp metabolism (Karobath et al., 1971).

It has been suggested that high dosage of NAM protected neuroblastoma cells from cell death and increased oxidant generation, DNA damage, and protein oxidation in a 1-methyl-4-phenylpyridinium (MPP^+)-induced cellular model of PD (Jia et al., 2008). In the *Drosophilia* PD model, climbing ability was improved. NAM at high doses decreased oxidative stress to improve both mitochondria and motor function in these PD models.

A more recent study has determined GPR109A is actually elevated in PD patients (Wakade et al., 2014). With niacin levels low in these patients, GPR109A is upregulated in the macrophages and CNS microglia in an attempt to compensate and restore the reduced NAD levels. However, despite the proper metabolites feeding into the niacin pathway, NAD levels remain low, resulting in impaired mitochondrial function and surprisingly disrupted rapid eye movement sleep.

These studies demonstrate that niacin and GPR109A activation promote antiinflammatory and antioxidant effects in neurons and may prove be a potential treatment to reduce PD progression. However, more research needs to be done into the scope of effects on mitochondrial physiology and what dosage of niacin will have to be considered to avoid negative effects on neuron physiology.

32.3.5 Colon

GPR109A has been previously reported to be the most highly expressed on immune cells and adipocytes, but recent work has determined the high level of expression of GPR109A in the colon and its importance to overall colonic health. GPR109A is expressed in the intestines, with the largest expression in the colon (Thangaraju et al., 2009). Butyrate has also been determined to be another endogenous ligand for GPR109A, with its endogenous effects restricted to the colon environment. Colonic bacteria ferment dietary fiber to generate short-chain fatty acids, which are responsible for the beneficial effects of gut bacteria on intestinal/colonic health (Hamer et al., 2008). Butyrate is one of the most commonly generated short-chain fatty acids and is present at high concentrations in the colon compared to plasma levels (10 mmol/L colon vs 10 μmol/L plasma). It will be remembered that the short-chain fatty acid β-hydroxybuturate is the accepted ligand for GPR109A; however, the same study noted that butyrate could also activate GPR109A (Taggart et al., 2005).

Short-chain fatty acids, butyrate in particular, in the colonic lumen have been demonstrated to improve inflammatory bowel disease and decrease the incidence of colorectal cancer in a variety of different studies (Clarke et al., 2012; Hung and Suzuki, 2016; Singh et al., 2014; Venkatraman et al., 2003; Vieira et al., 2012). This effect may be through the activation of GPR109A to act as a tumor suppressor in the colon. GPR109A was linked with the induction of apoptosis, increased GPR109A activity leading to an increase in caspase 3, 8, and 9, as well as an increase in proapoptotic genes (*FAS-L*, *FAS-R*, *FADD*, and *TNF-R1*) and a decrease in antiapoptotic genes (*Bcl-2*, *Blc-W*, *Bcl-xL*, and *Bfll-1*) in colon cancer cell lines (Thangaraju et al., 2009). This change in gene expression is believed to be mediated through the inhibition of histone deacetylase (HDAC) activity by butyrate, as the ability of butyrate to inhibit HDACs and its effect on cell growth and apoptosis has been well-documented (van der Beek et al., 2017). GPR109A was also determined to be a blocker of LPS-induced NF-κB activation following treatment with butyrate. The connection between butyrate and NF-κB inhibition had been confirmed years before by previous studies (Inan et al., 2000;

Segain et al., 2000), but GPR109A as a link between the two had not been proposed before this study.

Further examinations of colon tissues in normal and cancerous states have revealed the colon protective effects of the butyrate/GPR109A mechanism. The expression of GPR109A in human colon cancer samples was decreased compared to human normal colon samples (Thangaraju et al., 2009). Silencing of GPR109A was determined to occur through the increase of DNA methyltransferases (DNMT) 1 and DNMT3b activity in colon cancer cells. DNMT1 also silences a butyrate transporter on the apical membrane of the cell. Sodium-coupled monocarboxylate transporter (SMCT1 or SLC5A8) is the intracellular transporter for butyrate and other short-chain fatty acids that are silenced in human colon cancer samples (Cresci et al., 2010; Thangaraju et al., 2008). Butyrate was shown to induce apoptosis only when SLC5A8 was present in colon cancer cell lines, activation of caspases 3, 8, and 9 promoting the activation of death pathways. Therefore it has been speculated that the tumor seeks to silence SLC5A8 and GPR109A to keep butyrate in from the colonic lumen and out of the colon cells where they can affect apoptosis. GPR109A silencing in the tumor may be overcome, as a study demonstrated that IFNγ promotes GPR109A expression through p300 acetylation and pSTAT-activation of GPR109A transcription (Bardhan et al., 2015). Despite there already being methylation present on GPR109A, it is able to be activated. Therefore this may be a mechanism through which GPR109A silencing within the tumor may be overcome.

GPR109A expression on immune cells also contributes to the tumor suppressive effects and its activity (Singh et al., 2014). It was found that GPR109A signaling on dendritic cells and macrophages in the colon promote the differentiation of T regulatory cells and IL-10-producing $CD4^+$ T cells. Both NA and butyrate treatment promoted this phenotype, in addition to promoting the production of IL-18 from the colonic epithelium. Gpr109a-knockout mice were further shown to have increased susceptibility to azoxymethane-dextran sulfate sodium (DSS)-induced colitis and colon inflammation, promoted by the widespread production of proinflammatory molecules and reduction of antiinflammatory mediators without Gpr109a activity. However, bone marrow transplant from the WT mice to Gpr109a-knockout mice resulted in an improved phenotype. Furthermore, NA decreased colon inflammation, despite the absence of gut microbiota or dietary fiber, making a strong case for the necessity of Gpr109a activity in colonic protection against both inflammation and cancer. Another study has demonstrated GPR109A activation by butyrate can decrease inflammation in the colon by increasing NLRP3 inflammasome activation, which significantly improved DSS colitis outcomes in mice (Macia et al., 2015).

32.3.6 Breast

GPR109A has also been shown to have a role in tumor suppression in the mammary gland, another organ that naturally produces butyrate during lactation. Human breast milk contains a significant amount of butyrate (~0.75 mM) (Ochoa-Zarzosa et al., 2009; Parodi, 1997). Butyrate induces differentiation in normal mammary epithelial cells and apoptosis in breast cancer cells (Abe and Kufe, 1984; Berni Canani et al., 2012; Graham and Buick, 1988). In breast cancer models, butyrate administration decreases mammary tumor formation by reducing the levels of estrogen receptor α (ERα) and progesterone receptor (Belobrajdic and McIntosh, 2000; deFazio et al., 1992; Heerdt et al., 1999; Horwitz et al., 1982). Therefore butyrate is a protective compound against breast cancer. GPR109A was found to be expressed in the mammary epithelium at levels comparable with those in spleen and intestine (Elangovan et al., 2014). As in colon cancer, GPR109A expression is also silenced in human breast tumor tissues by DNA methylation. Reactivation of GPR109A in mammary tumor tissue could be achieved with the treatment of DNMT inhibitors 5-azacytidine and 5-aza-2′-deoxycytidine (5-AzaDC). Combined treatment of either 5-AzaDC and butyrate or 5-AzaDC and NA reduced breast tumor growth by inducing tumor cell-specific apoptosis. This increased the apoptosis observed in breast cancer cell lines via the increased expression of proapoptotic genes and caspases and decreased antiapoptotic and cell-cycle progression genes. Further investigation demonstrated that expression of GPR109A alone was able to inhibit cell growth and tumor formation in mouse xenograft, addition of NA augmenting the effect. Knockout of Gpr109a in the genetically engineered mouse model of breast cancer (MMTV-Neu-Tg) caused increased tumor incidence, lung metastasis, and tumor invasion with reduced overall survival.

32.4 Future perspective/clinical relevance

GPR109A has proven to be a unique G protein-coupled receptor since its discovery nearly 20 years ago, having many different effects in a wide array of different tissues. The previously described studies clearly demonstrate its pleiotropic potential, bringing this receptor to the forefront of consideration for potential therapeutic targets. GPR109A has long been the receptor through which niacin was able to act as an antidyslipidemic, which naturally has a considerable impact on cardiovascular health. However, the emerging role of GPR109A in inflammation regulation has been the focus of many studies in the past decade. This antiinflammatory potential also allows GPR109A to have a functional role in several different tissues and disease states. Most importantly, it has been demonstrated to date to be a tumor suppressor in two different types of cancer, breast and colon.

Determining the appropriate targeting strategy to harness GPR109A regulation of antiinflammatory molecules and pathways will be the area of research in the coming years. It is already known that niacin and its derivatives are very well-utilized pharmacological agonists that can activate GPR109A. What is not known is the exact dosing that is required to elicit the appropriate effects. Proper dosing applies to attempts to utilize the endogenous ligands β-hydroxybuturate and butyrate as well. Diet has been well-documented to play a huge role in preventing disease states and cancer development. Activation of GPR109A may be one of these added health benefits of diets high in fiber or those that promote a ketogenic state. However, diet is an environmental condition that cannot always be strictly adhered to by the patient. Therefore alternative therapeutics for GPR109A activation may have to be considered.

It must also be considered that GPR109A expression can be depleted in cancer by epigenetic regulation. However, reversing of this silencing has been documented. Gene regulation of GPR109A may also have to be considered in combination with its activation to develop effective pharmaceutics. Therefore despite certain hurdles that must be considered, there are options to determine the best method of activation, whether indirectly through inhibition or direct activation through its ligands.

References

Abe, M., Kufe, D.W., 1984. Effect of sodium butyrate on human breast carcinoma (MCF-7) cellular proliferation, morphology, and CEA production. Breast Cancer Res. Treat. 4, 269–274.

Aktories, K., Jakobs, K.H., Schultz, G., 1980. Nicotinic acid inhibits adipocyte adenylate cyclase in a hormone-like manner. FEBS Lett. 115, 11–14.

Alisky, J.M., 2005. Niacin improved rigidity and bradykinesia in a Parkinson's disease patient but also caused unacceptable nightmares and skin rash—a case report. Nutr. Neurosci. 8, 327–329.

Altschul, R., Hoffer, A., Stephen, J.D., 1955. Influence of nicotinic acid on serum cholesterol in man. Arch. Biochem. Biophys. 54, 558–559.

Anderson, D.W., Bradbury, K.A., Schneider, J.S., 2008. Broad neuroprotective profile of nicotinamide in different mouse models of MPTP-induced parkinsonism. Eur. J. Neurosci. 28, 610–617.

Bardhan, K., Paschall, A.V., Yang, D., Chen, M.R., Simon, P.S., Bhutia, Y.D., et al., 2015. IFNgamma induces DNA methylation-silenced GPR109A expression via pSTAT1/p300 and H3K18 acetylation in colon cancer. Cancer Immunol. Res. 3, 795–805.

Belobrajdic, D.P., McIntosh, G.H., 2000. Dietary butyrate inhibits NMU-induced mammary cancer in rats. Nutr. Cancer 36, 217–223.

Benyo, Z., Gille, A., Kero, J., Csiky, M., Suchankova, M.C., Nusing, R.M., et al., 2005. GPR109A (PUMA-G/HM74A) mediates nicotinic acid-induced flushing. J. Clin. Invest. 115, 3634–3640.

Berni Canani, R., Di Costanzo, M., Leone, L., 2012. The epigenetic effects of butyrate: potential therapeutic implications for clinical practice. Clin. Epigenet. 4, 4.

Bogan, K.L., Brenner, C., 2008. Nicotinic acid, nicotinamide, and nicotinamide riboside: a molecular evaluation of NAD^+ precursor vitamins in human nutrition. Annu. Rev. Nutr. 28, 115–130.

Butcher, R.W., Baird, C.E., Sutherland, E.W., 1968. Effects of lipolytic and antilipolytic substances on adenosine 3′,5′-monophosphate levels in isolated fat cells. J. Biol. Chem. 243, 1705–1712.

Carlson, L.A., 1963. Studies on the effect of nicotinic acid on catecholamine stimulated lipolysis in adipose tissue in vitro. Acta Med. Scand. 173, 719–722.

Carlson, L.A., 2005. Nicotinic acid: the broad-spectrum lipid drug. A 50th anniversary review. J. Intern. Med. 258, 94–114.

Carlson, L.A., Oro, L., 1962. The effect of nicotinic acid on the plasma free fatty acid; demonstration of a metabolic type of sympathicolysis. Acta Med. Scand. 172, 641–645.

Carlson, L.A., Hamsten, A., Asplund, A., 1989. Pronounced lowering of serum levels of lipoprotein Lp(a) in hyperlipidaemic subjects treated with nicotinic acid. J. Intern. Med. 226, 271–276.

Clarke, J.M., Young, G.P., Topping, D.L., Bird, A.R., Cobiac, L., Scherer, B.L., et al., 2012. Butyrate delivered by butyrylated starch increases distal colonic epithelial apoptosis in carcinogen-treated rats. Carcinogenesis 33, 197–202.

Cresci, G.A., Thangaraju, M., Mellinger, J.D., Liu, K., Ganapathy, V., 2010. Colonic gene expression in conventional and germ-free mice with a focus on the butyrate receptor GPR109A and the butyrate transporter SLC5A8. J. Gastrointest. Surg. 14, 449–461.

deFazio, A., Chiew, Y.E., Donoghue, C., Lee, C.S., Sutherland, R.L., 1992. Effect of sodium butyrate on estrogen receptor and epidermal growth factor receptor gene expression in human breast cancer cell lines. J. Biol. Chem. 267, 18008–18012.

Digby, J.E., McNeill, E., Dyar, O.J., Lam, V., Greaves, D.R., Choudhury, R.P., 2010. Anti-inflammatory effects of nicotinic acid in adipocytes demonstrated by suppression of fractalkine, RANTES, and MCP-1 and upregulation of adiponectin. Atherosclerosis 209, 89–95.

Digby, J.E., Martinez, F., Jefferson, A., Ruparelia, N., Chai, J., Wamil, M., et al., 2012. Anti-inflammatory effects of nicotinic acid in human monocytes are mediated by GPR109A dependent mechanisms. Arterioscler. Thromb. Vasc. Biol. 32, 669–676.

Eklund, B., Kaijser, L., Nowak, J., Wennmalm, A., 1979. Prostaglandins contribute to the vasodilation induced by nicotinic acid. Prostaglandins 17, 821–830.
Elangovan, S., Pathania, R., Ramachandran, S., Ananth, S., Padia, R.N., Lan, L., et al., 2014. The niacin/butyrate receptor GPR109A suppresses mammary tumorigenesis by inhibiting cell survival. Cancer Res. 74, 1166–1178.
Fall, P.A., Fredrikson, M., Axelson, O., Granerus, A.K., 1999. Nutritional and occupational factors influencing the risk of Parkinson's disease: a case-control study in southeastern Sweden. Mov. Disord. 14, 28–37.
Gambhir, D., Ananth, S., Veeranan-Karmegam, R., Elangovan, S., Hester, S., Jennings, E., et al., 2012. GPR109A as an anti-inflammatory receptor in retinal pigment epithelial cells and its relevance to diabetic retinopathy. Invest. Ophthalmol. Vis. Sci. 53, 2208–2217.
Graham, K.A., Buick, R.N., 1988. Sodium butyrate induces differentiation in breast cancer cell lines expressing the estrogen receptor. J. Cell Physiol. 136, 63–71.
Hamer, H.M., Jonkers, D., Venema, K., Vanhoutvin, S., Troost, F.J., Brummer, R.J., 2008. Review article: the role of butyrate on colonic function. Aliment. Pharmacol. Ther. 27, 104–119.
Heerdt, B.G., Houston, M.A., Anthony, G.M., Augenlicht, L.H., 1999. Initiation of growth arrest and apoptosis of MCF-7 mammary carcinoma cells by tributyrin, a triglyceride analogue of the short-chain fatty acid butyrate, is associated with mitochondrial activity. Cancer Res. 59, 1584–1591.
Hellenbrand, W., Boeing, H., Robra, B.P., Seidler, A., Vieregge, P., Nischan, P., et al., 1996. Diet and Parkinson's disease. II: a possible role for the past intake of specific nutrients. results from a self-administered food-frequency questionnaire in a case-control study. Neurology 47, 644–650.
Hoane, M.R., Tan, A.A., Pierce, J.L., Anderson, G.D., Smith, D.C., 2006. Nicotinamide treatment reduces behavioral impairments and provides cortical protection after fluid percussion injury in the rat. J. Neurotrauma 23, 1535–1548.
Horwitz, K.B., Mockus, M.B., Lessey, B.A., 1982. Variant T47D human breast cancer cells with high progesterone-receptor levels despite estrogen and antiestrogen resistance. Cell 28, 633–642.
Hung, T.V., Suzuki, T., 2016. Dietary fermentable fiber reduces intestinal barrier defects and inflammation in colitic mice. J. Nutr. 146, 1970–1979.
Inan, M.S., Rasoulpour, R.J., Yin, L., Hubbard, A.K., Rosenberg, D.W., Giardina, C., 2000. The luminal short-chain fatty acid butyrate modulates NF-kappaB activity in a human colonic epithelial cell line. Gastroenterology 118, 724–734.
Jia, H., Li, X., Gao, H., Feng, Z., Li, X., Zhao, L., et al., 2008. High doses of nicotinamide prevent oxidative mitochondrial dysfunction in a cellular model and improve motor deficit in a Drosophila model of Parkinson's disease. J. Neurosci. Res. 86, 2083–2090.
Karobath, M., Diaz, J.L., Huttunen, M.O., 1971. The effect of L-dopa on the concentrations of tryptophan, tyrosine and serotonin in rat brain. Eur. J. Pharmacol. 14, 393–396.
Macia, L., Tan, J., Vieira, A.T., Leach, K., Stanley, D., Luong, S., et al., 2015. Metabolite-sensing receptors GPR43 and GPR109A facilitate dietary fibre-induced gut homeostasis through regulation of the inflammasome. Nat. Commun. 6, 6734.
Maciejewski-Lenoir, D., Richman, J.G., Hakak, Y., Gaidarov, I., Behan, D.P., Connolly, D.T., 2006. Langerhans cells release prostaglandin D2 in response to nicotinic acid. J. Invest. Dermatol. 126, 2637–2646.
Ochoa-Zarzosa, A., Villarreal-Fernandez, E., Cano-Camacho, H., Lopez-Meza, J.E., 2009. Sodium butyrate inhibits *Staphylococcus aureus* internalization in bovine mammary

epithelial cells and induces the expression of antimicrobial peptide genes. Microb. Pathog. 47, 1–7.
Offermanns, S., 2006. The nicotinic acid receptor GPR109A (HM74A or PUMA-G) as a new therapeutic target. Trends Pharmacol. Sci. 27, 384–390.
Ogawa, T., Matson, W.R., Beal, M.F., Myers, R.H., Bird, E.D., Milbury, P., et al., 1992. Kynurenine pathway abnormalities in Parkinson's disease. Neurology 42, 1702–1706.
Parodi, P.W., 1997. Cows' milk fat components as potential anticarcinogenic agents. J. Nutr. 127, 1055–1060.
Puchalska, P., Crawford, P.A., 2017. Multi-dimensional roles of ketone bodies in fuel metabolism, signaling, and therapeutics. Cell. Metab. 25, 262–284.
Sadana, R., Dessauer, C.W., 2009. Physiological roles for G protein-regulated adenylyl cyclase isoforms: insights from knockout and overexpression studies. Neurosignals 17, 5–22.
Segain, J.P., Raingeard de la Bletiere, D., Bourreille, A., Leray, V., Gervois, N., Rosales, C., et al., 2000. Butyrate inhibits inflammatory responses through NFkappaB inhibition: implications for Crohn's disease. Gut 47, 397–403.
Shepherd, J., Packard, C.J., Patsch, J.R., Gotto Jr., A.M., Taunton, O.D., 1979. Effects of nicotinic acid therapy on plasma high density lipoprotein subfraction distribution and composition and on apolipoprotein A metabolism. J. Clin. Invest. 63, 858–867.
Singh, N., Gurav, A., Sivaprakasam, S., Brady, E., Padia, R., Shi, H., et al., 2014. Activation of Gpr109a, receptor for niacin and the commensal metabolite butyrate, suppresses colonic inflammation and carcinogenesis. Immunity 40, 128–139.
Soga, T., Kamohara, M., Takasaki, J., Matsumoto, S., Saito, T., Ohishi, T., et al., 2003. Molecular identification of nicotinic acid receptor. Biochem. Biophys. Res. Commun. 303, 364–369.
Srivastava, S., 2016. Emerging therapeutic roles for NAD(+) metabolism in mitochondrial and age-related disorders. Clin. Transl. Med. 5, 25.
Taggart, A.K., Kero, J., Gan, X., Cai, T.Q., Cheng, K., Ippolito, M., et al., 2005. D)-beta-Hydroxybutyrate inhibits adipocyte lipolysis via the nicotinic acid receptor PUMA-G. J. Biol. Chem. 280, 26649–26652.
Thangaraju, M., Cresci, G., Itagaki, S., Mellinger, J., Browning, D.D., Berger, F.G., et al., 2008. Sodium-coupled transport of the short chain fatty acid butyrate by SLC5A8 and its relevance to colon cancer. J. Gastrointest. Surg. 12, 1773–1781. discussion 1781–1772.
Thangaraju, M., Cresci, G.A., Liu, K., Ananth, S., Gnanaprakasam, J.P., Browning, D.D., et al., 2009. GPR109A is a G-protein-coupled receptor for the bacterial fermentation product butyrate and functions as a tumor suppressor in colon. Cancer Res. 69, 2826–2832.
Tunaru, S., Kero, J., Schaub, A., Wufka, C., Blaukat, A., Pfeffer, K., et al., 2003. PUMA-G and HM74 are receptors for nicotinic acid and mediate its anti-lipolytic effect. Nat. Med. 9, 352–355.
van der Beek, C.M., Dejong, C.H.C., Troost, F.J., Masclee, A.A.M., Lenaerts, K., 2017. Role of short-chain fatty acids in colonic inflammation, carcinogenesis, and mucosal protection and healing. Nutr. Rev. 75, 286–305.
Venkatraman, A., Ramakrishna, B.S., Shaji, R.V., Kumar, N.S., Pulimood, A., Patra, S., 2003. Amelioration of dextran sulfate colitis by butyrate: role of heat shock protein 70 and NF-kappaB. Am. J. Physiol. Gastrointest. Liver Physiol. 285, G177–G184.
Vieira, E.L., Leonel, A.J., Sad, A.P., Beltrao, N.R., Costa, T.F., Ferreira, T.M., et al., 2012. Oral administration of sodium butyrate attenuates inflammation and mucosal lesion in experimental acute ulcerative colitis. J. Nutr. Biochem. 23, 430–436.
Wakade, C., Chong, R., 2014. A novel treatment target for Parkinson's disease. J. Neurol. Sci. 347, 34–38.

Wakade, C., Chong, R., Bradley, E., Thomas, B., Morgan, J., 2014. Upregulation of GPR109A in Parkinson's disease. PLoS. One 9, e109818.
Westphal, S., Borucki, K., Taneva, E., Makarova, R., Luley, C., 2007. Extended-release niacin raises adiponectin and leptin. Atherosclerosis 193, 361–365.
Wise, A., Foord, S.M., Fraser, N.J., Barnes, A.A., Elshourbagy, N., Eilert, M., et al., 2003. Molecular identification of high and low affinity receptors for nicotinic acid. J. Biol. Chem. 278, 9869–9874.
Zellner, C., Pullinger, C.R., Aouizerat, B.E., Frost, P.H., Kwok, P.Y., Malloy, M.J., et al., 2005. Variations in human HM74 (GPR109B) and HM74A (GPR109A) niacin receptors. Hum. Mutat. 25, 18–21.

CHAPTER 33

Vitamin C: epigenetic roles and cancer

Sushmita Mustafi[1] **and Gaofeng Wang**[2]
[1]John P. Hussman Institute for Human Genomics, Miller School of Medicine, University of Miami, Miami, FL, United States
[2]John P. Hussman Institute for Human Genomics, Dr. John T. Macdonald Foundation Department of Human Genetics, Sylvester Comprehensive Cancer Center, Miller School of Medicine, University of Miami, Miami, FL, United States

Contents

Key facts of vitamin C and cancer

- Unlike mice, which are extensively used for cancer research, humans cannot synthesize vitamin C de novo due to a mutant and nonfunctional L-gulonolactone oxidase (Gulo), the enzyme catalyzing the last step of vitamin C biosynthesis. Therefore dietary supplementation of vitamin C is essential in humans.

Molecular Nutrition
DOI: https://doi.org/10 1016/B978-0-12-811907-5.00003-8

- In vitro culture of cancer cells is critical for analyzing the molecular mechanism of malignancy and for testing candidate cancer drugs. However, vitamin C is often not included in the formulation of media used for culturing cancer cells. On the other hand, standard mouse models for cancer research synthesize endogenous vitamin C in their livers and thus cannot model the differences in vitamin C bioavailability observed in human patients.
- Using vitamin C to treat cancer has a long controversial history of inconsistent outcomes.
- The recently uncovered function of vitamin C in regulating the epigenome, especially active DNA demethylation, once again revitalizes the hope for this easily accessible and inexpensive vitamin in cancer patient care.
- Vitamin C can be conveniently delivered through oral supplementation, which could help reprogram cancer cells toward noncancerous cells through epigenetic regulation.
- Vitamin C is also considered as a prodrug to deliver free radicals to damage cancer cells by intravenous infusion of high doses.

Summary points

- Inadequate vitamin C consumption, certain genetic variation in transporters, and cancer-associated oxidative stress collectively contribute to the intracellular vitamin C deficiency in cancer.
- Vitamin C deficiency may be associated with the risk of cancer, cancer recurrence, and cancer-related mortality.
- Recent research has discovered a novel function of vitamin C in promoting active DNA demethylation, which directly contributes to cancer cell reprogramming.
- By enhancing collagen cross-linking and hypoxia-inducible factor-1α degradation, and by generating free radicals, vitamin C may be helpful in cancer treatment.
- Vitamin C can be used for cancer treatment due to its epigenetic role and other functions.

Definitions of words and terms

DNA methylation: Methylation at the fifth carbon of cytosine is a major epigenetic modification of mammalian DNA, which is often associated with the suppression of gene transcription. This modification is established and maintained by DNA methyltransferases.

Active DNA demethylation: Active DNA demethylation is initiated by the conversion of 5-methylcytosine (5mC) to 5-hydroxymethylcytosine (5hmC), which is catalyzed by ten-eleven translocation (TET) methylcytosine dioxygenases. TETs can further oxidize 5hmC to 5-formylcytosine (5fC) and 5-carboxylcytosine (5caC), which are eventually replaced by unmodified cytosine, thus completing the process of demethylation.

Vitamin C as a cofactor: Without sufficient vitamin C, the enzymatic activity of collagen hydroxylases is affected, resulting in scurvy, which is characterized by insufficient collagen cross-linking. Sufficient vitamin C, which has the capacity to convert enzymatically inactive Fe(III) to active Fe(II) for collagen hydroxylases, cures the disease. Epigenetic enzymes, such as TET methylcytosine dioxygenases and JmjC domain-containing demethylases, like collagen hydroxylases, also require vitamin C as a cofactor.

Epigenetic reprogramming: Remodeling of epigenetic marks by adding new or erasing the existing ones, for example, DNA methylation. Loss of 5hmC is an epigenetic hallmark of most cancers. Vitamin C can help reprogram cancer cells toward nonmalignant cells by promoting 5hmC generation.

Vitamin C (L-ascorbic acid) is an essential dietary micronutrient with a growing list of biological functions in which it is implicated. Primarily known for its antiscorbutic properties, vitamin C has been characterized as a potent antioxidant and cofactor for enzymes including copper-dependent monooxygenases as well as iron and 2-oxoglutarate-dependent dioxygenases. The major known functions of vitamin C could be accounted for by a single chemical property, that is, it is an electron donor. Studies have shown that demethylation of both DNA and histones is catalyzed by iron and 2-oxoglutarate-dependent dioxygenases, which require vitamin C as a cofactor. In light of the recent discoveries regarding its participation in DNA and histone demethylation, the emerging role of vitamin C as an epigenetic modulator has put vitamin C once again in the spotlight of health and disease. In this chapter, we will discuss the various functions of vitamin C at the molecular and epigenetic levels, considering its therapeutic potential and impact on cancer.

33.1 Vitamin C intake and cancer

33.1.1 Cellular uptake of vitamin C in cancer

Most mammals synthesize vitamin C de novo in the liver from glucose through an evolutionarily conserved biosynthetic pathway. In contrast, humans no longer can synthesize vitamin C due to a loss-of-function mutation in the L-gulonolactone oxidase (Gulo) enzyme, which catalyzes the last step of biosynthesis. Due to this loss-of-function in humans, vitamin C must be supplied through dietary sources and supplements. Vitamin C enters cells primarily through sodium-dependent vitamin C transporters (SVCTs). The high-capacity, low-affinity SVCT1 is primarily responsible for vitamin C absorption and reabsorption in intestinal and renal epithelial cells. The high-affinity, low-capacity SVCT2 distributes vitamin C to most tissues and is expressed ubiquitously (Wilson, 2005). In the dbSNP database, there are ~60 nonsynonymous single nucleotide polymorphisms (SNP) in the SLC23A1 gene (encoding SVCT1), all of which are rare in the population (minor allele frequency <0.5%). Some of these SNPs, including rs35817838 (amino acid change M258V), rs33972313 (V264M), and rs34521685 (I218V), are associated with a 40% – 75% decline in human plasma vitamin C regardless of dietary intake (up to 2.5 g/day) (Corpe et al., 2010; Timpson et al., 2010). An intronic SNP rs4257763 is also correlated with a reduced serum vitamin C level (Cahill and El-Sohemy, 2009). There are about 40 nonsynonymous SNPs in the SLC23A2 gene (encoding SVCT2) in the dbSNP database. The impact of these variants on SVCT2 function is less clear. Although the functional analysis of the genetic variation in SVCT1 and SVCT2 is incomplete, individuals carrying certain genetic variants could have a higher risk of vitamin C deficiency (Handelman, 2007).

Genetic variation in SVCT1 and SVCT2 has been associated with the risk of certain types of cancer including advanced colorectal adenoma (Erichsen et al., 2008), muscle-invasive bladder cancer (Guey et al., 2010), gastric cancer (Wright et al., 2009), and non-Hodgkin lymphoma (Skibola et al., 2008). One should be cautious in interpreting these genetic associations which have not yet been independently validated in other cohorts. The potential functional consequences of these associated variants on vitamin C cellular uptake also remain largely unclear. A search of the COSMIC database (Catalogue of Somatic Mutations in Cancer) (http://cancer.sanger.ac.uk/cancergenome/projects/cosmic/) reveals that mutations in SVCTs have been identified in many types of cancer, such as breast cancer, colorectal adenoma, and brain tumors, although the frequency of these mutations is low (<8.81%). Furthermore, recurrent mutations in the splicing factor SF3B1 have been identified in chronic lymphocytic leukemia, uveal melanoma, and other cancers (Quesada et al., 2011; Harbour et al., 2013). In chronic lymphocytic leukemia the mutant SF3B1 causes a truncated, most likely nonfunctional, SVCT2 that can result in the intracellular deficiency of vitamin C in cancer cells (Quesada et al., 2011). Taken together, genetic variations in SVCT1 and SVCT2, which can potentially disrupt vitamin C cellular uptake, have been identified in a minority of cases of cancer.

The aberrant expression of SVCTs is also discovered in cancer. The SVCT2 expression is decreased in 72.5% cases by at least 1.5-fold compared to the matched normal breast tissues by analyzing RNA-Seq data of 113 matched pairs of breast cancer and normal breast tissue obtained from the same patients in The Cancer Genome Atlas (Sant et al., 2018). In a minority of breast cancer cases, the expression of SVCT2 is upregulated (Hong et al., 2013). The aberrant expression of SVCTs is also detected in breast cancer cell lines and melanoma cell lines (Sant et al., 2018; Gustafson et al., 2015). Furthermore, the uptake rate of ascorbate, the dominant form of vitamin C in the plasma, by melanoma cells is only ~50% of the uptake rate of the healthy melanocytes (Spielholz et al., 1997), which correlates the lower expression of SVCT2 in melanoma cells. Overall, available data suggest that in certain types of cancer, such as breast cancer, a majority of cases display lower expression of SVCT2, which could consequently disrupt vitamin C cellular uptake.

Cancer-associated genetic variants, somatic mutations, and the lower expression of SVCT2 collectively lead to intracellular vitamin C deficiency. Furthermore, cancer-associated oxidative stress could worsen this deficiency by attenuating vitamin C within cancer cells (Toyokuni et al., 1995). The average concentration of vitamin C in healthy human plasma is generally near the ~50 μM range. By diet and oral supplements, plasma vitamin C can reach up to ~200 μM (Levine et al., 2011). To obtain higher than 300 μM vitamin C in the plasma would require intravenous injection (Chen et al., 2007). Vitamin C is readily absorbed and distributed in the body with a constant turnover rate, creating a need for regular supplementation. It has been proposed for decades that the repletion of vitamin C may have a certain therapeutic value in decreasing malignancy by rectifying the intracellular vitamin C deficiency in cancer cells.

33.1.2 Vitamin C and cancer risk, recurrence, or mortality

Studies have observed a correlation between the occurrence of scurvy and certain types of cancer. For example, a higher incidence of scurvy or subclinical scurvy in cancer patients has been reported (Fain et al., 1998; Krasner and Dymock, 1974). Plasma vitamin C deficiency, which is correlated with low intake of vitamin C, is also seen in 30% of cancer patients (Mayland et al., 2005). Epidemiological studies further show an inverse association between dietary vitamin C intake and the risk of cancer. For instance, vitamin C supplementation is associated with a decreased risk, recurrence, and mortality of breast cancer (Greenlee et al., 2012; Poole et al., 2013; Harris et al., 2013; Hutchinson et al., 2012). A study investigating a cohort of 4877 women aged 20–75 years diagnosed with invasive breast cancer found that vitamin C supplementation shortly after breast cancer diagnosis is associated with reduced mortality and recurrence risk (Nechuta et al., 2011). An inverse association between dietary vitamin C supplements and the risk of melanoma has also been observed in population studies (Malavolti et al., 2013; Miura and Green, 2015). However, it remains largely unclear if the benefits of vitamin C in prevention and treatment are universal or limited to certain types of cancer only.

On the other hand, epidemiological evidence of vitamin C in decreasing the risk of cancer remains inconsistent. Many studies showed minimal or no benefit of vitamin C in cancer prevention and treatment. It is noteworthy that it is difficult, if not impossible, to control vitamin C quantitatively in human subjects, which may underlie the inconsistent epidemiological reports. For instance, vitamin C supplements in treatment groups can easily be confounded by consumption of vitamin C–rich fruits and vegetables in control/placebo groups. Most studies examined vitamin C consumption by questionnaire or other indirect self-report methods, but did not verify effects of vitamin C levels within cancer cells. Vitamin C measurements in the plasma or cancer tissue do not necessarily reflect the vitamin C level within the cancer cell. Furthermore, the effect of vitamin C can be complicated by other antioxidants or micronutrients. Even with these difficulties, recent meta-analyses of observational studies indicate a potential benefit of vitamin C in breast cancer survivors. One meta-analysis of epidemiological observational studies showed that higher plasma levels of vitamin C are associated with a reduced breast cancer risk (Hu et al., 2015). Another meta-analysis ($n = 17{,}696$ breast cancer patients) showed a statistically significant association between the use of vitamin C supplements and reduced breast cancer mortality (Harris et al., 2014). These studies suggest that vitamin C is beneficial for breast cancer prevention and treatment.

Animal studies with the advantage of controlling vitamin C clearly demonstrate the benefit of vitamin C in cancer treatment. Vitamin C depletion increases the growth and metastasis of melanoma (Cha et al., 2011). In contrast, vitamin C supplementation inhibits the growth and metastasis of melanoma, breast cancer, and colorectal cancer (Cha et al., 2013; Campbell et al., 2015, 2016). Corroborating human studies, the results of animal experiments indicate a therapeutic potential for vitamin C in cancer treatment. Available data suggest that it is likely that vitamin C exerts its anticancer action through different molecular mechanisms.

33.2 The epigenetic role of vitamin C in cancer treatment

33.2.1 Vitamin C promotes DNA demethylation

Methylation at the C (Handelman, 2007) position of cytosine (5-methylcytosine, 5mC) is the major covalent modification in mammalian DNA, which plays an essential role in promoter silencing, X chromosome inactivation, gene imprinting, and transposon silencing (Bestor et al., 2015). Catalyzed by DNA methyltransferases (DNMTs), the methyl group from the donor *S*-adenosyl methionine is transferred to the C (Handelman, 2007) position of cytosine, thus forming 5mC. De novo cytosine methylation is established by DNA methyltransferase 3 (DNMT3). Although 5mC is relatively stable, it can be lost due to the lack of maintenance by DNA methyltransferase 1 (DNMT1) during DNA replication, thus resulting in passive demethylation by dilution.

Active DNA demethylation is initiated by ten-eleven translocation (TET) methylcytosine dioxygenases, which catalyze a cascade oxidation by converting 5mC to 5-hydroxymethylcytosine (5hmC), and further to 5-formylcytosine (5fC) and 5-carboxylcytosine (5caC) (Kriaucionis and Heintz, 2009; Tahiliani et al., 2009; Ito et al., 2010). 5fC and 5caC are excised by the DNA repair enzyme thymine DNA glycosylase to produce an abasic site, which is eventually replaced by an unmodified cytosine (5C), thus completing the process of active DNA demethylation (He et al., 2011; Ito et al., 2011; Maiti and Drohat, 2011). In mammalian genomes, 5mC and 5hmC are abundant, while 5fC and 5caC are relatively rare. Within the framework of the CpG dinucleotide pattern, methyl-CpG-binding proteins can recognize and bind to these patterns of 5mC to mediate transcriptional regulation of the associated DNA. 5hmC also regulates transcription by recruiting a different set of binding proteins compared to 5mC. Hence, 5hmC is recognized as an epigenetic mark with unique regulatory capacities (Shen et al., 2014).

TETs belong to the iron and 2-oxoglutarate (2OG, alternatively termed α-ketoglutarate)-dependent dioxygenase superfamily. The cascade oxidation catalyzed by TETs requires 5mC as the initial substrate, labile Fe(II) as the cofactor, 2OG as the cosubstrate, and oxygen. 5mC is abundant in the genome of most mammalian cell types. Under physiological conditions, 2OG (an abundant intermediate in the Krebs cycle) and oxygen are accessible to TETs. In contrast, Fe(II) must be tightly controlled in the cell due to its active redox capacity, especially its ability to produce free radicals through the Fenton reaction. In cultured cells, active DNA demethylation is generally paused as shown by a very low or undetectable 5hmC signal. In each reaction catalyzed by TETs, Fe(II) is converted to Fe(III) or Fe(IV) along with the conversion of 5mC to 5hmC, then to 5fC and 5caC. Although the initial oxidation could be carried out by TETs, the accumulation of catalytically inactive Fe(III)/Fe(IV) would soon result in TET inactivation, which could explain the low basal levels of 5hmC in cultured cells. Initial studies identified that vitamin C, which has the capacity to reduce Fe(III)/Fe(IV) to Fe(II), promotes 5hmC generation in a cultured cell (Minor et al., 2013; Dickson et al., 2013). The role of vitamin C in promoting TET-mediated DNA demethylation has been confirmed in stem cells and vitamin C–deficient L-gulonolactone oxidase knockout (Gulo) mice (Yin et al., 2013; Blaschke et al., 2013; Chen et al., 2013). Thus a previously unrecognized function of vitamin C in regulating DNA demethylation has been discovered (Fig. 33.1).

33.2.2 Vitamin C suppresses malignancy by reestablishing 5-hydroxymethylcytosine

Aberrant epigenetic alterations, reflected at the interface of a dynamic microenvironment and the genome, are involved in malignant transformation (Dawson and Kouzarides, 2012). Loss of 5hmC has been recognized as an epigenetic hallmark of most, if not all, types of cancer (Huang and Rao, 2014). For example, the content of 5hmC is high in healthy melanocytes but is gradually lost during progression from benign nevi through malignant stages of primary and metastatic melanoma

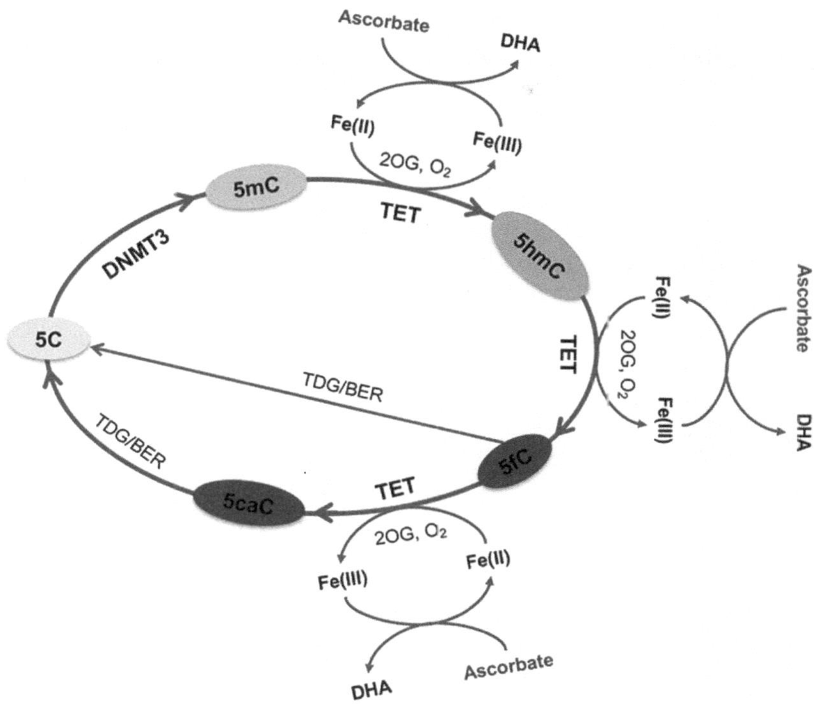

Figure 33.1 The role of vitamin C (ascorbate) in DNA methylation and demethylation dynamics.
Fe(II) is an essential cofactor for TET-mediated active demethylation. Vitamin C, which has the capacity to convert Fe(III) to Fe(II), promotes active DNA demethylation. *TET*, Ten-eleven translocation; *TDG/BER*, thymine DNA glycosylase/base excision repair.

(Lian et al., 2012). This global loss of 5hmC disrupts the dynamics of DNA methylation–demethylation and affects genome-wide gene expression, which could eventually lead to malignant transformation. The known mechanism underlying the loss of 5hmC in some melanoma cases is a decreased expression of TET2 or somatic mutations (Lian et al., 2012). Overexpressing TET2 partially reestablishes a normal 5hmC profile in melanoma cells and decreases their invasiveness (Lian et al., 2012). The cancer suppressing effect of the forceful expression of TETs has also been proven in other types of cancer, such as breast cancer (Hsu et al., 2012). While overexpressing TETs in patients might not be clinically feasible, this discovery suggests that finding a means of restoring normal 5hmC content may yield a novel therapy for cancer.

An alternative to TETs overexpression, vitamin C may enhance or even maximize the catalytic activity of existing TETs, including those from nonmutant alleles or isoforms in cancer. Initial in vitro studies showed that vitamin C treatment increases the content of 5hmC in melanoma cell lines derived from different stages toward the level of healthy melanocytes (Gustafson et al., 2015). The effect of vitamin C on 5hmC is comparable to the effect of overexpressing TET2. The promotion of 5hmC by vitamin C has been subsequently demonstrated in many types of cancer cells, including hepatocellular carcinoma (Sajadian et al., 2016), leukemia (Cimmino et al., 2017), breast cancer (Sant et al., 2018), kidney cancer (Ge et al., 2018), bladder cancer (Peng et al., 2018), and colon cancer (Gerecke et al., 2018). By compensating for the potential intracellular deficiency, vitamin C increases 5hmC content in various cancer cells, suggesting that there is a potential therapeutic value for vitamin C in treating different types of cancer.

The dosage of vitamin C used should be sufficient to meet the need of TETs. In vitro studies provide some clues as to an appropriate dosage. In the absence of vitamin C, 5hmC is barely detectable in cultured melanoma cells. Vitamin C at low concentrations dose-dependently increases 5hmC content, which plateaus after the application of 100 μM vitamin C. Higher concentrations, such as 500 μM, of vitamin C do not exert additional benefits in 5hmC restoration (Gustafson et al., 2015). A similar dose effect is also observed in other cancers, such as breast cancer (Sant et al., 2018). However, the required doses to be applied could be different in cancer types or even cases, which more or less rely on the relative expression of SVCTs in cancer cells. Overall, vitamin C can be used to increase 5hmC content in melanoma cells, thus reprogramming melanoma cells back toward healthy melanocytes (Fig. 33.2).

By increasing 5hmC content and changing genome-wide 5hmC profiles, vitamin C changes DNA methylation—demethylation dynamics, which subsequently affect gene expression profiles. Using high-throughput sequencing, studies have shown that vitamin C treatment shifts the transcriptome of different cancer cells. For instance, after the treatment of melanoma cells with 100 μM vitamin C, hundreds of genes are differentially transcribed, with some being upregulated and some being downregulated, which is consistent with the known bidirectional effects of 5hmC on transcription (Wu et al., 2011). Some of the most dramatically altered genes could underlie certain cellular phenotypes, including TNF-related apoptosis-inducing ligand (TRAIL). Vitamin C increases the

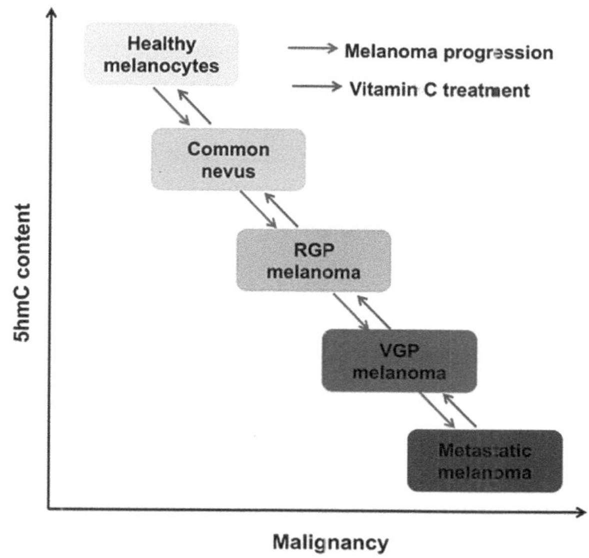

Figure 33.2 Treatment of melanoma by vitamin C via 5-hydroxymethylcytosine (5hmC) restoration.
5hmC is gradually lost as melanoma progresses from the radial growth phase (RGP) to the vertical growth phase and further to metastasis. Vitamin C helps to reestablish 5hmC content by promoting TET-mediated active demethylation and by epigenetically reprogramming melanoma cells toward healthy melanocytes. *TET*, Ten-eleven translocation.

transcription, translation, and secretion of TRAIL, a key apoptosis inducer, which causes apoptosis in breast cancer cells (Sant et al., 2018). Taken together, these results suggest a potential role of vitamin C in cancer treatment by increasing 5hmC and changing gene expression.

Vitamin C is a safe and well-tolerated micronutrient, suggesting that any potential "off-5hmC-target" effects might not be a concern for in vivo usage. To deliver vitamin C in vivo, one way is by oral delivery, which can be conveniently carried out multiple times per day in order to maintain plasma vitamin C at around 100 μM. The other way is through intravenous injection or intraperitoneal injection, which can raise plasma vitamin C to much higher levels for a relatively short period of time. Both methods have been applied in cancer modeling in animals. Murine melanoma tumor grafts are much smaller in vitamin C-sufficient mice than in vitamin C−deficient Gulo$^{-/-}$ mice, suggesting that endogenously produced vitamin C inhibits melanoma growth (Mustafi et al., 2018). Restoring physiological levels of vitamin C in Gulo$^{-/-}$ mice by dietary supplementation suppresses various tumor growth (Cha et al., 2013; Campbell et al., 2015, 2016). The intravenous injection of high doses of vitamin C also blocks leukemia progression by compensating for the loss of TET2 (Cimmino et al., 2017). Some of the anticancer effects of vitamin C are likely due to the enhanced activity of TETs, the restoration of 5hmC, and the subsequent altered expression of cancer-related genes, while the rest can be allocated to other mechanisms in which vitamin C is involved.

33.2.3 Vitamin C promotes histone demethylation

Methylation at lysine residues is a major posttranslational modification in histones. The addition of methyl groups to lysine residues is catalyzed by histone methyltransferases. There could be one, two, or three methyl groups added to a lysine residue resulting in monomethylated, dimethylated, or trimethylated lysine, respectively. Two types of enzymes remove methyl groups from the methylated lysine. The first type, termed lysine-specific histone demethylases, targets monomethylated and dimethylated lysines. The second type, named JmjC domain-containing demethylases of which there are more than 20 members, can demethylate tri-, di-, and monomethylated histone lysine residues.

JmjC domain-containing histone demethylases, like TETs, also belong to the Fe(II) and 2OG dioxygenase superfamily. Because the catalytic activity of JmjC domain-containing demethylases require labile Fe(II) as an essential cofactor, vitamin C may also have an impact on histone demethylation due to its capacity to convert Fe(III)/Fe(IV) to Fe(II). Initial studies demonstrated that vitamin C is required for optimal catalytic activity for different JmjC domain-containing histone demethylases (Tsukada et al., 2006; Klose et al., 2006). Subsequent studies showed that vitamin C induces H3K36me2/3 demethylation in mouse embryonic fibroblasts or H3K9me2 demethylation in mouse embryonic stem cells (Wang et al., 2011; Ebata et al., 2017). These suggest that vitamin C also promotes histone demethylation in the cell by enhancing the activity of JmjC domain-containing demethylases.

Impaired histone demethylation has been identified in certain types of cancer, especially leukemia. For example, frequent mutations in isocitrate dehydrogenases identified in leukemia and glioma could lead to histone hypermethylation (Lu et al., 2012). It remains unclear if vitamin C can play a role in rectifying the histone hypermethylation in cancer by enhancing demethylation. Future studies may help to determine if vitamin C exerts anticancer activity by promoting histone demethylation.

33.3 Other potential mechanisms in the anticancer action of vitamin C

33.3.1 Prevention of metastasis by collagen cross-linking

The tumor microenvironment, especially the stroma, plays an important role in tumor progression. Collagen is the most abundant constituent of the extracellular matrix which primarily constitutes stromal tissues. Vitamin C deficiency causes scurvy mainly due to insufficient collagen synthesis and cross-linking (May and Harrison, 2013). The hydroxylation of collagen is essential for procollagen cross-linking and further the assembly of collagen fibrils. As a cofactor, vitamin C is required for collagen hydroxylases, which also belong to the iron and 2OG-dependent dioxygenase superfamily. Furthermore, vitamin C appears to increase the expression of certain types of collagens while its mechanism remains elusive. It is shown that DNA hypermethylation at the promoters inhibits the transcription of various types of collagen (Thompson et al., 1991). After demethylation of promoter CpG sites, the transcription of collagens is activated (Zimmermann et al., 2008). Thus it could be that vitamin C promotes collagen synthesis and cross-linking by serving as a cofactor for TETs to demethylate the gene and for collagen hydroxylases to cross-link the protein.

Collagen in tissues is regarded as a physical barrier against cancer invasion. By increasing collagen synthesis and cross-linking, vitamin C is thought to be able to help prevent cancer metastasis (Cameron et al., 1979). However, later studies showed that strengthening collagen cross-linking for stiffer collagen fibrils by lysyl oxidase, a copper-dependent amine oxidase that requires vitamin C as cofactor, enhances malignancy (Levental et al., 2009). At this time, it remains uncertain if vitamin C could exert anticancer activity by promoting collagen synthesis and cross-linking.

33.3.2 Suppression of cancer progression by hypoxia-inducible factor-1α degradation

Higher expression of hypoxia-inducible factor-1α (HIF-1α) is associated with cancer cell survival, metastasis, angiogenesis, and poor prognosis. As a transcription factor, HIF-1α regulates the transcription of hundreds of genes which can be involved in malignancy. One well-studied gene targeted by HIF-1α is vascular endothelial growth factor which is necessary for angiogenesis in cancer. HIF-1α has long been regarded as a therapeutic target for cancer (Schito and Semenza, 2016), and inhibitors are currently being tested in clinical trials.

The degradation of HIF-1α starts with hydroxylation catalyzed by HIF hydroxylases. Since HIF hydroxylases are also iron and 2OG-dependent dioxygenases, vitamin C is essential for HIF-1α hydroxylation and further degradation. Thus vitamin C naturally targets HIF-1α. Indeed, vitamin C supplementation is shown to diminish HIF-1α and inhibit tumorigenesis in a lymphoma mouse model (Gao et al., 2007). Although more studies are required to understand its role in different types of cancer, it is highly likely that vitamin C has anticancer value through the enhancement of HIF-1α degradation.

33.3.3 Targeting cancer cells by free radicals

Cancer cells are shown to be more sensitive to vitamin C than normal cells. Under culture conditions, the EC_{50} of vitamin C in damaging cancer cells is <4 mM while nonmalignant cells remain unaffected by 20 mM vitamin C (Chen et al., 2005). Intravenous infusion can elevate plasma vitamin C concentration to the mM range which cannot be achievable by oral delivery (Levine et al., 2011). At mM concentrations, vitamin C selectively generates ascorbate radicals and hydrogen peroxide (H_2O_2) in the extracellular milieu, suggesting that vitamin C could be a prodrug to deliver H_2O_2 to the cell (Chen et al., 2007). Cancer cells may have an impaired capacity to metabolize H_2O_2, such as a lower activity of catalase, which could explain the sensitivity of cancer cells to pharmacological doses of vitamin C compared to nonmalignant cells (Doskey et al., 2016). The intravenous infusion of high doses of vitamin C may also drastically increase intracellular labile Fe(II), which can produce free radicals to harm cells through the Fenton reaction (Schoenfeld et al., 2016). These studies suggest that pharmacological doses of vitamin C are prooxidant, which could be used for cancer treatment.

A single pharmacological dose of vitamin C could produce sustained ascorbate radicals and H_2O_2 in the interstitial fluids. It has been showed that intravenous injection of a pharmacological dose of vitamin C inhibits cancer xenografts in mice (Chen et al., 2008). Instead of SVCTs, the oxidized form of vitamin C, dehydroascorbic acid (DHA), enters the cell via facilitated glucose transporters (GLUTs). In various cancers, GLUTs are overexpressed in a fraction of cases according to the COSMIC database. DHA is either very low or undetectable in the plasma of humans and DHA may also be easily converted to ascorbate in the plasma. To take advantage of the overexpressed GLUTs, high doses of vitamin C via intraperitoneal injection are shown to selectively kill colorectal cancer cells by causing oxidative stress (Yun et al., 2015). These studies have fueled clinical trials involving intravenous administration of high doses of vitamin C to achieve mM levels in the circulation to treat various types of cancer, often in combination with other chemotherapy drugs.

33.4 Summary

There is a long controversial history of using vitamin C to treat cancer. Mechanistically, vitamin C serves as a cofactor for TETs to increase 5hmC and for HIF hydroxylases to degrade HIF-1α, which are beneficial in cancer treatment. Oral supplementation could largely meet the requirements of these enzymes by compensating for the intratumoral vitamin C deficiency in many cancer cases caused by lower SVCT2 and cancer-associated oxidative stress. On the other hand, vitamin C is regarded as a prodrug for generating H_2O_2 to preferentially damage cancer cells, which requires the intravenous injection of a pharmacological dose of vitamin C. Due to its easy accessibility, low toxicity, and convincing molecular mechanisms, the value of vitamin C in cancer treatment should not be simply overlooked. Rather, additional basic and clinical research could help to establish the doses and method of delivery of vitamin C for individualized treatment in order to obtain a much better outcome for cancer patients.

Acknowledgments

We apologize to colleagues whose work we were not able to cite here due to space limitations. We thank Tyler Huff for his assistance in editing the manuscript. The work on the epigenomic regulation by vitamin C in the Wang lab is supported by grants (R01NS089525, R21CA191668) from the National Institutes of Health.

References

Bestor, T.H., Edwards, J.R., Boulard, M., 2015. Notes on the role of dynamic DNA methylation in mammalian development. Proc. Natl. Acad. Sci. U.S.A. 112, 6796–6799.

Blaschke, K., Ebata, K.T., Karimi, M.M., Zepeda-Martínez, J.A., Goyal, P., Mahapatra, S., et al., 2013. Vitamin C induces TET-dependent DNA demethylation and a blastocyst-like state in ES cells. Nature 500, 222–226.

Cahill, L.E., El-Sohemy, A., 2009. Vitamin C transporter gene polymorphisms, dietary vitamin C and serum ascorbic acid. J. Nutrigenet. Nutrigenomics 2, 292–301.

Cameron, E., Pauling, L., Leibovitz, B., 1979. Ascorbic acid and cancer: a review. Cancer Res. 39, 663–681.

Campbell, E.J., Vissers, M.C., Bozonet, S., Dyer, A., Robinson, B.A., Dachs, G.U., 2015. Restoring physiological levels of ascorbate slows tumor growth and moderates HIF-1 pathway activity in Gulo (−/−) mice. Cancer Med. 4, 303–314.

Campbell, E.J., Vissers, M.C., Dachs, G.U., 2016. Ascorbate availability affects tumor implantation-take rate and increases tumor rejection in Gulo −/− mice. Hypoxia (Auckl) 4, 41–52.

Cha, J., Roomi, M.W., Ivanov, V., Kalinovsky, T., Niedzwiecki, A., Rath, M., 2011. Ascorbate depletion increases growth and metastasis of melanoma cells in vitamin C deficient mice. Exp. Oncol. 33, 226–230.

Cha, J., Roomi, M.W., Ivanov, V., Kalinovsky, T., Niedzwiecki, A., Rath, M., 2013. Ascorbate supplementation inhibits growth and metastasis of B16FO melanoma and 4T1 breast cancer cells in vitamin C-deficient mice. Int. J. Oncol. 42, 55–64.

Chen, Q., Espey, M.G., Krishna, M.C., Mitchell, J.B., Corpe, C.P., Buettner, G.R., et al., 2005. Pharmacologic ascorbic acid concentrations selectively kill cancer cells: action as a pro-drug to deliver hydrogen peroxide to tissues. Proc. Natl. Acad. Sci. U.S.A. 102, 13604–13609.

Chen, Q., Espey, M.G., Sun, A.Y., Lee, J.H., Krishna, M.C., Shacter, E., et al., 2007. Ascorbate in pharmacologic concentrations selectively generates ascorbate radical and hydrogen peroxide in extracellular fluid in vivo. Proc. Natl. Acad. Sci. U.S.A. 104, 8749–8754.

Chen, Q., Espey, M.G., Sun, A.Y., Pooput, C., Kirk, K.L., Krishna, M.C., et al., 2008. Pharmacologic doses of ascorbate act as a prooxidant and decrease growth of aggressive tumor xenografts in mice. Proc. Natl. Acad. Sci. U.S.A. 105, 11105–11109.

Chen, J., Guo, L., Zhang, L., Wu, H., Yang, J., Liu, H., et al., 2013. Vitamin C modulates Tet1 function during somatic cell reprogramming. Nat. Genet. 45, 1504–1509.

Cimmino, L., Dolgalev, I., Wang, Y., Yoshimi, A., Martin, G.H., Wang, J., et al., 2017. Restoration of TET2 function blocks aberrant self-renewal and leukemia progression. Cell 170, 1079–1095.

Corpe, C.P., Tu, H., Eck, P., Wang, J., Faulhaber-Walter, R., Schnermann, J., et al., 2010. Vitamin C transporter Slc23a1 links renal reabsorption, vitamin C tissue accumulation, and perinatal survival in mice. J. Clin. Invest. 120, 1069–1083.

Dawson, M.A., Kouzarides, T., 2012. Cancer epigenetics: from mechanism to therapy. Cell 150, 12–27.

Dickson, K.M., Gustafson, C.B., Young, J.I., Züchner, S., Wang, G., 2013. Ascorbate-induced generation of 5-hydroxymethylcytosine is unaffected by varying levels of iron and 2-oxoglutarate. Biochem. Biophys. Res. Commun. 439, 522–527.

Doskey, C.M., Buranasudja, V., Wagner, B.A., Wilkes, J.G., Du, J., Cullen, J.J., et al., 2016. Tumor cells have decreased ability to metabolize H_2O_2: implications for pharmacological ascorbate in cancer therapy. Redox Biol. 10, 274–284.

Ebata, K.T., Mesh, K., Liu, S., Bilenky, M., Fekete, A., Acker, M.G., et al., 2017. Vitamin C induces specific demethylation of H3K9me2 in mouse embryonic stem cells via Kdm3a/b. Epigenetics Chromatin 10, 36.

Erichsen, H.C., Peters, U., Eck, P., Welch, R., Schoen, R.E., Yeager, M., et al., 2008. Genetic variation in sodium-dependent vitamin C transporters SLC23A1 and SLC23A2 and risk of advanced colorectal adenoma. Nutr. Cancer 60, 652–659.

Fain, O., Mathieu, E., Thomas, M., 1998. Scurvy in patients with cancer. BMJ 316, 1661–1662.

Gao, P., Zhang, H., Dinavahi, R., Li, F., Xiang, Y., Raman, V., et al., 2007. HIF-dependent antitumorigenic effect of antioxidants in vivo. Cancer Cell 12, 230–238.

Ge, G., Peng, D., Xu, Z., Guan, B., Xin, Z., He, Q., et al., 2018. Restoration of 5-hydroxymethylcytosine by ascorbate blocks kidney tumour growth. EMBO Rep. 19, e45401.

Gerecke, C., Schumacher, F., Edlich, A., Wetzel, A., Yealland, G., Neubert, L.K., et al., 2018. Vitamin C promotes decitabine or azacytidine induced DNA hydroxymethylation and subsequent reactivation of the epigenetically silenced tumour suppressor CDKN1A in colon cancer cells. Oncotarget 9, 32822–32840.

Greenlee, H., Kwan, M.L., Kushi, L.H., Song, J., Castillo, A., Weltzien, E., et al., 2012. Antioxidant supplement use after breast cancer diagnosis and mortality in the Life After Cancer Epidemiology (LACE) cohort. Cancer. 118, 2048–2058.

Guey, L.T., García-Closas, M., Murta-Nascimento, C., Lloreta, J., Palencia, L., Kogevinas, M., et al., 2010. Genetic susceptibility to distinct bladder cancer subphenotypes. Eur. Urol. 57, 283–292.

Gustafson, C.B., Yang, C., Dickson, K.M., Shao, H., Van Booven, D., Harbour, J.W., et al., 2015. Epigenetic reprogramming of melanoma cells by vitamin C treatment. Clin. Epigenetics 7, 51.

Handelman, G.J., 2007. Vitamin C deficiency in dialysis patients—are we perceiving the tip of an iceberg? Nephrol. Dial. Transplant. 22, 328–331.

Harbour, J.W., Roberson, E.D., Anbunathan, H., Onken, M.D., Worley, L.A., Bowcock, A.M., 2013. Recurrent mutations at codon 625 of the splicing factor SF3B1 in uveal melanoma. Nat. Genet. 45, 133–135.

Harris, H.R., Bergkvist, L., Wolk, A., 2013. Vitamin C intake and breast cancer mortality in a cohort of Swedish women. Br. J. Cancer 109, 257–264.

Harris, H.R., Orsini, N., Wolk, A., 2014. Vitamin C and survival among women with breast cancer: a meta-analysis. Eur. J. Cancer 50, 1223–1231.

He, Y.F., Li, B.Z., Li, Z., Liu, P., Wang, Y., Tang, Q., et al., 2011. Tet-mediated formation of 5-carboxylcytosine and its excision by TDG in mammalian DNA. Science 333, 1303–1307.

Hong, S.W., Lee, S.H., Moon, J.H., Hwang, J.J., Kim, D.E., Ko, E., et al., 2013. SVCT-2 in breast cancer acts as an indicator for L-ascorbate treatment. Oncogene 32, 1508–1517.

Hsu, C.H., Peng, K.L., Kang, M.L., Chen, Y.R., Yang, Y.C., Tsai, C.H., et al., 2012. TET1 suppresses cancer invasion by activating the tissue inhibitors of metalloproteinases. Cell Rep. 2, 568–579.

Hu, F., Wu, Z., Li, G., Teng, C., Liu, Y., Wang, F., et al., 2015. The plasma level of retinol, vitamins A, C and alpha-tocopherol could reduce breast cancer risk? A meta-analysis and meta-regression. J. Cancer Res. Clin. Oncol. 141, 601–614.

Huang, Y., Rao, A., 2014. Connections between TET proteins and aberrant DNA modification in cancer. Trends Genet. 30, 464–474.

Hutchinson, J., Lentjes, M.A., Greenwood, D.C., Burley, V.J., Cade, J.E., Cleghorn, C. L., et al., 2012. Vitamin C intake from diary recordings and risk of breast cancer in the UK Dietary Cohort Consortium. Eur. J. Clin. Nutr. 66, 561–568.

Ito, S., D'Alessio, A.C., Taranova, O.V., Hong, K., Sowers, L.C., Zhang, Y., 2010. Role of Tet proteins in 5mC to 5hmC conversion, ES-cell self-renewal and inner cell mass specification. Nature 466, 1129–1133.

Ito, S., Shen, L., Dai, Q., Wu, S.C., Collins, L.B., Swenberg, J.A., et al., 2011. Tet proteins can convert 5-methylcytosine to 5-formylcytosine and 5-carboxylcytosine. Science 333, 1300–1303.

Klose, R.J., Yamane, K., Bae, Y., Zhang, D., Erdjument-Bromage, H., Tempst, P., et al., 2006. The transcriptional repressor JHDM3A demethylates trimethyl histone H3 lysine 9 and lysine 36. Nature 442, 312–316.

Krasner, N., Dymock, I.W., 1974. Ascorbic acid deficiency in malignant diseases: a clinical and biochemical study. Br. J. Cancer 30, 142–145.

Kriaucionis, S., Heintz, N., 2009. The nuclear DNA base 5-hydroxymethylcytosine is present in Purkinje neurons and the brain. Science 324, 929–930.

Levental, K.R., Yu, H., Kass, L., Lakins, J.N., Egeblad, M., Erler, J.T., et al., 2009. Matrix crosslinking forces tumor progression by enhancing integrin signaling. Cell 139, 891–906.

Levine, M., Padayatty, S.J., Espey, M.G., 2011. Vitamin C: a concentration-function approach yields pharmacology and therapeutic discoveries. Adv. Nutr. 2, 78–88.

Lian, C.G., Xu, Y., Ceol, C., Wu, F., Larson, A., Dresser, K., et al., 2012. Loss of 5-hydroxymethylcytosine is an epigenetic hallmark of melanoma. Cell 150, 1135–1146.

Lu, C., Ward, P.S., Kapoor, G.S., Rohle, D., Turcan, S., Abdel-Wahab, O., et al., 2012. IDH mutation impairs histone demethylation and results in a block to cell differentiation. Nature 483, 474–478.

Maiti, A., Drohat, A.C., 2011. Thymine DNA glycosylase can rapidly excise 5-formylcytosine and 5-carboxylcytosine: potential implications for active demethylation of CpG sites. J. Biol. Chem. 286, 35334–35338.

Malavolti, M., Malagoli, C., Fiorentini, C., Longo, C., Farnetani, F., Ricci, C., et al., 2013. Association between dietary vitamin C and risk of cutaneous melanoma in a population of Northern Italy. Int. J. Vitam. Nutr. Res. 83, 291–298.

May, J.M., Harrison, F.E., 2013. Role of vitamin C in the function of the vascular endothelium. Antioxid. Redox Signal. 19, 2068–2083.

Mayland, C.R., Bennett, M.I., Allan, K., 2005. Vitamin C deficiency in cancer patients. Palliat. Med. 19, 17–20.

Minor, E.A., Court, B.L., Young, J.I., Wang, G., 2013. Ascorbate induces ten-eleven translocation (TET) methylcytosine dioxygenase-mediated generation of 5-hydroxymethylcytosine. J. Biol. Chem. 288, 13669–13674.

Miura, K., Green, A.C., 2015. Dietary antioxidants and melanoma: evidence from cohort and intervention studies. Nutr. Cancer 67, 867–876.

Mustafi, S., Camarena, V., Volmar, C.H., Huff, T.C., Sant, D.W., Brothers, S.P., et al., 2018. Vitamin C sensitizes melanoma to BET inhibitors. Cancer Res. 78, 572–583.

Nechuta, S., Lu, W., Chen, Z., Zheng, Y., Gu, K., Cai, H., et al., 2011. Vitamin supplement use during breast cancer treatment and survival: a prospective cohort study. Cancer Epidemiol. Biomarkers Prev. 20, 262–271.

Peng, D., Ge, G., Gong, Y., Zhan, Y., He, S., Guan, B., et al., 2018. Vitamin C increases 5-hydroxymethylcytosine level and inhibits the growth of bladder cancer. Clin. Epigenetics 10, 94.

Poole, E.M., Shu, X., Caan, B.J., Flatt, S.W., Holmes, M.D., Lu, W., et al., 2013. Postdiagnosis supplement use and breast cancer prognosis in the After Breast Cancer Pooling Project. Breast Cancer Res. Treat. 139, 529–537.

Quesada, V., Conde, L., Villamor, N., Ordóñez, G.R., Jares, P., Bassaganyas, L., et al., 2011. Exome sequencing identifies recurrent mutations of the splicing factor SF3B1gene in chronic lymphocytic leukemia. Nat. Genet. 44, 47–52.

Sajadian, S.O., Tripura, C., Samani, F.S., Ruoss, M., Dooley, S., Baharvand, H., et al., 2016. Vitamin C enhances epigenetic modifications induced by 5-azacytidine and cell cycle arrest in the hepatocellular carcinoma cell lines HLE and Huh7. Clin. Epigenetics 8, 46.

Sant, D.W., Mustafi, S., Gustafson, C.B., Chen, J., Slingerland, J.M., Wang, G., 2018. Vitamin C promotes apoptosis in breast cancer cells by increasing TRAIL expression. Sci. Rep. 8, 5306.

Schito, L., Semenza, G.L., 2016. Hypoxia-inducible factors: master regulators of cancer progression. Trends Cancer 2, 758–770.

Schoenfeld, J.D., Sibenaller, Z.A., Mapuskar, K.A., Wagner, B.A., Cramer-Morales, K.L., Furqan, M., et al., 2016. O_2- and H_2O_2-mediated disruption of Fe metabolism causes the differential susceptibility of NSCLC and GBM cancer cells to pharmacological ascorbate. Cancer Cell 31, 487–500.

Shen, L., Song, C.X., He, C., Zhang, Y., 2014. Mechanism and function of oxidative reversal of DNA and RNA methylation. Annu. Rev. Biochem. 83, 585–614.

Skibola, C.F., Bracci, P.M., Halperin, E., Nieters, A., Hubbard, A., Paynter, R.A., et al., 2008. Polymorphisms in the estrogen receptor 1 and vitamin C and matrix metalloproteinase gene families are associated with susceptibility to lymphoma. PLoS One 3, e2816.

Spielholz, C., Golde, D.W., Houghton, A.N., Nualart, F., Vera, J.C., 1997. Increased facilitated transport of dehydroascorbic acid without changes in sodium-dependent ascorbate transport in human melanoma cells. Cancer Res. 57, 2529–2537.

Tahiliani, M., Koh, K.P., Shen, Y., Pastor, W.A., Bandukwala, H., Brudno, Y., et al., 2009. Conversion of 5-methylcytosine to 5-hydroxymethylcytosine in mammalian DNA by MLL partner TET1. Science 324, 930–935.

Thompson, J.P., Simkevich, C.P., Holness, M.A., Kang, A.H., Raghow, R., 1991. In vitro methylation of the promoter and enhancer of pro alpha 1 (I) collagen gene leads to its transcriptional inactivation. J. Biol. Chem. 266, 2549–2556.

Timpson, N.J., Forouhi, N.G., Brion, M.J., Harbord, R.M., Cook, D.G., Johnson, P., et al., 2010. Genetic variation at the SLC23A1 locus is associated with circulating concentrations of L-ascorbic acid (vitamin C): evidence from 5 independent studies with >15,000 participants. Am. J. Clin. Nutr. 92, 375–382.

Toyokuni, S., Okamoto, K., Yodoi, J., Hiai, H., 1995. Persistent oxidative stress in cancer. FEBS Lett. 358, 1–3.

Tsukada, Y., Fang, J., Erdjument-Bromage, H., Warren, M.E., Borchers, C.H., Tempst, P., et al., 2006. Histone demethylation by a family of JmjC domain-containing proteins. Nature 439, 811–816.

Wang, T., Chen, K., Zeng, X., Yang, J., Wu, Y., Shi, X., et al., 2011. The histone demethylases Jhdm1a/1b enhance somatic cell reprogramming in a vitamin-C-dependent manner. Cell Stem. Cell 9, 575–587.

Wilson, J.X., 2005. Regulation of vitamin C transport. Annu. Rev. Nutr. 25, 105–125.

Wright, M.E., Andreotti, G., Lissowska, J., Yeager, M., Zatonski, W., Chanock, S.J., et al., 2009. Genetic variation in sodium-dependent ascorbic acid transporters and risk of gastric cancer in Poland. Eur. J. Cancer 45, 1824–1830.

Wu, H., D'Alessio, A.C., Ito, S., Xia, K., Wang, Z., Cui, K., et al., 2011. Dual functions of Tet1 in transcriptional regulation in mouse embryonic stem cells. Nature 473, 389–393.

Yin, R., Mao, S.Q., Zhao, B., Chong, Z., Yang, Y., Zhao, C., et al., 2013. Ascorbic acid enhances Tet-mediated 5-methylcytosine oxidation and promotes DNA demethylation in mammals. J. Am. Chem. Soc. 135, 10396–10403.

Yun, J., Mullarky, E., Lu, C., Bosch, K.N., Kavalier, A., Rivera, K., et al., 2015. Vitamin C selectively kills KRAS and BRAF mutant colorectal cancer cells by targeting GAPDH. Science 350, 1391–1396.

Zimmermann, P., Boeuf, S., Dickhut, A., Boehmer, S., Olek, S., Richter, W., 2008. Correlation of COL10A1 induction during chondrogenesis of mesenchymal stem cells with demethylation of two CpG sites in the COL10A1 promoter. Arthritis Rheum. 58, 2743–2753.

Author Index

Note: Page numbers followed by "*f*" and "*t*" refer to figures and tables, respectively.

B

C

E

F

G

H

N

O

Q

R

S

T

U

X

Y

Z

Subject Index

Note: Page numbers followed by "*f*," "*t*," and "*b*" refer to figures, tables, and boxes, respectively.

B

D

H

M

N

Q

R

S

T

U

V

Kolibri 360 GmbH
Ferdinand-Jühlke-Straße 7
99095 Erfurt, Deutschland
produktsicherheit@kolibri360.de